1999
YEAR BOOK OF
FAMILY PRACTICE®

Statement of Purpose

The YEAR BOOK Service

The YEAR BOOK series was devised in 1901 by practicing health professionals who observed that the literature of medicine and related disciplines had become so voluminous that no one individual could read and place in perspective every potential advance in a major specialty. In the final decade of the 20th century, this recognition is more acutely true than it was in 1901.

More than merely a series of books, YEAR BOOK volumes are the tangible results of a unique service designed to accomplish the following:

- to *survey* a wide range of journals of proven value
- to *select* from those journals papers representing significant advances and statements of important clinical principles
- to provide *abstracts* of those articles that are readable, convenient summaries of their key points
- to provide *commentary* about those articles to place them in perspective

These publications grow out of a unique process that calls on the talents of outstanding authorities in clinical and fundamental disciplines, trained literature specialists, and professional writers, all supported by the resources of Mosby, the world's preeminent publisher for the health professions.

The Literature Base

Mosby and its editors survey approximately 500 journals published worldwide, covering the full range of the health professions. On an annual basis, the publisher examines usage patterns and polls its expert authorities to add new journals to the literature base and to delete journals that are no longer useful as potential YEAR BOOK sources.

The Literature Survey

The publisher's team of literature specialists, all of whom are trained and experienced health professionals, examines every original, peer-reviewed article in each journal issue. More than 250,000 articles per year are scanned systematically, including title, text, illustrations, tables, and references. Each scan is compared, article by article, to the search strategies that the publisher has developed in consultation with the 270 outside experts who form the pool of YEAR BOOK editors. A given article may be reviewed by any number of editors, from one to a dozen or more, regardless of the discipline for which the paper was originally published. In turn, each editor who receives the article reviews it to determine whether the article should be included in the YEAR BOOK. This decision is based on the article's inherent quality, its probable usefulness to readers of that YEAR BOOK, and the editor's goal to represent a balanced picture of a given field in each volume of the YEAR BOOK. In addition, the editor indicates when to include figures and tables from the article to help the YEAR BOOK reader better understand the information.

Of the quarter million articles scanned each year, only 5% are selected for detailed analysis within the YEAR BOOK series, thereby assuring readers of the high value of every selection.

The Abstract

The publisher's abstracting staff is headed by a seasoned medical professional and includes individuals with training in the life sciences, medicine, and other areas, plus extensive experience in writing for the health professions and related industries. Each selected article is assigned to a specific writer on this abstracting staff. The abstracter, guided in many cases by notations supplied by the expert editor, writes a structured, condensed summary designed so that the reader can rapidly acquire the essential information contained in the article.

The Commentary

The YEAR BOOK editorial boards, sometimes assisted by guest commentators, write comments that place each article in perspective for the reader. This provides the reader with the equivalent of a personal consultation with a leading international authority—an opportunity to better understand the value of the article and to benefit from the authority's thought processes in assessing the article.

Additional Editorial Features

The editorial boards of each YEAR BOOK organize the abstracts and comments to provide a logical and satisfying sequence of information. To enhance the organization, editors also provide introductions to sections or individual chapters, comments linking a number of abstracts, citations to additional literature, and other features.

The published YEAR BOOK contains enhanced bibliographic citations for each selected article, including extended listings of multiple authors and identification of author affiliations. Each YEAR BOOK contains a Table of Contents specific to that year's volume. From year to year, the Table of Contents for a given YEAR BOOK will vary depending on developments within the field.

Every YEAR BOOK contains a list of the journals from which papers have been selected. This list represents a subset of approximately 500 journals surveyed by the publisher and occasionally reflects a particularly pertinent article from a journal that is not surveyed on a routine basis.

Finally, each volume contains a comprehensive subject index and an index to authors of each selected paper.

The 1999 Year Book Series

Year Book of Allergy, Asthma, and Clinical Immunology: Drs. Rosenwasser, Boguniewicz, Borish, Routes, Spahn, and Weber

Year Book of Anesthesiology and Pain Management®: Drs. Tinker, Abram, Chestnut, Roizen, Rothenberg, and Wood

Year Book of Cardiology®: Drs. Schlant, Collins, Gersh, Graham, Kaplan, and Waldo

Year Book of Chiropractic®: Dr. Lawrence

Year Book of Critical Care Medicine®: Drs. Parrillo, Balk, Calvin, Franklin, and Shapiro

Year Book of Dentistry®: Drs. Meskin, Berry, Jeffcoat, Leinfelder, Roser, Summitt, and Zakariasen

Year Book of Dermatology and Dermatologic Surgery™: Drs. Thiers and Lang

Year Book of Diagnostic Radiology®: Drs. Osborn, Dalinka, Groskin, Maynard, Pentecost, Ros, Smirniotopoulos, and Young

Year Book of Emergency Medicine®: Drs. Wagner, Dronen, Davidson, King, Niemann, and Hamilton

Year Book of Endocrinology®: Drs. Bagdade, Braverman, Horton, Kannan, Landsberg, Molitch, Morley, Odell, Poehlman, Rogol, and Fitzpatrick

Year Book of Family Practice®: Drs. Berg, Bowman, Davidson, Dexter, and Scherger

Year Book of Gastroenterology: Drs. Aliperti and Fleshman

Year Book of Hand Surgery®: Drs. Amadio and Hentz

Year Book of Medicine®: Drs. Klahr, Frishman, Malawista, Mandell, Jett, Young, Barkin, and Bagdade

Year Book of Neonatal and Perinatal Medicine®: Drs. Fanaroff, Maisels, and Stevenson

Year Book of Nephrology, Hypertension, and Mineral Metabolism: Drs. Schwab, Bennett, Emmett, Hostetter, and Moe

Year Book of Neurology and Neurosurgery®: Drs. Bradley and Gibbs

Year Book of Nuclear Medicine®: Drs. Gottschalk, Blaufox, Coleman, Strauss, and Zubal

Year Book of Obstetrics, Gynecology, and Women's Health: Drs. Mishell, Herbst, and Kirschbaum

Year Book of Oncology®: Drs. Ozols, Eisenberg, Glatstein, Loehrer, and Urba

Year Book of Ophthalmology®: Drs. Wilson, Augsburger, Cohen, Eagle, Grossman, Laibson, Maguire, Nelson, Penne, Rapuano, Sergott, Spaeth, Tipperman, Ms. Gosfield, and Ms. Salmon

Year Book of Orthopedics®: Drs. Morrey, Beauchamp, Currier, Tolo, Trigg, and Swiontkowski

Year Book of Otolaryngology–Head and Neck Surgery®: Drs. Paparella, Holt, and Otto

Year Book of Pathology and Laboratory Medicine®: Drs. Raab, Cohen, Dabbs, Olson, and Stanley

Year Book of Pediatrics®: Dr. Stockman

Year Book of Plastic, Reconstructive, and Aesthetic Surgery®: Drs. Miller, Bartlett, Garner, McKinney, Ruberg, Salisbury, and Smith

Year Book of Psychiatry and Applied Mental Health®: Drs. Talbott, Ballenger, Frances, Lydiard, Meltzer, Jensen, and Tasman

Year Book of Pulmonary Disease®: Drs. Jett, Castro, Maurer, Peters, Phillips, and Ryu

Year Book of Rheumatology, Arthritis, and Musculoskeletal Disease™: Drs. Panush, Hadler, Hellman, LeRoy, Pisetsky, and Simon

Year Book of Sports Medicine®: Drs. Shephard, Drinkwater, Eichner, Torg, Alexander, and Mr. George

Year Book of Surgery®: Drs. Copeland, Bland, Deitch, Eberlein, Howard, Luce, Seeger, Souba, and Sugarbaker

Year Book of Urology®: Drs. Andriole and Coplen

Year Book of Vascular Surgery®: Dr. Porter

1999
The Year Book of
FAMILY PRACTICE®

Editor
Alfred O. Berg, M.D., M.P.H.

Associate Editors
Marjorie A. Bowman, M.D., M.P.A.
Robert C. Davidson, M.D., M.P.H.
William W. Dexter, M.D.
Joseph E. Scherger, M.D., M.P.H.

Mosby

St. Louis Baltimore Boston Carlsbad Naples New York Philadelphia Portland London
Madrid Mexico City Singapore Sydney Tokyo Toronto Wiesbaden

M Mosby
Dedicated to Publishing Excellence

Associate Publisher: Gretchen C. Murphy
Developmental Editor: Jaime Pendill
Manager, Periodical Editing: Kirk Swearingen
Manuscript Editor: Pat Costigan
Project Supervisor, Production: Joy Moore
Production Assistant: Karie House
Manager, Literature Services: Idelle L. Winer
Illustrations and Permissions Coordinator: Chidi C. Ukabam

1999 EDITION
Copyright © 1999 by Mosby, Inc.

All rights reserved. No part of this publication may be reproduced, stored in a retrieval system, or transmitted, in any form or by any means, electronic, mechanical, photocopying, recording, or otherwise, without prior written permission from the publisher.

Permission to photocopy or reproduce solely for internal or personal use is permitted for libraries or other users registered with the Copyright Clearance Center, provided that the base fee of $4.00 per chapter plus $.10 per page is paid directly to the Copyright Clearance Center, 21 Congress Street, Salem, MA 01970. This consent does not extend to other kinds of copying, such as copying for general distribution, for advertising or promotional purposes, for creating new collected works, or for resale.

Printed in the United States of America
Composition by Reed Technology and Information Services, Inc.
Printing/binding by Maple–Vail

Editorial Office:
Mosby, Inc.
11830 Westline Industrial Drive
St. Louis, MO 63146
Customer Service: customer.support@mosby.com
www.mosby.com/Mosby/CustomerSupport/index.html

International Standard Serial Number: 0147–1996
International Standard Book Number: 0–8151–9630–X

Editorial Board

Editor
Alfred O. Berg, M.D., M.P.H.
Professor and Acting Chair, Director, Affiliated Residency Network, Department of Family Medicine, University of Washington, Seattle, Washington

Associate Editors
Marjorie A. Bowman, M.D., M.P.A.
Professor and Chair, Department of Family Practice and Community Medicine, University of Pennsylvania Health System, Philadelphia, Pennsylvania

Robert C. Davidson, M.D., M.P.H.
Associate Professor, Department of Family and Community Medicine, University of California, Davis, California

William W. Dexter, M.D.
Director, Sports Medicine; Assistant Director, Family Practice Residency, Maine Medical Center, Portland, Maine; Assistant Professor, Department of Family Medicine, University of Vermont, Burlington, Vermont

Joseph E. Scherger, M.D., M.P.H.
Professor and Chair, Department of Family Medicine; Associate Dean for Clinical Affairs, University of California, Irvine, California

Table of Contents

JOURNALS REPRESENTED	xv
1. Cardiovascular Disease	1
Overview	1
Hypertension	2
Coronary Artery Disease Risk	7
Myocardial Infarction	19
Secondary Prevention of Coronary Artery Disease	24
Miscellaneous	25
2. Vascular Disease	33
Overview	33
Carotid Artery Disease	33
Deep Vein Thrombosis and Pulmonary Embolism	37
Anticoagulation	40
3. Metabolism and Endocrinology	45
Overview	45
Lipids	46
Obesity	54
Insulin-Dependent Diabetes Mellitus	61
Diabetes Mellitus Type 2	66
Diabetes Mellitus—Miscellaneous	76
Endocrine—Miscellaneous	85
4. Infectious Diseases	91
Overview	91
Lyme Disease	92
Sexually Transmitted Disease	96
HIV Infection and AIDS	102
Urinary Tract Infection	110
Miscellaneous	112
5. Asthma and Allergy	121
Overview	121
Asthma and Reactive Airways Disease	121
Miscellaneous	127

6. Gastroenterology ... 131
Overview ... 131
Upper Gastrointestinal Problems ... 131
Lower Gastrointestinal Problems ... 137
Miscellaneous ... 141

7. Skin Conditions ... 149
Overview ... 149
Sun Exposure ... 149
Therapeutics ... 152
Miscellaneous ... 158

8. Urological Conditions ... 163
Overview ... 163
Prostate Disease ... 163
Circumcision ... 170
Miscellaneous ... 172

9. Musculoskeletal Conditions and Fibromyalgia ... 175
Overview ... 175
Back Pain ... 176
Fibromyalgia ... 179
Miscellaneous ... 182

10. Mental Health and Psychiatry ... 193
Overview ... 193
Dementia and Alzheimer's Disease ... 194
Drug and Alcohol Use ... 198
Marital Distress and Domestic Violence ... 205
Mental Health Services and Insurance ... 210
Miscellaneous ... 212

11. Preventive Medicine ... 223
Overview ... 223
Fitness and Physical Activity ... 224
Smoking ... 231
Antioxidants ... 239
Garlic ... 243

12. Neurologic Conditions	247
Overview	247
Stroke	247
Headache	254
13. Eye, Ear, Nose, and Throat Conditions	259
Overview	259
14. Children's Health	265
Overview	265
Immunization	266
Infectious Diseases	272
Sudden Infant Death Syndrome	283
Injury	288
Preparticipation Examinations	292
Miscellaneous	296
15. Women's Health	309
Overview	309
Breast Cancer	310
Cervical Cancer	320
Polycystic Ovary Syndrome	329
Premenstrual Syndrome	331
Emergency Contraception and Abortion	336
Menopause	339
Hormone Replacement Therapy	341
Miscellaneous	347
16. Pregnancy	353
Overview	353
Prenatal Issues	354
Gestational Diabetes	361
Labor and Delivery	365
Pregnancy Outcomes	370
Miscellaneous	374
17. Other Clinical Issues	377
Overview	377
Cancer	378

    Ethics and End-of-Life Issues 383
    Patient Compliance 388
    Alternative and Complementary Medicine 391
    Miscellaneous 393

18. Health Policy and Economics 401
    Overview 401
    Issues in Primary Care 402
    Health System Issues 409
    Quality, Outcomes, and Peer Review 414

SUBJECT INDEX. 421
AUTHOR INDEX 457

Journals Represented

Mosby and its editors survey approximately 500 journals for its abstract and commentary publications. From these journals, the editors select the articles to be abstracted. Journals represented in this YEAR BOOK are listed below.

Acta Anaesthesiologica Scandinavica
Acta Cytologica
Acta Obstetricia et Gynecologica Scandinavica
Acta Ophthalmologica Scandinavica
Acta Oto-Laryngologica
Acta Paediatrica
Acta Paediatrica Supplement
Age and Ageing
Alzheimer Disease and Associated Disorders
American Family Physician
American Journal of Cardiology
American Journal of Clinical Nutrition
American Journal of Emergency Medicine
American Journal of Epidemiology
American Journal of Gastroenterology
American Journal of Kidney Diseases
American Journal of Medicine
American Journal of Obstetrics and Gynecology
American Journal of Preventive Medicine
American Journal of Public Health
American Journal of Sports Medicine
Annals of Allergy, Asthma, & Immunology
Annals of Epidemiology
Annals of Internal Medicine
Archives of Dermatology
Archives of Disease in Childhood
Archives of Family Medicine
Archives of Neurology
Archives of Orthopaedic and Trauma Surgery
Archives of Otolaryngology-Head and Neck Surgery
Archives of Pediatrics and Adolescent Medicine
Archives of Surgery
Australian and New Zealand Journal of Obstetrics and Gynaecology
British Journal of General Practice
British Journal of Surgery
British Medical Journal
Canadian Journal of Cardiology
Canadian Journal of Physiology and Pharmacology
Canadian Medical Association Journal
Cancer
Cephalalgia
Circulation
Clinical Infectious Diseases
Clinical Pediatrics
Contraception
Diabetes Care

Diabetic Medicine
Diseases of the Colon and Rectum
European Respiratory Journal
Fertility and Sterility
Gastroenterology
Gut
Hypertension
International Journal of Dermatology
International Journal of Geriatric Psychiatry
International Journal of Obesity
International Journal of Sports Medicine
Journal of Allergy and Clinical Immunology
Journal of Athletic Training
Journal of Clinical Epidemiology
Journal of Clinical Oncology
Journal of Clinical Pathology
Journal of Consulting and Clinical Psychology
Journal of Developmental and Behavioral Pediatrics
Journal of Emergency Medicine
Journal of Epidemiology and Community Health
Journal of Family Practice
Journal of General Internal Medicine
Journal of Gerontology
Journal of Human Hypertension
Journal of Manipulative and Physiological Therapeutics
Journal of Maternal-Fetal Medicine
Journal of Occupational and Environmental Medicine
Journal of Otolaryngology
Journal of Pediatric Gastroenterology and Nutrition
Journal of Pediatrics
Journal of Reproductive Medicine
Journal of Rheumatology
Journal of Ultrasound in Medicine
Journal of Urology
Journal of the American Academy of Child and Adolescent Psychiatry
Journal of the American Academy of Dermatology
Journal of the American Board of Family Practice
Journal of the American College of Cardiology
Journal of the American Geriatrics Society
Journal of the American Medical Association
Journal of the National Cancer Institute
Lancet
Mayo Clinic Proceedings
Medical Care
Medicine and Sciences in Sports and Exercise
Neurology
New England Journal of Medicine
New Zealand Medical Journal
Obstetrics and Gynecology
Otolaryngology — Head and Neck Surgery
Pain
Pediatric Infectious Disease Journal

Pediatrics
Scandinavian Journal of Work, Environment and Health
Sleep
Southern Medical Journal
Stroke

STANDARD ABBREVIATIONS

The following terms are abbreviated in this edition: acquired immunodeficiency syndrome (AIDS), cardiopulmonary resuscitation (CPR), central nervous system (CNS), cerebrospinal fluid (CSF), computed tomography (CT), deoxyribonucleic acid (DNA), electrocardiography (ECG), health maintenance organization (HMO), human immunodeficiency virus (HIV), intensive care unit (ICU), intramuscular (IM), intravenous (IV), magnetic resonance (MR) imaging (MRI), and ribonucleic acid (RNA).

NOTE

The YEAR BOOK OF FAMILY PRACTICE is a literature survey service providing abstracts of articles published in the professional literature. Every effort is made to assure the accuracy of the information presented in these pages. Neither the editors nor the publisher of the YEAR BOOK OF FAMILY PRACTICE can be responsible for errors in the original materials. The editors' comments are their own opinions. Mention of specific products within this publication does not constitute endorsement.

To facilitate the use of the YEAR BOOK OF FAMILY PRACTICE as a reference tool, all illustrations and tables included in this publication are now identified as they appear in the original article. This change is meant to help the reader recognize that any illustration or table appearing in the YEAR BOOK OF FAMILY PRACTICE may be only one of many in the original article. For this reason, figure and table numbers will often appear to be out of sequence within the YEAR BOOK OF FAMILY PRACTICE.

Foreword

Never before have more sources of medical information crowded the landscape in hopes of attracting the attention of family physicians. It is a myth, however, to imagine that the quality and usefulness of the information have grown at the same rate as its quantity and availability. Indeed, it is a paradox that the flood of print, computer-based, and Internet medical information has made the family physician's task of finding the "good stuff" more, rather than less, difficult.

Any physician who has ever searched the MEDLINE database knows that the most important predictor of a successful search is the knowledge, thought, care, and skill of the searcher—not the speed of your computer or the "power" of the software search engine. Think of the editors of the YEAR BOOK OF FAMILY PRACTICE as your agents in scanning for the year's most interesting, provocative, and useful 325 or so articles out of thousands published in scores of the best biomedical journals. For most of the editors, we have had 10 years' experience in the process of selecting and commenting on the articles.

The process the editors used in selecting and presenting the articles in this volume from among the 10,000 articles in nearly 1,000 journals that we reviewed has not changed. We have grouped articles in chapters and sections and cross-referenced other articles of interest.

The index of the YEAR BOOK is a good indicator of recent developments in biomedicine. This year's volume has expanded sections on diabetes, lipids, and many womens' health issues reflecting the significant advances made during the last year.

The overviews appearing at the beginning of each chapter can be scanned quickly to locate articles of interest, and they also list the randomized controlled trials (RCTs) in each section that will be the most reliable guidance for interventions. Readers will note that RCTs are a small minority of the articles presented. Many important clinical topics will never be subjected to an RCT. The 1999 YEAR BOOK OF FAMILY PRACTICE also presents the best descriptive studies we could find, along with provocative case series, case reports, rigorous reviews, and thoughtful editorials. Each entry that follows presents a detailed abstract and commentary written by the editorial staff and medical editors. Full-text copies of articles can be obtained through your local medical library.

The editors can look back with satisfaction that many of the articles chosen for earlier volumes have proved useful, and more than a few are recognized as landmarks for medical practice. The findings from many articles abstracted have even turned up on various board and certifying examinations! We are confident that prospects for the 1999 YEAR BOOK OF FAMILY PRACTICE are equally bright. We hope readers share the enthusiasm of the editors for this unique publication enterprise.

Alfred O. Berg, M.D., M.P.H.

1 Cardiovascular Disease

Overview

Randomized controlled trials: Abstracts 1–1, 1–4, 1–14, 1–17, 1–21, and 1–22

Hypertension

- A meta-analysis of randomized controlled trials showing the effect of exercise on lowering blood pressure
- Two articles discussing blood pressure and sleep
- Side effects of antihypertensives on sexual functioning in men *and* women

Coronary Artery Disease Risk

- Three articles on overall risk from Framingham, Bogalusa, and France
- Two articles on the effects of fish consumption, folate, and vitamins on risk
- Hyperinsulinemia and risk
- Two articles on *Helicobacter pylori* and risk, including a meta-analysis

(See related articles in Chapter 3: Lipids.)

Coronary Artery Disease and Myocardial Infarction

- Invasive vs. conservative therapy
- Comparative outcomes in hospitals with and without catheterization facilities
- Outcomes on reperfusion in right ventricular infarction

Secondary Prevention of Coronary Artery Disease

- Effects of pravastatin on further cardiac events in women

Miscellaneous

- Spontaneous conversion of atrial fibrillation to sinus rhythm
- Calcium channel blockers and risk of cancer
- Lovastatin and the immune system

- Reduction of plasma homocysteine levels with fortified cereals
- Intermittent transdermal nitroglycerin and ischemia

Hypertension

The Effectiveness of Exercise Training in Lowering Blood Pressure: A Meta-analysis of Randomised Controlled Trials of 4 Weeks or Longer

Halbert JA, Silagy CA, Finucane P, et al (Flinders Univ of South Australia, Bedford Park; Repatriation Gen Hosp, Daw Park, South Australia; Royal Adelaide Hosp, South Australia)

J Hum Hypertens 11:641–649, 1997

Introduction.—Because physical inactivity is an independent risk factor for coronary heart disease, exercise programs are recommended as a means of reducing morbidity and mortality from coronary heart disease. To identify the features of an optimal program, researchers reviewed the results of randomized controlled trials involving an aerobic or resistance training program.

Methods.—Studies included in the analysis had to be of at least 4 weeks' duration and to have blood pressure (BP) as either the primary or secondary outcome measure. English language studies were identified through a search of electronic databases, previous review articles, and examination of references of relevant trials. A 3-point rating scale was used to assess the methodological quality of the studies.

Results.—Twenty-nine trials involving 1,533 participants, both hypertensive and normotensive, were included in the review. Five studies had a crossover design and 24 a parallel group design. The mean number of participants was 53 per study. Analysis of methodological quality found that most studies made little or no effort to control selection bias at entry. Most training programs used a combination of exercise techniques; all but 3 involved aerobic exercise training. Compared with nonexercising controls, participants in aerobic exercise training reduced systolic BP by a mean of 4.7 mm mercury and diastolic BP by a mean 3.1 mm mercury. Reductions in BP attributed to aerobic exercise training were independent of exercise intensity and the number of exercise sessions per week. Only 3 small trials examined the effectiveness of resistance exercise, and pooled results found no statistically significant effects.

Conclusion.—Hypertensive patients who participated in aerobic exercise training had a small but statistically significant reduction in systolic and diastolic BP. This effect was independent of intensity of exercise and number of sessions per week. No definitive conclusions could be drawn about the value of resistance training.

▶ This article reports a meta-analysis of the literature related to exercise and the lowering of blood pressure. The authors reviewed all studies which met their criteria of being randomized, controlled trials of aerobic or resistance exercise training with a minimum of 4 weeks' or greater duration. There are no surprises in their conclusions. The authors found a small but significant effect in reducing both systolic and diastolic blood pressure by aerobic exercise. The amount of this aerobic exercise, however, seemed to have little effect in increasing the reduction in blood pressure. There was no conclusive evidence that resistance exercise (weight training) affected blood pressure either positively or negatively.

I routinely recommend aerobic exercise 3–4 times per week for my patients with hypertension. However, family physicians know well the low percentage of patients who will maintain this type of program, and its effect seems to be small in comparison to other therapies. I don't think we should discard exercise therapy, but we can't rely upon it alone.

R.C. Davidson, M.D., M.P.H.

Avoiding the Supine Position During Sleep Lowers 24 H Blood Pressure in Obstructive Sleep Apnea (OSA) Patients
Berger M, Oksenberg A, Silverberg DS, et al (Loewenstein Rehabilitation Hosp, Roonana, Israel; Tel Aviv Med Ctr, Israel)
J Hum Hypertens 11:657–664, 1997 1–2

Background.—Studies have shown that patients with essential hypertension are more likely to have obstructive sleep apnea (OSA) than is the general population. Likewise, half of patients with OSA have hypertension. One treatment for OSA is avoiding the supine position during sleep.

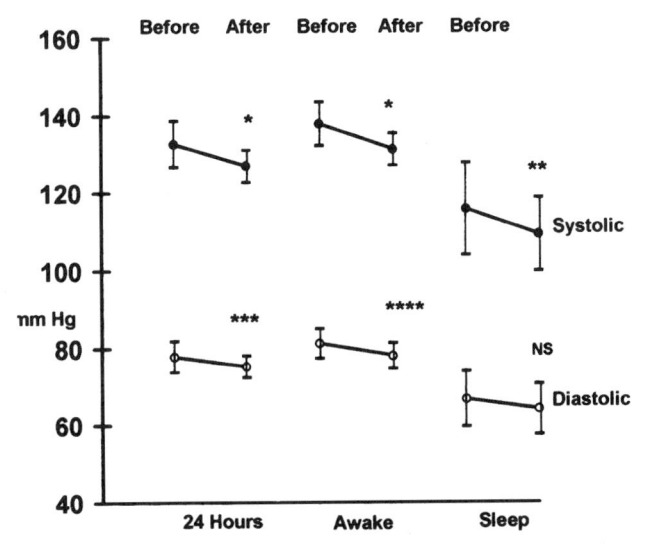

FIGURE 1.—Graphic demostration of the effect of avoiding the supine position during sleep for a 1-month period on 24-hour awake and sleep systolic (*black circles*) and diastolic (*white circles*) blood pressure in 13 patients with obstructive sleep apnea. *Single asterisk* indicates $P = 0.001$; *double asterisk* indicates $P = 0.022$; *triple asterisk* indicates $P = 0.006$; *quadruple asterisk* indicates $P = 0.002$. Values are mean ± standard deviation. *Abbreviation: NS,* non-significant. (Courtesy of Berger M, Oksenberg A, Silverberg DS, et al: Avoiding the supine position during sleep lowers 24 h blood pressure in obstructive sleep apnea (OSA) patients. *J Hum Hypertens* 11:657–664, 1997.)

This study examines the effect of supine position avoidance on 24-hour blood pressure (BP) in patients with OSA.

Method.—Seven normotensive and 6 hypertensive patients with OSA—all with breathing problems related to the supine position as determined by polysomnography—underwent 1 month of sleep position intervention by the tennis ball technique. At the beginning and end of the month, BP was measured for 24-hour periods using an ambulatory device.

Results.—All 13 patients had significant (P less than 0.05) reduction in 24-hour mean BP in all areas but sleeping diastolic BP (Fig 1). The overall systolic/diastolic BP was reduced by 6.4/2.9 mm Hg. Patients' mean sleeping BP fell by 6.5/2.7 mm Hg. For the 24-hour mean and waking hours BP, hypertensive patients showed a significantly greater reduction compared with the normotensive group. Researchers also noted reduced variability and load of BP.

Conclusion.—Avoidance of the supine position could be used as a treatment for hypertension.

Essential Hypertension and Abnormal Upper Airway Resistance During Sleep

Silverberg DS, Oksenberg A (Tel Aviv Med Ctr, Israel)
Sleep 20:794–806, 1997   1–3

Background.—Patients with obstructive sleep apnea (OSA) have a very high prevalence of essential hypertension. Even after adjustment for confounding factors, OSA appears to be an independent risk factor for hypertension; treatment for OSA may reduce daytime and nighttime blood pressure. The available evidence linking hypertension and OSA was reviewed.

Increased Upper Airway Resistance and Hypertension.—The prevalence of hypertension appears to be increased not only in patients with OSA but also in nonapneic snorers. If this is true, it would mean that most cases of "essential" hypertension actually result from sleep-disordered breathing. Both OSA and nonapneic snoring are characterized by increased upper airway resistance during sleep. These conditions have other similarities as well, including certain craniofacial abnormalities, daytime sleepiness, sleep arousals, and pathologic changes of the pharyngeal area. Some patients with apneic snoring have upper airway resistance syndrome, with symptoms including excessive daytime sleepiness, snoring, frequent increased upper airway resistance during sleep, absence of hypoxia, and increased brief arousals during sleep. These patients are often clinically indistinguishable from those with OSA syndrome. The assembled evidence strongly suggests that some nonapneic snorers and nonsnorers have persistent hypertension caused by recurrent episodes of increased upper airway resistance during sleep. Treating the sleep disturbances may reduce blood pressure as well.

Mechanism and Characteristics.—Although the mechanism of this relationship is unclear, episodes of upper airway collapse may lead to hypoxia, hypercapnia, increased breathing effort, increased arousals, and increased sympathetic activity. All of these factors may increase blood pressure toward the end of the apneic period, which persists even after the resumption of normal breathing. As time goes by, persistent elevations of sympathetic activity and blood pressure may lead to permanent systemic hypertension. This would suggest that OSA syndrome and essential hypertension have similar characteristics, which appears to be the case. Both conditions are most common in obese, young and middle-aged men. Both improve with weight loss, in addition to other clinical similarities. Consistent hematologic, biochemical, physiologic, and hereditary characteristics are noted as well.

Discussion.—There is strong evidence that many or most cases of essential hypertension are associated with sleep-related breathing disturbances caused by intermittent, partial, or complete upper airway obstruction during sleep. Detailed studies would be needed to test this hypothesis; if it holds, most patients with essential hypertension would be expected to show increased upper airway resistance during sleep. Treatment of increased upper airway resistance would be expected to reduce blood pressure.

▶ These 2 articles (Abstracts 1–2 and 1–3) complement one another and, combined, present a very interesting and compelling picture of the relationship between essential hypertension and OSA and airway resistance during sleep. The article by Silverberg and Oksenberg is a conceptual and literature review of the relationship between essential hypertension and abnormally high upper airway resistance during sleep. The authors go so far as to suggest that most essential hypertension is mainly caused by increased upper airway resistance during sleep.

The second article, by the same authors, reports on the effect of sleeping position on 24-hour blood pressure in patients with OSA. This study had more objective evidence that airway resistance during sleep does affect BP. The authors were able to show a significant reduction in both systolic and diastolic blood pressure by avoidance of the supine position.

I included these articles because they provide an interesting insight into at least 1 of the causes of what we had previously thought to be essential hypertension or hypertension not attributable to any known cause. I suspect that we will need significant more study on this subject, and I am not yet ready to accept the authors' hypothesis that most essential hypertension is related to increased upper airway resistance during sleep. However, there may well be more to this relationship than what we have previously thought. Stay tuned.

R.C. Davidson, M.D., M.P.H.

Long-term Effects on Sexual Function of Five Antihypertensive Drugs and Nutritional Hygienic Treatment in Hypertensive Men and Women: Treatment of Mild Hypertension Study (TOMHS)

Grimm RH Jr, for the TOMHS Research Group (Shapiro Ctr for Evidence-Based Medicine, Minneapolis, Minn)
Hypertension 29:8–14, 1997

Introduction.—The relationship between hypertensive drugs and sexual dysfunction has been addressed in only a few placebo-controlled trials. Some have questioned whether the sexual dysfunction is caused by drug treatment for hypertension or by the hypertension itself. Data from the Treatment of Mild Hypertension Study (TOMHS) were used to explore the relationship between 5 antihypertensive drugs and placebo on sexual function in men and women aged 45–69 years with stage I diastolic hypertension.

Methods.—The TOMHS was a double-blind, placebo-controlled, randomized trial with 902 patients with hypertension. The effect of placebo and 5 active drugs (acebutolol, amlodipine maleate, chlorthalidone, doxazosin maleate, and enalapril maleate) on sexual function was evaluated at baseline and at annual follow-up visits by means of physician interview.

Results.—Baseline interviews revealed 14.4% of men and 4.9% of women had problems with sexual function. Problems maintaining or obtaining an erection were reported by 12.2% of men at baseline; 2% of women reported problems with achieving orgasm. For men, problems with erection were positively associated with age, systolic pressure, and previous antihypertensive drug use. At 24- and 48-month follow-up, 9.5% and 14.7% of men, respectively, experienced erection dysfunction related to the type of antihypertensive therapy. Compared with placebo, patients randomized to receive chlorthalidone reported a significantly higher incidence of erection dysfunction through 24 months (8.1% vs. 17.1%). At 48 months, the incidence rates of erection dysfunction were similar among treatment groups. The lowest rate for drugs was observed in the doxazosin group, but it was not significantly different from that of the placebo group. The incidence rate was similar for placebo, acebutolol, amlodipine, and enalapril. Erection dysfunction did not require medication withdrawal for most patients.

Conclusion.—The incidence of erection dysfunction in men treated for hypertension was low in all treatment groups but higher for men in the chlorthalidone group. The rate of sexual problems was even lower for women, and did not seem to differ by type of drug. The similar dysfunction rates for drug and placebo groups indicate that problems should not automatically be attributed to antihypertensive medications.

▶ Sexual dysfunction in men using antihypertensive drugs is a commonly perceived problem. Fewer studies have been done on sexual dysfunction in hypertensive women taking various therapies. This interesting prospective study was designed to look at the efficacy of various drugs on mild hypertension. As part of the study, the authors ascertained a baseline of sexual dysfunction problems and followed these men and women through a minimum of 4 years. The authors found that, in both men and women, the overall incidence of sexual dysfunction exacerbated by antihypertensive drugs was quite low. The 1 exception seemed to be chlorothalidone, which accounted for a significantly higher rate of erectile dysfunction in men than did the placebo in the control group. The authors found little incidence of increased sexual dysfunction in women in regard to any of the antihypertensive medications.

R.C. Davidson, M.D., M.P.H.

Coronary Artery Disease Risk

Prediction of Coronary Heart Disease Using Risk Factor Categories
Wilson PWF, D'Agostino RB, Levy D, et al (Natl Heart, Lung, and Blood Inst, Framingham, Mass; Boston Univ, Framingham, Mass)
Circulation 97:1837–1847, 1998   1–5

Background.—Coronary heart disease (CHD) is a major cause of morbidity and mortality in the United States. Many CHD risk factors have been defined. This report presents a simplified CHD prediction model based on Joint National Committee blood pressure and National Cholesterol Education Program cholesterol categories. A large Framingham Heart Study sample was followed for 12 years to examine the accuracy and usefulness of this predictive model.

Study Design.—The population based sample included 2,489 men and 2,856 women, aged 30 to 74 years, at time of entry (1971 to 1974) into the Framingham Heart Study. A medical history and physical examination were performed at baseline. Those with CHD at entry were excluded. Participants were then followed prospectively for 12 years for the development of CHD. Separate prediction score sheets were developed by sex.

Findings.—During the 12 years of follow-up, 383 men and 227 women developed CHD. Development of CHD was significantly associated with blood pressure, total cholesterol, low-density lipoprotein cholesterol, and high-density lipoprotein cholesterol. Sex-specific prediction equations were created to predict CHD risk by age, diabetes, smoking, Joint National Committee blood pressure categories and National Cholesterol Education Program total cholesterol and low-density lipoprotein cholesterol categories. This category approach was as accurate as the use of continuous variables. After adjustment for other factors, 28% of CHD events in men and 29% in women were attributable to blood pressure levels in excess of 130/85 and 27% of CHD events in men and 34% in women were attributable to cholesterol in excess of 200 mg/dL (Table 4).

Conclusions.—A model based on risk factor categories of blood pressure and cholesterol levels accurately predicted CHD risk in a large mid-

TABLE 4.—Multivariable-Adjusted Relative Risks for CHD According to TC Categories

	Men Relative Risk	95% CI	Women Relative Risk	95% CI
Age, y	1.05‡	1.04–1.06	1.04‡	1.03–1.06
Blood pressure				
Normal (including optimal)	1.00	Referent	1.00	Referent
High normal	1.31	0.98–1.76	1.30	0.86–1.98
Hypertension stage I	1.67†	1.28–2.18	1.73†	1.19–2.52
Hypertension stage II–IV	1.84‡	1.37–2.49	2.12†	1.42–3.17
Cigarette use (y/n)	1.68‡	1.37–2.06	1.47†	1.12–1.94
Diabetes (y/n)	1.50*	1.06–2.13	1.77†	1.16–2.69
TC, mg/dL				
<200	1.00	Referent	1.00	Referent
200–239	1.31*	1.01–1.68	1.51*	1.01–2.24
≥240	1.90‡	1.47–2.47	1.72†	1.15–2.56
HDL-C, mg/dL				
<35	1.47†	1.16–1.86	2.02†	1.29–3.15
35–59	1.00	Referent	1.00	Referent
≥60	0.56†	0.37–0.83	0.58†	0.43–0.79

Note: The multivariate models were performed separately for men and women. Each model included simultaneously all variables listed in the table. All analyses used categorical variables.
*0.01<P<0.05
†0.001<P<0.01
‡P<0.001
(Courtesy of Wilson PWF, D'Agostino RB, Levy D, et al: Prediction of Coronary Heart Disease Using Risk Factor Categories *Circulation* 97:1837–1847, copyright 1998, American Heart Association.)

dle-aged white population sample. This simplified CHD prediction algorithm permits physicians to predict patients' multivariate CHD risk.

▶ There were no surprises in the finding of this research program. I included it because of its strength by using a large cohort of both men and women in a prospective 12-year follow-up study. Using recognized national standards for blood pressure and cholesterol, the authors showed a high correlation of prediction for risk of CHD related to the common variables of blood pressure and elevated total cholesterol. I know I am preaching to the choir when I speak to the readers of the YEAR BOOK OF FAMILY PRACTICE. However, continuing to do everything possible in our patients to reduce risk factors for coronary artery disease is of the highest importance.

R.C. Davidson, M.D., M.P.H.

Longitudinal Changes in Cardiovascular Risk From Childhood to Young Adulthood in Offspring of Parents With Coronary Artery Disease: The Bogalusa Heart Study

Bao W, Srinivasan SR, Valdez R, et al (Tulane Ctr for Cardiovascular Health, New Orleans, La)
JAMA 278:1749–1754, 1997

1–6

Background.—The association between parental coronary artery disease (CAD) and its risk factors in the offspring has been determined.

However, the timing and course of the development of risk factors from childhood to adulthood have not been delineated.

Methods.—Two hundred seventy-one individuals with a verified parental history of CAD and 1,253 with no such history were included in this longitudinal study. Mean ages at first CAD event among fathers and mothers were 50 and 52 years, respectively.

Findings.—Individuals with a parental history of CAD were consistently overweight, beginning in childhood. At older ages, these individuals had significantly greater levels of total serum cholesterol, low-density lipoprotein cholesterol (LDL-C), plasma glucose, and insulin because of a higher rate of increase in these risk factors over time. Adults with a parental history of CAD had a higher level of obesity, increased cholesterol and LDL-C levels, hyperglycemia, and coexistence of these conditions. Also significantly greater in adults with a parental history of CAD was the prevalence of dyslipidemia, involving LDL-C alone or combined with HDL-C and/or triglycerides.

Conclusions.—The offspring of parents with early CAD tend to be overweight, beginning in childhood and to develop an adverse cardiovascular risk factor profile at an increased rate. These findings have implications for preventing and treating CAD in individuals with a positive parental history.

▶ From the literature as well as from our own practices, we know that the children of parents with CAD, especially with a myocardial infarction at a relatively young age, are at increased risk for their own cardiovascular disease. This was an interesting substudy of a longitudinal heart study in Bogalusa, Louisiana. The authors attempted to look at the age onset of risk factors for CAD in the children of parents with known CAD.

It is disturbing but not surprising that the authors found that an adverse cardiovascular risk factor profile develops at an earlier age and at an increased rate in children of parents with CAD when compared with children of parents with no CAD. Most disturbing was the significant increase in adolescent obesity. Unfortunately, the authors were unable to determine whether this had a genetic basis or was predominantly environmental. In any case, as family physicians we should not forget the children of our patients with CAD, and should try our best to assist the families in reducing risk factors in these children.

R.C. Davidson, M.D., M.P.H.

Pulse Pressure: A Predictor of Long-term Cardiovascular Mortality in a French Male Population

Benetos A, Safar M, Rudnichi A, et al (INSERM, Paris; State Univ of New York, Syracuse)
Hypertension 30:1410–1415, 1997

Objective.—Previous studies have examined the value of blood pressure (BP)—measured as diastolic or systolic—as a prognostic factor in patients with cardiovascular disease. Blood pressure may also be measured as steady pressure, i.e., mean pressure, and pulsatile pressure, i.e., pulse pressure (PP). A growing body of evidence suggests that PP could be a valuable predictor of cardiac risk. This longitudinal study evaluated PP as a long–term predictor of cardiovascular mortality.

Methods.—The study used data on 19,083 men undergoing systematic health checkups in the French Public Health System. The men were age 40 to 69 when examined in the 1970s. The subjects were followed up for a mean of 19.5 years. For analysis of the effects of initial PP on long-term risk of cardiovascular mortality, the men were grouped by age (40–54 years vs. 55–69 years) and by mean arterial pressure (<107 mm Hg vs. ≥107 mm Hg). These groups were then subdivided according to PP.

Results.—A widened PP was a significant, independent predictor of all–cause mortality, total cardiovascular mortality, and coronary mortality. This was so whether PP was evaluated according to quartile group or as a continuous quantitative variable, and for all age and mean pressure groups. PP did not affect risk of cerebrovascular death.

Conclusions.—Increased PP is a strong, independent predictor of general and cardiovascular morbidity among men, independent of mean arterial pressure and other prognostic factors. PP has a particularly strong impact on coronary mortality, but not cerebrovascular mortality. Widening of PP may be considered an indicator of increased arterial stiffness, which may lead to both decreased diastolic BP and increased systolic BP.

▶ Usually when I think about blood pressure and its relation to morbidity predictions, I think of elevated systolic, diastolic, or both blood pressures. This interesting study raises a different question.

The authors studied a cohort of more than 19,000 men age 40 to 69 who were otherwise healthy in relationship to cardiovascular disease. These men were followed for 20 years. The population was divided into four quartiles, depending on the mean arterial pressure (the average intra-arterial pressures) and further divided into subgroups depending on the pulse pressure difference between systolic and diastolic pressures. The authors found men who showed a wider pulse pressure had a significantly higher all-cause and total cardiovascular mortality experience. This was especially true for coronary artery mortality in all ages. Interestingly enough, no significant association was noted between the pulse pressure and cerebrovascular mortality.

After rereading the article and thinking about this, it does make sense. Men with wider pulse pressures are more likely to have a valvular disease or myocardial injury, or a higher resistance in the peripheral arterial tree. The authors did not suggest any minimum pulse pressure to be considered "normal;" however, a wide pulse pressure in addition to an elevation of either the systolic or diastolic pressure ought to stimulate physician concern.

R.C. Davidson, M.D., M.P.H.

Dietary Sodium Intake and Mortality: The National Health and Nutrition Examination Survey (NHANES I)
Alderman MH, Cohen H, Madhaven S (Albert Einstein College of Medicine, Bronx, NY)
Lancet 351:781–785, 1998

Introduction.—Studies have shown that a restricted-sodium diet is associated with lower blood pressure. A restriction of daily sodium intake to 2,400 mg has been recommended because of the associations with intermediate physiologic variables. There is an expectation that any harmful effects are outweighed by the beneficial changes in intermediate physiologic variables and that the net effect would be lower mortality and cardiovascular morbidity. These expectations, however, have not been supported by empirical data. The relationship of sodium intake to death from all causes and from cardiovascular disease was examined to find out whether dietary sodium is associated with mortality in a general population.

Methods.—There were 20,729 adults, aged 25 to 75, for whom baseline information was obtained during 1971 to 1975 through the first National Health and Nutrition Examination Survey. In 1992, the vital status of 11,346 participants was followed through interview, tracing, and searches of the national death index. Mortality data were examined in sex-specific quartiles of sodium intake, calorie intake, and sodium/calorie ratio. To assess the relations with mortality, multiple regression analyses were done.

Results.—There were 3,923 deaths, of which 1,970 were due to cardiovascular disease. There was an inverse association with sex-specific quartiles of sodium intake and total calorie intake to all-cause mortality rates. There was a weak positive association with quartiles of sodium/calorie ratio and all-cause mortality figures. There was a similar pattern for deaths due to cardiovascular disease. Sodium intake was inversely associated with all-cause mortality rates and cardiovascular-disease mortality rates. All-cause and cardiovascular-disease mortality rates were directly associated with sodium/calorie ratio. Mortality was not independently associated with calorie intake in the presence of the 2 measures of sodium intake.

Conclusion.—A particular dietary recommendation could not be justified. Current recommendations for routine reduction of sodium consumption could not be supported. Advice to increase salt intake or to decrease its concentration in the diet could not be supported either.

▶ I am becoming a real fan of the National Health and Nutrition Examination Survey. Over the past several decades, this survey has produced excellent data on nutritional patterns, specific food intake, and disease. The study size is large, the data often compelling. Presented here are data that challenge the current dogma on sodium intake. Reduction of dietary salt has become a standard instruction to our patients. In fact, patients seem to bring it up more frequently than we do. This study does not draw any conclusions about optimal sodium intake or relationship to other disease processes. However, at least for cardiovascular disease, the conclusion that we need not be so concerned with sodium intake is well supported. Note carefully the limits of this study though. This study does not infer causality; nor is there any suggestion that increasing sodium intake will be beneficial. Given these admonishments, I will include this study in my discussions with my patients.

W.W. Dexter, M.D.

▶ There is a common perception among physicians and patients that the U.S. diet is too high in sodium. The relationship of sodium intake to hypertension risk has been documented in numerous studies. However, this very interesting article of a well-designed large population group study revealed no relationship between sodium intake and overall mortality.

I am not sure what to conclude regarding salt intake. This is a powerful study with a large population and good data. However, there is other evidence, particularly in relationship to hypertension, that urges us to reduce salt in our diets. I don't think I'm going to change my clinical behavior from this study. The large amount of salt in the American diet seems intuitively to be of little health value, and it certainly can increase the risk for certain diseases.

R.C. Davidson, M.D., M.P.H.

Fish Consumption and Risk of Sudden Cardiac Death
Albert CM, Hennekens CH, O'Donnell CJ, et al (Harvard School of Public Health, Boston; Natl Heart, Lung, and Blood Inst, Framingham, Mass)
JAMA 279:23–28, 1998
1–9

Background.—Fish consumption has been thought to reduce risk of sudden cardiac death through a selective benefit on fatal arrhythmias. This study investigates the relationship between eating fish and sudden cardiac death.

Methods.—As part of the U.S. Physicians' Health Study, male U.S. physicians aged 40 to 84 years were observed for up to 11 years after completion, in 1982, of a semiquantitative questionnaire on the frequency of fish consumption. Test subjects had no history of cancer, transient ischemic attack, or myocardial infarction at baseline. The physicians were also randomly assigned to take aspirin, beta-carotene, or placebos. Follow-up questionnaires on food consumption were administered at 12 and 18 months and at 5 years. Sudden cardiac death was determined through medical records and reports from relatives of test subjects.

Results.—During the study period, 133 sudden deaths occurred. Researchers controlled for coronary risk factors, age and assignments for aspirin and beta-carotene and determined that the intake of dietary fish was associated with a decreased risk of sudden death. The threshold for this effect was consumption of one fish per week (P for trend $= 0.03$). In comparison with test subjects who ate fish less than once a month, among men who ate fish at least once a week the multivariate relative risk of sudden death was 0.48 (0.24–0.96; $P = 0.04$, 95% confidence interval. However, increasing intake beyond one serving per week did not further decrease the risk of sudden death. Dietary n-3 fatty acid is suspected to provide these preventive effects. However, the effects were not consistent when dark-meat fish was consumed, and yet dark-meat fish have a higher n-3 fatty acid content. Thus, some other unidentified nutrient may actually play a role. Eating fish was not correlated with decreased risk of nonsudden cardiac death, myocardial infarction, or total cardiovascular mortality. However, reduced risks of total mortality were found with threshold fish consumption.

Conclusion.—This cohort study has several possible flaws and is not clear cut. For example, individuals with a family or personal history of hypertension, hypercholesterolemia, or coronary heart disease are more likely to eat fish. This complicates the relationship examined in this study. Nevertheless, the study shows that men who eat fish at least once per week have reduced risk of sudden cardiac death.

▶ The Physicians' Health Study is providing a wealth of data on cardiovascular disease risk factors and risk factor modification. Observational data accumulated on such a focused population (male, largely white, educated) may not be widely generalizable to the population at large. Nevertheless, the statistical analysis applied to the relationship between fish consumption and sudden cardiac death is well done. Interestingly, no other food groups were found to have an impact on sudden cardiac death. This includes intake of fruits and vegetables, which is quite surprising and a bit dismaying. It is also intriguing to note that the incidence of myocardial infarction did not show the same relationship to fish consumption, although the authors cite other studies that have shown such a relationship. The authors equate fish intake to intake of n-3 fatty acids. Perhaps. I am not convinced. As with other food and supplement investigations, I suspect the benefits lie in much more complex interactions between nutrients and perhaps other factors (lifestyle, genetic factors, environment). These concerns aside, including fish in our recommendations regarding a balanced diet seems to make sense. Here's hoping that the fishing industry can sustain stocks and provide this important food for us!

W.W. Dexter, M.D.

Folate and Vitamin B₆ From Diet and Supplements in Relation to Risk of Coronary Heart Disease Among Women
Rimm EB, Willett WC, Hu FB, et al (Harvard School of Public Health, Boston; Harvard Med School, Boston)
JAMA 279:359–364, 1998

Background.—Hyperhomocysteinemia is associated with increased incidence of vascular disease. Increased levels of homocysteine can be caused by low intakes of folate and vitamin B₆. The relationship between folate and vitamin B₆ intakes and the risk of coronary heart disease (CHD) was examined prospectively among 80,082 women participating in the Nurses' Health Study.

Methods.—The Nurses' Health Study cohort was established in 1976. Every 2 years, participants complete a medical history and lifestyle questionnaire. In 1980, a food frequency questionnaire was added. Food composition values were derived from the Harvard University Food Composition Database. All nutrients were energy-adjusted using the residual method. The 1980 diet questionnaire was returned by 98,462 women. This study excluded women with previously diagnosed cancer, cardiovascular disease, hypercholesterolemia, or diabetes. The final baseline population consisted of 80,082 women. These women were divided into quintiles based on folate and vitamin B₆ intakes. The primary study outcome was defined as documented symptomatic fatal or nonfatal CHD after 1980 but before 1994.

Results.—During the 14 years of follow-up, there were 658 documented incident cases of nonfatal myocardial infarction and 281 cases of fatal CHD. After controlling for the cardiovascular risk factors smoking; hypertension; alcohol intake; fiber intake; vitamin E intake; and saturated, polyunsaturated, and *trans*fat intake, the relative risks of CHD between extreme quintiles were 0.69 for folate and 0.67 for vitamin B₆. Controlling for the above variables, the relative risk was 0.55 for women in the highest quintile of both folate and vitamin B₆ intake compared with women in the lowest quintile. The risk of CHD was reduced for women who regularly ingested multiple vitamins and for women with higher dietary intake of folate and vitamin B₆. This association was strongest among women who consumed at least 1 alcoholic beverage each day.

Conclusions.—In this large group of women prospectively followed for 14 years, higher intakes of folate from either food or supplements, alone or in combination with vitamin B₆, were associated with significantly lower risk of CHD. The lowest risk was among women with folate intake above 400 µg/day and vitamin B₆ intake above 3 mg/day, which are both substantially above current recommended daily allowances. Intake of folate and vitamin B₆ above current recommended daily allowances may be useful in the prevention of CHD among women.

▶ This article on folate and vitamin B₆ intake in women and the women's risk of coronary heart disease adds evidence to the argument that we have traditionally underestimated recommended intake of certain vitamins. The authors looked at the intake of folate and vitamin B₆ in a large longitudinal study of over 80,000 women in the Nurses Health Study. The study found a strong inverse association between a high folate diet and coronary heart disease. The authors also found that this relationship was strongest among women who consumed 1 alcoholic beverage per day.

The authors conclude that we should increase the recommended daily allowance of folic acid to 400 mg/dL. Since there seems to be no evidence of increased risk, I am routinely recommending that women take a multivitamin which includes folic acid and vitamin B₆.

R.C. Davidson, M.D., M.P.H.

Hyperinsulinemia Predicts Coronary Heart Disease Risk in Healthy Middle-aged Men: The 22-Year Follow-up Results of the Helsinki Policemen Study
Pyörälä M, Miettinen H, Laakso M, et al (Univ of Kuopio, Finland)
Circulation 98:398–404, 1998   1–11

Background.—The Helsinki Policemen Study was one of the first prospective studies to demonstrate an association between high plasma insulin levels and coronary heart disease (CHD), but this association remains controversial. Follow-up of the Helsinki Policemen Study has been extended to 22 years and the predictive value of hyperinsulinemia for CHD was evaluated during this time period.

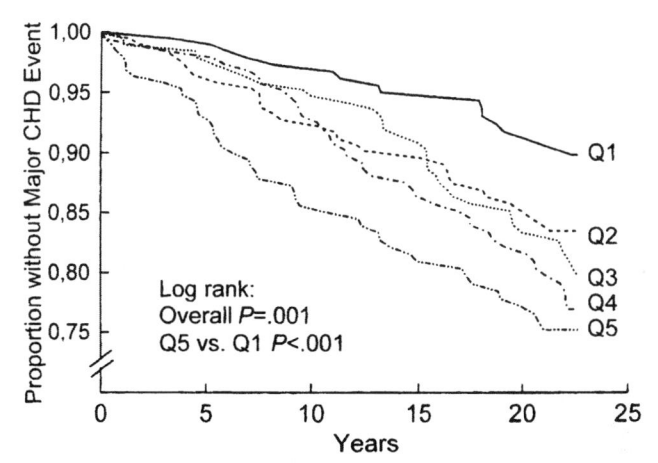

FIGURE 2.—Kaplan-Meier survival curves for remaining free of major CHD events during 22-year follow-up by quintiles of AUC insulin. The risk of having a major CHD event was significantly higher in men in the highest quintile than in those in the lowest quintile. (P <0.0001; age-adjusted P <0.001). The overall trend for the risk of a major CHD event tested over all AUC insulin quintiles was also statistically significant (P=0.001; age-adjusted P=0.006). (Courtesy of Pyörälä M, Miettinen H, Laakso M, et al: Hyperinsulinemia Predicts Coronary Heart Disease Risk in Healthy Middle-Aged Men: The 22-Year Follow-Up Results of the Helsinki Policemen Study *Circulation* 98:398–404, copyright 1998, American Heart Association.)

Study Design.—The study group consisted of 970 men from the Helsinki Policemen Study cohort aged 34–64 years and free of cardiovascular disease and diabetes in 1971 and 1972. Baseline measurements included a health history questionnaire, Rose cardiovascular questionnaire, anthropometric measurements, clinical examination, physical fitness assessment and laboratory tests. The follow-up period extended until the beginning of 1994. The median follow-up for survivors was 22.3 years.

Findings.—During a follow-up of 22 years, 164 participants had a CHD death or nonfatal myocardial infarction. Age-adjusted hazard ratios for a major CHD event of men in the highest area under the plasma insulin response curve (AUC insulin) during an oral glucose tolerance test was 3.29 at 5 years, 2.72 at 10 years, 2.14 at 15 years and 1.61 at 22 years compared to participants in the lower quintiles (Fig 2). The risk of having a major CHD event was significantly higher in men in the highest quintile than those in the lowest quintile.

Conclusions.—Hyperinsulinemia was independently associated with increased risk of CHD during 22 years of follow-up of the Helsinki Policemen Study cohort. The predictive power of this association decreased over time, but was similar to that of cholesterol.

▶ Interest has been increasing in the scientific literature regarding insulin levels and risk for coronary heart disease and hypertension. The link between high insulin levels and risk for hypertension has been established more strongly than a link with coronary heart disease risk. This is a well-designed, prospective, longitudinal epidemiologic study of 970 middle-aged men. As the data shows, there appears to be a strong predictive value for future coronary events in relationship to serum insulin levels.

Unfortunately, there seems little that we can do with this information. These men were not diabetic and their glucose metabolism was within the parameters of what we consider normal limits. The risks of trying to reduce serum insulin levels raise all kinds of problems and would not seem to be an efficacious research project. The only value would be to identify men at high risk for coronary events because of their elevated serum insulin and attempt to reduce secondary risk factors such as smoking and serum lipids.

R.C. Davidson, M.D., M.P.H.

***Helicobacter pylori* Infection and Mortality From Ischaemic Heart Disease: Negative Result From a Large, Prospective Study**
Wald NJ, Law MR, Morris JK, et al (St. Bartholomew's and the Royal London School of Medicine and Dentistry)
BMJ 315:1199–1201, 1997
1–12

Background.—An association has been proposed between *H. pylori* stomach infection and ischemic heart disease. A large prospective study was designed to assess this relationship.

Study Design.—The British United Provident Association study is a prospective study of 21,520 professional British men aged 35–64 who attended the British United Provident Association medical center between 1975 and 1982 for a routine medical examination. Risk factors for ischemic heart disease were assessed and serum samples were stored. This study is based on follow-up until the end of 1994, an average of 15.6 years of follow-up for study participants. During this period, 684 men without a history of ischemic heart disease died of ischemic heart disease. For each case, 2 controls without ischemic heart disease, but matched for age and duration of serum sample storage were selected. Antibody titers specific for *H. pylori* were measured by enzyme-linked immunosorbent assay kit for the stored serum samples.

Findings.—The presence of *H. pylori* infection did not differ significantly between the men who died of ischemic heart disease and the controls. Risk factors were identical between these 2 groups, indicating that the study population avoided confounding variables. There was no association detected between *H. pylori* infection and ischemic heart disease risk in this study population.

Conclusions.—This study is the largest, prospective study without confounding variables of ischemic heart disease and *H. pylori* infection. There was no significant association detected. This result indicates that screening and treating for *H. pylori* infection, while it may reduce the incidence of stomach cancer, will do little to prevent ischemic heart disease.

▶ I have read with curiosity some of the previously published results raising the possibility that infection with *H. pylori* increases the risk for ischemic heart disease. Although it is intriguing to think of a reversible risk factor for ischemic heart disease, this well-designed large cohort study showed no relationship between infection and ischemic heart disease. I think the power of this study puts to rest the controversy regarding *H. pylori* and ischemic heart disease. However, this does not reduce the need to treat these patients with *H. pylori* to reduce their gastrointestinal complications.

R.C. Davidson, M.D., M.P.H.

Risk Factors for Coronary Heart Disease and Infection with *Helicobacter pylori*: Meta-analysis of 18 Studies
Danesh J, Peto R (Univ of Oxford, England)
BMJ 316:1130–1132, 1998   1–13

Introduction.—There are epidemiologic data linking chronic gastric infection with *Helicobacter pylori* to coronary heart disease. It is uncertain whether *H. pylori* infection is correlated with risk factors for coronary heart disease, such as body mass index, blood pressure, and blood lipid levels. Correlations between *H. pylori* seropositivity and risk factors for coronary heart disease were assessed.

Methods.—The meta-analysis included 18 epidemiologic studies reporting on correlations between serum antibody titers to *H. pylori* and specific vascular risk factors, including blood pressure, body mass index, plasma viscosity, white blood cell count, and lipid levels. Data on 10,000 patients were included.

Results.—Absolute differences between patients who were *H. pylori* seropositive and seronegative were small, including differences in plasma viscosity, blood glucose concentration, body mass index, and high-density lipoprotein cholesterol. The only highly significant differences between groups were in body mass index, which was slightly higher (0.37) in seropositive patients; and high-density lipoprotein cholesterol, which was slightly lower (0.032 mmol/L) in seropositive patients. Some studies of certain risk factors gave heterogeneous results, mainly between the initial studies proposing the associations and the later studies that failed to confirm them.

Conclusions.—Few important correlations were found between *H. pylori* infection and risk factors for coronary heart disease. Previous reports of such correlations may have resulted from chance and/or preferential publication. If there is any link between *H. pylori* infection and coronary heart disease, it does not operate through the risk factors examined in this study.

▶ The past year has shown a flurry of interest around a possible link between *H. pylori* infection and coronary artery disease. A retrospective study published in the *Lancet* suggested a link, and theorized that the increased leukocytes from the chronic infection might be the causative factor.

However, these authors did a meta-analysis of 18 studies involving 10,000 patients comparing serum antibody titers to *H. pylori* and risk factors for coronary artery disease. They could find no relationship between *H. pylori* seropositivity and risk factors for coronary heart disease.

Wouldn't it be nice to find some type of easily treatable condition whose amelioration would reduce a patient's risk for myocardial infarction? However, *H. pylori* infection does not seem to be this condition.

R.C. Davidson, M.D., M.P.H.

Myocardial Infarction

Outcomes in Patients With Acute Non–Q-Wave Myocardial Infarction Randomly Assigned to an Invasive as Compared With a Conservative Management Strategy

Boden WE, for the Veterans Affairs Non–Q-Wave Infarction Strategies in Hospital (VANQWISH) Trial Investigators (State Univ of New York, Syracuse; Veterans Affairs Med Ctr, San Antonio, Tex; Veterans Affairs Med Ctr, Albuquerque, NM; et al)
N Engl J Med 338:1785–1792, 1998
1–14

Background.—The majority of acute myocardial infarctions in the United States are non–Q-wave myocardial infarctions, but the management of this type of infarction remains controversial. Early invasive management of the non–Q-wave myocardial infarction patient is common. A multicenter, randomized, controlled clinical trial was performed to prospectively compare invasive with conservative therapy in a large group of acute non–Q-wave myocardial infarction patients.

Methods.—The Veterans Affairs Non–Q-Wave Infarction Strategies in Hospital trial began enrollment at 15 sites in 1993. Participants were randomly assigned to invasive or conservative management within 72 hours after onset of non–Q-wave infarction, according to the adaptive-allocation procedure to maximize the similarity of the 2 treatment groups. Patients randomly assigned to the early invasive strategy group underwent coronary angiography and then the Thrombolysis in Myocardial Infarction trial management guidelines for revascularization were followed. Patients randomly assigned to the conservative strategy group underwent radionuclide ventriculography and a symptom-limited treadmill exercise test with thallium scintigraphy. Coronary angiography was only performed in this group if there was recurrent postinfarction angina with ischemic electrocardiographic changes, ST-segment depression of at least 2 mm on peak exercise electrocardiogram, redistribution defects in at least 2 vascular regions on thallium scintigraphy or a redistribution defect plus increased lung uptake of thallium. Patients could receive any standard medical therapy. Trial enrollment ended at the end of 1995. Patients were followed up 1 month after discharge and then at 3-month intervals until the end of 1996. The primary trial end point was death or myocardial infarction. Overall mortality and major procedural complications were also examined.

Results.—During a mean follow-up of 23 months, there were 80 deaths and 72 nonfatal myocardial infarctions in 138 patients in the invasive strategy group and 59 deaths and 80 nonfatal myocardial infarctions in 123 patients in the conservative strategy group. Patients in the invasive strategy group had worse clinical outcomes during the first year of follow-up. The number of patients with either death or myocardial infarction at discharge, at 1 month and at 1 year was significantly higher in the invasive strategy group. Overall mortality during follow-up did not differ significantly between these 2 groups.

Conclusions.—In a predominantly male moderate-to-high risk population of non–Q-wave myocardial infarction patients, conservative management had better outcomes at all time points examined than early invasive treatment. This suggests that most non–Q-wave myocardial infarction patients will not benefit from routine management with early invasive treatment. A conservative strategy based on ischemia-guided management is both safe and effective for these patients.

▶ There is a current emphasis nationwide on physicians relying more on "evidenced-based medicine" in their decision-making. As I reviewed the literature on numerous studies, I am always amazed at the large number of "truths" in medicine that have never been studied in a controlled manner. That is why articles such as this study are so important to our decision-making.

This is a nicely designed random assignment of 920 patients into an invasive or conservative therapy program for non–Q-wave myocardial infarction. Surprising to many, and probably controversial to many, is the finding that conservative therapy at least equaled if not exceeded both event-based occurrence and overall survival of patients with this condition.

Even with the improvements in technique and survival for invasive procedures, there is still an inherent risk in these procedures. I was very pleased that the authors did not use cost as a major criteria in this study. Certainly the conservative management program is less expensive than the invasive program. However, they base their recommendations purely on the science of a well controlled study.

R.C. Davidson, M.D., M.P.H.

Long-term Outcome in Acute Myocardial Infarction Patients Admitted to Hospitals With and Without On-site Cardiac Catheterization Facilities
Every NR, Parsons LS, Fihn SD, et al (Univ of Washington, Seattle; Henry Ford Health Care System, Detroit)
Circulation 96:1770–1775, 1997   1–15

Introduction.—Limiting the availability of technology can reduce costs, but this strategy may not be appropriate in many conditions. Several recent studies, however, suggest that not all hospitals need catheterization facilities for optimal management of patients with acute myocardial infarction (AMI). A cohort of patients with AMI was followed to determine the long-term consequences of admission to hospitals with and without on-site cardiac catheterization laboratories.

Methods.—Patients included in the study had been admitted to 19 hospitals in the Seattle area: 7,985 patients to hospitals with and 4,346 patients to hospitals without on-site catheterization laboratories. Patient

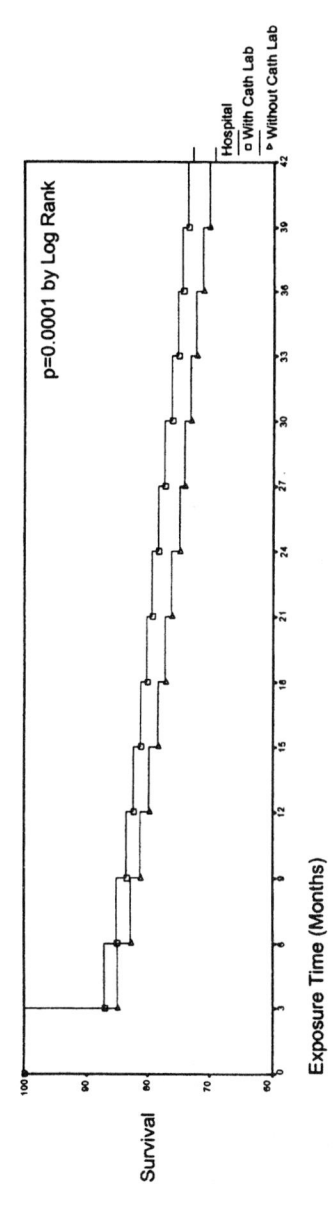

FIGURE 3.—Survival rates during follow-up in patients admitted to hospitals with and without on-site cardiac catheterization labs. In this unadjusted comparison, patients admitted to hospitals with on-site catheterization labs had higher long-term survival (74% vs. 71% at 3 years, P=.0001). *Abbreviation: Cath*, catheterization. (Courtesy of Every NR, Parsons LS, Fihn SD, et al: Long-term outcome in acute myocardial infarction patients admitted to hospitals with and without on-site cardiac catheterization facilities. *Circulation* 96:1770–1775, 1997.)

records were examined within 3 months of discharge or death for demographic data, admission status, hospital course, and procedural information.

Results.—The 2 groups were generally similar in medical history. Those admitted to hospitals with on-site catheterization were younger and more likely to be male than those admitted to hospitals without an on-site facility. During the index hospitalization, patients at hospitals with on-site catheterization were significantly more likely to undergo coronary angiography than those at hospitals without on-site catheterization (67.1% vs. 39.3%). Patients with access to on-site laboratories also had a higher rate of coronary angioplasty (32.5% vs. 13.2%) and coronary bypass surgery (12.5% vs. 9.5%). Thirty percent of those admitted to the hospitals without on-site catheterization were transferred during the index hospitalization; 90% subsequently underwent coronary angiography. Patients who were not transferred were significantly more likely to die during hospitalization. Total cumulative costs at 3 years were higher for patients admitted to hospitals with on-site catheterization, and these patients had higher unadjusted long-term survival (Fig 3) than patients admitted to hospitals without such facilities. With multivariate adjustments, however, long-term mortality did not differ in the 2 groups.

Conclusion.—Patients with AMI who were admitted to a hospital without on-site catheterization facilities were managed with fewer procedures than similar patients admitted to a hospital with such facilities. In an urban area with access to transfer, this conservative approach was not associated with increased long-term mortality.

▶ As I read this article, I was reminded of the popular movie about the building of a baseball field in the middle of a cornfield in Iowa. The key phrase in this movie was, "If you build it, they will come." We might paraphrase that to summarize this article by saying, "If you have a cath lab, they will use it."

It is not my intent to poke fun at the excellent cardiologists who are working diligently to reduce the mortality from coronary artery disease and acute myocardial infarction. However, the invasive cardiologists seem absolutely convinced that immediate transfer to a facility with catheterization capability is "best" for the patient. This large study of over 12,000 acute myocardial infarction patients showed no difference in immediate or 3-year morbidity or mortality between patients cared for in a cardiac center with catheterization capability and patients cared for in a community hospital without this capability. Of course the corollary of this was true also. Facilities with coronary angiography capability used this procedure much more frequently, at an increased average cost per case of $2,500.

The simple message is that we cannot accept at face value any new technology. We must apply the same rigorous well-controlled studies to cardiac catheterization that we do to all other proposed treatments.

R.C. Davidson, M.D., M.P.H.

Effect of Reperfusion on Biventricular Function and Survival After Right Ventricular Infarction
Bowers TR, O'Neill WW, Grines C, et al (William Beaumont Hosp, Royal Oak, Mich)
N Engl J Med 338:933–940, 1998

Background.—Although the beneficial effects of reperfusion in patients with left ventricular infarction have been well documented, the benefits for patients with acute right ventricular infarction are more controversial. The effects of primary percutaneous transluminal coronary angioplasty (PTCA) of the occluded right coronary artery on right ventricular function and clinical outcome were assessed in patients with acute ischemic right ventricular dysfunction.

Methods.—The study group consisted of 53 patients who were seen between 1994 and 1996 with acute inferior myocardial infarction and ischemic right ventricular dysfunction, and who underwent emergency cardiac catheterization and primary PTCA. To evaluate ventricular function, serial echocardiograms were obtained before PTCA and 1 hour, 24 hours, 3–5 days, and 1 month after PTCA. To evaluate perfusion, coronary angiograms were also obtained. Adverse clinical events were recorded.

Results.—Complete reperfusion was achieved in 77% of the patients. Reperfusion was associated with rapid, significant recovery of right ventricular function. Reperfusion was unsuccessful in 12 of 53 patients. Reperfusion failure was associated with a lack of recovery of right ventricular function, persistent hypotension, low cardiac output, and a high mortality rate.

Conclusions.—The results of this study of reperfusion in patients with acute right ventricular infarction demonstrate that complete reperfusion improves right ventricular function and clinical outcome. Reperfusion failure is associated with impaired right ventricular function recovery, persistent hemodynamic compromise, and a high rate of mortality.

▶ Common sense leads one to conclude that if we were able to reestablish the blood supply to infarcted heart muscle safely, we might improve the function of that heart muscle, compared to the function of infarcted muscle that has not been successfully reperfused. This has certainly been shown in a number of trials on left ventricular function. This article describes a similar effect on survival after right ventricular infarction in patients who were successfully reperfused, compared to survival in patients who did not have this reperfusion. The authors found a significant improvement in right ventricular function after reperfusion.

The improving statistics on reduction of morbidity and mortality for coronary artery disease are encouraging. Certainly much of this improvement can be attributed to lifestyle and dietary changes, as well as to medications that affect adverse lipid profiles. However, we should not neglect the significant improvement that can occur with modern reparative surgery immediately following myocardial infarction.

R.C. Davidson, M.D., M.P.H.

Secondary Prevention of Coronary Artery Disease

Effect of Pravastatin on Cardiovascular Events in Women After Myocardial Infarction: The Cholesterol and Recurrent Events (CARE) Trial
Lewis SJ, for the CARE Investigators (Legacy Good Samaritan Hosp, Portland, Ore; Brigham and Women's Hosp, Boston; Baylor Univ, Dallas; et al)
J Am Coll Cardiol 32:140–146, 1998
1–17

Introduction.—Previous studies of cardiovascular risk and cholesterol levels often have been limited to male patients. The Cholesterol and Recurrent Events (CARE) trial also included a large number of women in its investigation of the effect of pravastatin on recurrent cardiovascular events. The 576 postmenopausal women in this article had average cholesterol levels after myocardial infarction (MI).

Methods.—Patients eligible for the multicenter trial were younger than 75 years, had an acute MI between 3 and 20 months before randomization, a plasma total cholesterol level less than 240 mg/dL, a low density lipoprotein (LDL) cholesterol level 115 to 174 mg/dL, and a fasting triglyceride level less than 350 mg/dL. Randomization was to pravastatin (40 mg/day) or matching placebo for a median follow-up period of 5 years. Men and women were compared for their response to drug therapy as indicated by reductions in total coronary events.

Results.—Women were older than men at randomization and were more likely than men to have multiple risk factors for coronary heart disease (CHD). Some baseline risk factors were significantly greater in women than in men: hypertension, diabetes, current smoking, and family history of CHD. Women also had a higher mean total cholesterol concentration than men. Men were more likely to have received thrombolytic therapy for their MI and to have undergone coronary artery bypass graft (CABG) surgery between MI and randomization. Treatment with pravastatin was beneficial in both men and women, but the magnitude of risk reduction was greater in women: 43% for the primary end point, 46% for combined coronary events, 40% for CABG, and 56% for stroke. Pravastatin improved plasma lipids similarly in both men and women.

Conclusion.—Cardiovascular disease is the leading cause of death in women, and there is need for information about cholesterol treatment for women after MI. Women with an MI showed strong and early reductions in recurrent coronary events during pravastatin therapy, despite having some greater risks than men and higher mean total cholesterol levels before treatment.

▶ After my negative comments on several of the studies that included male subjects only, I felt it only fair to include a research project on women and their risk for coronary events. The authors showed a reduction in risk for coronary events by use of a statin drug in women who have had myocardial infarction.

There are no surprises here. The cardiovascular systems of men and women are almost identical. It makes sense that women who have known coronary artery disease and have had a myocardial infarction will be helped by secondary prevention of future events by reduction of their cholesterol levels. I do feel compelled to identify that this research project was funded by a major drug company with secondary gain from the sale of their statin drug.

R.C. Davidson, M.D., M.P.H.

Miscellaneous

Likelihood of Spontaneous Conversion of Atrial Fibrillation to Sinus Rhythm
Danias PG, Caulfield TA, Weigner MJ, et al (Univ of Connecticut, Farmington; Harvard Med School, Boston)
J Am Coll Cardiol 31:588–592, 1998

Background.—Up to 2% of the population experiences atrial fibrillation, a condition which often spontaneously converts to a sinus rhythm. Early therapy for this state often includes pharmacologic or direct current cardioversion. However, these procedures are expensive, time-consuming, and have a number of related risks. This study investigated the predictive factors for and likelihood for spontaneous conversion from atrial fibrillation (symptoms less than 72 hours) to sinus rhythm.

Methods.—Researchers identified 356 patients with atrial fibrillation lasting less than 72 hours before presentation from among 1,822 adults consecutively admitted with atrial fibrillation (45% men; mean age, 68 ± 16 years). Patient charts were reviewed for spontaneous conversion to sinus rhythm. Researchers also noted echocardiographic and clinical data.

Results.—Sixty eight percent of the test group exhibited spontaneous conversion to sinus rhythm (n = 242; 95% confidence interval [CI], 63% to 73%). Among these 242 patients, 159 (66%) experienced atrial fibrillation for less than 24 hours, 42 (17%) had atrial fibrillation for from 24 to 48 hours, and 41 (17%) had atrial fibrillation for more than 48 hours. The only predictor of spontaneous conversion identified through logistic regression analysis was early (24 hours) patient presentation after onset of symptoms (odds ratio, 1.8; 95% CI; 1.4 to 2.4, P less than 0.0001). Although patients who experienced spontaneous conversion were more likely to have normal systolic function of the left ventricle, this was not a predictive factor ($P = 0.03$).

Conclusion.—The best predictor for spontaneous conversion from atrial fibrillation in patients seen with less than 72 hours of symptoms is early patient presentation (less than 24 hours) after onset of symptoms.

▶ The potential adverse effects of atrial fibrillation on cardiovascular hemodynamics as well as embolic sequelae is well known. Conversion to a normal rhythm is certainly preferable than long-term anticoagulation therapy. This interesting study looks at the spontaneous conversion rate of almost 2,000 consecutive adults admitted to hospital for recent onset atrial fibrillation. They found that almost 70% of these patients spontaneously converted to sinus rhythm. They also found that most of these spontaneous conversions occurred within the first 24 hours of hospitalization. It seemed to me a logical conclusion from this study that, barring other factors, a waiting period of 24 hours before any type of electroconversion is attempted would be prudent. However, these cardiology authors make no such recommendation.

R.C. Davidson, M.D., M.P.H.

Calcium Channel Blockers and the Risk of Cancer
Rosenberg L, Rao S, Palmer JR, et al (Boston Univ, Brookline, Mass; Univ of Pennsylvania, Philadelphia; Univ of Maryland, Baltimore; et al)
JAMA 279:1000–1004, 1998

Objective.—Epidemiologic studies have suggested that calcium channel blockers (CCBs) increase the risk of cancer overall as well as of specific cancers. Results of a case-control drug surveillance study investigating this and whether β-blockers and angiotensin-converting enzyme (ACE) inhibitors also increase cancer risk were reported.

Methods.—Between 1976 and 1996, nurses at participating hospitals in Baltimore, New York, and Philadelphia interviewed 9,513 patients, aged 40 to 69 years, who had been admitted for first occurrences of cancer, and 6,492 case controls with nonmalignant conditions regarding their medical and lifestyle histories. Primary cancers affecting at least 20 patients were recorded. Use of CCBs, β-blockers, and ACE inhibitors was assessed.

Results.—Use of CCBs averaged 3.8 years for patients with malignancies and 3.7 years for controls. There was no increase in either overall or specific cancer incidence with CCB use, with the exception of kidney cancer (relative risk, 1.8). The duration of CCB use, specific CCB use, and recent CCB use were unrelated to cancer incidence. The use of β-blockers or ACE inhibitors also did not increase overall or specific cancer incidence except for kidney cancer (relative risk, 1.8 and 1.9, respectively).

Conclusion.—Whereas CCB, β blocker, and ACE inhibitor use did not increase the incidence of overall cancer, each approximately doubled the risk of kidney cancer.

▶ A number of studies over the past 2 years have raised significant questions regarding the efficacy of CCBs as a primary drug for hypertension.

Several studies have shown all-cause mortality to be higher in patients taking these agents. There was a suggestion that this may be the result of an increased risk of cancer in patients taking CCBs. This study did an in-depth analysis of 9,513 cases of patients with new-onset cancer admitted to hospital. From this population, the authors took a case-control drug history, specifically investigating the use of CCBs.

With the exception of kidney cancer, they found no relationship between the use of CCBs and the overall risk of cancer. Because calcium channel blockers are predominantly used in the treatment of hypertension and hypertension is a known risk factor for renal cancer, the link is most probably this confounding variable rather than the drug itself.

We have certainly not heard the last of studies on CCBs. We still do not have an explanation for a demonstrable rise in all-cause mortality. However, this well-designed study was unable to demonstrate an increased cancer risk for patients using CCBs.

R.C. Davidson, M.D., M.P.H.

Effects of Lovastatin on the Immune System
Muldoon MF, Flory JD, Marsland A, et al (Univ of Pittsburgh, Pa)
Am J Cardiol 80:1391–1394, 1997   1–20

Introduction.—Evidence suggests that the 3-hydroxy-3-methaglutaryl coenzyme A (HMG-CoA) reductase inhibitors—the "statin" cholesterol-lowering drugs—could affect immune function. Clinical trials of these drugs have found no increase in deaths from noncoronary heart disease; however, the incidence of infections and the possible long-term effects on cancer are unknown. The effects of lovastatin on immune cell function in humans were studied.

Methods.—The study included 67 otherwise healthy adults with hypercholesterolemia, defined as a low-density lipoprotein (LDL) cholesterol level of 160 mg/dL or more. They were randomized to receive 6 months of treatment with either lovastatin, 20 mg/day, or placebo. Blood samples were taken for immune testing before and after treatment.

Results.—Compared with the placebo group, patients treated with lovastatin had a 17% reduction in total cholesterol and a 25% reduction in LDL cholesterol, with a slight increase in high-density lipoprotein cholesterol. Total lymphocyte number, and all lymphocyte subset populations, were unaffected by lovastatin treatment. Neither were there any differences in proliferative responses to phytohemagglutinin, natural killer cell cytotoxicity, or interleukin 2 production.

Conclusions.—These findings indicate lovastatin treatment has no adverse effects on immune function in healthy patients with hypercholesterolemia. The results are not consistent with those of some laboratory studies. Long-term studies of the effects of statin drugs on the immune system are needed.

▶ The HMG-CoA reductase inhibitors, commonly known as the "statin" drugs, have become the first line drug therapy for the common condition of hypercholesterolemia. It is well known that some individuals demonstrate elevated liver function tests when taking the statin drugs. We commonly check for this on a periodic basis. There has been concern that the statin drugs might lower the body's immune response. Some laboratory studies have demonstrated a lower immune cell response in the serum of patients on statin drugs.

However, the large trials of the efficacy of the statin drugs have shown no increase in noncardiac mortality. This in vivo study attempted to look at the effect on the immune response of a cohort of 67 adult patients started on lovastatin. The authors found no reduction in immune function during the 6-month clinical trial.

Those of us in practice for awhile have seen other "wonder drugs" come and go because of unexpected side effects of the medication. The statin drugs seem to be a remarkable drug in lowering overall mortality from coronary artery disease and myocardial infarction. It is comforting to find that, at least in this trial, the authors could find no evidence of a lowered immune response as one of the potential side effects of the statin drugs. I certainly hope we don't find any unexpected bad effects from these drugs, but I'm glad our research industry continues to look.

R.C. Davidson, M.D., M.P.H.

Reduction of Plasma Homocyst(e)ine Levels by Breakfast Cereal Fortified With Folic Acid in Patients With Coronary Heart Disease
Malinow MR, Duell PB, Hess DL, et al (Oregon Regional Primate Research Ctr, Beaverton; Oregon Health Sciences Univ, Portland; Providence St Vincent Med Ctr, Portland, Ore; et al)
N Engl J Med 338:1009–1015, 1998   1–21

Objective.—The research finding that folic acid supplementation can prevent congenital neural tube defects has led to folic acid supplementation of cereal-grain products in the U.S. food supply. At the fortification level recommended by the Food and Drug Administration (FDA), folic acid intake would increase by 80–100 µg/day in women of childbearing age and by 70–120 µg/day in adults more than 50 years of age. Plasma homocysteine is commonly elevated in patients with arterial occlusive disease and can be reduced by folic acid supplementation. This study sought to determine whether folic acid fortification can reduce plasma homocysteine levels in patients with coronary artery disease.

Methods.—The randomized, controlled trial included 75 adult patients with coronary artery disease. They were randomized to receive breakfast cereals fortified with 3 levels of folic acid—127, 499, and 665 µg—along with the recommended daily allowances of vitamins B_6 and B_{12}. The subjects ate cereal containing 1 of the 3 folic acid levels or placebo for the first 5 weeks; after a 5-week washout period, they were switched to the alternate cereal. The effects of the different levels of folic acid fortification on plasma folic acid and homocysteine levels were assessed.

Results.—As the level of folic acid fortification increased, so did plasma folic acid and plasma homocysteine. The 127–µg folic acid level, chosen to approximate the results of the FDA's recommended fortification level, produced a 31% increase in plasma folic acid, but only a 4% decrease in plasma homocysteine. The 499-µg level of folic acid increased plasma folic acid by 65% and reduced plasma homocysteine by 11%. The 665-µg level increased plasma folic acid by 106% while reducing plasma homocysteine by 14%.

Conclusions.—Fortification of cereal grains with folic acid could lead to increased plasma folic acid levels and reduced plasma homocysteine levels. To achieve this effect, higher levels of folic acid supplementation than those currently recommended by the FDA may be required. Additional studies will be needed to determine whether folic acid fortification can prevent vascular disease.

▶ There is increasing evidence that diets deficient in folic acid can lead to multiple health problems. The neural tube defects in children born to women with folic acid deficiency are well known. More recently, evidence is mounting that folic acid is related to levels of plasma homocysteine, which is a known risk factor for coronary artery disease. This study was designed to test the hypothesis put forward by the Food and Drug Administration (FDA) that we should recommend that breakfast cereal grain products be fortified with additional folic acid. In a well-designed, randomized, double-blind, placebo-controlled crossover trial, the authors were able to demonstrate that cereal fortified with folic acid has the potential to increase plasma folic acid levels and reduce plasma homocysteine levels.

There is an inevitable debate whenever the government attempts to add a substance in food or water supply. Our community continues to debate fluoride in the water system. However, vitamin D supplementation of most milk products seems to be universally accepted. This study shows compelling evidence of the value of folic acid fortification of morning breakfast cereals. Whether this will be accepted by the manufacturers and consumers is yet to be seen.

R.C. Davidson, M.D., M.P.H.

Effects of Intermittent Transdermal Nitroglycerin on Occurrence of Ischemia After Patch Removal: Results of the Second Transdermal Intermittent Dosing Evaluation Study (TIDES-II)

Pepine CJ, Lopez LM, Bell DM, et al (Univ of Florida, Gainesville; West Virginia Univ, Morgantown)
J Am Coll Cardiol 30:955–961, 1997

Introduction.—Transdermal nitroglycerin (TD-NTG) patches, initially applied continuously over 24 hours, were found to be associated with partial or complete tolerance, and a 10- to 12-hour "patch-off" period was recommended. Some patients, however, had more ischemia during this nitrate-free interval. In a multicenter study, the effects of intermittent TD-NTG on the occurrence of ischemia during patch-off hours were evaluated in patients with stable angina who were taking other agents to suppress angina.

Methods.—Period 1 of the study assessed tolerability to TD-NTG during a 3-week period in which patients were instructed to wear the patch for 14 hours a day. In period 2, 72 patients received either double-blind transdermal placebo or maximally tolerated TD-NTG for 2 weeks, then they crossed over to the alternate treatment for an additional 2 weeks during period 3. The patch was applied daily at 8 AM and removed at 10 PM; symptoms and sublingual nitroglycerin use were recorded in a diary. Ischemia during patch-on and patch-off periods was assessed by patients' perceptions of angina, a symptom-limited exercise treadmill test (ETT), and 48-hour ambulatory ECG (AECG) monitoring.

Results.—Compared with placebo, TD-NTG (0.2–0.4 mg/hr) significantly reduced the magnitude of ST-segment depression at angina onset during ETT. The active and placebo patch groups did not differ significantly in total angina frequency, but angina frequency increased with TD-NTG compared with placebo during patch-off hours. The AECG analyses also yielded similar trends for an increase in ischemia after TD-NTG. The frequency of ischemia tended to be higher during patch-on hours but lower during patch-off hours for placebo. The ischemia frequency decreased 58% from patch-on to patch-off periods in the placebo condition, whereas the TD-NTG condition resulted in a 14% increase in ischemia frequency. The frequency of ischemic episodes during TD-NTG therapy did not vary during 6-hour periods, but with placebo, there was a highly significant difference in the 6-hour period after midnight compared with the morning and afternoon periods.

Conclusions.—The normal diurnal pattern of ischemia appears to be disrupted with intermittent TD-NTG. Patients using intermittent TD-NTG have an increase in ischemia during patch-off hours, which is a subjective finding supported by a similar trend for increased AECG ischemia during this period.

▶ The use of continuous nitrate dosing by transdermal nitroglycerin patches remains controversial. It has been proven that this is an effective way to provide steady-state nitrate blood levels. However, previous studies have raised the issue of the development of partial or complete tolerance when these patches are used continuously. More commonly, patients are advised to use them for 10–12 hours per day.

This was a well-designed, double-blind, placebo-controlled crossover study watching for signs of myocardial ischemia during periods of use of the transdermal patch or drug-free periods. The authors found an increase in ischemic frequency during the periods when the patches were not being used. They raised the question of whether the risks of ischemia during these off-patch hours overcomes the risks of drug tolerance development. Obviously, more studies will need to be done on this issue. For now, I think we need to follow our best judgment regarding clinical symptoms in our patients.

R.C. Davidson, M.D., M.P.H.

2 Vascular Disease

Overview

Randomized controlled trial: Abstract 2–5

Carotid Artery Disease

- Outcomes in asymptomatic carotid disease
- Outcomes for carotid endarterectomy related to provider volumes
- Increase in carotid endarterectomy following publication of the ACAS study

Deep Vein Thrombosis and Pulmonary Embolism

- Diagnosis of deep vein thrombosis
- Vena caval filters in the prevention of pulmonary embolism
- Pulmonary embolism presenting as syncope

Anticoagulation

- An algorithm for administering subcutaneous heparin
- Cost effectiveness of a nurse specialist anticoagulation service
- Acetaminophen and other risks for excessive warfarin anticoagulation

Carotid Artery Disease

Outcome of Asymptomatic Patients With Carotid Disease
Mackey AE, and the Asymptomatic Cervical Bruit Study Group (Laval Univ, Quebec; McGill Univ, Montreal; Montreal Gen Hosp)
Neurology 48:896–903, 1997   2–1

Background.—A variable risk of vascular events is associated with asymptomatic cervical atherosclerosis. The current study attempted to identify patients with asymptomatic cervical bruits in whom the risk of ischemic events may be increased.

Methods.—Seven hundred fifteen patients with a cervical bruit but no neurologic symptoms were enrolled in the prospective, multicenter cohort study. Mean patient age was 65 years. Neurologic and carotid duplex assessments were done biannually. Mean follow-up was 3.6 years.

Findings.—Three hundred fifty-seven patients had stenoses of 50% or greater at the initial visit. Overall, 177 patients had a total of 237 events. The annual rates of all primary vascular events were 11% in those with

50% stenosis or greater and 4.2% in those with less than 50% stenosis. The annual rates of stroke and vascular death were 5.5% and 1.9%, respectively. Patients with stenoses of 80% or greater had an annual unheralded ischemic stroke rate of 4.2%, compared with 1.4% in those with stenoses of less than 80%. In 66% of the patients, a stroke or transient ischemic attack was ipsilateral to a stenosis of 80% or more. Progression of carotid stenosis, especially to more than 80%, was correlated with a greater rate of ipsilateral neurologic events and overall combined vascular events.

Conclusions.—Severity of carotid stenosis is the primary risk factor predicting the occurrence of neurologic and other vascular events. The annual rate of ipsilateral stroke in patients with 50% or greater carotid stenosis is low, and most of these strokes are not disabling. Outcomes are worse when disease progresses to 80% or greater occlusion.

▶ This is an important study in the debate on screening and treatment of asymptomatic carotid artery disease. The findings are consistent with earlier (and smaller) studies showing that asymptomatic patients generally have good outcomes without intervention. Even in the group with the highest grade of stenosis, annual stroke rates were less than 3%. In their 1995 report, the U.S. Preventive Services Task Force found insufficient evidence to recommend screening for asymptomatic carotid artery stenosis. The best means of prevention is to control risk factors such as hypertension and smoking. This study reinforces that conclusion.

A.O. Berg, M.D., M.P.H.

Indications, Outcomes, and Provider Volumes for Carotid Endarterectomy
Cebul RD, Snow RJ, Pine R, et al (Case Western Reserve Univ, Cleveland, Ohio; Cleveland Clinic Found, Ohio; Peer Review Systems, Inc, Westerville, Ohio)
JAMA 279:1282–1287, 1998

Introduction.—Several controlled trials have provided evidence that carotid endarterectomy is superior to best medical therapy in reducing subsequent stroke rates among patients at risk. The importance of patient selection relative to surgical or institutional proficiency has not been adequately studied, because measurements of surgical indications or patients' comorbid illness have not been adequately taken. The use and outcomes of carotid endarterectomy over a 1-year period were profiled. The relationships between surgeon-specific and hospital-specific volumes and 30-day stroke or death rate were examined, while the researchers controlled for surgical indications and other factors predictive of adverse outcomes.

Methods.—There were 678 charts retrospectively reviewed. The patients were non-health maintenance organization Medicare beneficiaries who had carotid endarterectomy in a 1-year period. They were similar to all eligible patients in sociodemographic characteristics and 30-day mortality rates.

Results.—Indications for surgery were asymptomatic carotid stenosis in 24.6% of patients, transient ischemic attack for 43.4% of patients, completed stroke in 9.1% of patients, and nonspecific symptoms in 22.9% of patients. By 30 days postoperatively, 32 patients (4.7%) died or suffered nonfatal strokes. Rates did not vary by surgeons' volume, but they did vary by hospital volume; however, the power to detect this difference was limited. Similar indications and distributions of comorbidities were found among patients at higher- and lower-volume hospitals. Being operated on in a higher-volume hospital conferred a 71% reduction in risk for 30-day stroke or death, in analyses controlling for indications, comorbid conditions, and surgeon's volume.

Conclusion.—Patients who are asymptomatic or who have nonspecific symptoms constitute almost half (47.5%) of the patients who receive carotid endarterectomies. It is important to identify patients and providers having the most favorable outcome profiles. Further investigation into the higher rate of adverse outcomes seen in lower-volume hospitals is merited, because the difference does not appear to be caused by differences in patient selection.

▶ As a member of the 1995 U.S. Preventive Services Task Force, I had responsibility for supervising and writing the chapter on screening for asymptomatic carotid artery stenosis. We concluded that there was insufficient evidence to recommend for or against routine screening, and were further concerned about the documented variations in outcomes with carotid endarterectomy. This article confirms that the concern about variation was well founded; but, more significantly, the study shows that surgery for patients with no or only mild symptoms accounts for nearly half of the procedures. These 2 findings add up to a potentially dangerous situation. Where screening is of uncertain benefit, and surgery is known to cause harm (at least occasionally) in the wrong hands, could we be doing more harm than good? I, for one, recommend a conservative approach that does not routinely screen asymptomatic individuals.

A.O. Berg, M.D., M.P.H.

Effect of the Asymptomatic Carotid Atherosclerosis Study on Carotid Endarterectomy in Florida
Huber TS, Wheeler KG, Cuddeback JK, et al (Univ of Florida, Gainesville; Duke Univ, Durham, NC)
Stroke 29:1099–1105, 1998   2–3

Background.—The value of carotid endarterectomy (CEA) for both symptomatic and asymptomatic patients has recently been defined by several clinical trials. The effect of the release of the Asymptomatic Carotid

Atherosclerosis Study (ACAS) Clinical Advisory in September 1994 on the number of CEAs performed in non-federal Florida hospitals was retrospectively examined.

Study Design.—Data were obtained from the Florida Agency for Healthcare Administration database on all patients undergoing CEA from 1992 (before Advisory) through 1996 (after Advisory) in all 202 non-federal, general, acute-care hospitals in Florida. Over this period, there were 46,741 CEAs performed in these hospitals. The number of CEAs, severity of illness, risk of mortality, and costs were compared by year and demographic group to determine the effect of the ACAS results.

Findings.—The number of CEAs increased 68% in 1995–1996 as compared with 1992–1994. This increase exceeded increases in total hospital discharges, surgical discharges, and state population. The increase included all demographic groups. There was a significant decrease in mortality, Risk of Mortality Scale, Severity of Illness Scale, and percentage of patients discharged more than 7 days postoperatively after release of the Clinical Advisory. The average length of hospital stay declined 28% and average adjusted charges declined 7% in this period. Despite the decline in average cost per patient, the overall increase in patient number resulted in an estimated $56 million increase in annual hospital payments.

Conclusion.—There was a large, sustained increase in the number of CEAs performed in non-federal Florida hospitals immediately after the release of the ACAS Clinical Advisory in September 1994. This increase could not be explained by increased hospital discharges, surgical discharges, or population increases. The increased volume was detected in all regions of Florida and in all demographic groups. This increase was associated with decreased procedure-associated in-hospital mortality, complication rates, and overall severity. The temporal relationship between the release of the Clinical Advisory and the increased CEA volume suggests a causal relationship. The estimated increases in hospital payments associated with this increased volume suggests a need for further cost-benefit analysis.

▶ I follow this issue closely because I did the primary review on asymptomatic carotid artery stenosis for the last United States Preventive Services Task Force report in 1995. I am unpersuaded that the ACAS study cited here which precipitated all the extra surgery really settles the issue, but no matter. The study shows that trials reporting results of a certain kind can have an enormous and rapid effect on the provision of services. "Of a certain kind" here means the suggestion that a surgical procedure has more indications. Unfortunately, we have more examples of the rapid introduction of new technologies (or extensions of old ones, as in this study) than we have examples of the withdrawal of interventions that have been proven not to work. It is a statement of the times.

A.O. Berg, M.D., M.P.H.

Deep Vein Thrombosis and Pulmonary Embolism

Does This Patient Have Deep Vein Thrombosis?
Anand SS, Wells PS, Hunt D, et al (McMaster Univ, Hamilton, Ontario, Canada; Ottawa Civic Hosp, Ontario, Canada)
JAMA 279:1094–1099, 1998

Objective.—Deep vein thrombosis (DVT) is the third most common cardiovascular disease in the United States. Unfortunately, because clinical symptoms and signs have low specificity, most symptomatic patients will not have DVT. A clinical scenario was presented to test the validity of the clinical assessment and diagnostic tests for suspected DVT.

Methods.—A MEDLINE computer search identified 68 articles published between 1966 and April 1997 dealing with the diagnosis of DVT.

Results.—The sensitivity and specificity of the clinical examination were 60% and 72%, respectively. Combining results of the clinical examination with independent predictive factors gave a sensitivity of 96% and a specificity of 20%. When clinical examination data, predictive factors, and noninvasive compression US results were combined into a clinical model, it was possible to stratify patients with suspected DVT into low-, moderate-, or high-probability groups.

Conclusion.—Using clinical examination data, independent predictive factors, and noninvasive tests such as compression US in a clinical predictive guide makes it possible to stratify patients into low-, moderate-, and high-risk groups for DVT and simplifies management of these patients.

▶ These authors completed a very thorough review of the literature over a 20-year period covering all research articles regarding DVT. From these, they developed a prediction model for the probability of patients actually having DVT. The authors suggest a point rating scale with 7 clinical parameters, each contributing 1 point. If the patient score is equal to or greater than 3, they predict a high probability of DVT and suggest additional testing, even in the case of normal US test results.

The most interesting part of this article, from my perspective, is the 7 risk factors identified in the medical literature. The authors' suggested clinical model for patients with a low, moderate, or high probability of DVT constitutes a rational approach to this difficult diagnostic issue.

R.C. Davidson, M.D., M.P.H.

A Clinical Trial of Vena Caval Filters in the Prevention of Pulmonary Embolism in Patients With Proximal Deep-Vein Thrombosis

Decousus H, for the Prévention du Risque d'Embolie Pulmonaire par Interruption Cave Study Group (Bellevue Hosp, Saint-Etienne, France; Cardiological Hosp, Lyons, France; Antoine Béclère Hosp, Clamart, France; et al)
N Engl J Med 338:409–415, 1998

Background.—The safety and efficacy of vena caval filters in preventing pulmonary embolism in patients with proximal deep-vein thrombosis have not been definitively established. The current study further investigated these issues.

Methods.—In a 2-by-2 factorial design, 400 patients with proximal deep-vein thrombosis at risk for pulmonary embolism were assigned to receive a vena caval filter or no filter and to receive low–molecular weight heparin or unfractionated heparin. On day 12 and at 2 years, the rates of recurrent venous thromboembolism, death, and major bleeding were determined.

Findings.—By day 12, symptomatic or asymptomatic pulmonary embolism had occurred in 1.1% of the patients with filters and in 4.8% of those with no filters. By 2 years, 20.8% and 11.6%, respectively, had had recurrent deep-vein thrombosis. Mortality and other outcomes did not differ significantly between groups. By day 12, 1.6% of the patients receiving low–molecular weight heparin and 4.2% given unfractionated heparin had had symptomatic or asymptomatic pulmonary embolism.

Conclusions.—The initial benefits of vena caval filter use for preventing pulmonary embolism in high-risk patients with proximal deep-vein thrombosis is counterbalanced by an excess of recurrent deep-vein thrombosis, with no difference in mortality. Low–molecular weight heparin is as safe and effective as unfractionated heparin for preventing pulmonary embolism.

▶ I intend to add this article to the cases I use when teaching evidence-based medicine. Here is another example of a time-honored treatment—making perfect mechanical and physiological sense—that turns out to confer no net benefit on important outcomes that patients would care about: recurrent deep-vein thrombosis and overall mortality. It takes a randomized clinical trial to prove efficacy, and it is especially hard to perform randomized trials in cases like this where usual care and common sense suggest that the status quo is just fine. Despite the many uncontrolled reports suggesting that filters are a good thing (and that up to 40,000 filters are inserted annually in the United States), in my view this single high-quality randomized controlled trial should change practice in the direction of discouraging their use.

A.O. Berg, M.D., M.P.H.

Syncope as an Emergency Department Presentation of Pulmonary Embolism
Wolfe TR, Allen TL (Univ of Utah, Salt Lake City; Univ of Pittsburgh, Pa)
J Emerg Med 16:27–31, 1998
2–6

Background.—Venous thromboembolism causes about 50,000 deaths per year in the United States and is responsible for more than 250,000 hospitalizations. Although the actual incidence of pulmonary embolism is estimated at 650,000 cases per year, the actual incidence is unknown because it is difficult to diagnosis. The cases of 3 patients with pulmonary embolism–induced syncope are described.

Case 2.—Man, 38, suddenly felt dizzy while walking into his bathroom. His wife reported that he sat down, shook his head, and was unresponsive for about 20 seconds. She called the paramedics, but on their arrival, the patient was alert, oriented, and denied any continuing symptoms. The patient had a history of hypertension and was taking diltiazem, atenolol, and chlorthalidone. About twenty minutes after the paramedics had left, they were called back for cardiopulmonary arrest. The patient had no pulse, was apneic, and had a Glasgow coma score of 3. The monitor showed bradycardic pulseless electrical activity. The patient died in spite of the use of standard advanced cardiac life support measures. Autopsy showed a massive pulmonary embolus. The patient had no risk factors for venous thrombosis (Table 1) and no other medical history.

TABLE 1.—Risk Factors for Pulmonary Embolism

Current deep venous thrombosis
Trauma (especially to lower extremity, pelvis)
Postoperative period
Prolonged immobilization
Previous thrombophlebitis, venous thrombosis, or pulmonary emboli
Pregnancy or postpartum <3 months
Oral estrogen therapy
Underlying malignancy
Polycythemia
Burns
Obesity
Stroke
Heart disease (especially congestive heart failure)
Protein C or S deficiency
Resistance to activated protein C
Antithrombin III deficiency

(Reprinted with permission from Wolfe TR, Allen TL: Syncope as an emergency department presentation of pulmonary embolism. *J Emerg Med* 16:27–31. Copyright 1998, Elsevier Science.)

Discussion.—Clinicians are encouraged to consider pulmonary embolism in every patient with syncope. Patients with pulmonary embolism and syncope often seek treatment after the clot has dispersed and they are relatively asymptomatic. Identifying pulmonary embolism as the underlying cause of syncope is difficult and becomes more difficult when patients delay seeking treatment. Recommendations are also discussed.

▶ Pulmonary embolism is often a fatal condition and frequently a missed diagnosis. When it causes an untimely death, a lawsuit frequently arises. I have never considered syncope as a presentation for pulmonary embolism, but this article has sensitized me to this possibility. The table from this article is a handy reference and a reminder that pulmonary embolism should be considered in a wide range of patients with acute illness.

J.E. Scherger, M.D., M.P.H.

Anticoagulation

Use of an Algorithm for Administering Subcutaneous Heparin in the Treatment of Deep Venous Thrombosis
Prandoni P, Bagatella P, Bernardi E, et al (Univ of Padua, Italy)
Ann Intern Med 129:299–302, 1998   2–7

Introduction.—An initial course of unfractionated or low–molecular-weight heparin, followed by long-term oral anticoagulation therapy, is the usual initial treatment for patients with deep venous thrombosis. In previous studies, subcutaneous heparin has been shown to be as effective as intravenous heparin. The early discharge of patients from the hospital may be facilitated by low–molecular-weight heparins. However, no accepted guidelines exist to achieve adequate degrees of anticoagulation with the subcutaneous administration of heparin.

Methods.—Seventy patients with proximal venous thrombosis received an intravenous bolus of heparin followed by a subcutaneous injection of heparin in doses adjusted for body weight (Table). Twice daily, subsequent adjustments of the subcutaneous dose of heparin were scheduled according to the algorithm. In the mid-interval, the activated partial thromboplastin time was measured, with a target range of 50–90 seconds.

Results.—The therapeutic threshold activated partial thromboplastin time of more than or equal to 50 seconds was achieved within 24 hours in 61 patients (87%) and within 48 hours in 69 patients (99%). A supratherapeutic activated partial thromboplastin time lasted more than 12 hours in 7 patients (10%). Patients had early mobilization and early discharge. No patient had heparin-induced thrombocytopenia or major bleeding episodes. During 3 months of follow-up, recurrent thromboembolism was found in 3 patients (4.3%).

Conclusion.—An effective and safe degree of anticoagulation in patients with deep venous thrombosis is rapidly achieved with heparin subcutaneously administered according to a weight-based algorithm. The initial treatment of venous thromboembolic disorders may be greatly simplified

TABLE.—Algorithm for the Adjustment of Subcutaneous Heparin Doses

aPTT	Adjustment of Heparin Dose†	Time To Peform Next aPTT
≤120 s		
<50 s	One step up	After 6 hours
50–90 s	Same step	After 6 hours
91–120 s	One step down	After 6 hours
>120 s: Withhold heparin treatment, perform aPTT, and proceed as follows:		
<50 s	Same step	After 6 hours
50–90 s	One step down	After 6 hours
91–120 s	Two steps down	After 6 hours
>120 s	Withhold heparin treatment	After 3 hours‡

Body weight < 50 kg, 4,000 U intravenously and 12,500 U subcutaneously; body weight 50–70 kg, 5,000 U intravenously and 15,000 U subcutaneously; and body weight > 70 kg, 6,000 U intravenously and 17,500 U subcutaneously.
†Steps (in U): 10,000–12,500–15,000–17,500–21,500–25,000–30,000.
‡Repeat aPTT until a value < 120 seconds is obtained, then adjust heparin dose according to the schedule given for aPTT > 120 seconds.
Abbreviation: aPTT, activated partial thromboplastin time.
(Courtesy of Prandoni P, Bagatella P, Bernardi E, et al: Use of an algorithm for administering subcutaneous heparin in the treatment of deep venous thrombosis. Ann Intern Med 129:299–302, 1998.)

by the use of a weight-based algorithm for the subcutaneous administration of unfractionated heparin. In comparison α with the use of low–molecular-weight heparins, the relatively low cost of unfractionated heparin makes this approach attractive. This strategy has major implications for the short-term treatment of a broad spectrum of conditions, such as unstable angina and myocardial infarction, for which heparin is indicated.

▶ This welcome algorithm should be retained as a handy reference. The clinical application is common in any sort of general hospital practice. It comes up at least once a month in our residency teaching practice.

A.O. Berg, M.D., M.P.H.

Cost and Effectiveness of a Nurse Specialist Anticoagulant Service

Taylor FC, Gray A, Cohen H, et al (Royal Free Hosp School of Medicine, London; Wolfson College, Oxford, England; St Albans and Hemel Hempstead NHS Trust, St Albans, England; et al)
J Clin Pathol 50:823–828, 1997   2–8

Objective.—Chronic anticoagulation therapy is cost effective for individuals at risk of blood clots so long as the risk of bleeding is low. Differing methods for achieving safe levels of anticoagulation have met with variable rates of success. The costs and effectiveness of a nurse specialist anticoagulant service were retrospectively evaluated in 2 hospitals in northwest Hertfordshire, England.

Methods.—Two groups of patients were studied sequentially. Group A included 206 consecutive patients referred over a 3-month period and assigned to a consulting service (n = 100) or to a nurse specialist service (n = 106). Group B included 224 randomly selected patients attending the anticoagulation clinic for 1 year or more and assigned to a consulting service (n = 111) or to a nurse specialist service (n = 113). Group A was followed for 3 months or less and group B for 6 months or less. Total costs and effectiveness were measured and compared. Patient and practitioner satisfaction were assessed by questionnaire.

Results.—Average visit costs were £4.75 in the consulting service and £4.99 in the nurse specialist service. All other per patient costs were similar for both services. Significantly more group A patients in the consulting service were aged 66 to 75 years, and significantly fewer were over 76 years than in the nurse specialist service. Significantly fewer group B patients in the consulting service were receiving anticoagulation for cardiac conditions and significantly more were receiving anticoagulation for thromboembolic conditions than in the nurse specialist service. The average time patients spent in the therapeutic range was similar for both services. Compared with group A patients in the consulting service, group A patients in the nurse specialist service were taking significantly fewer drugs that would interfere with the anticoagulant regimen, and significantly more of them were satisfied with the service. Satisfaction rates for responding practitioners and nurses were similar.

Conclusion.—Costs, safety, and effectiveness of consulting and nurse specialist anticoagulation services were similar. Fewer patients in the nurse specialist service were taking drugs that interfered with anticoagulation therapy, and a higher percentage were satisfied with the service. Both nurses and practitioners were satisfied with the nurse specialist service.

▶ Although a cost-effectiveness study performed in England may have limited applicability to the United States, I include this study because it describes a growing disease management program. Patients on continuous anticoagulant medications require careful monitoring, and they frequently "fall through the cracks" in a busy physician's practice, The consequences is potentially life-threatening bleeding complications or the danger of inadequate anticoagulation. Having a dedicated nurse specialist or manager monitoring patients on anticoagulant medications such as warfarin makes sense and probably saves lives. I would suspect that, given a large enough patient population, such programs are cost-effective for many medical groups.

J.E. Scherger, M.D., M.P.H.

Acetaminophen and Other Risk Factors for Excessive Warfarin Anticoagulation
Hylek EM, Heiman H, Skates SJ, et al (Harvard Med School, Boston)
JAMA 279:657–662, 1998

Introduction.—The major complication of warfarin anticoagulation is hemorrhage, and major hemorrhage is strongly associated with the intensity of anticoagulation (international normalized ratio [INR] levels higher than 4.0). A prospective case-control study examined factors associated with an INR higher than 6.0 among outpatients taking warfarin whose target INR was between 2.0 and 3.0.

Methods.—Study participants were identified from a daily log of INR tests. Case participants had an INR higher than 6.0, reported within 24 hours of the blood draw. This level is unlikely to be the result of usual intraindividual fluctuations and indicates a markedly increased risk of major hemorrhage. Control participants were randomly selected patients whose target INR was also between 2.0 and 3.0, and whose actual INR value recorded in the daily log was between 1.7 and 3.3. Interviewers contacted a total of 93 case participants and 196 control participants and asked them to record medications they were currently taking, diet changes, consumption of foods high in vitamin K content, recent illnesses, and compliance with warfarin therapy.

Results.—Case participants and control participants did not differ in age, indication for warfarin or warfarin dose, length of therapy, number of prescription medications, or previous INR. Fifty-two case participants (56%) and 70 control participants (36%) reported taking acetaminophen during the week before INR testing. Sixty-one case participants (66%) and 79 control participants (40%) reported routine consumption of 1 or none of the 12 listed foods with high vitamin K content. Diarrhea was reported by 22% of case participants and 8% of control participants during the preceding week. Factors independently associated with an INR higher than 6.0 were acetaminophen ingestion, a new medication known to potentiate warfarin, advanced malignancy, recent diarrheal illness, decreased oral intake, and taking more than the prescribed dose of warfarin. There was an association of both higher vitamin K intake and habitual alcohol consumption (from 1 drink every other day to 2 drinks daily) with a decreased risk of having an INR higher than 6.0.

Conclusion.—There was a highly significant dose-response relationship between acetaminophen use and having an INR higher than 6.0, and this relationship was independent of other factors that alter response to anticoagulation. With ingestion of more than 9,100 mg/week, the odds of having an INR higher than 6.0 were increased 10-fold. The risk of warfarin-related hemorrhage could be reduced by knowledge of factors that increase INR and by careful monitoring of patients who regularly take acetaminophen.

▶ In the dosing range which is normal for the patient's age and weight, acetaminophen is thought to be a "safe" drug. This study of patients on chronic warfarin therapy, however, showed that acetaminophen use was a common factor in increases in anticoagulability as measured by INR. There are certainly other causes for patients in this study to have INRs above the maximum limit of 60. Concurrent illnesses, malignancies, alcohol intake, and aspirin and other NSAIDs all are known causes of increased INR. However, it is interesting to find that acetaminophen was the most common cause found in this study population.

R.C. Davidson, M.D., M.P.H.

3 Metabolism and Endocrinology

Overview

Randomized controlled trials: Abstracts 3–2, 3–3, 3–10, 3–14, 3–15, 3–16, 3–17, 3–18, 3–19, 3–21, 3–22, and 3–30

Lipids

- Dietary fat and coronary heart disease risk in women
- Fat-restricted diets and changes in hyperlipidemic men
- Lovastatin for primary prevention of acute coronary events in men and women with average cholesterol levels
- Fasting insulin and apolipoprotein B levels as risk factors for ischemic heart disease
- The value of C-reactive protein in determining risk of myocardial infarction

Obesity

- Two articles on dietary fat and obesity
- Predictors of weight change in men
- Energy expenditure in overweight women
- Weight maintenance and carbohydrates, chromium, fiber, and caffeine
- The effects of ketogenic diets in morbidly obese adolescents

Insulin-Dependent Diabetes Mellitus

- The economics of ACE inhibitors and renal failure in IDDM
- Microalbuminuria and dietary saturated fat
- Insulin lispro and reduced hypoglycemia and coma
- Effect of excessive weight gain on lipids and blood pressure

Diabetes Mellitus Type 2

- Comparative outcomes using sulfonylurea, insulin, and metformin in newly diagnosed NIDDM
- Troglitazone
- Enalapril and renal function

- Outcomes in the FACET trial (fosinopril vs. amlodipine)
- Safety and efficacy of insulin in NIDDM
- Comparison of acarbose, metformin, and placebo
- Simvastatin and renal function

Diabetes Prevention, Follow-up, and Complications

- Unrecognized diabetes in hospitalized patients
- Physical activity and insulin resistance
- High blood glucose as an overall mortality risk factor
- Fish oil and glycemic control
- Effect of diabetes on outcome in patients presenting with chest pain
- A computer aid for diabetes control
- Hyperbaric oxygen and lasers for diabetic foot ulcers

Endocrine—Miscellaneous

- Therapy for hyperthyroidism and the course of Graves' ophthalmopathy
- Morbidity in Turner syndrome

Lipids

Dietary Fat Intake and the Risk of Coronary Heart Disease in Women
Hu FB, Stampfer MJ, Manson JE, et al (Harvard Med School, Boston)
N Engl J Med 337:1491–1499, 1997   3–1

Purpose.—The effects of specific types of dietary fat intake on coronary disease risk are unclear. Some studies suggest saturated fat is related to coronary disease, but others find no such association. Most previous studies of this issue have been performed in men. Data from the Nurses' Health Study were used to analyze the relationship between dietary intake of trans unsaturated fat and risk of coronary disease.

Methods.—The prospective analysis included 80,082 female nurses, aged 34 to 59 years when enrolled in the study in 1980. At that time, the women were free of known coronary disease, stroke, cancer, hypercholesterolemia, or diabetes. Dietary information was assessed at baseline and updated by questionnaire throughout the 14-year follow-up period. Nine hundred thirty-nine subjects had a nonfatal myocardial infarction or died of coronary heart disease during follow-up. Multivariate analysis, with adjustment for other dietary and nondietary risk factors, assessed the effects of trans unsaturated fat and other types of fat intake.

Results.—With each 5% increase in energy intake from saturated fat versus carbohydrates, the risk of coronary disease increased by 17%. For each 2% increase in energy intake from trans unsaturated fat, relative risk was 1.93, compared with equivalent energy from carbohydrates (Fig 1). Relative risks were 0.81 for a 5% increase in energy from monounsaturated fat and 0.62 for a 5% increase in energy from polyunsaturated fat.

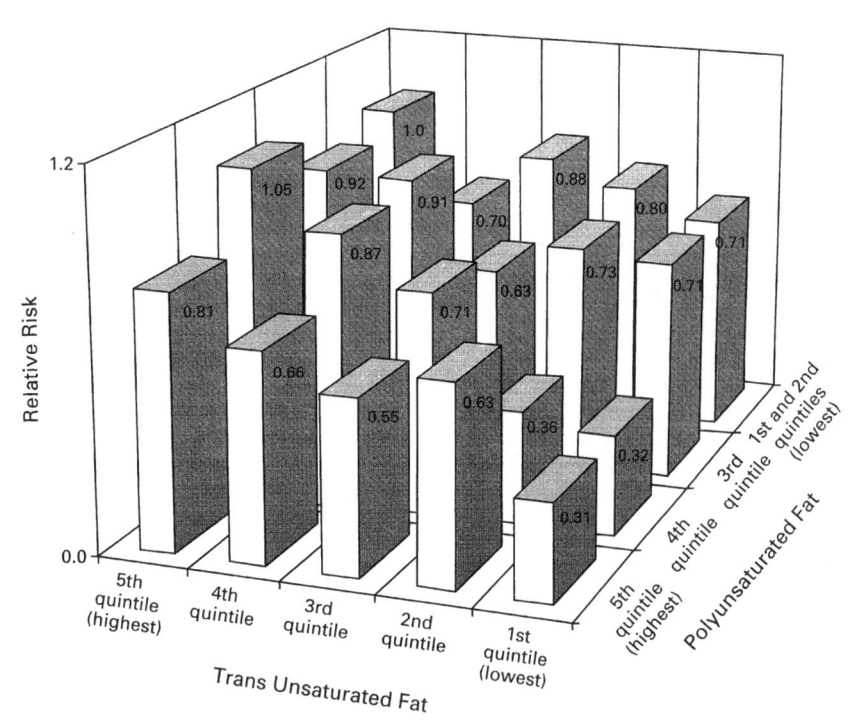

FIGURE 1.—Multivariate relative risk of coronary heart disease according to dietary intake of trans unsaturated and polyunsaturated fats. The first and second quintiles for polyunsaturated-fat intake were combined to provide a sufficient number of women in each of the categories. The relative risks have been adjusted for age, time interval, body-mass index, cigarette smoking, menopausal status, parental history of premature myocardial infarction, use of multivitamins, use of vitamin E supplements, alcohol consumption, history of hypertension, aspirin use, physical activity, percentage of energy obtained from protein, saturated fat, and monounsaturated fat, dietary cholesterol, and total energy intake. The reference group for all comparisons was the women with the highest intake of trans unsaturated fat and the lowest intake of polyunsaturated fat. (Reprinted by permission of *The New England Journal of Medicine* from Hu FB, Stampfer MJ, Manson JE, et al: Dietary fat intake and the risk of coronary heart disease in women. *N Engl J Med* 337:1491–1499. Copyright 1997, Massachusetts Medical Society. All rights reserved.)

There was no association between total fat intake and coronary disease risk. The authors calculated that replacing 5% of energy from saturated fat with energy from unsaturated fats would lead to a 42% reduction in risk. Replacing 2% of energy from trans fat with energy from unhydrogenated, unsaturated fats would lead to a 53% risk reduction.

Conclusions.—Risk of coronary disease appears to increase with a higher intake of saturated and trans unsaturated fat, and to decrease with a higher intake of monounsaturated and polyunsaturated fats. The results are consistent with metabolic studies showing that reducing overall fat has little effect on lipid profile, but replacing saturated and trans unsaturated fats with unhydrogenated, monounsaturated, and polyunsaturated fats has a significant effect.

▶ This is a very important study published in the NEJM. The authors studied 80,000 women during a 14-year period who were enrolled in the Nurses'

Health Study. The study found each 5% increase of energy intake from saturated fat, compared to either carbohydrates or unsaturated fats, was associated with a significant increase in the risk of coronary disease. From the data of this large cohort, the authors estimated we would reduce the overall risk of coronary artery disease by 42% by reducing 5% of the energy intake from saturated fats and replacing it with unsaturated fats.

The strength of the methodology of this study is in its large numbers (80,000) and the length of follow-up (14 years). It is common knowledge that saturated fats are not good for you. However, the extraordinary difference in mortality risks by a reduction as small as 5% of energy intake from saturated to unsaturated fats should lead all of us to redouble our efforts in diet counseling with our patients.

R.C. Davidson, M.D., M.P.H.

Long-term Cholesterol-lowering Effects of 4 Fat-restricted Diets in Hypercholesterolemic and Combined Hyperlipidemic Men: The Dietary Alternatives Study
Knopp RH, Walden CE, Retzlaff BM, et al (Univ of Washington, Seattle)
JAMA 278:1509–1515, 1997   3–2

Background.—Diet is the first step in hypercholesterolemia management, but the ideal, sustainable diet has not been ascertained. The effect of 1 year of 4 fat-restricted diets on hypercholesterolemia was examined in a large, randomized, parallel comparison trial.

Methods.—The study group consisted of 444 employed men with a spouse or partner and 2 low-density lipoprotein cholesterol measurements greater than the age-specific 75% value. Those with triglyceride (TG) values less than the age-specific 75% value were classified as hypercholesterolemic (HC) and those with TG more than the 75% value were classified as combined hyperlipidemic (CHL). The study diets were designed to contain 30%, 26%, 22%, and 18% of energy from fat and 300, 200, 100, and 100 mg/d of cholesterol, respectively. The ratio of polyunsaturated fat to saturated fat was 1.0. There were fewer CHL participants who were only randomized to diets 1, 2, and 3. The 4 diets were taught to participants and their partners during 8 weekly 2-hour classes. At baseline and 5 times during the year, lifestyle data, medical history, vital signs, anthropometric measurements, psychological data, behavioral data, and 4-day food records were obtained. Lipoprotein, apoprotein, glucose, and insulin concentrations and the percent of total plasma lipid fatty acid composition were measured on fasting plasma at baseline and at 1 year.

Results.—Fat intake declined during the year from an average of 35% of energy at baseline to 27%, 26%, 25%, and 22% in the 4 HC diet groups. It declined to 28%, 26%, and 25% in the 3 CHL diet groups. Average low-density lipoprotein cholesterol reductions were approximately 5.3%, 13.4%, 8.4%, and 13.0% in the 4 HC diet groups and 7.0%, 2.8%, and 4.6% in the 3 CHL diet groups. Apoprotein B levels decreased an average of approximately 8.6%, 10.7%, 4.3%, and 5.3% in the 4 HC diet groups and 14.6%, 11.4%, and 9.9% in the 3 CHL diet groups. TG levels increased significantly in those on HC diets 3 and 4, but not in any CHL participants. HDL cholesterol decreased 2.8% and 3.2% in those on HC diets 3 and 4.

Conclusions.—The results of this study of reduced fat diets on hypercholesterolemia in men demonstrated that moderate restriction of dietary fat is both feasible and effective over the long term. Aggressive dietary fat restriction offers no additional benefit and may have some adverse effects on this population.

▶ Reduction of saturated fat in the diet continues to be the first step in the therapy of patients with hyperlipidemia. I selected this article because it has two major good news findings. The first is that reduction of saturated fat in the diet does sustain a significant reduction in total cholesterol. Depending on the amount of saturated fat in the diet, the authors found a 5% to 13% reduction in serum cholesterol. Previous studies have shown that a reduction in cholesterol of this magnitude would have a significant reduction of coronary artery disease risk.

The second good news finding in this study is that moderate reduction of saturated fat in the diet was as effective as a much more restricted diet. All of us have had the frustration with our patients, and probably with ourselves, of the difficulty of reducing saturated fat in the diet to 18%. However, these authors found that reductions to the range of 22%–26% saturated fat in the diet still held significant reductions in total cholesterol. At these levels, a sane approach to reduction of saturated fat in the diet is much more attainable and sustainable in the long run.

R.C. Davidson, M.D., M.P.H.

Primary Prevention of Acute Coronary Events With Lovastatin in Men and Women With Average Cholesterol Levels: Results of AFCAPS/TexCAPS

Downs JR, for the AFCAPS/TexCAPS Research Group (Wilford Hall Med Ctr, Lackland Air Force Base, San Antonio, Tex; Univ of North Texas, Fort Worth; Heart and Vascular Inst of Texas, San Antonio; et al)
JAMA 279:1615–1622, 1998   3–3

Objective.—Although the connection between plasma total cholesterol (TC) and incidence of coronary heart disease (CHD) is well known, the effect of reducing low-density lipoprotein cholesterol (LDL-C) in men and women with normal serum cholesterol levels, below-average high-density lipoprotein cholesterol (HDL-C) levels, and without CHD is not known.

Methods.—Either lovastatin (20 to 40 mg/d) or placebo was administered in a double-blind, randomized fashion to 5,608 men, aged 45 to 73, and 997 postmenopausal women, aged 55 to 73, with average TC and LDL-C and below-average HDL-C enrolled in the AFCAPS/TexCAPS study conducted at 2 Texas sites. Lipid profile averages were TC=5.71 mmol/L, LDL-C=3.89 mmol/L, and HDL-C=0.94 mmol/L for men and 1.03 mmol/L for women. Median triglyceride levels were 1.78 mmol/L. All participants were placed on a low-saturated fat, low-cholesterol diet. The outcome measure was the first acute major coronary event.

Results.—Participants were followed for an average of 5.2 years. Lovastatin was administered to 2,805 men and 499 women, and placebo was administered to 2,803 men and 498 women. Lovastatin significantly reduced LDL-C levels by 25%, TC levels by 18%, triglyceride levels by 15%, and HDL-C levels by 6%. TC/HDL-C and LDL-C/HDL-C ratios were reduced by 22% and 28%, respectively. The lovastatin group had 37% fewer first acute major coronary events than the placebo group (Relative Risk, 0.63). The relative risks for the lovastatin group compared with the placebo group were 0.60 for myocardial infarction, 0.68 for unstable angina, 0.67 for coronary revascularization procedures, 0.75 for coronary events, and 0.75 for cardiovascular events. The treatment was well tolerated for the most part. Mortality rates, deaths, and incidences of cancer were similar for the 2 groups.

Conclusion.—The fact that lovastatin lowers the risk of cardiac events in individuals with average cholesterol levels, illustrates the importance of including HDL-C in the risk factors for first acute major coronary events and for reexamining the National Cholesterol Education Program guidelines for drug therapy.

▶ This is an important article that extends our knowledge of the prevention of coronary disease with one of the reductase inhibitors. The amount of event reduction in middle-aged men and women with no known coronary disease and cholesterol levels not usually considered high is quite impressive. The study was large and well-designed. The lovastatin group appeared to do better no matter what the other risk factors (smoking, age) were, although some of the differences by subgroup (such as patients with non-insulin-dependent diabetes) were not statistically significant. This is the first trial to include a large number of women, and they benefited as well, although the amount of benefit was less than for the men. The lovastatin was well tolerated throughout 7 years. The improved rate of events seemed to be greater for patients with higher LDL cholesterol and lower HDL cholesterol before the trial. Thus, I agree with the authors that the results suggest we revise our cutoffs for treatment of cholesterol. While some may question the cost-effectiveness of this action, the cost is relatively dependent on how much the drug itself costs. I believe the costs should drop and may well do so when lovastatin becomes generic.

M.A. Bowman, M.D., M.P.A.

▶ After reading this article, I envisioned a statewide initiative to add one of the statin drugs to the water supply in order to reduce risk of coronary artery disease. However, in fairness to the authors, their study really looked at patients with average or "normal" total and LDL cholesterol levels but with low HDL levels. In this population, they showed a clear risk reduction using a statin drug.

There is a message from this study that we need to consider. Quite often we screen for total cholesterol, and if this is in a "normal" range we do not do further screening. This would suggest that we should routinely screen for both total and HDL levels. For patients with low HDL, we need further study to determine their cardiac and lipid profile risk factors.

I included this study even though it broke one of my primary tenets for inclusion of a study. I will just identify for the readers that this project was funded by a major drug company whose bottom-line profits are dependent upon a high sales volume of its statin drug.

R.C. Davidson, M.D., M.P.H.

Fasting Insulin and Apolipoprotein B Levels and Low-density Lipoprotein Particle Size as Risk Factors for Ischemic Heart Disease
Lamarche B, Tchernof A, Mauriège P, et al (Laval Univ, Ste-Foy, Québec; Univ of Montréal)
JAMA 279:1955–1961, 1998
3–4

Background.—The relationship between cholesterol and low-density lipoprotein cholesterol (LDL-C) levels and risk of ischemic heart disease (IHD) has been established. However, as many as half the patients with IHD may have cholesterol levels in the normal range. The predictive value of a cluster of nontraditional metabolic risk factors—increased fasting insulin, apolipoprotein B levels, and small, dense LDL particles—in IHD risk was determined.

Methods and Findings.—In this nested case-control study, incident IHD cases and matched IHD-free controls were identified from a population-based cohort of men initially free of IHD and followed up for 5 years. The risk of IHD was significantly increased in men with increased fasting plasma insulin and apolipoprotein B levels and small, dense LDL particles compared with men with normal levels of 2 of these 3 parameters. In a multivariate analysis, adjustment for LDL-C, triglycerides, and high-density lipoprotein cholesterol (HDL-C) did not affect the relationship between these risk factors and IHD. However, the risk of IHD in men with combined increases in LDL-C and triglyceride levels and decreased HDL-C levels did not remain significant after adjustment for fasting plasma insulin levels, apolipoprotein B levels, and LDL particle size.

Conclusions.—Measuring fasting plasma insulin levels, apolipoprotein B levels, and LDL particle size may provide useful additional information on the risk of IHD. These data also underscore that the etiology of IHD is multifactorial.

▶ The past decade might be characterized as the decade of identifying risk factors for coronary artery disease. This research project takes 3 known risk factors for coronary artery disease and studies the combined predictive value with 1 or more of these risk factors.

There are no surprises here. Risk factors are additive. What is interesting about this article is that the 3 risk factors studied are not ones that we routinely use in our screening activities. Apolipoprotein B levels are becoming more common in secondary identification of patients with hyperlipidemia. Low-density lipoprotein particle size is still basically a research measure. It is not commonly available in most laboratories. Fasting insulin levels are readily available in most laboratories but are not commonly used by primary care physicians in risk identification. I'm not ready to begin routinely screening for these risk factors. However, for a patient with some known risk factors for which the decision is not clear regarding medication for reduction of lipids, these additional factors may be helpful in assisting the patient and the physician in this decision.

R.C. Davidson, M.D., M.P.H.

C-Reactive Protein Adds to the Predictive Value of Total and HDL Cholesterol in Determining Risk of First Myocardial Infarction
Ridker PM, Glynn RJ, Hennekens CH (Brigham and Women's Hosp, Boston; Harvard Med School, Boston)
Circulation 97:2007–2011, 1998 3–5

Background.—C-reactive protein (CRP), a marker of systemic inflammation, has recently been associated with myocardial infarction (MI) risk. Data from the Physicians' Health Study were reexamined to assess whether measurement of CRP added to the predictive power of total cholesterol (TC) and high-density lipoprotein cholesterol (HDL-C) levels in determining risk of first MI.

Study Design.—The participants in the U.S. Physicians' Health Study were 14,916 men initially free of cardiovascular disease, cancer or chronic illness, who provided a baseline plasma sample. The current study focused on 246 of these men who had a first MI and 543 controls who remained free of cardiovascular disease during an average follow-up period of 9 years. Baseline blood samples from these men were assayed for CRP, TC, and HDL-C. The predictive power of the levels of these 3 prognostic indicators for first MI was evaluated.

Findings.—Univariate analysis indicated that high baseline levels of CRP, TC, and TC:HDL-C ratio were individually associated with significantly increased risk of first MI. Multivariate analysis indicated models that incorporated CRP level with lipid parameters had significantly more predictive power for first MI than models that employed lipid parameters alone (Fig 2). Stratified analysis indicated that baseline CRP level was predictive of risk of first MI for those participants with low or high levels of TC or TC:HDL-C ratio. These findings were unchanged by controlling for smoking and other cardiovascular risk factors.

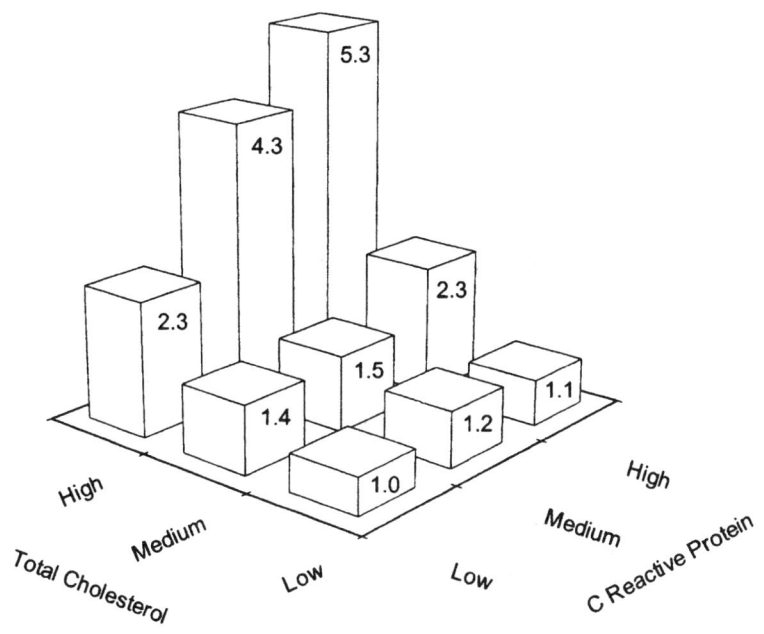

FIGURE 2.—Relative risks of first MI among apparently healthy men associated with high (>223 mg/dL), middle (191 to 223 mg/dL), and low (<191 mg/dL) tertiles of TC and high (>1.69 mg/L), middle (0.72 to 1.69 mg/L), and low (<0.72 mg/L) tertiles of CRP. (Courtesy of Ridker PM, Glynn RJ, Hennekens CH: C-reactive protein adds to the predictive value of total and HDL cholesterol in determining risk of first myocardial infarction. *Circulation* 97:2007–2011. Copyright 1998, American Heart Association.)

Conclusions.—Baseline C-reactive protein level increased the predictive value of lipid parameters for determining the risk of first MI in a prospective study based on data from a large cohort of initially healthy men. Assessment of CRP level may be particularly useful in the assessment of risk of first MI among apparently low-risk individuals.

▶ When the first reports of a relationship between CRP and MI risk were published, I became curious—why would a marker for systemic inflammatory processes predict coronary artery disease? However, this and other studies now provide powerful evidence of a relationship. An inflammatory process must clearly be part of the development of coronary artery disease.

This study shows that CRP adds additional information when combined with either total or HDL-C levels. Since CRP is readily available in most laboratories, it seems to make sense to use it as a risk factor stratification test for patients suspected of coronary artery disease. Unfortunately, this research project again was limited to men. Come on, guys—when are we going to learn!

R.C. Davidson, M.D., M.P.H.

Obesity

Dietary Fat and Obesity: An Epidemiologic Perspective
Seidell JC (Natl Inst of Public Health and the Environment, Bilthoven, The Netherlands)
Am J Clin Nutr 67:546S–550S, 1998   3–6

Background.—The notion that high-fat diets are more likely to result in weight gain and obesity than isoenergetic low-fat diets is controversial. The epidemiologic evidence that high-fat diets lead to obesity in populations independent of total energy intake was reviewed.

Review.—Evidence for the effect of dietary fat on weight gain and obesity is primarily experimental. Methodological flaws in existing epidemiologic studies cast doubt on observed associations between dietary fat intake and obesity. Important methodological issues include underreporting of energy and fat intakes, dieting behavior, insufficient control of variables such as energy expenditure, and limited between-subject variation in fat intake in developed countries. Different types of epidemiologic studies, especially ecologic and cross-sectional studies, have different types and magnitudes of bias that result in conflicting findings. More appropriate types of studies are prospective studies of fat intake and subsequent weight gain. Although such studies have been conducted in several countries, findings have been conflicting. In general, observed associations appear to depend on the stage of cultural transition of the population investigated. Current epidemiologic techniques are not sufficient for conducting valid research on the relationship between percentage of energy from dietary fat and obesity.

Conclusions.—Currently no conclusive epidemiologic evidence exists that, under isoenergetic conditions, dietary fat intake results in obesity more than other macronutrients do. Future research should incude specifically designed prospective studies of the association between percentage of energy from dietary fat and obesity, appropriate control for confounding variables, and an emphasis on the possible role of genetic predisposition.

Is Dietary Fat a Major Determinant of Body Fat?
Willett WC (Harvard Med School, Boston)
Am J Clin Nutr 67:556S–562S, 1998   3–7

Background.—Dietary fat composition may be an important determinant of body fat. Evidence for the role of dietary fat as a major determinant of body fat was discussed.

Discussion.—Comparisons of diets and obesity prevalence in affluent and poor countries have been used to support a causal relationship. However, these contrasts are seriously confounded by differences in physical activity levels and food availability. Regional intake of fat and obesity

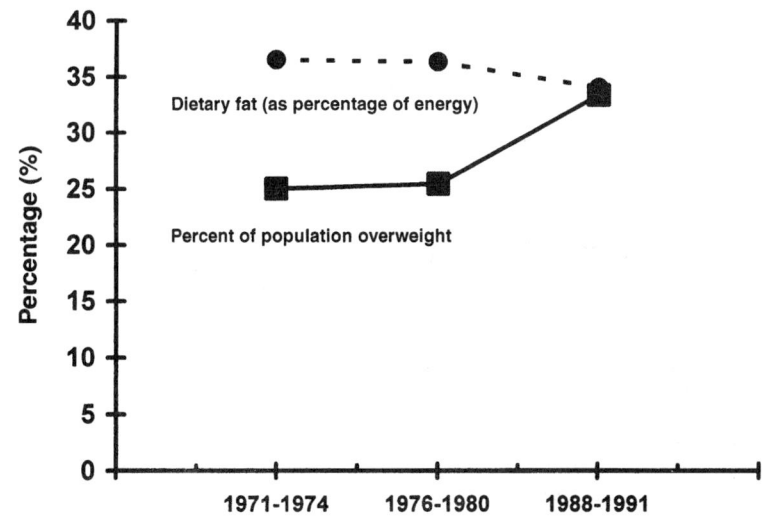

FIGURE 2.—Changes in dietary fat (as percentage of energy) and the percentage of population that is overweight. (Courtesy of Willett WC: Is dietary fat a major determinant of body fat? *Am J Clin Nutr* 67:556S–562S. Copyright 1998, American Society for Clinical Nutrition.)

prevalence have not been correlated positively in areas of similar economic development. Randomized studies, which are preferred for assessing the effect of dietary fat on adiposity, are feasible because the number of subjects needed for such trials is not great. Short-term studies have shown that individuals randomly assigned to diets with a lower percentage of energy from fat have modest weight reductions. However, trials lasting a year or more suggest that compensatory mechanisms operate, as fat intake in the 18% to 40% range of energy appears to have little if any effect on body fat. In addition, a marked decrease in the percentage of energy from fat consumed in the past 2 decades in the United States has corresponded with a massive increase in obesity (Fig 2).

Conclusions.—High-fat diets do not seem to be the main cause of the high prevalence of excess body fat in the United States. Thus, decreasing fat is not a solution to increasing prevalences in obesity.

▶ Calories in=calories out: a basic equation that is pretty immutable. Often, the focus on the "calories in" side of the equation is on calories from fat. These studies by Seidell (Abstracts 3–6 and 3–7) and Willett put this thinking in a new perspective. In the end, though, these 2 investigations do not allow us to draw any hard conclusions other than the oft-used "more study is necessary." However, the data as presented are intriguing. Reduction in fat intake may be beneficial for a variety of reasons; weight loss, it would seem, might not be among them. Theoretical rationale and observational evidence relating intake and obesity are compelling. In my work with patients regarding weight loss, reducing fat intake has been an easy target objective to set and is readily agreed upon. The evidence as presented here, particularly the inverse relationship between fat intake and obesity (see Fig 2), makes me question my practice. However, do not lose sight of the fact that the increase in adiposity in our society has also mirrored an increase in sedentary behavior. Take-home message from these 2 analyses? Fat intake is only one piece of one side of the basic equation. Both sides need to be addressed in efforts to aid our patients in their goals of weight loss and better health.

W.W. Dexter, M.D.

Predictors of Weight Change in Men: Results From the Health Professionals Follow-up Study
Coakley EH, Rimm EB, Colditz G, et al (Harvard Med School, Boston)
Int J Obes 22:89–96, 1998
3–8

Introduction.—The association of increased levels of body mass with the increase lifetime risks of heart disease, diabetes, osteoarthritis, hypertension, and other illnesses has been well-defined. About 33% of adult males meet the definition for obesity. About 25% of adult males are attempting to lose weight at any given time. The impact of ordinary lifestyle factors on weight change were assessed during 1988 to 1992 in a cohort of middle to older aged male health professionals.

Methods.—The Health Professionals Follow-up Study is a prospective investigation that was initiated in 1986 in 51,529 health professional men aged 40 to 75 years. At baseline, participants completed a questionnaire regarding diet, exercise, and medical history. Questionnaires were mailed in 1988 and 1992 for updated information. Body weight was self-reported and was an average of 1.0 kg lower than when measured by a technician. The association between 4-year change in body weight from 1988 to 1992 and common habits (exercise, smoking, TV/VCR viewing, dieting, and eating) was analyzed after adjusting for baseline age, hypertension, and hypercholesterolemia.

Results.—Complete data were available for 19,478 men. For middle-aged men, vigorous activity was correlated with weight reduction. Eating between meals and TV/VCR viewing were associated with weight gain. Weight increase was consistently related to quitting smoking and a history of voluntary weight loss before baseline assessment. In older men, dieting was strongly correlated with weight loss. During the 4-year assessment period, middle-aged men who increased exercise, reduced TV viewing, and ceased eating between meals lost an average weight of 1.4 kg, compared with a weight gain of 1.4 kg among the overall population. Compared to participants who were relatively sedentary, those middle-aged men who maintained a relatively high level of vigorous physical activity had the lowest prevalence of obesity.

Conclusion.—Improved health habits, particularly increasing vigorous activity, decreasing TV use, and changing eating habits results in weight maintenance or a modest weight loss over a 4-year period in middle- and older-aged health professionals.

▶ I accept the premise of the study: we are too sedentary and too heavy. Exercise and weight loss are goals I spend a lot of time working toward with my patients. I am not at all surprised at the findings presented here. For instance, I certainly would expect that one would find less obesity in folks who routinely exercise vigorously. Looking at this data, I question whether there is a significant selection bias regarding sedentary and exercise behaviors. Note that the average weight loss (or gain) over 4 years was only about 3 pounds. I find this discouraging, particularly as I fight my own battles toward (hopefully not inevitably upward) middle-age weight creep. Nevertheless, I continue to see advocacy of the basic healthy lifestyle habits described as an important component of health care maintenance.

W.W. Dexter, M.D.

Differences in Resting Energy Expenditure in African-American vs Caucasian Overweight Females
Jakicic JM, Wing RR (Univ of Pittsburgh, Pa)
Int J Obes 22:236–242, 1998   3–9

Background.—Nearly half of African-American women are classified as overweight. This may result partly from cultural, socioeconomic, and behavioral factors. However, metabolic factors may also contribute to the higher rates of obesity among African-American women. Recent research has suggested that the rate of resting energy expenditure (REE), accounting for about 65% of total energy expenditure, may be lower in African-American women than in white women.

Methods.—Resting energy expenditure was assessed in 22 African-American and 19 white women. Mean age and body mass index were 36.4 years and 32.6 kg/m^2 in the fomer group, and 35.4 years and 31.3 kg/m^2, in the latter. The dilution method after an overnight fast was used to determine REE.

Findings.—African-American women had an REE of 7,279 kJ/d, compared with an REE of 7,807 kJ/d among white women. This difference remained significant after adjustment for body weight and lean body mass. Ethnicity did not affect respiratory quotient.

Conclusions.—Resting energy expenditure differs significantly between African-American and white overweight women. This difference may contribute to the greater rates of obesity among African-American women and may explain the smaller weight losses reported in African-American women enrolled in weight loss programs.

▶ Obesity is more common in African-Americans than in white Americans. The causes are likely to be multifactorial. This article suggests that a significant difference in the resting energy expenditure—a difference in 120 kcal/day, enough to account for 10–15 pounds a year—is at least 1 reason. Unfortunately, it is difficult for me to translate this into the best action in the office. Do I tell my overweight African-American women it may be harder for them, but that it is still important to maintain weight control? (Answer: Yes.) Do we admit defeat? (Hopefully, no.) Weight is not easy to manage in our food-plenty society, but it is still a major determinant of health, and we should continue to encourage our patients to improve diet and to exercise regularly.

M.A. Bowman, M.D., M.P.A.

The Effectiveness of Long-term Supplementation of Carbohydrate, Chromium, Fibre and Caffeine on Weight Maintenance
Pasman WJ, Westerterp-Plantenga MS, Saris WHM (Maastricht Univ, The Netherlands; Open Univ, Heerlen, The Netherlands)
Int J Obes 21:1143–1151, 1997   3–10

Objective.—Weight loss is difficult to maintain long-term. Lowering insulin resistance and decreasing fat consumption have been suggested as ways to help maintain weight loss. The effect on weight maintenance of food supplements rich in carbohydrates (CHO), chromium-picolinate, caffeine, and dietary fiber was examined in weight-reduced individuals with respect to body composition, fasting plasma insulin, glucose, and serum cholesterol concentrations, and energy percentage (En%) of macronutrient intake.

Methods.—There were 33 obese women (average body weight [BW] 85.5 kg, average body mass index [BMI] 31.2 kg/m^2), average age 34.8 years, who completed a longitudinal, double-blind, randomized study.

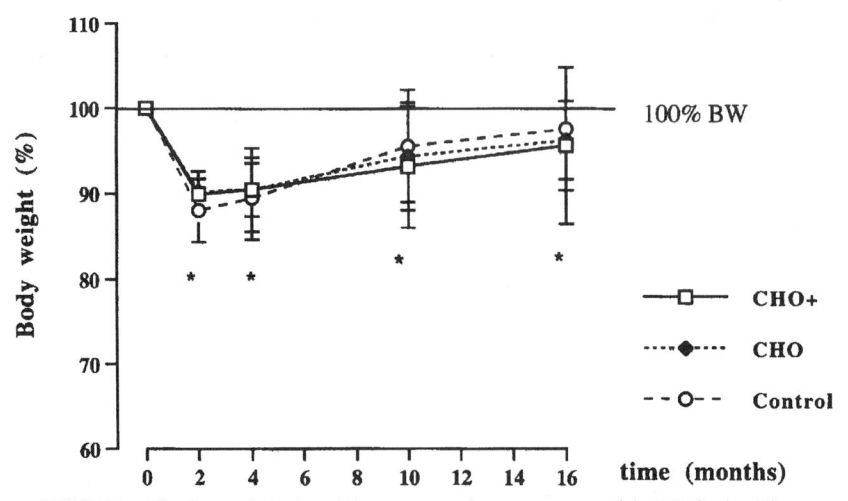

FIGURE 2.—The changes in body weight are expressed as a percentage of the initial value. The mean and standard deviation are presented at different time points measured, for the CHO+ group (*open squares*), CHO group (*filled diamonds*), and control group (*open circles*). *Abbreviations:* CHO, carbohydrate; CHO+, soluble fiber plus caffeine. (Courtesy of Pasman WJ, Westerterp-Plantenga MS, Saris WHM: The effectiveness of long-term supplementation of carbohydrate, chromium, fibre and caffeine on weight maintenance. *Int J Obes* 21:1143–1151, 1997.)

Thirteen patients received a 50 g CHO supplement plus 200 µg of chromium-picolinate, 20 g of soluble fiber and 100 mg of caffeine (CHO+) or 50 g of CHO for 16 months. All patients were assigned a very low energy diet (VLED) for the first 2 months. Body composition, BW, energy intake, and blood parameters were measured at baseline and at 2, 4, 10, and 16 months.

Results.—The women lost an average of 9 kg during the VLED (Fig 2). Whereas all women had significantly lower BW at 16 months than at baseline, they had regained an average of 66.1% of the weight they had lost. Body compositions were similar among groups. Energy percentage CHO intake was significantly higher in both the CHO-supplemented groups compared to the placebo group. Increases in BW were significantly correlated with fat intake at 16 months ($r = -0.40$). There was a significant correlation between En% CHO daily intake and less regain ($r = -0.40$). Blood parameters and body composition were unaffected by chromium intake.

Conclusion.—A high En% CHO intake and low-fat intake helped to maintain weight loss after 16 months. Addition of dietary chromium had no significant effect on blood parameters and body composition.

▶ More hopes are dashed. In patients who had lost weight through a very low calorie diet, the authors were unable to prevent weight regain compared to control patients given a combination of commonly recommended amounts of caffeine, CHO, chromium-picolinate, and fiber. Although the numbers of patients were small, they were close to what the power analysis recommended as needed. Body composition analysis, probably more accurate than the skin fold measurements used in other studies, suggested no difference, nor were there differences in fasting or insulin concentrations—more blows to the hopes for chromium.

M.A. Bowman, M.D., M.P.A.

The Effects of a High-protein, Low-fat, Ketogenic Diet on Adolescents With Morbid Obesity: Body Composition, Blood Chemistries, and Sleep Abnormalities
Willi SM, Oexmann MJ, Wright NM, et al (Univ of South Carolina, Charleston)
Pediatrics 101:61–67, 1998
3–11

Objective.—The incidence of childhood obesity is growing, and obesity in childhood is strongly linked to obesity in adulthood. Seventy percent of obese adolescents will be obese as adults. The prognosis for adolescent obesity is poor; the most effective approach to weight loss for this age group may be the very low calorie ketogenic diet (K diet). Supplemented with 2 carbohydrates (30 g) at each meal (K+2 diet), this diet provides a low-calorie, low-fat, ketogenic diet. The metabolic consequences and efficacy of the K and K+2 diets were evaluated in adolescents with morbid obesity.

Methods.—The study included 6 adolescents with morbid obesity, defined as greater than 200% of ideal body weight. There were 3 males and 3 females, aged 12 to 15 years; average weight was 148 kg and average body mass index 51 kg/m^2. For 8 weeks, the participants followed the K diet. This diet provided a daily intake of 650 to 725 calories. It included 80 to 100 g of protein, with only 25 g each of carbohydrates and fat. The participants then followed the K +2 diet, which added 30 g of carbohydrates per meal, for 12 weeks. Outcome measures included anthropometric data, blood and urine studies, resting energy expenditure, estimates of body composition, and sleep studies.

Results.—Mean weight loss was 15 kg on the K diet and an additional 2 kg on the K+2 diet. Mean reduction in body mass was 6 and 1 kg/m^2, respectively. Weight loss, mostly fat, appeared to come from all areas of the body equally. Percentage body fat, as estimated by dual-energy radiographic absorptiometry, decreased from 51% at baseline to 44% during the K diet to 42% during the K+2 diet. There was no significant change in lean body mass. Resting energy expenditure decreased by 5 kcal/kg of fat-free mass/day. No blood chemistry abnormalities were noted. During the first 4 weeks of the K diet, serum cholesterol decreased from 162 to 121 mg/dL. Calcium excretion increased as bone mineral content decreased. Baseline sleep studies showed little rapid eye movement sleep and excessive slow-wave sleep in all patients. These abnormalities improved significantly as the patients lost weight.

Conclusions.—In adolescents with morbid obesity, the K diet is an effective means of rapid weight loss. The diet achieves rapid and consistent weight loss, almost exclusively of body fat, with little change in lean body mass. Weight loss occurs with no blood chemistry abnormalities. The diet lowers serum cholesterol and significantly reduces sleep abnormalities.

▶ At first glance, I was intrigued by the stated success of this approach to morbid obesity in adolescents. On further reflection, though, I had more questions than answers from this study. It certainly was effective, but the subjects (few) were intensively scrutinized and spent significant time in the hospital. I suspect that the dramatic weight loss, and concomitant improvement in symptoms and laboratory parameters would not bear out under less structured circumstances. I am also skeptical about the persistence of the effects. I agree that obesity in kids (adults, too) is a significant national health problem; the data from my state (Maine) are tragic and discouraging. We need to address this problem on multiple fronts: from individually in the office to nationally on a policy level. I am not convinced that this approach is the answer.

W.W. Dexter, M.D.

Insulin-Dependent Diabetes Mellitus

Routine Treatment of Insulin-Dependent Diabetic Patients With ACE Inhibitors to Prevent Renal Failure: An Economic Evaluation
Kiberd BA, Jindal KK (Dalhousie Univ, Halifax, Nova Scotia, Canada)
Am J Kidney Dis 31:49–54, 1998
3–12

Objective.—Angiotensin-converting enzyme (ACE) inhibitors delay progression from microalbuminuria to macroalbuminuria and progressive loss of renal function in patients with diabetic nephropathy. The efficacy of routine administration of ACE inhibitors to insulin-dependent diabetic patients or to a group at high risk for development of diabetic nephropathy was assessed.

Methods.—The cost-effectiveness of 3 strategies was determined. Strategy I tested the current recommendation of annual screening for microalbuminuria in patients who had had diabetes for more than 5 years and of treatment with ACE inhibition if 2 or 3 tests are positive. Strategy II tested routine treatment of all patients with an ACE inhibitor 5 years after diagnosis. Strategy III tested a hybrid approach of treating high-risk patients as in Strategy II, screening low-risk patients for hypertension and macroalbuminuria, and treating those low-risk patients who have hypertension and/or macroalbuminuria with an ACE inhibitor. Strategy outcomes were compared as quality-adjusting life-years, using a Markov model.

Results.—Strategy II produced the longest life expectancy and the greatest number of quality-adjusting life-years at the lowest cost (Table 3). Strategy III would perform better than Strategy I if high- and low-risk groups could be identified and if the rate of development of microalbuminuria could be reduced by 20% in the high-risk group. Strategy II would perform almost as well as Strategy I if active treatment reduced the annual rate of development of microalbuminuria by 26%.

TABLE 3.—Predictions for Life Expectancy, Quality of Life-Years, and Costs for the Three Strategies

Strategy	Life Expectancy	Quality-Adjusting Life-Years	Costs (Constant $)
I	42.9 yr	19.15 yr	$29,350
II*	44.2 yr	19.34 yr	$29,180
III*	43.2 yr	19.17 yr	$29,236

*Assumes that routine ACE inhibition reduces the rate of progression from normoalbuminuria to microalbuminuria in all patients by 26% in Strategy II and by 20% in high-risk patients only in Strategy III.

(Courtesy of Kiberd BA, Jindal KK: Routine treatment of insulin-dependent diabetic patients with ACE inhibitors to prevent renal failure: An economic evaluation. *Am J Kidney Dis* 31:49–54, 1998.)

Conclusion.—Routine ACE inhibitor therapy for high-risk diabetic patients would be a cost-effective way to prevent or delay progression to diabetic nephropathy if these patients could be identified.

▶ I was impressed with the overall model, and variations in the cost of the drugs led to the conclusion that treatment with ACE inhibitors after 5 years of insulin-dependent diabetes mellitus is preferable to yearly testing for microalbuminuria before starting ACE inhibitors. Any of these computer models depends on many assumptions and the conclusions show small change in the life expectancy; thus many physicians will dismiss these results. Yet more physicians will dismiss them because they prefer the "hard data" (yearly tests for microalbuminuria) before starting drug therapy. This analysis suggests we rethink our threshold for starting ACE inhibitors in insulin-dependent diabetes mellitus. There is not sufficient evidence to apply these results to non–insulin-dependent diabetes mellitus.

M.A. Bowman, M.D., M.P.A.

Microalbuminuria Is Positively Associated With Usual Dietary Saturated Fat Intake and Negatively Associated With Usual Dietary Protein Intake in People With Insulin-Dependent Diabetes Mellitus
Riley MD, Dwyer T (Univ of Tasmania, Hobart, Australia)
Am J Clin Nutr 67:50–57, 1998   3–13

Objective.—Most of the deaths from insulin-dependent diabetes mellitus (IDDM) occur in diabetic patients with an increased urinary albumin excretion rate (UAER) that leads to renal disease. Whereas attention had been focused on dietary protein as a cause of hyperfiltration and loss of nephron units, some researchers now blame fat intake. The association between dietary macronutrient intake and the presence of early stages of UAERs in people with IDDM was examined in a cross-sectional population-based IDDM case series on Tasmania.

Methods.—A food-frequency questionnaire was mailed to 358 registrants in the Tasmanian Insulin-Treated Diabetes Register who had had IDDM for 7 or more years but no diagnosis of microalbuminuria (UAER of 20 to 200 µg albumin/min in at least 2 of 3 timed overnight urine collections). Protein and fat intake was determined in addition to age, sex, duration of diabetes, daily number of injections, body mass index, glycated hemoglobin, serum high-density lipoprotein cholesterol, frequency of exercise, and smoking status. The relation between microalbuminuria and dietary macronutrient intake was compared by logistic regression modeling.

Results.—There were 210 patients who provided samples and responses. On the basis of the analysis, there were 48 patients with microalbuminuria and 130 with normoalbuminuria. Patients in the highest quintile of energy-adjusted saturated fat had a significantly greater likelihood of having microalbuminuria than did individuals in the lowest quintile,

TABLE 5.—Odds Ratios and 95% CIs Microalbuminuria in Subjects With Insulin-dependent Diabetes Mellitus According to Quintile of Energy-adjusted Macronutrient Intake

Dietary quintile	Unadjusted Odds ratio	95% CI (P)	Adjusted Odds ratio	95% CI (P)
Saturated fat				
1 (lowest)	1.0	Referent	1.0	Referent
2	1.9	0.51, 6.7 (0.34)	2.2	0.54, 9.0 (0.27)
3	1.0	0.25, 4.0 (1.00)	0.6	0.14, 3.0 (0.57)
4	1.3	0.33, 4.8 (0.74)	1.1	0.26, 4.6 (0.91)
5 (highest)	3.0	0.87, 10.6 (0.08)	4.9	1.2, 20.0 (0.03)
Protein				
1 (lowest)	1.0	Referent	1.0	Referent
2	0.85	0.28, 2.6 (0.78)	0.88	0.25, 3.2 (0.85)
3	0.49	0.15, 1.6 (0.24)	0.58	0.16, 2.2 (0.42)
4	0.72	0.23, 2.3 (0.56)	0.81	0.23, 2.9 (0.75)
5 (highest)	0.14	0.03, 0.71 (0.02)	0.10	0.02, 0.56 (0.01)
Carbohydrate				
1 (lowest)	1.0	Referent	1.0	Referent
2	0.41	0.11, 1.6 (0.20)	0.31	0.06, 1.5 (0.13)
3	1.0	0.31, 3.3 (1.00)	0.98	0.25, 3.9 (0.98)
4	0.83	0.25, 2.8 (0.76)	0.49	0.12, 2.0 (0.32)
5 (highest)	1.0	0.31, 3.3 (1.00)	0.81	0.22, 3.0 (0.75)

Adjusted for sex, age at diagnosis, smoking status, duration of diabetes, body mass index, glycated hemoglobin, serum HDL cholesterol, frequency of exercise, and number of daily insulin injections.

(Courtesy of Riley MD, Dwyer T: Microalbuminuria is positively associated with usual dietary saturated fat intake and negatively associated with usual dietary protein intake in people with insulin-dependent diabetes mellitus. *Am J Clin Nutr* 67:50–57. Copyright 1998, American Society for Clinical Nutrition.)

after demographic and laboratory parameters were taken into account (odds ratio, 4.9) (Table 5). Patients in the highest quintile of energy-adjusted usual protein intake had a significantly lower likelihood of having microalbuminuria than did individuals in the lowest quintile (odds ratio, 0.10). There was no relationship between microalbuminuria and energy-adjusted mono- or polyunsaturated fats.

Conclusion.—Patients with IDDM who eat a diet high in saturated fat are significantly more likely to develop an insulin-resistant state than are those who eat a diet low in saturated fat. High protein intake is not associated with development of microalbuminuria.

▶ It seemed so logical—protein in (the mouth), protein out (the urine). This study suggests that this logic does not prevail; rather, it is high saturated fat in, diabetic nephropathy begins, protein out. How this works remains a mystery, but it is consistent with other known facts, such as that urinary albumin excretion rate is associated with mortality in diabetics and nondiabetics. I doubt that the results apply only to the Tasmanians who were studied. This appears to be the first study to consider saturated fat intake specifically, and it needs to be replicated, but these results are enough for me to incorporate this addition into my patient education.

M.A. Bowman, M.D., M.P.A.

Reduced Frequency of Severe Hypoglycemia and Coma in Well-controlled IDDM Patients Treated With Insulin Lispro

Holleman F, Schmitt H, Rottiers R, et al (Diakonessenhuis, Utrecht, The Netherlands; Eli Lilly, Indianapolis, Ind; Univ Hosp, Gent, Belguim; et al)
Diabetes Care 20:1827–1832, 1997
3–14

Background.—Previous research indicates that insulin lispro, an insulin analogue that is short-acting, can reduce risk for hypoglycemia when used in multiple injection therapy. Glycemic control associated with using this drug in patients with well-controlled insulin-dependent diabetes mellitus (IDDM) was investigated.

Method.—One hundred ninety-nine patients with IDDM were treated in this randomized, open-label, crossover trial. After being normalized with NPH insulin and regular insulin during a 4-week period, patients were treated for 12 weeks with NPH insulin and regular insulin or with NHP insulin and insulin lispro. Insulin lispro was to be injected directly before meals, whereas regular insulin was to be injected 30 minutes before meals. Results were monitored at baseline, after the initial 4-week period, and at 4 and 12 weeks. In addition, patients monitored blood glucose starting 2 weeks before each study visit and completed a questionnaire at the end of the study.

Results.—Severe hypoglycemia (58 vs. 36, $P = 0.037$) occurred less in the insulin lispro test group (Table 3). The HbA_{1c} did not fluctuate during the course of the study ($\approx 7.3\%$). Significantly lower digressions in meal-related glucose were noted using insulin lispro as well as more constant within-day variability.

TABLE 3.—Hypoglycemic Events During the Study Periods

	Total	Regular insulin	Insulin lispro	P value
Total	4,593	2,344	2,249	NS
Nonsevere				
Total	4,499	2,286	2,213	NS
Severe				
Total	94	58	36	0.037*
Coma	19	16	3	0.004*
Symptomatic				
Total	3,617	1,846	1,771	NS
<3.0 mmol/l	2,095	1,055	1,040	NS
Asymptomatic				
Total	976	498	478	NS
<3.0 mmol/l	924	479	445	NS
12:00–6:00 A.M.	488	312	176	<0.001†
6:00 A.M.–12:00 P.M.	1,395	612	783	0.015†
12:00–6:00 P.M.	1,510	790	720	NS
6:00 P.M.–12:00 A.M.	1,150	604	546	NS

Note: Data are n.
*X^2 test.
†X^2 approximation to the Wilcoxon's rank-sum test.
(Courtesy of Holleman F, Schmitt H, Rottiers R, et al: Reduced frequency of severe hypoglycemia and coma in well-controlled IDDM patients treated with insulin lispro. *Diabetes Care* 20:1827–1832, 1997.)

Conclusion.—In this study, insulin lispro treatment caused fewer cases of severe hypoglycemia than regular insulin in patients with well-controlled IDDM. Insulin lispro was also determined by patients to encourage a more flexible lifestyle.

▶ Lispro insulin is relatively new and its place in treatment strategies not fully clear. Its main apparent advantage is that it can be given immediately before a meal, rather than 30 minutes before the meal. This study confirms this advantage—the rate of severe hypoglycemia was much decreased, and only one third of the patients said they gave the regular insulin 30 minutes in advance. With its overall shorter length of activity than regular insulin, the pattern of blood glucose values differed, but the glycated hemoglobin values remained the same. In practice, this suggests that for patients with recurrent severe or problematic hypoglycemic episodes, lispro insulin is worth trying, particularly if patients note they have difficulty injecting the regular insulin 30 minutes before the meal.

M.A. Bowman, M.D., M.P.A.

Effect of Excessive Weight Gain With Intensive Therapy of Type 1 Diabetes on Lipid Levels and Blood Pressure: Results From the DCCT
Purnell JQ, Hokanson JE, Marcovina SM (Univ of Washington, Seattle; George Washington Univ, Rockville, Md; Univ of Minnesota, Minneapolis)
JAMA 280:140–146, 1998   3–15

Introduction.—With the institution of insulin therapy, patients with type 1 diabetes characteristically gain weight. Improvement in hemoglobin A_{1c} correlates inversely with continued weight gain with intensification of diabetes therapy. Compared with the conventionally treated group, lipid levels for the intensively treated group improved, including lower levels of dense low-density lipoprotein, despite their weight gain. A leading cause of death in adults with type 1 diabetes is coronary artery disease. The effect of weight gain on lipid levels and blood pressure was determined.

Methods.—There were 1,168 patients, aged 18 or older, with type 1 diabetes who participated in a randomized controlled trial. Patients received either intensive or conventional diabetes treatment. There was a mean follow-up of 6.1 years. In each treatment group, plasma lipid levels and blood pressure were measured and categorized by quartile of weight gain.

Results.—The highest body mass index, blood pressure, and levels of triglyceride, total cholesterol, low-density lipoprotein cholesterol, and apolipoprotein B were found in patients in the fourth quartile of weight gain who had intensive treatment as compared with patients in the first quartile of weight gain. For example, body mass index was 31 kg/m² for the fourth quartile and 24 kg/m² for the first quartile. Blood pressure was 120/77 Hg for those in the fourth quartile compared with 113/73 Hg for those in the first quartile. Triglyceride was 0.99 mmol/L in the fourth quartile and 0.79 mmol/L in the first quartile. The fourth-quartile group also had more cholesterol in the very low density lipoprotein, a higher waist-to-hip-ratio, intermediate dense lipoprotein, and dense low-density lipoprotein fractions. Compared with the first quartile, they also had lower high-density lipoprotein cholesterol and apolipoprotein A-I levels. Between the first and fourth quartiles of weight gain with intensive therapy, baseline characteristics were not different, except for a higher hemoglobin A_{1c} in the fourth quartile. Smaller increases in body mass index, lipids, and systolic blood pressure were the results of weight gain with conventional therapy.

Conclusion.—In this subset of patients, the risk of coronary artery disease may be increased with time because of the changes in lipid levels and blood pressure that occur with excessive weight gain with intensive therapy and are similar to those seen in the insulin-resistance syndrome.

▶ More trade-offs. Intensive insulin therapy for type 1 diabetics lowers some diabetic complications, such as eye and kidney disease, but increases others, including hypoglycemia and now, according to this article, weight, lipids, and blood pressure. The authors suggest this means that more coronary artery disease will occur over the years. The patients who had the most weight gain actually started to have a major feature of type 2 diabetes—insulin resistance. This may mean that tight control trades off microvascular complications for macrovascular complications. This study is further proof that we do not fully understand diabetes, and even patients with type 1 diabetes can become obese.

M.A. Bowman, M.D., M.P.A.

Diabetes Mellitus Type 2

United Kingdom Prospective Diabetes Study 24: A 6-Year, Randomized, Controlled Trial Comparing Sulfonylurea, Insulin, and Metformin Therapy in Patients With Newly Diagnosed Type 2 Diabetes That Could Not Be Controlled With Diet Therapy
Wright A, and the United Kingdom Prospective Diabetes Study Group (Radcliffe Infirmary, Oxford, England)
Ann Intern Med 128:165–175, 1998   3–16

Background.—The value of oral hypoglycemic drugs and insulin treatment for patients with newly diagnosed type 2 diabetes is uncertain. Responses of such patients to 6-year treatment with sulfonylurea, insulin, or metformin were assessed.

Methods.—Two groups were studied. The primary diet failure group (group 1) included 458 patients with newly diagnosed type 2 diabetes that was not controlled with diet. These patients had hyperglycemic symptoms or fasting plasma glucose levels exceeding 15 mmol/L during the first 3 months of diet therapy. Group 2 consisted of 1,620 patients in whom diet therapy controlled disease, fasting glucose levels ranged from 6 to 15 mmol/L, and no hyperglycemic symptoms occurred during diet therapy alone.

Findings.—Group 1 patients were younger, were less obese, and had more retinopathy, lower fasting plasma insulin levels, and decreased β-cell function compared with group 2 patients. At 6 years, fasting plasma glucose levels were lower in patients given insulin than in those given oral agents. However, hemoglobin A_{1c} concentrations were similar. Forty-eight percent of group 1 patients maintained hemoglobin A_{1c} levels of less than 0.08. By 6 years, 51% of patients given ultralente insulin needed additional short-acting insulin, and 66% given sulfonylurea needed additional treatment with metformin or insulin to control symptoms and maintain fasting plasma glucose levels at less than 15 mmol/L. Compared with patients given sulfonylurea, those given insulin gained more weight and had more hypoglycemic attacks. Obese patients receiving metformin gained the least weight and had the fewest hypoglycemic attacks. With any treatment, control achieved at 6 years was worse in group 1 than in group 2.

Conclusions.—Initial insulin therapy induced more hypoglycemic reactions and weight gain without necessarily providing better control. Thus, beginning with oral agents and changing to insulin may be reasonable when glycemic level goals are not attained.

▶ This is a complicated long-term study with a large amount of data. After looking at all that was presented, I took away a few helpful points. At 6 years, control as measured by HbA_{1c} in the various groups was similar. However, insulin was associated with more hypoglycemia, and insulin and sulfonylureas were associated with more weight gain. Thus, metformin appeared to be preferable. All groups had a significant failure rate of initial therapy, and younger and less obese patients needed more changes of therapy. Metformin was used only in patients who were obese at baseline. I would say that the glyburide patients fared better than chlorpropamide patients—at least there was less need for additional therapy with glyburide. This paper did not report any substantial differences in major morbidity or mortality, although I suspect the numbers were potentially too small to detect potentially real differences.

M.A. Bowman, M.D., M.P.A.

Effect of Troglitazone in Insulin-treated Patients With Type II Diabetes Mellitus
Schwartz S, for the Troglitazone and Exogenous Insulin Study Group (Diabetes and Glandular Diseases Clinic, San Antonio, Tex; Univ of Texas, Dallas; Univ of Arkansas, Little Rock; et al)
N Engl J Med 338:861–866, 1998 3–17

Introduction.—The thiazolidinediones are a class of compounds that reduce insulin resistance in animals with hyperglycemia and hyperinsulinemia. Administration of the thiazolidinedione troglitazone increased insulin-stimulated glucose disposal in human obese patients and patients with type 2 diabetes. The ability of troglitazone to improve glycemic control, as reflected primarily in changes in glycosylated hemoglobin values and fasting serum glucose concentrations, was evaluated in patients who had poorly controlled type 2 diabetes despite insulin therapy.

Methods.—There were 350 patients with poorly controlled type 2 diabetes mellitus who were studied to determine the effect of troglitazone. The patients had glycosylated hemoglobin values of 8% to 12%, despite therapy with at least 30 U of insulin daily. The patients were randomly assigned to receive placebo, 600 mg of troglitazone, or 200 mg of troglitazone for 26 weeks. Insulin doses were reduced only to prevent hypoglycemia, and they were not increased. During an 8-week baseline period, measurements of glycosylated hemoglobin, serum glucose while fasting, serum total cholesterol, high-density lipoprotein cholesterol, low-density lipoprotein cholesterol, and triglycerides were taken 5 times. The study was completed by 90% of the patients. These same measurements were repeated 10 times during the 26-week treatment period. During both periods, daily insulin doses were recorded.

Results.—In the group given 200 mg of troglitazone, the adjusted mean glycosylated hemoglobin values decreased by 0.8%, and in the group given 600 mg of troglitazone, there was a decrease of 1.4%. In the group given 200 mg of troglitazone, fasting serum glucose concentrations decreased by 35 mg/dL or 1.9 mmol/L, despite a decrease of 11% in the insulin dose. In the group given 600 mg of troglitazone, fasting serum glucose concentrations decreased by 49 mg/dL or 2.7 mmol/L, despite a decrease of 29% in the insulin dose. There were slight increases in serum total cholesterol, low-density lipoprotein cholesterol, and high-density lipoprotein cholesterol concentrations. In the troglitazone-treated patients, there was a slight decrease in serum triglyceride concentrations.

Conclusion.—Troglitazone improves glycemic control in patients with type 2 diabetes mellitus, when given with insulin.

▶ Troglitazone appears to be a useful drug in practice. This article notes the increases in cholesterol, which can be concerning in patients with diabetes. Another recent article by Inzucchi, et al.,[1] found similar reductions in HbA$_{1c}$—a decrease of 1.2% with 400 mg daily troglitazone. The same article found that troglitazone (400 mg daily) and metformin (100 mg twice a day) led to similar improvements in diabetes control, and that troglitazone and metformin combined had approximately twice the effect of either alone. We do not know the side effects of long-term combination therapy. Patients on troglitazone need liver-function test monitoring.

M.A. Bowman, M.D., M.P.A.

Reference

1. Inzucchi SE, Maggs DG, Spollett GR, et al: Efficacy and metabolic effects of metformin and troglitazone in type II diabetes mellitus. N Engl J Med 338:867–872, 1998.

Use of Enalapril to Attenuate Decline in Renal Function in Normotensive, Normoalbuminuric Patients With Type 2 Diabetes Mellitus: A Randomized, Controlled Trial

Ravid M, Brosh D, Levi Z, et al (Tel-Aviv Univ, Israel; Meir Hosp, Kfar-Sava, Israel)
Ann Intern Med 128:982–988, 1998   3–18

Background.—Angiotensin-converting enzyme (ACE) inhibitors decrease nephropathy progression in diabetics with microalbuminuria. A randomized, double-blind, placebo-controlled trial of the effect of ACE inhibitors on nephropathy was conducted with patients with type 2 diabetes, normal blood pressure, and normal urinary albumin excretion.

Methods.—The study group consisted of 156 type 2 diabetic patients from 8 outpatient clinics who had been given their diagnosis after the age of 40 years and who had normal blood pressure and albuminuria at baseline. Their diabetes duration was 0 to 9 years. After a 2-month observation period, patients were randomly assigned in a double-blind fashion to receive enalapril or placebo. Patients were followed by their family physicians and seen semiannually for blood pressure, hemoglobin A_{1c}, serum creatinine, serum electrolytes, 24-hour albumin excretion, and urinary creatinine evaluations. Follow-up was for a 6-year period for each patient.

Results.—Enalapril administration decreased urinary albumin excretion at 2 years, followed by a slow increase. In the placebo group, albumin excretion was significantly higher at 6 years. Transition to microalbuminuria occurred in 15% of those taking placebo and in 6.5% of those in the enalapril group. Enalapril treatment was associated with a 12.5% absolute risk reduction for the development of microalbuminuria. Hemoglobin A_{1c} values decreased slightly in both groups. Average blood pressure remained normal in both groups.

Conclusion.—This 6-year randomized, placebo-controlled, double-blind study of the effect of the ACE-inhibitor, enalapril, on normotensive, normoalbuminuric, low-risk type 2 diabetics, showed that enalapril had a significant renal-protective effect. Further long-term research is required to determine whether treatment with ACE inhibitors can prevent the development of overt nephropathy.

▶ This excellent randomized, controlled trial with long-term follow-up (6 years) shows an impressive reduction in the progression to microalbuminuria and less reduction in creatinine clearance when enalapril, 10 mg per day, was used prophylactically in patients with type 2 diabetes and normal blood pressure. One potential disadvantage of this study was that the study population was probably primarily Jewish, as it was done in Israel. The enalapril was only partially preventive, i.e., the mean renal function still declined and microalbuminuria still developed in some.

Another finding of potentially great importance is that there were substantially fewer new cases of retinopathy, although the study was not designed to test this and did not objectively test for retinopathy. The authors theorize that the retinopathy was lower because of better control of blood pressure.

M.A. Bowman, M.D., M.P.A.

Outcome Results of the Fosinopril Versus Amlodipine Cardiovascular Events Randomized Trial (FACET) in Patients With Hypertension and NIDDM

Tatti P, Pahor M, Byington RP, et al (Univ of Tennessee, Memphis; Wake Forest Univ, Winston-Salem, NC; Istituto Nazionale di Ricerca e Cura per gli Anziani, Rome)
Diabetes Care 21:597–603, 1998   3–19

Background.—Calcium antagonists and angiotensin converting enzyme inhibitors may positively affect serum lipids and glucose metabolism. The effects of fosinopril and amlodipine on serum lipids and diabetes control

Follow-up time (years)

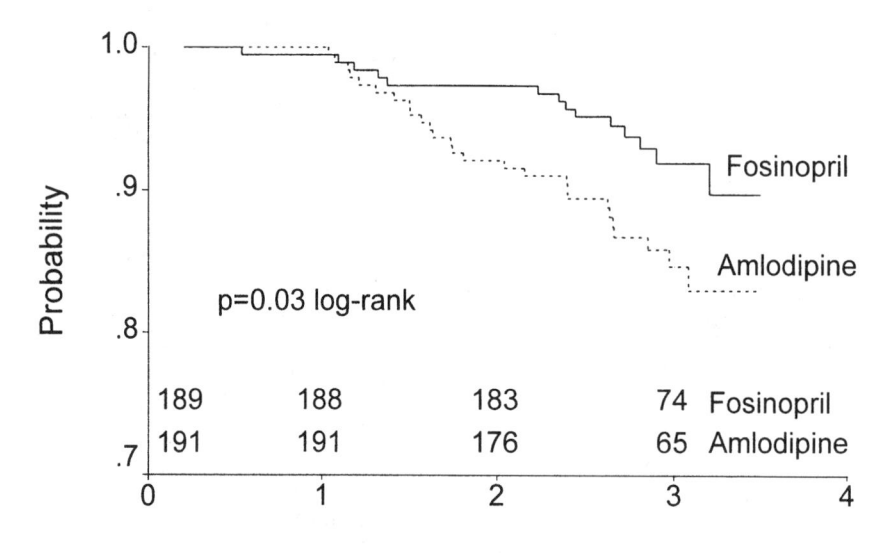

FIGURE 2.—Probability, according to treatment, of remaining free of stroke, acute myocardial infarction, and hospitalized angina. The number of participants receiving each treatment at each time is indicated at the bottom of the graph. (Courtesy of Tatti P, Pahor M, Byington RP, et al: Outcome results of the fosinopril versus amlodipine cardiovascular events randomized trial (FACET) in patients with hypertension and NIDDM. *Diabetes Care* 21:597–603, 1998.)

in patients with NIDDM and hypertension were studied in the Fosinopril Versus Amlodipine Cardiovascular Events Randomized Trial (FACET).

Methods.—Three hundred eighty hypertensive patients with NIDDM were included in the randomized study. None had a history of coronary heart disease or stroke, serum creatinine levels exceeding 1.5 mg/dL, or albuminuria exceeding 40 µg/min. None of the patients used lipid-reducing drugs, aspirin, or antihypertensive agents other than β-blockers or diuretics. The patients were assigned to open-label fosinopril, 20 mg/day, or amlodipine, 10 mg/day, and studied for 3.5 years. The other study drug was added to treatment for patients in whom blood pressure was not controlled.

Findings.—Both treatments effectively reduced blood pressure. At the end of follow-up, the groups did not differ significantly in total serum cholesterol, HDL cholesterol, HbA_{1c}, fasting serum glucose, or plasma insulin.The risk of the combined outcome of acute myocardial infarction, stroke, or angina requiring hospitalization was significantly lower in patients given fosinopril than in those given amlodipine (Fig 2).

Conclusions.—The effects of fosinopril and amlodipine on biochemical measures were comparable. However, the risk of major vascular events was significantly lower with fosinopril than with amlodipine.

▶ In this group of middle-aged patients with hypertension and well-controlled NIDDM, the angiotensin converting enzyme inhibitor fosinopril was associated with far fewer vascular events in the approximately 3 years of the trial than the long-acting calcium channel blocker amlodipine. The patients' diabetes remained well controlled. Lipid values were similar. Hypertension was slighter better controlled by amlodipine. Approximately one third of the group received the other study drug as an addition to achieve blood pressure control, and some patients were also on a diuretic. However, statistically speaking, the vascular events were considered secondary outcome measures, and were not the primary outcome measure of the study. My bottom line: angiotensin converting enzyme inhibitors are clearly a preferred drug for patients with diabetes.

M.A. Bowman, M.D., M.P.A.

Starting Insulin Therapy in Patients With Type 2 Diabetes: Effectiveness, Complications, and Resource Utilization
Hayward RA, Manning WG, Kaplan SH, et al (Univ of Michigan, Ann Arbor; Univ of Minnesota, Minneapolis; New England Med Ctr, Boston; et al)
JAMA 278:1663–1669, 1997   3–20

Introduction.—Insulin therapy has been shown to be safe and efficacious in enhancing glycemic control in type 2 diabetes under optimal conditions, but not much is known about the effectiveness, complication rates, and associated resource use in actual clinical practice. The effectiveness of insulin therapy and the associated resource use was examined in a large staff-model HMO.

Methods.—Clinical, survey, and administrative information systems data were used to assess hospitalizations, outpatient visits, laboratory testing, home glucose monitoring, and glycemic control in 8,668 patients with type 2 diabetes. A subsample of 1,738 patients was used to determine total illness and Burden index via detailed case-mix data.

Results.—In patients beginning insulin therapy, the level of Hb A10 dropped 0.9 percentage point at 1 year compared with patients receiving stable medication regimens. At 2 years after initiation of insulin therapy, 60% still had Hb A10 levels of 8% or higher. Notably greater Hb A10 reductions were observed in patients with the poorest baseline glycemic control. Patients with a baseline Hb A10 level of 13% had a threefold greater decrease in Hb A10, compared with patients with baseline Hb A10 levels of 9%. In the subset of patients for whom detailed case-mix data were collected, insulin users had a higher resource use than patients taking sulfonylureas, regardless of the illness severity. Patients taking insulin had slightly more laboratory tests, 2.4 more outpatient visits per year, and about 300 more fingersticks for home glucose testing per year compared with patients taking sulfonylureas. Patients taking insulin had about 15% more weekly symptoms of hypoglycemia. Patients taking insulin had nonsignificantly more (0.5) hypoglycemia-related hospitalizations per 100 patient-years.

Conclusion.—Patients with type 2 diabetes with poor glycemic control, managed by generalist physicians who initiated insulin therapy, were able to achieve safe and effective moderate glycemic control. Insulin therapy was associated with a higher resource use and was rarely effective in achieving tight glycemic control, even for patients with moderate control.

▶ Insulin helped patients with type 2 diabetes control blood sugar a little bit but took a lot of resources and a lot of effort on the part of the patients. It appeared to be more worthwhile for the patients with poorer control. Very few of these patients were receiving a combination of oral hypoglycemics and insulin, which I often use for patients with type 2 diabetes. Patients were all primarily managed by primary care physicians. Three fourths were using 2 or 3 insulin shots a day. A new measure of diabetes severity was used to adjust the data; this measure has face validity (i.e., looks reasonable to me) and good statistics but has not withstood use in various settings for various purposes. I agree with the authors' conclusions: it is difficult to obtain good control for many patients with diabetes. Lack of patient motivation, concurrent patient issues, and lack of adequate health resource use (such as visits or individualized attention and education) contribute to this lack of control far more than physician indifference or lack of knowledge. The question remains as to whether the total costs and problems of insulin therapy are worth the small amount of improvement in glucose control. I do think the newer oral medications are helping us to improve average glycemic control and may be at least a partial answer.

M.A. Bowman, M.D., M.P.A.

Efficacy of 24-Week Monotherapy With Acarbose, Metformin, or Placebo in Dietary-treated NIDDM Patients: The Essen-II Study
Hoffman J, Spengler M (Clinical Research Collaborative Study Group, Essen, Germany; Bayer AG, Leverkusen, Germany)
Am J Med 103:483–490, 1997   3–21

Objective.—Whereas clinical trials have confirmed the therapeutic potential of acarbose or metformin in the treatment of patients with non–insulin-dependent diabetes mellitus (NIDDM), there have been no studies directly comparing efficacy of the 2 drugs. The efficacies of acarbose, metformin, and placebo were compared in patients with NIDDM previously treated with diet alone.

Methods.—The study, double-blind with respect to acarbose-placebo treatment and single-blind with respect to metformin treatment, was conducted in 4 internal medicine practices in Essen, Germany for 24 weeks. Patients aged 35–70 years received 1 placebo tablet (n = 32, 38% male), 1 100-mg tablet of acarbose 3 times daily with meals (n = 31, 19% male), or 1 850-mg tablet of metformin twice daily after meals (n = 31, 45% male). Compliance, adverse events, and blood parameters were assessed every 6 weeks. The efficacy criteria were glycated HbA_{1c} hemoglobin value, fasting blood glucose (BG) and insulin, 1-hour postprandial BG and insulin (after standard meal test), postprandial insulin increase, and fasting plasma lipids. Diet consisted of 50% carbohydrates, 35% fat, and 15%

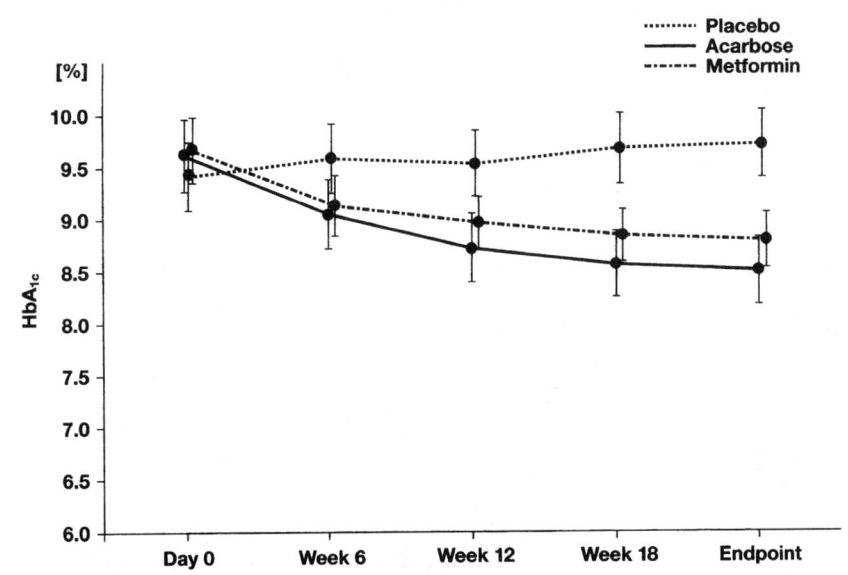

FIGURE 2.—Hemoglobin A_{1c} values before, during, and at the end of 24 weeks of treatment with placebo, acarbose, and metformin (means with 95% confidence intervals). (Reprinted by permission of the publisher, from Hoffman J, Spengler M: Efficacy of 24-week monotherapy with acarbose, metformin, or placebo in dietary-treated NIDDM patients: The Essen-II Study. *Am J Med* 193:483–490. Copyright 1997 by Excerpta Medica, Inc.)

protein. There were 94 patients assessable for efficacy and 96 for tolerability.

Results.—There were no significant changes in fasting and postprandial BG or HbA$_{1c}$ level after 24 weeks in the placebo group, whereas all 3 values decreased significantly in both treatment groups (Fig 2). There were no significant differences between the metformin and acarbose treatment groups. Neither drug had an effect on fasting insulin but both lowered the postprandial insulin increase significantly with respect to placebo but not with respect to each other. Acarbose lowered the low-density lipoprotein high-density lipoprotein cholesterol ratio significantly by 26.7% with respect to metformin, which had no effect, and to placebo, which increased the ratio by 14.4%. The difference between metformin and placebo was not significant. Patients taking metformin and acarbose but not placebo lost a slight amount of weight. Sixteen (50%) patients taking acarbose reported mild to moderate gastrointestinal complaints during the first 4 weeks. During weeks 21 to 24, the figure dropped to 13.8%. No patient experienced hypoglycemia.

Conclusion.—Metformin and acarbose are equally effective in controlling NIDDM in patients previously insufficiently treated with diet alone. Fasting and postprandial BG, HbA$_{1c}$, and postprandial insulin increase were significantly reduced. Patients on both drugs lost a slight amount of weight. Acarbose but not metformin significantly reduced the low-density lipoprotein high-density lipoprotein cholesterol ratio.

▶ Personally, I have been more impressed with metformin than acarbose for glucose control in patients with type 2 diabetes, based on what I had read in the literature and what I had seen with patients. Metformin has the distinct disadvantage of potential lactic acidosis and many more contraindications, such as renal disease, than acarbose. This article finds that metformin (1,700 mg/day) was similar to acarbose (300 mg/day) in controlling glucose, but that acarbose had better effect on cholesterol (total, low-density lipoprotein, and high-density lipoprotein), an attractive drug effect in diabetic patients. The amount of decrease in the glycated hemoglobin with metformin was about 1.0%, less than recently reported for 1,500 mg of metformin (about 1.6% drop) or 2,000 mg of metformin (about 2.0% drop) in another study.[1] Higher doses of the metformin may have produced greater drops in glycated hemoglobin. Both acarbose and metformin decreased postprandial hyperinsulinemia. Acarbose may treat both hypercholesterolemia and diabetes for some patients, meaning one drug rather than two.

M.A. Bowman, M.D., M.P.A.

Reference

1. Garber AJ, Duncan TG, Goodman AM, et al: Efficacy of metformin in type II diabetes: Results of a double-blind, placebo-controlled, dose-response trial. *Am J Med* 102:491–497, 1997.

Reduction of Albumin Excretion Rate in Normotensive Microalbuminuric Type 2 Diabetic Patients During Long-term Simvastatin Treatment
Tonolo G, Ciccarese M, Brizzi P, et al (Univ of Sassari, Italy)
Diabetes Care 20:1891–1895, 1997   3–22

Introduction.—Patients with type 2 diabetes who have microalbuminuria are at elevated risk of cardiovascular disease. However, the effects of plasma glucose, blood pressure, and cholesterol level on the progression of microalbuminuria are unclear. There is debate over the effects of pharmacologic cholesterol reduction on kidney function. The long-term effects of simvastatin treatment on albuminuria in hypercholesterolemic patients with type 2 diabetes were studied.

Methods.—The two-year, double-blind, crossover trial included 19 patients with type 2 diabetes who had microalbuminuria and hypercholesterolemia. All were normotensive and had good metabolic control. The patients received each treatment for one year, simvastatin 20 mg/day and placebo. The effects of simvastatin treatment on urinary albumin excretion rate and creatinine clearance were assessed.

Results.—Plasma total and low-density cholesterol significantly decreased with simvastatin treatment. High-density lipoprotein cholesterol, creatinine clearance, blood pressure, and glucose control were unaffected.

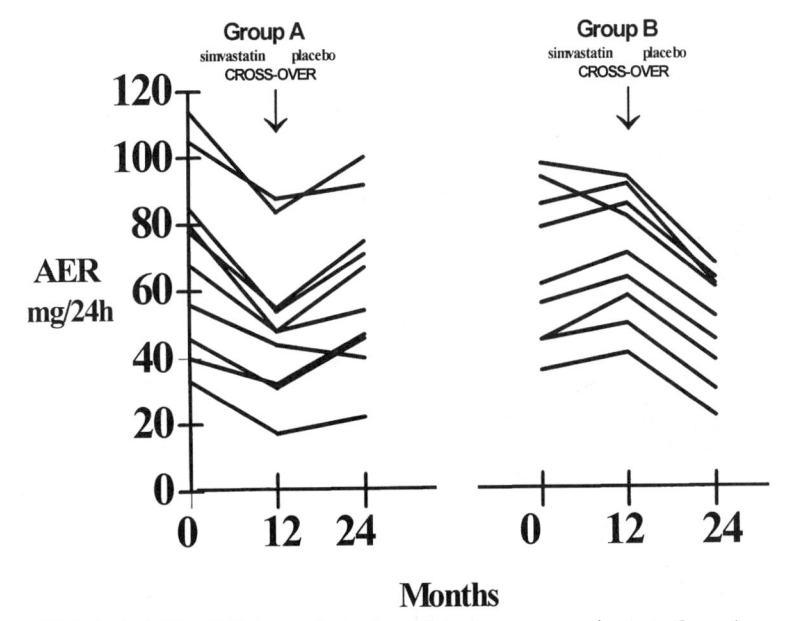

FIGURE 1.—Individual AER changes during the study in the two groups of patients. Group A: n = 10, 20 mg/day simvastatin for 12 months and then placebo after the crossover for an additional 12 months; group B: n = 9, placebo for 12 months and then 20 mg/day simvastatin after the crossover for an additional 12 months. (Courtesy of Tonolo G, Ciccarese M, Brizzi P, et al: Reduction of albumin excretion rate in normotensive microalbuminuric type 2 diabetic patients during long-term simvastatin treatment. *Diabetes Care* 20:1891–1895, 1997.)

Simvastatin was also associated with a significant reduction in urinary albumin excretion rate (AER), a mean decrease of 25% from baseline (Fig 1).

Conclusions.—In hypercholesterolemic, microalbuminuric patients with type 2 diabetes, cholesterol-lowering treatment with simvastatin also appears to reduce urinary AER. Simvastatin might offer an additional approach to protecting renal function for such patients. More research is needed to confirm the findings and evaluate possible mechanisms.

▶ This article provides convincing data that simvastatin reduces microalbuminuria in type 2 diabetic patients who have hypercholesterolemia, are well controlled, and are without hypertension or overt kidney disease. The data are consistent between the early and delayed treatment groups, although the number of patients was small. The patients were highly selected so that the effect of simvastatin alone could be identified. This may mean that the results cannot be generalized to all type 2 diabetic patients, but there is indirect rationale for this effect because microalbuminuria is known to be associated with negative arteriosclerotic outcomes in diabetes. What should this mean for practice? Well, we should be aggressive with lipid-lowering in diabetes as already recommended, but it may mean we do not start that new patient with microalbuminuria and hypercholesterolemia on an ACE inhibitor and a HMG CoA reductase inhibitor until we see the effect of the HMG CoA reductase inhibitor alone.

M.A. Bowman, M.D., M.P.A.

Diabetes Mellitus—Miscellaneous

Unrecognized Diabetes Among Hospitalized Patients
Levetan CS, Passaro M, Jablonski K, et al (Medlantic Research Inst, Washington, DC; Washington Hosp Ctr, Washington, DC)
Diabetes Care 21:246–249, 1998
3–23

Introduction.—About 50% of the 16 million Americans with diabetes are undiagnosed. The diagnosis of type 2 diabetes may be delayed by an average of 10 years after actual disease onset. Not much is known about the prevalence of hyperglycemia among hospitalized patients with no diagnosis of diabetes. Hospital care given to hyperglycemic hospitalized patients with no diagnosis of diabetes was assessed to determine whether these patients are appropriately evaluated and treated.

Methods.—All 1,034 consecutively hospitalized adult patients at a 750-bed inner-city teaching hospital during a 1-week period were evaluated. On a daily basis, the laboratory data system identified all patients with 1 or more plasma glucose values greater than 200 mg/dL. Patients with hyperglycemia and no diagnosis of diabetes were followed up to determine whether they were given a diagnosis during hospitalization and whether medical records reflected follow-up to address hyperglycemia.

Results.—A total of 37.5% and 33%, respectively, of all medical and surgical patients with hyperglycemia had no diagnosis of diabetes at the time of admission. The mean peak glucose in these patients was 299 mg/dL. Sixty-six percent had 2 or more elevations during hospitalization. Of these, 54% received insulin therapy and 59% received bedside glucose monitoring. The presence of hyperglycemia or diabetes was not documented in 66% of patient medical records. The medical records of only 3 patients (7.3%) documented possible diagnosis of diabetes in the progress notes.

Conclusions.—The failure to address the possibility of diabetes is a missed opportunity for making an earlier diagnosis and initiating interventions that could delay the harmful complications of this disease. It is recommended that physicians assume that hyperglycemia is diabetes until a diagnostic work-up can be performed.

▶ About 3% of the hospitalized adults had substantial hyperglycemia during hospitalization (glucose level of greater than 200 mg/dL) without mention, discussion, or treatment of diabetes by physicians. It is likely that many of these patients had diabetes and that the physicians wrongly attributed the glucose levels to stress hyperglycemia or concurrent medications. This level of glucose strongly suggests diabetes. We should notice these elevated glucose levels, check a HbA_{1c}, and treat appropriately. It is likely that even more unrecognized diabetic patients had high glucose levels not discovered by this study because of the cutoff of 200 mg/dL.

M.A. Bowman, M.D., M.P.A.

Intensity and Amount of Physical Activity in Relation to Insulin Sensitivity: The Insulin Resistance Atherosclerosis Study
Mayer-Davis EJ, for the IRAS Investigators (Univ of South Carolina, Columbia; Wake Forest Univ, Winston-Salem, NC; Permanente Med Group Inc, Oakland, Calif; et al)
JAMA 279:669–674, 1998

3–24

Objective.—Whereas exercise has been shown to reduce the incidence of non–insulin-dependent diabetes mellitus (NIDDM), the benefit of moderate exercise on NIDDM risk is unclear. Whether self-reported participation in physical activity of moderate or vigorous intensity was associated with improved insulin sensitivity was evaluated in a multicultural epidemiologic study.

Methods.—Intravenous glucose tolerance tests were performed in 1,467 individuals (45% men and 38% white, 28% Hispanic, and 34% black). Glucose function was normal in 46% and impaired in 22%; NIDDM was diagnosed in 32%. Patients rated their physical activity level. Insulin sensitivity was compared with exercise level.

Results.—There were 446 patients who did not participate in vigorous activities. Two percent of total time was spent in vigorous activities and

7% in moderate activities. Patients who exercised vigorously 5 or more times a week had an adjusted insulin sensitivity of 1.59, whereas those who rarely or never exercised had an insulin sensitivity of 0.90. Insulin sensitivity and estimated energy expenditure (EEE) for regular physical activity were significantly correlated ($\kappa = 0.14$). For both vigorous and nonvigorous activities, EEEs were significantly associated with insulin sensitivity. Body mass index and waist-to-height ratio were associated with, but did not entirely account for, the significant predicted increase in insulin sensitivity with higher EEE. Results were similar for all subgroups.

Conclusions.—Both vigorous and nonvigorous activity increased insulin sensitivity in a large cohort of individuals with glucose tolerance ranging from normal to mild NIDDM. The results were similar across all racial and ethnic subgroups tested and for males and females.

▶ My impression is that it is much easier to get nonexercising patients to begin to participate in nonvigorous activity than vigorous activity. Thus, it is very helpful to know that nonvigorous activity also improves insulin sensitivity, which in turn probably means less diabetes and heart disease in the long run. Vigorous activity was still better, and total energy expenditure is important. The improvements were also fairly linear, i.e., the more the better. One of the strengths of the study is that almost two thirds of the patients were Hispanic or African American.

M.A. Bowman, M.D., M.P.A.

High Blood Glucose Concentration Is a Risk Factor for Mortality in Middle-aged Nondiabetic Men: 20-Year Follow-up in the Whitehall Study, the Paris Prospective Study, and the Helsinki Policemen Study
Balkau B, Shipley M, Jarrett RJ, et al (INSERM, Villejuif, France; Univ of Kuopio, Finland; Univ College Med School, London; et al)
Diabetes Care 21:360–367, 1998

Objective.—Whether high but nondiabetic glucose levels were associated with increased risk of death from all causes, coronary heart disease (CHD), cardiovascular disease, and neoplasms was examined in 3 cohorts of nondiabetic men, aged 44–55 years at baseline after 20 years of follow-up.

Methods.—Mortality during a 20-year period was studied in 10,025 men in the Whitehall Study, 6,629 in the Paris Prospective Study, and 631 in the Helsinki Policemen Study who had high but nondiabetic glucose levels by the 2-hour oral glucose tolerance test. Mortality was analyzed using fasting glucose distributions according to Cox proportional hazards model, and survival curves were calculated using the Kaplan-Meier method.

Results.—Policemen had the highest "all causes" death rate and the highest death rates from all individual causes except neoplasms. Men in the highest 20% of the 2-hour glucose distribution had a significantly

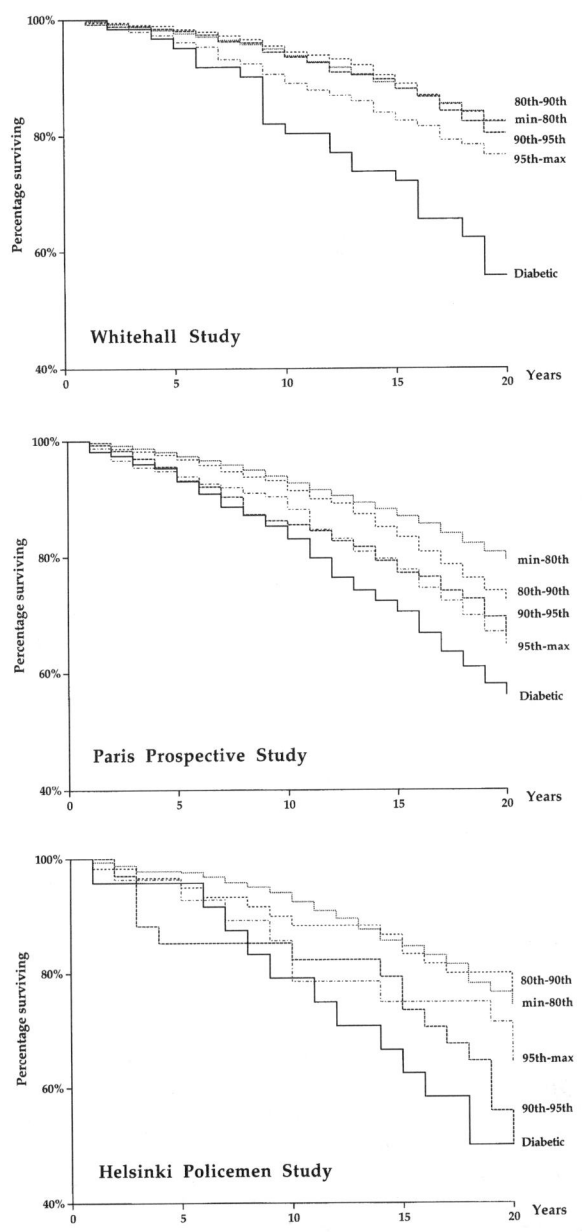

FIGURE 2.—Survival curves for death from all causes for nondiabetic men, by risk classes formed according to percentiles of the 2-hour blood glucose concentrations: the Whitehall Study, the Paris Prospective Study, and the Helsinki Policemen Study. (Courtesy of Balkau B, Shipley M, Jarrett RJ, et al: High blood glucose concentration is a risk factor for mortality in middle-aged nondiabetic men: 20-year follow-up in the Whitehall Study, the Paris Prospective Study, and the Helsinki Policemen Study. *Diabetes Care* 21:360–367, 1998.)

higher "all causes" mortality than the men in the remaining 80% (age-adjusted hazard ratio 1.6) (Fig 2). Men in the highest 2.5% of the 2-hour glucose distribution had an even higher risk (age-adjusted hazard ratio 2.0). Men in the highest 2.5% also had a significantly increased risk for cardiovascular disease and CHD (age-adjusted hazard ratios 1.8 and 2.7, respectively).

Conclusions.—Nondiabetic men with high 2-hour blood glucose levels are at increased risk for all causes mortality and for death from cardiovascular disease and CHD specifically. If efforts to lower blood glucose levels can be shown to decrease mortality, such intervention may be justified.

▶ Given that middle-aged men who have high glucose concentrations, but not the levels used to diagnose diabetes, had a substantially higher risk of death than men with lower glucose concentrations, we should implement preventive measures and treatment earlier. This higher rate of death was primarily related to cardiovascular disease and remained even after accounting for some other variables, such as total cholesterol. Many of these men would become overtly diabetic in future years, but it would appear they are at risk before the diabetes occurs. Perhaps providing this information to patients will encourage more aggressive self-care before diabetes develops.

M.A. Bowman, M.D., M.P.A.

Fish Oil and Glycemic Control in Diabetes

Friedberg CE, Janssen MJEM, Heine RJ, et al (Ziekenhuis de Vrije Universiteit, Amsterdam; Vrije Universiteit, Amsterdam; Het Rijnland Ziekenhuis, Leiderdorp, The Netherlands; et al)
Diabetes Care 21:494–500, 1998

Introduction.—The net benefit of administering fish oil to diabetics is still being debated. The effectiveness in reducing diabetes and cardiovascular disease is not fully studied, and there is a theory that fish consumption may be inversely related to cardiovascular mortality and to glucose intolerance. An unfavorable lipoprotein profile may be linked to the high cardiovascular mortality rate in diabetes. A decrease in serum triglycerides has been seen with fish oil. A meta-analysis to estimate the size and direction of the effects of fish oil administration on glycemic control and lipid parameters in non–insulin-dependent diabetics and insulin-dependent diabetics was conducted.

Methods.—A meta-analysis was conducted in which 26 trials were chosen, and all trials included more than 5 diabetes patients, insulin-dependent and non-insulin dependent. The trials also addressed the effects of fish oil and docosahexaenoic acid on serum lipids and glucose tolerance.

Results.—A decrease in mean triglyceride concentrations in association with fish oil was seen in all studies, as was a slight but significant increase in serum LDL cholesterol at 0.18 mmol/L (Table 2). The findings were

TABLE 2.—Combined (Weighted) Results of All 26 Studies and of NIDDM and IDDM Studies Considered Separately

	Fasting blood glucose (mmol/l)	HbA$_{1c}$ (%)	Triglycerides (mmol/l)	Total cholesterol (mmol/l)	LDL cholesterol (mmol/l)	HDL cholesterol (mmol/l)
All studies						
Mean baseline level (range)	9.7 (7.11–15.4)	9.4 (7.4–12.1)	2.02 (0.93–4.91)	5.6 (4.5–7.1)	3.6 (2.44–4.64)	1.17 (0.79–1.64)
Mean change on	−0.06	0.16	−0.60*	0.02	0.18*	0.03
intervention (95% CI)	(−0.71 to 0.59)	(−0.10 to 0.41)	(−0.84 to −0.37)	(−0.09 to 0.14)	(0.04–0.32)	(−0.02 to 0.08)
NIDDM studies						
Mean baseline level (range)	9.11 (7.11–13.1)	8.8 (7.7–12.1)	2.6 (1.73–4.91)	5.8 (4.94–7.13)	3.7 (2.8–4.64)	1.01 (0.79–1.18)
Mean change on	0.43	0.14	−0.81*	−0.07	0.20*	−0.01
intervention (95% CI)	(0.0–0.87)	(−0.41 to 0.68)	(−1.16 to −0.46)	(−0.24 to 0.09)	(0.0–0.40)	(−0.08 to 0.05)
IDDM studies						
Mean baseline level (range)	11.9 (9.9–15.4)	9.8 (7.4–11.1)	1.17 (0.93–1.47)	5.1 (4.48–6.26)	3.3 (4.48–4.53)	1.38 (1.08–1.64)
Mean change on	−1.86*	0.17	−0.29*	0.19*	0.13	0.08*
intervention (95% CI)	(−3.1 to −0.61)	(−0.09 to 0.43)	(−0.50 to −0.07)	(0.04–0.33)	(−0.14 to 0.41)	(0.01–0.16)

*P less than 0.05.
(Courtesy of Friedberg CE, Janssen MJEM, Heine RJ, et al: Fish oil and glycemic control in diabetes. *Diabetes Care* 21:494–500, 1998.)

most prominent in the non–insulin-dependent diabetics. In diabetics treated with fish oil, no significant changes were seen in HbA_{1c} percentages. In the non–insulin-dependent diabetics, fasting blood glucose levels were increased with borderline significance at 0.43 mmol/L, and were significantly lower in the insulin-dependent diabetics, at −1.86 mmol/L. Only in the non–insulin-dependent diabetics, significant dose-response effects of eicosapentaenoic acid on HbA_{1c}, as well as significant effects of triglycerides of docosahexaenoic acid on fasting blood glucose levels, HBA_{1c}, and triglycerides, were demonstrated.

Conclusion.—No adverse effects on HbA1c in diabetics were seen with the use of fish oil. Triglyceride levels were lowered effectively by almost 30%. A slight increase in LDL cholesterol concentration was seen. In treating dyslipidemia in diabetes, fish oil may be useful.

▶ Generally, these results apply to supplements of fish oil and not fish oil components, and the results are not all positive. Fish oil supplements were associated with improvements in triglycerides, but at the expense of increased LDL cholesterol in NIDDM patients, and of worsened glucose control and increased total cholesterol in IDDM patients. So, should we encourage or discourage fish oil use? The authors suggest that fish oil be combined with statin treatment of mixed hyperlipidemia when there are significant elevations of both triglycerides and LDL cholesterol, because the alternative—combined use of fibrates and statins (HMG-CoA reductase inhibitors)—may increase the risk of myopathy. This makes some sense, but we will need to follow fasting lipid levels carefully.

M.A. Bowman, M.D., M.P.A.

Rate and Mode of Death During Five Years of Follow-up Among Patients With Acute Chest Pain With and Without a History of Diabetes Mellitus
Herlitz J, Karlson BW, Lindqvist J, et al (Sahlgrenska Univ, Göteborg, Sweden)
Diabetic Med 15:308–314, 1997

Introduction.—An increased risk of coronary artery disease and increased mortality and morbidity after acute myocardial infarction are found in patients with diabetes mellitus. The prognosis among diabetic patients admitted to the emergency department for acute chest pain has not been adequately examined. In diabetic and nondiabetic patients admitted to the emergency department with acute chest pain, or other symptoms raising a suspicion of acute myocardial infarction, the rate and mode of death during 5 years of follow-up are reported.

Methods.—There were 5,230 patients studied, and 8% or 402 had a history of diabetes. These patients were retrospectively reviewed through interviews and information in their charts. They were admitted to the emergency room for chest pain, acute heart failure, arrhythmia, loss of consciousness, or other symptoms thought to potentially portend acute myocardial infarction.

Results.—Patients with diabetes were older, had a higher prevalence of previously diagnosed cardiovascular disease, had fewer symptoms of chest pain, more symptoms of acute severe heart failure, and more electrocardiographic abnormalities upon admission than nondiabetic patients. Nondiabetic patients had a 5-year mortality of 23.3%, whereas diabetic patients had a 5-year mortality of 53.5%. Independent predictors of death among diabetic patients were ST-segment elevation on admission, a history of myocardial infarction, and a nonpathological electrocardiogram on admission.

Conclusion.—More than 50% of diabetic patients admitted to the emergency department with acute chest pain or other symptoms suggestive of acute myocardial infarction are dead 5 years later. Interventions to reduce mortality should be the focus of future research. At the time these patients were treated, thrombolytic agents, aspirin, acute coronary event inhibitors, lipid lowering drugs, and revascularization procedures were seldom used, which may have affected the long-term prognosis.

▶ I chose this article because half (!) of the diabetic patients it describes were dead 5 years after coming to an emergency room with chest pain or other symptoms suggestive of acute myocardial infarction—twice the mortality rate of those patients without diabetes. And 4 out of 5 patients who had a final diagnosis of myocardial infarction were dead after 5 years. We know that diabetes worsens the prognosis, but this is astonishing and should be a call-to-arms for both physicians and patients to be very aggressive with all known forms of secondary prevention—glucose, blood pressure, lipid lowering, diet control, exercise, tobacco cessation, and surgical intervention—if appropriate.

M.A. Bowman, M.D., M.P.A.

An Electronic Case Manager for Diabetes Control
Meneghini LF, Albisser AM, Goldberg RB, et al (Univ of Miami, Fla)
Diabetes Care 21:591–596, 1998   3–28

Background.—Sustained improvement in blood glucose control can decrease the long-term complications of diabetes. The use of an electronic case manager (ECM) system designed to facilitate glycemic control was reported.

Methods.—A customized microcomputer system located at the clinic was actively used by 107 patients for daily diabetes care. The voice-interactive system could be contacted by touch-tone phone 24 hours a day. Patients reported daily self-measured glucose levels or hypoglycemic symptoms as well as lifestyle events.

Findings.—The ECM received more than 45,000 telephone calls in the first year. A total of 788 patient-months of follow-up were accumulated.

The prevalence of diabetes-associated crises declined about threefold. Concurrently, HbA$_{1c}$ declined significantly by 0.8% at 6 months and by 0.9% at 12 months. The ECM assisted patients with adjustments in daily insulin and/or tablet treatment, automatically generated standardized medical reports, and kept electronic medicolegal documents. Clinic visits for managing complex diabetes were decreased by about twofold.

Conclusion.—Diabetic patients accessing this ECM system received timely, cost-effective, reliable medical care. The ECM system decreased the incidence of diabetic crises and the need for clinic visits. This system empowers case managers to improve diabetes care.

▶ This is the most advanced technology I have read about for the day-to-day management of diabetes. There is a health care professional interface, a patient interface, and an individually programmed expert subsystem for insulin dosage. The diabetic patients who chose to use this system improved their glycemic control. They interacted with the system most days, averaging almost 2 calls a day. With time and system use, the number of hypoglycemic and hyperglycemic events fell. This intensive management still required a significant amount of physician and case manager time (average, 33 minutes per patient per month). Visits to the office decreased.

Many insurance companies provided at least partial payment, and the authors note than an office would only need 20 patients with reasonable payment to make it viable. Unfortunately, the authors did not give the cost of the system. The system appears to be very attractive for more widespread use and trials.

M.A. Bowman, M.D., M.P.A.

Topical Hyperbaric Oxygen and Low Energy Laser for the Treatment of Diabetic Foot Ulcers

Landau Z (Kaplan Hosp, Rehovot, Israel)
Arch Orthop Trauma Surg 117:156–158, 1998   3–29

Background.—The value of systemic hyperbaric oxygen in the treatment of difficult wounds such as diabetic foot ulcers has not been definitively established. However, many clinicians feel that such treatment can be effective. In the current study, topical hyperbaric oxygen was used alone or with a low energy laser to treat chronic diabetic foot ulcers unresponsive to antibiotics, débridement, and weight reduction.

Methods and Findings.—Fifteen patients were given topical hyperbaric oxygen alone, and 35 received topical hyperbaric oxygen with a low energy laser. Ulcers had been present for a mean of 9 months before this treatment. The average number of treatments was 25. The mean duration of therapy was 3 months. Ulcers were cured in 43 patients. No adverse reactions were seen.

Conclusions.—In this series of patients with diabetic foot ulcers refractory to conventional treatment, topical hyperbaric oxygen administered alone or with a low power laser was successful. These modalities should be considered for patients with chronic diabetic foot ulcers.

▶ Those nasty, chronic, nonhealing diabetic foot ulcers can be very difficult to treat without amputation. Rumors have floated around for a long time that hyperbaric oxygen might work. This article provides good evidence that hyperbaric oxygen (perhaps with added laser therapy) may be effective. This was not a randomized, controlled trial, and it is the work of 1 investigator at 1 institution. It was not designed specifically to test laser therapy, either. However, almost all of the previously recalcitrant ulcers healed in a group of 50 patients. So, hyperbaric oxygen, if reasonably accessible, may well be worth a try before sending a patient under the knife.

M.A. Bowman, M.D., M.P.A.

Endocrine—Miscellaneous

Relation Between Therapy for Hyperthyroidism and the Course of Graves' Ophthalmopathy
Bartalena L, Marcocci C, Bogazzi F, et al (Istituto di Endocrinologia, Pisa, Italy; Clinica Oculistica, Pisa, Italy; Univ of Pisa, Italy; et al)
N Engl J Med 338:73–78, 1998   3–30

Objective.—The effects of radioiodine therapy for treatment of hyperthyroidism on Graves' ophthalmopathy are unknown. Results of a prospective, randomized study of the effects of the treatment of Graves' hyperthyroidism with methimazole or radioiodine therapy, and the effects of corticosteroids in patients with mild or moderate Graves' ophthalmopathy or none, are presented.

Methods.—After 3 or 4 months of treatment with methimazole, 443 patients with Graves' disease were randomly allocated to receive radioiodine therapy (120 to 150 µCi) for 18 months, radioiodine therapy plus prednisone (0.4 to 0.5 mg/kg) for 3 months, or continuing methimazole. Ocular examinations were performed every 2 months. Thyroid function was evaluated every 1 or 2 months for 1 year. Hypothyroidism or persistent hyperthyroidism was corrected.

Results.—Within 6 months ophthalmopathy developed or worsened in 23 (15%) of 150 patients treated with radioiodine. Smokers were significantly more likely than nonsmokers to have ophthalmopathy or worsened ophthalmopathy (83% versus 50%). In the 145 patients treated with radioiodine and prednisone, 50 of 75 patients with ophthalmopathy at baseline had regression, and those without ophthalmopathy at baseline did not change (Fig 1). Of the 148 patients receiving methimazole, 3 of 74 with ophthalmopathy improved, 4 had new or worsened ophthalmopathy, and 141 had no change. The frequency of development or progression in the radioiodine group was significantly higher than in either the radioiodine-prednisone group or the methimazole group.

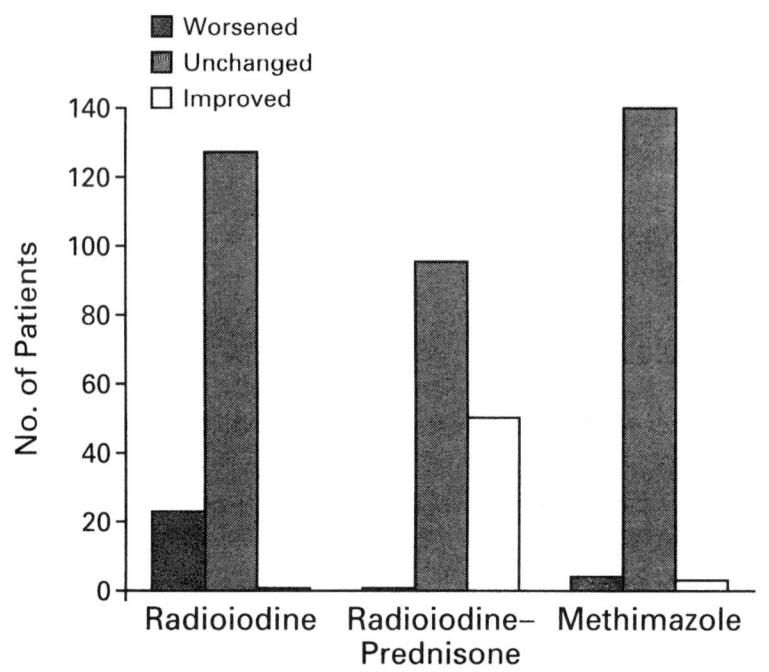

FIGURE 1.—Changes in the degree of ophthalmopathy in patients with hyperthyroidism who were treated with radioiodine, radioiodine and prednisone, or methimazole. Patients in whom ophthalmopathy developed are included in the group with patients whose condition worsened. The determination of patients' status was based on an overall evaluation of ocular changes, variations in the ophthalmopathy-activity score, and the patients' own evaluations, as described in the Methods section. (Reprinted by permission of *The New England Journal of Medicine* from Bartalena L, Marcocci C, Bogazzi F, et al: Relation between therapy for hyperthyroidism and the course of Graves' ophthalmopathy. *N Engl J Med* 338:73-78. Copyright 1998, Massachusetts Medical Society. All rights reserved.)

Conclusion.—Patients with Graves' hyperthyroidism, treated with radioiodine only, may show new or worsened ophthalmopathy to a greater extent than patients treated with methimazole. The ophthalmopathy is transient and regresses or can be prevented with prednisone therapy.

▶ As the ophthalmopathy of hyperthyroidism is probably autoimmune in origin, it makes sense that prednisone would both prevent and help treat the ophthalmopathy. Patients who smoked were more likely to develop ophthalmopathy, or to have it worsen if it already existed, and such patients should be counseled to quit smoking. Much of the ophthalmopathy was transient. Prednisone should be considered for all patients undergoing radioactive iodine treatment for hyperthyroidism. There are two alternatives. The prednisone can be held until ophthalmopathy is found with careful, frequent observation. Alternatively, as the rate of development of severe ophthalmopathy in those not given prednisone was low (5%), the prednisone could be given to all, and stopped in those with substantial side effects, who would be observed carefully.

M.A. Bowman, M.D., M.P.A.

Morbidity in Turner Syndrome
Gravholt CH, Juul S, Naeraa RW, et al (Aarhus Univ, Denmark)
J Clin Epidemiol 51:147–158, 1998   3–31

Background.—Turner's syndrome involves absence of at least part of an X chromosome, reduced height, reduced levels of female sex hormones,

TABLE 5.—Relative Risk of Disease in Turner's Syndrome (Other Than Endocrine Disease and Cancer)

Diagnoses (ICD-8)	Observed	Expected	RR (95% CI)
Anemia and other diseases of the blood (280–289)	7	4.19	1.67 (0.67–3.44)
Rheumatic heart diseases (390–398)	2	0.43	4.62 (0.56–16.67)
Hypertension (400–404)	7	2.40	2.91 (1.17–6.00)
Heart diseases and arteriosclerosis (410–429, 440–448)	16	7.58	2.11 (1.21–3.43)
Vascular diseases of the brain (430–438)	7	2.71	2.71 (1.04–5.33)
Venous diseases (450–458)	8	10.02	0.80 (0.34–1.57)
Ulcerotic colitis and Crohns disease (563)	4	1.78	2.25 (0.61–5.75)
Diseases of the liver, gall system, and pancreas (570–577)	11	6.31	1.74 (0.87–3.12)
Cirrhosis of the liver (571)	4	0.70	5.69 (1.55–14.56)
Gallstone diseases (574)	6	3.73	1.61 (0.59–3.50)
Selected diseases affecting the skin (696, 704, 709)	3	0.93	3.22 (0.66–9.40)
Psoriasis (696)	1	0.45	2.25 (0.06–12.51)
Bone, locomotive system, and connective tissue (710–718)	10	10.56	0.95 (0.45–1.74)
Rheumatic arthritis (712)	4	1.26	3.18 (0.87–8.15)
Osteoporosis* (723.09)	3	0.28	10.12 (2.18–30.93)
Fractures, combined (800–829)	35	16.23	2.16 (1.50–3.00)
Fractures of the spine (805)	2	0.82	2.44 (0.30–8.82)
Fractures of the humeral bone (812)	3	1.33	2.26 (0.47–6.60)
Fractures of the ulnar and radial bones (813)	6	2.89	2.08 (0.76–4.52)
Fractures of the metacarpal bones (815)	5	0.23	22.00 (7.14–51.33)
Fractures of the phalangeal bones (816)	2	0.47	4.24 (0.51–15.32)
Fractures of the femoral neck (820)	4	0.81	4.93 (1.34–12.61)
Fractures of the femoral bone (821)	6	0.60	9.93 (3.64–21.61)
Fractures of the tibial and fibular bone (823)	3	1.86	1.61 (0.33–4.72)
Potential osteoporotic fractures† (805, 813, 820)	12	4.52	2.66 (1.37–4.64)
Myasthenia gravis* (733.09)	0	0.07	—
Congenital malformation of the heart (746)	14	1.05	13.35 (7.30–22.40)
Coarctation of the aorta* (747.19)	21	0.06	367.13 (227.26–561.20)
Congenital malformations of the urinary system (753)	5	0.57	8.78 (2.85–20.48)
Congenital malformations of the face, ears, and neck (745)	7	2.10	3.34 (1.34–6.88)
Pterygium colli* (745.59)	3	0.003	1158 (239–3385)

*Based on diagnosis on the 5-digit level.
†These fractures include fractures of the spine, fractures of the ulnar and radial bones (including Colles' fracture), and fractures of the femoral neck.
(Reprinted by permission of the publisher from Gravholt CH, Juul S, Naeraa RW, et al: Morbidity in Turner syndrome. *J Clin Epidemiol* 51:147–158. Copyright 1998 by Elsevier Science Inc.)

TABLE 4.—Relative Risk of Endocrine Diseases in Turner Syndrome

Diagnoses (ICD-8)	Observed	Expected	RR (95% CI)
Endocrine diseases, overall (240–258)	51	10.47	4.87 (3.63–6.41)
Thyroid diseases, overall (240–246)	10	4.98	2.00 (0.96–3.69)
Thyrotoxicosis (242)	3	1.50	2.01 (0.41–5.86)
Hypothyrosis (244)	3	0.52	5.80 (1.20–16.94)
Thyroiditis (245)	3	0.81	16.60 (3.42–48.50)
Insulin dependent diabetes mellitus (IDDM) (249)	9	0.78	11.56 (5.29–21.95)
Non-insulin dependent diabetes mellitus (NIDDM) (250)	13	2.88	4.38 (2.40–7.72)
Miscellaneous endocrine diseases (251–258 (−251.13–15))	15	1.72	8.71 (4.87–14.36)
Parathyroid disease (252)	1	0.14	7.25 (0.18–40.37)
Hypoglycemia* (251.00)	2	0.57	3.51 (0.43–12.69)

*Based on diagnosis on the 5-digit level.
(Reprinted by permission of the publisher from Gravholt CH, Juul S, Naeraa RW, et al: Morbidity in Turner syndrome. J Clin Epidemiol 51:147–158. Copyright 1998 by Elsevier Science Inc.)

and decreased fertility. Turner's syndrome is associated with diseases such as diabetes, hypothyroidism, skeletal abnormalities, and congenital malformations. Data from the Danish Cytogenetic Central Register and the Danish National Registry of patients were used to estimate the incidence of other chronic diseases in patients with Turner's syndrome.

Study Design.—The study included all 2,594,036 women living in Denmark between 1983 and 1993. There were 594 women with Turner's syndrome identified in this group. Incident disease cases, defined as the first primary discharge diagnosis, were tallied for all women in the study group.

Findings.—Women with Turner's syndrome had an increased incidence of fractures, both osteoporotic fractures in adulthood and nonosteoporotic fractures in childhood (Table 5). Turner's syndrome was also associated with increased incidence of diabetes, ischemic heart disease, hypertension, and stroke. The risk of cancer of the bowel was also elevated in this group.

Conclusions.—This large population-based study of women with Turner's syndrome indicated that these women have an increased incidence of fractures, diabetes, ischemic heart disease, hypertension, and stroke (Table 4). This suggests that women with Turner's syndrome have a risk profile similar to that for postmenopausal women. This may explain the decreased life span of women with Turner's syndrome.

▶ This study finds an increased risk for all known patients with Turner's syndrome in Denmark to have multiple diseases based on hospitalization rates over a 10-year period. Several findings were already well known—higher congenital heart disease, coarctation of the aorta, diabetes, hypertension, vascular heart disease, and thyroid disease. Some were not, such as cirrhosis and colon cancer (although numbers were small). The increased incidence of childhood fractures was fascinating to me; the authors suggest that perhaps this is from the various bone abnormalities that occur in addition to osteoporosis. It is not known how many of the problems could be prevented by early and appropriate hormone therapy.

M.A. Bowman, M.D., M.P.A.

4 Infectious Diseases

Overview

Randomized controlled trials: Abstracts 4–3, 4–4, 4–5, and 4–7

Lyme Disease

- Cost-effectiveness of diagnostic strategies
- Problems with testing and prophylaxis
- Two articles on recombinant vaccines

Sexually Transmitted Disease

- Trovafloxacin and ofloxacin for single-dose treatment of gonorrhea
- Herpes simplex virus in the United States
- An immune-response modifier as a treatment for genital warts
- Isotretinoin treatment for condyloma

HIV Infection and AIDS

- Declining morbidity and mortality due to HIV infection
- Exercise and HIV infection
- Two articles on screening pregnant women for HIV infection
- Improved survival and early antiretroviral therapy
- Plasma viral load and CD4+ counts as prognostic indicators

Urinary Tract Infection

- Screening dipstick
- Sampling in elderly women

Miscellaneous

- A computer aid to diagnosing fever in hospitalized patients
- Switching acyclovir to over-the-counter use
- Safety and efficacy of oral ciprofloxacin to treat chronic otitis media in adults
- A consensus statement on treating pulmonary tuberculosis
- Outcomes of patients hospitalized with community-acquired pneumonia
- Antibiotics and lower respiratory infection
- Climatic changes and malaria

Lyme Disease

Test-Treatment Strategies for Patients Suspected of Having Lyme Disease: A Cost-Effectiveness Analysis
Nichol G, Dennis DT, Steere AC, et al (Univ of Ottawa, Ont, Canada; Ottawa Gen Hosp, Ont, Canada; Natl Ctr for Infectious Diseases, Fort Collins, Colo; et al)
Ann Intern Med 128:37–48, 1998
4–1

Objective.—Because of the difficulty in diagnosing Lyme disease, patients with positive serology tests but no clinical manifestations have been treated with expensive parenteral therapy that can sometimes cause adverse reactions. Guidelines for the management of Lyme disease are necessary to lower health costs and provide appropriate therapy for patients who have the disease. A cost-effectiveness analysis was performed to guide test-treatment strategies for patients who are suspected of having Lyme disease. The results were tested for sensitivity.

Methods.—Four test-treatment strategies were evaluated: no test-no treatment; enzyme-linked immunosorbent assay (ELISA) testing, with treatment for patients with positive results; ELISA testing followed by Western blot testing of ELISA-equivocal results, with treatment for patients with positive results; and antibiotic treatment for all patients sus-

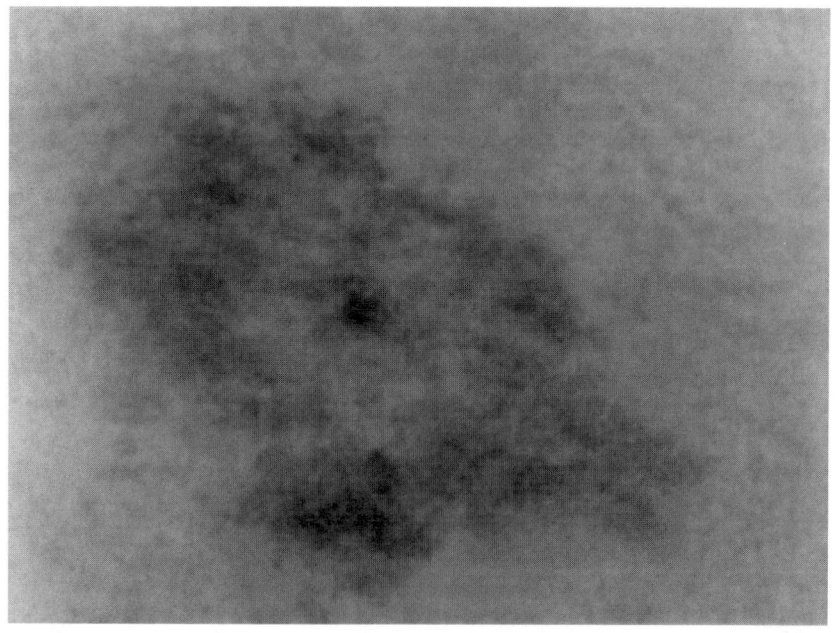

FIGURE 2.—Erythema migrans. (Courtesy of Nichol G, Dennis DT, Steere AC, et al: Test-treatment strategies for patients suspected of having Lyme disease: A cost-effectiveness analysis. *Ann Intern Med* 128:37–48, 1998.)

pected of having Lyme disease. Three common symptom scenarios were considered: A, myalgic symptoms; B, rash resembling erythema migrans (Fig 2); and C, recurrent oligoarticular inflammatory arthritis. The decision tree consisted of a model representing the natural history of patients with the disease. Costs per quality-adjusted life-year (QALY) were calculated and subjected to sensitivity analysis.

Results.—The no test-no treatment strategy for patients with myalgic symptoms with or without tick bite had the lowest cost-effectiveness ratio. Two-step testing added $7,000 per QALY. The 2-step test was the most cost-effective scenario for patients with myalgic symptoms, rash, and tick bite. Empirical therapy with antibiotics was the most cost-effective strategy for patients with a rash resembling erythema migrans. For patients with oligoarthritis with or without rash and tick bite, 2-step testing was the most cost-effective strategy, adding $10,000 per QALY. Use of ELISA testing and empirical antibiotic therapy, respectively, added $880,000 and $34,000 per QALY.

Conclusion.—No test-no treatment for Lyme disease is the most cost-effective strategy for patients with only myalgic symptoms. For patients with intermediate symptoms and clinical manifestations, 2-step testing is the most cost-effective method. For patients with a rash resembling erythema migrans, antibiotic therapy is recommended.

▶ Consideration or fear of Lyme disease seems to be consuming more time and money than the disease itself. Evidence-based clinical guidelines for different patient scenarios are much needed. This study presents a decision analysis model which gives excellent clarity for appropriate actions, given certain circumstances. Empirical antibiotic therapy for a rash similar to that shown in Figure 2 will be the easiest to follow. Two-step testing in the presence of arthralgias will be important to remember. Convincing physicians and patients not to test or treat in the presence of only myalgic symptoms will be the most difficult guideline to accept in clinical practice.

J.E. Scherger, M.D., M.P.H.

Tick Bites and Lyme Disease in an Endemic Setting: Problematic Use of Serologic Testing and Prophylactic Antibiotic Therapy
Fix AD, Strickland GT, Grant J, et al (Univ of Maryland, Baltimore; Kent County Health Dept, Chestertown, Md)
JAMA 279:206–210, 1998
4–2

Background.—There is little agreement as to the appropriate management of patients with suspected Lyme disease. Some physicians draw blood at the first visit for serologic testing, and some give prophylactic antibiotics even before a diagnosis is confirmed. This study examined whether these measures have an impact on the course of therapy and disease.

Methods.—The medical records of 232 patients with tick bites were divided into those having a tick bite alone (142 patients, or 61%), a tick bite plus suspected Lyme disease (50, or 22%), or a tick bite plus diagnosed Lyme disease (40, or 17%). The diagnostic tests used and the therapy prescribed were the main measures of interest in the chart review.

Findings.—Of the 142 patients with tick bite alone, two thirds (95 patients) underwent serologic testing, and only 3 patients had positive or equivocal results. Of the remaining 92 patients, 24 underwent repeat serologic testing an average of 42 days later; of these, 1 patient had seroconversion. None of the 142 patients underwent Western blot testing. More than half of this group (78 patients) received prophylactic antibiotics.

Of the 40 patients diagnosed with Lyme disease, 90% underwent serologic testing; of these 36 patients, 31 (86%) had a positive result. Only 5 patients in this group underwent Western blot testing, and 95% received prophylactic antibiotics. Of the 50 patients with suspected Lyme disease, 92% underwent serologic testing; of these 46 patients, only 4 (8.7%) had a positive result. Only 1 patient in this group underwent Western blot testing, and 38% received prophylactic antibiotics.

Conclusions.—Serologic testing was done in three fourths of the patients; yet the recommended confirmation by Western blot was performed only 6 times. Furthermore, more than half the patients received antibiotic therapy, typically even before results of any serologic tests were known. Thus, the use of serologic testing had little effect on the decision to institute antibiotic therapy.

▶ Folks are headed back into the woods here in the Northeast and tick season is right around the corner. I am sure we will soon be dealing with patients who have been bitten by ticks and who are worried about contracting Lyme disease, and this is a nonendemic area. This surveillance study is a terrific exercise in pointing out the discrepancies between well-considered guidelines in both diagnosis and treatment and well-intentioned practitioners. Lyme serologic studies are expensive ($40 for the routine study and $90 for the IgM study in our institution) and do not offer much help in the decision to treat. Treatment should be geared toward educating our patients and ourselves, not toward antibiotics.

W.W. Dexter, M.D.

A Vaccine Consisting of Recombinant *Borrelia burgdorferi* Outer-Surface Protein A to Prevent Lyme Disease
Sigal LH, and the Recombinant Outer-Surface Protein A Lyme Disease Vaccine Study Consortium (Univ of Medicine and Dentistry of New Jersey, New Brunswick; Pasteur Mérieux Connaught, Switftwater, Pa; Boston Biostatistics; et al)
N Engl J Med 339:216–222, 1998   4–3

Introduction.—Early clinical trials have shown that recombinant outer-surface protein A (OspA) is immunogenic and well tolerated, even in individuals with a history of Lyme disease. The protective efficacy of a 30-µg dose of vaccine without adjuvant in adults at risk for *Borrelia burgdorferi* infection was prospectively assessed in a multicenter, randomized, double-blind, placebo-controlled trial in areas of the United States in which Lyme disease is endemic.

Methods.—A total of 10,305 individuals 18 years of age and older were recruited at 14 sites in Connecticut, Massachusetts, New York, and Wisconsin. Participants were randomly assigned to receive either 30 µg of OspA vaccine (5,156 individuals) or placebo (5,149 individuals). The second injection was administered 1 month after the first injection. A booster was administered at 12 months. Participants were observed for 2 seasons in which the risk of Lyme disease transmission was high. Patient groups were followed up for the number of new clinically and serologically confirmed cases of Lyme disease.

Results.—Overall vaccine efficacy for the first year was 68%. Among the 3,745 recipients of the third injection, efficacy was 92%. The vaccine was well tolerated with mild, self-limited local and systemic reactions that lasted no longer than 7 days after injection. Recipients had no significant rise in the frequency of arthritis or neurologic events.

Conclusions.—The OspA vaccine was safe and effective in preventing Lyme disease in a large series of patients from areas endemic for the disease.

Vaccination Against Lyme Disease With Recombinant *Borrelia burgdorferi* Outer-Surface Lipoprotein A With Adjuvant

Steere AC, and the Lyme Disease Vaccine Study Group (Tufts Univ, Boston; SmithKline Beecham Pharmaceuticals, Collegeville, Pa; Yale Univ, New Haven, Conn; et al)
N Engl J Med 339:209–215, 1998   4–4

Introduction.—Lyme disease is currently the most common vector-borne disease in the United States. The risk of acquiring this disease in areas in which the disease is endemic is high, making the development of a safe and effective vaccine a priority. The efficacy, safety, and immunogenicity of the vaccine was examined in a multicenter, double-blind, randomized trial.

Methods.—A total of 10,936 individuals from 31 sites in 10 states in which Lyme disease is endemic were randomly assigned to receive either an injection of recombinant *Borrelia burgdorferi* outer-surface lipoprotein A (OspA) with adjuvant or placebo at baseline and 1 and 12 months later. In individuals with suspected Lyme disease, culture of skin lesions, polymerase chain reaction testing, or serologic testing was performed. Individuals underwent serologic testing at 12 and 20 months after baseline to detect asymptomatic infections.

Results.—In the first year after 2 injections, 1,109 of 10,936 (10%) individuals were examined for suspected Lyme disease. Of these, 22 individuals in the vaccine group and 43 in the placebo group had definite Lyme disease. In the second year, after the third injection, 16 recipients of the vaccine contracted definite Lyme disease, compared with 66 placebo recipients. Vaccine efficacy for the first and second years was 49% and 76%, respectively. The efficacy of the vaccine in preventing asymptomatic infection was 83% and 100% in the first and second years, respectively. Vaccine injection was associated with mild-to-moderate local or systemic reactions of a median duration of 3 days.

Conclusions.—A high level of protection from *B. burgdorferi* infection was able to be achieved with a series of 3 injections of OspA with adjuvant. The rate of local and systemic side effects was acceptable. This vaccine provides an important new public health tool for preventing Lyme disease.

▶ These 2 articles from *The New England Journal of Medicine* describe investigations of a vaccine for Lyme disease. In both studies, the vaccines appear effective, and I suspect we will see a Lyme vaccine on the market in the near future. In the meantime, we must still identify patients with this entity and treat appropriately. (See Abstract 4–2 for a discussion of diagnosis and treatment options.) There is no word yet regarding when to administer the vaccine and to whom. While the incidence of this disease is indeed climbing, Lyme disease—perhaps the most common vector-borne disease in the United States—is still not frequently seen even in endemic areas. Stay tuned—still unanswered are questions regarding whether the vaccine does not prevent illness but simply alters the natural history of disease, and on the duration of immunity.

W.W. Dexter, M.D.

Sexually Transmitted Disease

Randomized Trial of Trovafloxacin and Ofloxacin for Single-Dose Therapy of Gonorrhea
Jones RB, and the Trovafloxacin Gonorrhea Study Group (Indiana Univ, Indianapolis; Univ of Alabama, Birmingham; Memphis Women's Ctr, Tenn; et al)
Am J Med 104:28–32, 1998
4–5

Background.—A single dose of a broad-spectrum cephalosporin or a quinolone antibiotic has been recommended for the treatment of uncomplicated gonococcal infections. Presumptive treatment with a regimen effective against *Chlamydia trachomatis* is also recommended for patients with gonorrhea. In the current study, the efficacies of single-dose trovafloxacin, 100 mg, and ofloxacin, 400 mg, were compared in patients with uncomplicated gonorrhea.

Methods.—Six hundred twenty-five women and men with uncomplicated gonococcal urethritis or cervicitis were enrolled in a multicenter, double-blind study. The patients were randomly assigned to trovafloxacin or ofloxacin to be taken under direct supervision.

TABLE 2.—Eradication Rate by Source in Evaluable Patients

Gender	Source	Trovafloxacin 100 mg	Ofloxacin 400 mg
Males (%)	Urethra	103/104 (99)	111/111
	Pharynx	5/5	4/4
Females (%)	Cervix	93/94 (99)	112/116 (96)
	Urethra	2/2	0/0
	Rectum	27/27	18/18
	Pharynx	9/9	8/8

(Reprinted by permission of the publisher from Jones RB, and the Trovafloxacin Gonorrhea Study Group: Randomized trial of trovafloxacin and ofloxacin for single-dose therapy of gonorrhea. *Am J Med* 104:28–32. Copyright 1998 by Excerpta Medica, Inc.)

Findings.—Trovafloxacin treatment was bacteriologically and clinically comparable to ofloxacin. *Neisseria gonorrhoeae* was eradicated in 99% of assessable trovafloxacin recipients and in 98% of assessable ofloxacin recipients. Both treatments were well tolerated. The most common adverse effect was vaginitis, occurring in 4% and 7% of the trovafloxacin and ofloxacin groups, respectively (Table 2).

Conclusions.—In this large, randomized trial, single-dose oral therapy with trovafloxacin, 100 mg, was as bacteriologically and clinically effective as single-dose ofloxacin, 400 mg, in both women and men with uncomplicated gonorrhea. These drugs were effective against urogenital infections as well as infections at sites more difficult to treat.

▶ I always ask the question, "Was this drug study supported by the company that manufactures the drug?" If so, my skepticism antennae are immediately raised, and I look more carefully at the methodology and ask, "Was it sound?" In this study, the answer to both questions is yes. I will certainly consider adding trovafloxacin (100 mg orally) to my treatment options for uncomplicated gonorrhea.

W.W. Dexter, M.D.

Herpes Simplex Virus Type 2 in the United States, 1976 to 1994

Fleming DT, McQuillan GM, Johnson RE, et al (Ctrs for Disease Control and Prevention, Atlanta, Ga; Emory Univ, Atlanta, Ga)
N Engl J Med 337:1105–1111, 1997   4–6

Introduction.—Herpes simplex virus type 2 (HSV-2) infections typically affect the genital area and are usually sexually transmitted. In newborn infants, the infection may cause severe systemic disease and death. It is difficult to assess the extent of HSV-2 infection in the United States because most of those affected are unaware of the disease and few states require cases to be reported. Serologic methods were used to study the epidemiology of HSV-2 and to examine changes in HSV-2 seroprevalence during a 13-year period.

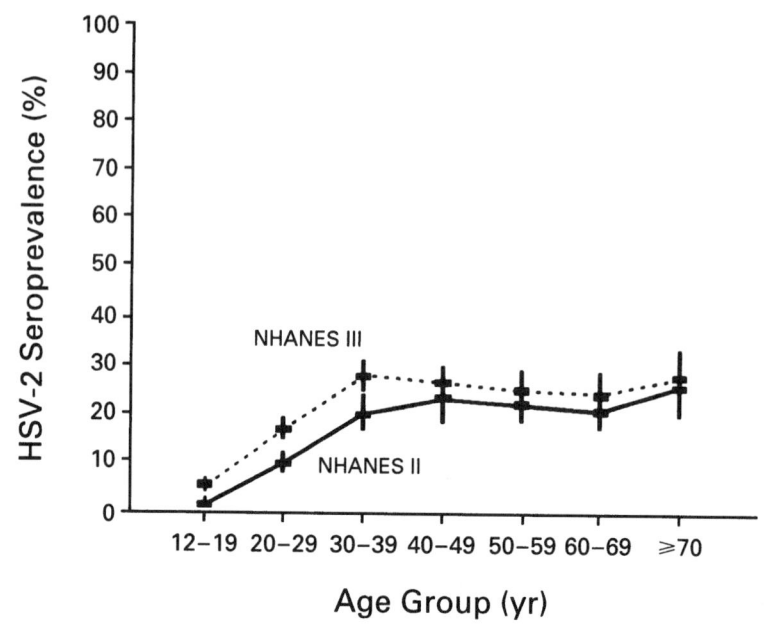

FIGURE 2.—Herpes simplex virus type 2 (*HSV-2*) seroprevalence according to age in National Health and Nutrition Examination Survey (*NHANES*) II (1976–1980) and NHANES III (1988–1994). Bars indicate 95% confidence intervals. (Courtesy of Fleming DT, McQuillan GM, Johnson RE, et al: Herpes simplex virus type 2 in the United States, 1976 to 1994. *N Engl J Med* 337:1105–1111. Copyright 1997, Massachusetts Medical Society. Reproduced by permission of *The New England Journal of Medicine*. All rights reserved.)

Methods.—A nationally representative serologic survey of HSV-2 was done as part of the third National Health and Nutrition Examination Survey (NHANES III), conducted from 1988 to 1994. This survey included information on behavioral risk factors for HSV-2 infection and the effects of an increased public awareness of genital herpes and other sexually transmitted diseases. Findings of NHANES III were compared with those of NHANES II, conducted between 1976 and 1980. An immunodot assay specific for glycoprotein gG-2 of HSV-2 was used to assess HSV-2 antibody.

Results.—Among study participants aged 12 years or older, the seroprevalence of HSV-2 was 21.9%, corresponding to 45 million infected individuals in the noninstitutionalized civilian U.S. population. The female-to-male prevalence ratio was 1.4, and the black-to-white prevalence ratio was 2.6. Fewer than 10% of seropositive individuals reported a history of genital herpes infection. Independent predictors of seropositivity in multivariate analysis were female sex, black race, Mexican-American ethnic background, older age, less education, poverty, cocaine use, and a greater lifetime number of sexual partners. The age-adjusted seroprevalence of HSV-2 rose 30% during the period from 1988 to 1994, compared with the period from 1976 to 1980. Among white teenagers, the seroprevalence quintupled; whites in their 20s had double the seroprevalence compared with the earlier period (Fig 2).

Conclusions.—The seroprevalence of HSV-2 in the U.S. population has increased by 30% since the late 1970s, and the greatest relative increases were among young whites. Findings emphasize the ongoing need to prevent HSV-2 and other sexually transmitted infections, especially because transmission of HIV may be facilitated by the presence of genital ulcers.

▶ Are you as taken aback at the data presented here as I? Seroprevalence of HSV-2 of up to 46% in some populations and 20% on average in this country! Several thoughts occur to me. I am certainly glad that acyclovir (a reasonably effective treatment for early disease and prophylaxis) is now off patent and more affordable. Reading this firms up my resolve to make my patients aware of these data, particularly as I counsel them to consider abstinence and monogamy, as well as condom use.[1] These data should help to focus our discussions about local, regional, and national policy, and of course, to increase our individual efforts in the office as well.

W.W. Dexter, M.D.

Reference

1. Schuster MA, Bell RM, Berry SH, et al: Students' acquisition and use of school condoms in a high school condom availability program. *Pediatrics* 100:689–694, 1997.

Treatment of Genital Warts With an Immune-response Modifier (Imiquimod)

Beutner KR, Spruance SL, Hougham AJ, et al (Univ of California, San Francisco; Sutter-Solano Med Ctr, Vallejo, Calif; Univ of Utah, Salt Lake City; et al)
J Am Acad Dermatol 38:230–239, 1998
4–7

Objective.—Imiquimod is a new nonnucleoside heterocyclic amine for treating genital warts. Belonging to a new class of immune-response modifiers, imiquimod induces interferon-α. In mice, imiquimod induces tumor necrosis factor-α and interleukins 1, 6, and 8. In animals it has shown antiviral, antitumor, and adjuvant activity. The safety and efficacy of topical imiquimod for the treatment of genital warts were evaluated in a double-blind, randomized, placebo-controlled, parallel design study.

Methods.—Either 5% imiquimod (n = 51) or placebo (n = 57) cream was applied topically 3 times per week for up to 8 weeks by 108 patients, predominantly white men, with external genital warts. Patients were followed up for 10 weeks after cessation of treatment.

Results.—Seven imiquimod and 12 placebo patients did not complete the study. Eighteen (40%) of 45 imiquimod patients or 19 of 51 in the intent-to-treat group had complete clearance. No placebo patients in the intent-to-treat group had complete clearance. Median time to clearance was 7 weeks (Fig 2). In the imiquimod group, 62% had an 80% or greater

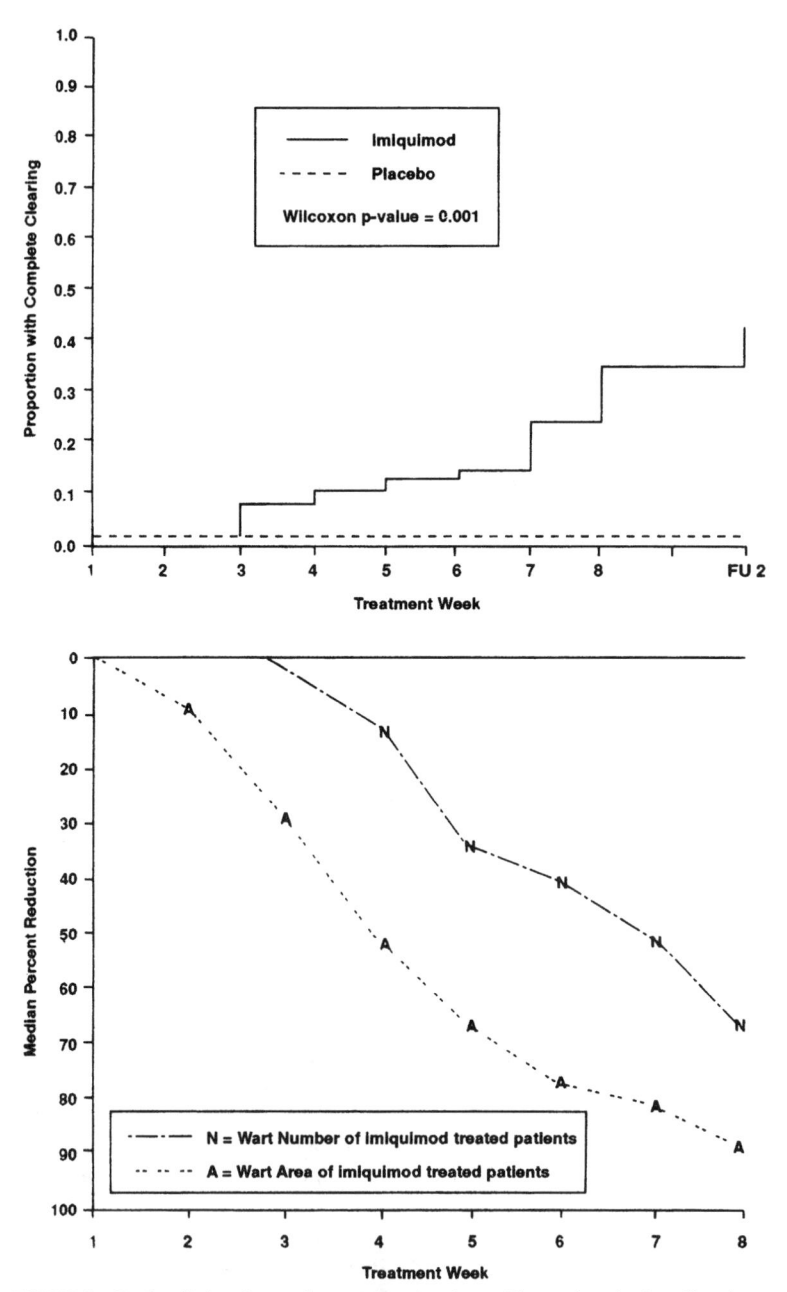

FIGURE 2.—Product limit estimate of proportion of patients with complete clearing of baseline warts during treatment period (**upper panel**). Median percent reduction in baseline wart area and wart count for imiquimod-treated patients (**lower panel**). (Courtesy of Beutner KR, Spruance SL, Hougham AJ, et al: Treatment of genital warts with an immune-response modifier (imiquimod). *J Am Acad Dermatol* 38:230–239, 1998.)

reduction and 76% had a 50% or greater reduction in wart area compared with 4% and 8%, respectively, in the placebo group. These differences were significant. Three of 16 imiquimod patients with complete clearance had a recurrence at week 2 (n = 2) and at week 6 of the follow-up period. Significantly more imiquimod than placebo patients had inflammation of the wart site. Compared with placebo patients, significantly more imiquimod patients reported side effects, including itching (54.2%), erythema (33.3%), burning (31.3%), irritation (16.7%), tenderness (12.5%), ulceration (10.4%), erosion (10.4%), and pain (8.3%). Wart area reduction and intensity of wart-site inflammation were significantly correlated.

Conclusions.—Patients taking imiquimod had a 40% complete response rate, which is comparable to other therapies for genital warts. An additional 35.6% of imiquimod patients had a greater than 50% reduction in wart area. Compared with placebo patients, imiquimod patients had significantly more side effects, including inflammation of the wart site, than did placebo patients.

▶ This novel approach to treating genital warts is a real breakthrough and is analogous to new emerging cancer therapies. Direct destruction of warts and tumors does little to the host response to the disease, and hence is often partial therapy. Treatment that mobilizes a host response against the disease is not only more effective but also may enhance the health of the patient.

J.E. Scherger, M.D., M.P.H.

Treatment of Condylomata Acuminata With Oral Isotretinoin
Tsambaos D, Georgiou S, Monastirli A, et al (Univ of Patras, Greece; Heinrich-Heine Univ, Düsseldorf, Germany)
J Urol 158:1810–1812, 1997   4–8

Background.—Many different techniques have been used for the treatment of condyloma acuminatum, but none has been completely effective. Topical treatments, because they do not completely eradicate the human papillomavirus, are associated with high relapse rates. The synthetic retinoid isotretinoin is a potent immunomodulator with dramatic effects on epithelial cell differentiation and proliferation. The efficacy and safety of oral isotretinoin for the treatment of condyloma acuminatum were evaluated.

Methods.—A total of 56 men with clinically visible condyloma acuminatum on the external genitalia and/or perianal area were studied. In each patient, at least 1 form of standard therapy had been tried unsuccessfully. All patients received 3 months of treatment with oral isotretinoin, 1 mg/kg/day. The treatment was evaluated for safety and efficacy.

Results.—There were 53 evaluable patients at the end of treatment. Oral isotretinoin was associated with a complete response rate of 40% and a partial response rate of 13%. Thus, 47% of patients had no response.

Lesion age and area were inversely related to the response to oral isotretinoin. Among complete responders, the rate of recurrence during 1 year of follow-up was 9.5%.

Conclusions.—Oral isotretinoin has significant effectiveness for the treatment of condyloma acuminatum, with a low recurrence rate and acceptable toxicity. It offers a noninvasive treatment alternative for immature and small condyloma acuminatum.

▶ Caveat emptor, here. (Buyer beware.) This study had no control group, was not blinded, and most importantly, particularly for this disease, was not placebo controlled. Why include it? There is a theoretical basis for the treatment, and if you get to the lesions soon enough it seems effective. Isotretinoin use is fraught with side effects, and one needs to be careful in patient selection. Nevertheless, in our patients who are seen early in the course of the disease (within a few months of appearance of lesions) and who either do not relish the use of or respond to topical therapy, oral isotretinoin might be worth a try.

W.W. Dexter, M.D.

HIV Infection and AIDS

Declining Morbidity and Mortality Among Patients With Advanced Human Immunodeficiency Virus Infection
Palella FJ Jr, and the HIV Outpatient Study Investigators (Northwestern Univ, Chicago; Health Research Network of Apache Med Systems, Chicago; Ctrs for Disease Control and Prevention, Atlanta, Ga; et al)
N Engl J Med 338:853–860, 1998   4–9

Introduction.—Specific therapeutic regimens have not been linked to reductions in mortality and in the rate of hospitalization of HIV-infected patients. Data collected over 42 months were analyzed to determine the rate of chemoprophylaxis against opportunist infection, even while patterns of antiretroviral therapy were changing. Changes in death rate and incidence of opportunistic infections in a large group of HIV-infected outpatients were reported.

Methods.—Data on 1,255 patients, each of whom had at least 1 CD4+ count below 100 cells per cubic millimeter during a 3-year period, were analyzed. Morbidity and mortality were compared for the antiretroviral-therapy categories, adjusted for chemoprophylaxis against opportunistic infection and demographic factors, CD4+ count at the first study visit, and method of payment.

Results.—There was a decline in mortality among the patients, from 29.4 per 100 person-years in 1995 to 8.8 per 100 person-years in the second quarter of 1997. Regardless of sex, race, age, and risk factors for transmission of HIV, there were reductions in mortality. There was also a decrease in the incidence of any of the 3 major opportunistic infections, from 21.9 per 100 person-years in 1994 to 3.7 per 100 person-years by mid-1997. The infections referred to were *Mycobacterium avium* complex

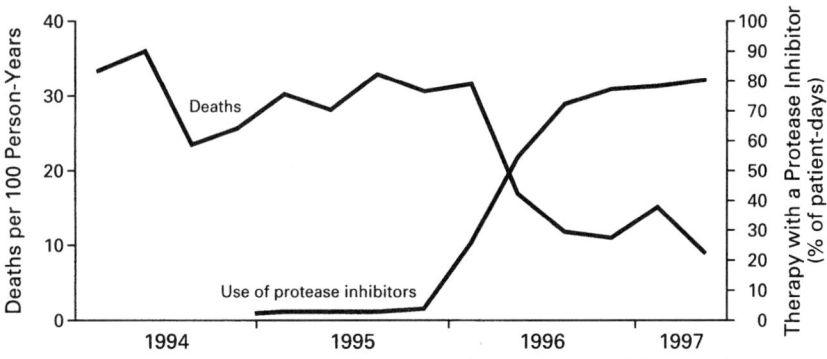

FIGURE 1.—Mortality and frequency of use of combination antiretroviral therapy including a protease inhibitor among HIV-infected patients with fewer than 100 CD4+ cells per cubic millimeter, according to calendar quarter, from January 1994 through June 1997. (Reprinted by permission of Palella FJ Jr, and the HIV Outpatient Study Investigators: Declining morbidity and mortality among patients with advanced human immunodeficiency virus infection *N Engl J Med* 338:853–860. Copyright 1998, Massachusetts Medical Society. All rights reserved.)

disease, *Pneumocystis carinii* pneumonia, and cytomegalovirus retinitis. Stepwise reductions in morbidity and mortality were associated with increases in the intensity of antiretroviral therapy in a failure-rate model. The anti-retroviral therapy was classified as none, monotherapy, combination therapy without a protease inhibitor, or combination therapy with a protease inhibitor. The most benefit was associated with combination antiretroviral therapy. Additional benefit was conferred with the inclusion of protease inhibitors in such regimens (Fig 1). Protease inhibitors were more often prescribed for patients with private insurance, who also had lower mortality rates than those insured by Medicare or Medicaid.

Conclusion.—The use of more intensive antiretroviral therapies is the cause of the recent declines in AIDS-related morbidity and mortality.

▶ This article describes an extremely careful study collecting information from several credible sources. The figure tells you everything you need to know, documenting the astonishing 70% reduction in mortality in the last 3 years. A subtext message here is that physicians caring for patients with AIDS must be absolutely committed to staying up-to-date with current medication protocols, so that their patients can receive the benefits of this revolution in therapy.

A.O. Berg, M.D., M.P.H.

The Effect of Exercise Training on Aerobic Fitness, Immune Indices, and Quality of Life in HIV+ Patients

Stringer WW, Berezovskaya M, O'Brien WA, et al (Harbor–Univ of California, Los Angeles Med Ctr, Torrance)
Med Sci Sports Exerc 30:11–16, 1998   4–10

Objective.—Whether regular aerobic exercise would benefit HIV+ patients is not known. An ethnically and sex-diverse population of HIV+

individuals with intermediate-stage disease was randomly assigned to exercise or not exercise and effects on aerobic fitness, immune indices, and quality of life were assessed.

Methods.—The CD4 count, Candida skin test results, HIV RNA virologic measurements, and cardiopulmonary fitness were determined in 34 HIV+ individuals who were randomly assigned to heavy or moderate exercise training for 1 hour 3 times a week for 6 weeks or to a no-regular-exercise control group. Participants completed a quality-of-life questionnaire and a physical activity recall questionnaire before and after the study.

Results.—Eight individuals dropped out of the study. Participants, average age 36 years, were 11% female, 29% Hispanic, and 20% black, and had had HIV+ for an average of 39 months. Lactic acidosis threshold increased significantly in both exercise groups but not in the control group. Peak oxygen uptake and work rate maximum increased significantly only in the heavy exercise group. There were minimal changes in CD4 counts in all groups at the end of the study. The *Candida albicans* antigen skin test reactivity increased significantly only, in the moderate exercise group. The number of plasma HIV RNA copies decreased insignificantly in all groups. Quality of life increased in both exercise groups but not in the control group.

Conclusion.—Moderate to heavy exercise training in HIV+ individuals improved exercise tolerance and aerobic function.

Clinical Significance.—Moderate to heavy aerobic exercise training should be promoted for HIV+ patients in the intermediate stages of their disease to improve aerobic function and exercise tolerance.

▶ Ah, the benefits of exercise! I am sure that most physicians caring for patients with HIV infection have patients who, after the diagnosis is made, use the opportunity to change their lives in the direction of making healthier personal health choices. This study quantifies the benefits from exercise. It was too much to hope that exercise would increase CD4+ counts, but at least patients felt better and had a more positive outlook on life. It is also important to note that there were no *adverse* effects documented, a potential concern with high-intensity conditioning programs.

A.O. Berg, M.D., M.P.H.

Effect of HIV Counseling and Testing on Sexually Transmitted Diseases and Condom Use in an Urban Adolescent Population

Clark LR, Brasseux C, Richmond D, et al (George Washington Univ, Washington, DC; Children's Natl Med Ctr, Washington, DC)
Arch Pediatr Adolesc Med 152:269–273, 1998

Objective.—Whether counseling and testing for HIV infection reduces the incidence of sexually transmitted diseases (STDs) and whether self-reported condom use is correlated with the acquisition of STDs over time was evaluated in a group of teens in an urban adolescent medicine clinic.

Methods.—Of the 8,000 teens who visit the clinic annually, 500 were thought to be at high risk for HIV. The 149 randomly selected teens (97% black, 21% male), whose average age was 16 years, were assigned to 1 of 3 groups based on condom use (frequently [F], sometimes [S], and rarely [R]) and variability of use over time. Teens were given a questionnaire, and their medical records were reviewed. The number of STDs acquired before and after HIV counseling and testing was compared.

Results.—Reported condom use at enrollment was 24% for the F group, 40% for the S group, and 36% for the R group. Males were less likely than females to use condoms. Teens became sexually active at 13–14 years of age. The average number of partners was 2.24 in the F group, 2.91 in the S group, and 3.83 in the R group. Before testing there was no correlation between reported condom use and number of monthly visits to the clinic or rate of STDs. There were 126 teens who returned within 1 year of enrollment. In the posttest period, there was no significant decrease in STD diagnosis.

Conclusions.—As with adults, a single counseling and testing session did not change risk behaviors or incidence of STDs in sexually active high-risk teens. Incidence of condom use was unrelated to incidence of STDs.

▶ I include this article merely to remind us (once again) that we cannot assume that our well-intentioned and well-constructed counseling interventions will have the intended effect of changing behavior. I view the effectiveness of office-based counseling—whether for condom use, exercise, diet, or smoking cessation—as one of the great frontiers of clinical research. Family physicians spend an enormous amount of time in "counseling" mode; we deserve better-quality research showing us how to make it effective. In today's managed care environment, there is increasing pressure to make every minute count. If we can't find ways to make counseling effective and prove it, we might find no one willing to pay for the time we spend on it.

A.O. Berg, M.D., M.P.H.

Cost-Effectiveness of Mandatory Compared With Voluntary Screening for Human Immunodeficiency Virus in Pregnancy

Myers ER, Thompson JW, Simpson K (Beth Israel Deaconess Med Ctr, Boston; US Public Health Service, Washington, DC; Univ of North Carolina, Chapel Hill)
Obstet Gynecol 91:174–181, 1998   4–12

Objective.—Most pediatric AIDS cases result from maternal transmission. Whether mandatory HIV screening for pregnant women is cost-effective is debatable. A decision-analysis model was used to compare the potential economic impact of voluntary and mandatory testing for HIV during pregnancy based on varying assumptions about behavior.

Methods.—Direct and indirect medical costs associated with prevention and treatment of pediatric HIV infections were accumulated. The 2 strategies evaluated were testing of pregnant women who volunteer after counseling and mandatory screening of all pregnant women after counseling. Posttest counseling was provided to all women. Zidovudine treatment was offered to all women who tested positive. Sensitivity analysis was used to test the potential effects of changes in patient behavior before and after mandatory testing.

Results.—The average cost per case prevented was lower for mandatory screening than for voluntary screening at low ($837,905 vs. $1,221,561), medium ($255,158 vs. $367,998), and high ($53,625 vs. $72,808) prevalences. The incremental cost per case prevented under mandatory testing was $70,594 at a low prevalence, $29,478 at medium prevalence, and $15,259 at high prevalence. Assuming a medium prevalence and an estimated cost for pediatric HIV of more than $129,250, mandatory testing was less expensive and more effective than voluntary testing. Assuming a 40% refusal rate for voluntary testing increases the incremental cost-effectiveness of the mandatory testing program to $112,434. The impact of refusal increased as the prevalence of HIV increased.

Conclusions.—Assuming no refusals, mandatory screening will prevent more pediatric AIDS cases but at a higher cost per case. Lack of acceptance of zidovudine treatment by HIV-positive women who refused to be voluntarily tested made the mandatory program increasingly more cost-effective as the prevalence of HIV increased.

▶ I chose this article to illustrate some issues about efficacy, effectiveness, costs, and cost-effectiveness—issues that are becoming more rather than less confusing as the literature proliferates and the terms are used imprecisely. We begin with efficacy, the scientific assessment of whether something "works"—in this case whether treating the HIV-positive pregnant woman with antiretrovirals prevents vertical transmission. The answer is "yes," so we move on to determine effectiveness: can a group of pregnant women be tested and treated in typical clinical settings? A "yes" answer then moves us to questions of cost, and finally, cost-effectiveness. In this context cost-effectiveness is judged from the societal perspective and compares the costs of competing strategies.

In this article, mandatory screening "wins" over voluntary screening, but the analysis cannot tell us whether *either* strategy is "worth" doing. Cost-effectiveness also has little to do with actual costs: something that is very inexpensive can be cost ineffective, and something that is very expensive can be cost-effective. In this study we have a costly intervention—mandatory screening—that is cost-effective compared with voluntary screening, which is also expensive.

This topic is also a good example of where a strategy to screen everyone, irrational as it may seem in some settings, makes sense when viewed from the point of view of society as a whole. A universal screening approach is more efficient than one individualized to a patient's risk (similar arguments are made for universal sickle cell screening).

A.O. Berg, M.D., M.P.H.

A Decision Analysis of Mandatory Compared With Voluntary HIV Testing in Pregnant Women

Nakchbandi IA, Longenecker JC, Risksecker MA, et al (Abington Mem Hosp, Pa; Allegheny Univ, Philadelphia; Columbia Univ, New York)
Ann Intern Med 128:760–767, 1998   4–13

Introduction.—The use of zidovudine to treat HIV-infected women during pregnancy could significantly reduce the number of infants born with HIV infection. This finding has led to a public policy debate on the value of mandatory vs. voluntary HIV screening in pregnant women. A decision analysis model was used to quantitatively evaluate the relative benefits and risks of the 2 strategies.

Methods.—Under a mandatory policy, all women who receive prenatal care would be tested for HIV infection. Under the current voluntary system, women who receive prenatal care are given the opportunity to be tested. Variables included in the decision analysis were the acceptance and benefit of prenatal care, the acceptance and benefit of zidovudine therapy in HIV-infected women, the prevalence of HIV infection, and mandatory compared with voluntary HIV testing. The model was used to calculate the absolute number of infants who would be spared HIV infection under a mandatory vs. voluntary testing policy. The difference in perinatal mortality was compared for the 2 policies.

Results.—With a baseline threshold deterrence rate of 0.4%, a voluntary testing policy is preferred in the model if more than 4 per 1,000 women were deferred from seeking prenatal care because of a mandatory HIV testing policy. With a deterrence rate of 0.5%, 167 infants would be spared HIV infection annually but 189 would die because of a lack of prenatal care. If no woman would be deterred from seeking medical care by a mandatory screening policy, the maximum number of infants spared HIV infection would be 34 if acceptance of voluntary testing were 97% and 173 if acceptance of voluntary testing were 85%.

Conclusion.—Over a broad range of variables used in the analysis, voluntary testing for HIV infections is preferable to mandatory testing of women seeking prenatal care. The most effective strategy for reducing maternal-fetal transmission of HIV is educational and outreach efforts to increase acceptance of voluntary testing during pregnancy.

▶ This is an important article that might seem of interest only to health policy makers, but it has direct relevance to family physicians offering prenatal care. This study shows that there are two characteristics of your patient population that will determine which strategy works best: the percentage of pregnant women who agree to voluntary testing and the percentage of women who might be deterred from prenatal care if a mandatory testing policy were in place. In most family practices, the latter characteristic is unknowable, so the issue of compliance with a voluntary testing program is the key. A very high level of voluntary compliance (greater than 97%) renders the issue of deterrence from prenatal care inconsequential. For me, the conclusion for most family practices is clear: aim to increase compliance with voluntary testing, a goal that we know from other studies is achievable.

A.O. Berg, M.D., M.P.H.

Improved Survival Among HIV-Infected Individuals Following Initiation of Antiretroviral Therapy
Hogg RS, Heath KV, Yip B, et al (St Paul's Hosp, Vancouver, BC, Canada; Univ of British Columbia, Canada)
JAMA 279:450–454, 1998   4–14

Background.—Clinical trials have demonstrated the efficacy of antiretroviral treatment with double- and triple-drug regimens for patients with HIV infection. However, the efficacy of these regimens in patients not enrolled in clinical trials is unknown. In the current prospective, population-based cohort study, survival was analyzed after the initiation of antiretroviral therapy among HIV-infected residents of British Columbia.

Methods.—All 1,178 HIV-positive adults who were first prescribed antiretroviral treatment between October 1992 and June 1996 and who had $CD4^+$ cell counts of less than 0.350×10^9/L were included. Median follow-up was 21 months. Treatment denoted as ERA 1 consisted of zidovudine-, didanosine-, or zalcitabine-based treatment. Treatment denoted as ERA 2 consisted of regimens including lamivudine or stavudine.

Findings.—During follow-up, 390 patients died, for a crude mortality of 33.1%. Patients treated in ERA 1 were nearly twice as likely to die as those treated in ERA 2. The former group had a mortality risk ratio of 1.86. Patients treated in ERA 1 were 1.93 times more likely to die than those treated in ERA 2 after adjustment for *Pneumocystis carinii* and *Mycobacterium avium* prophylaxis use, AIDS diagnosis, $CD4^+$ cell count, sex, and age. Among patients without a diagnosis of AIDS at the start of treatment, those treated in ERA 1 were 2.5 times more likely to progress to AIDS or death than those treated in ERA 2.

Conclusions.—Persons with HIV infection initially treated with regimens including stavudine or lamivudine had significantly lower mortality and longer AIDS-free survival than persons initially given regimens limited to zidovudine, didanosine, and zalcitabine. These findings remained significant even after adjustment for confounding variables.

▶ The field of HIV/AIDS infection changes so rapidly that I hesitate to include articles like this even in a rapid-publication resource like the YEAR BOOK OF FAMILY PRACTICE. However, this is one of those studies that serves as a useful milepost measuring how far we have come in treating HIV infection. It is not a randomized controlled trial, but rather a use-effectiveness study documenting what is actually achievable for an entire population of HIV-infected individuals. The survivals documented here using the newer antiretrovirals (and other interventions) are truly amazing. More needs to be done, but we need to pause occasionally to recognize how much is already being accomplished.

A.O. Berg, M.D., M.P.H.

Prognostic Indicators for AIDS and Infectious Disease Death in HIV-Infected Injection Drug Users: Plasma Viral Load and CD4+ Cell Count
Vlahov D, Graham N, Hoover D, et al (Johns Hopkins School of Hygiene and Public Health, Baltimore, Md; Ctrs for Disease Control and Prevention, Atlanta, Ga)
JAMA 279:35–40, 1998   4–15

Introduction.—Viral load is known to be a prognostic factor in patients with HIV-1 disease, and higher titers of the virus in peripheral blood mononuclear cells and plasma are associated with lower CD4+ cell counts. A cohort study was conducted to determine whether reports of the prognostic value of viral load and CD4+ cell counts, most of which were based upon findings in white homosexual men and patients with hemophilia, could be extended to HIV-infected injection drug users (IDUs).

Methods.—Study participants were recruited from the community in Baltimore, Md. Those eligible were at least 18 years of age, had used injection drugs within the previous 11 years, and had no AIDS-defining illness. Of 2,960 IDUs recruited, 664 were HIV-1-sero-positive and agreed to return for follow-up, consisting of interviews, physical examinations, and venipuncture, at 6-month intervals.

Results.—Of the 664 enrolled IDUs, 142 were excluded from analysis because of inadequate data. Most of the participants were male (80%), African American (96%), and current active drug injectors. The median age of the group was 33 years. During a median follow-up of 6.4 years, 146 cases of AIDS were diagnosed; 119 of the 182 deaths were from infectious disease. Plasma HIV-1 RNA and CD4+ cell counts measured at baseline were compared with time to first clinical AIDS diagnosis and infectious disease death. Both time-fixed baseline levels of viral load and CD4+ cell count were independent predictors of these 2 outcomes, but viral load had a better predictive value in proportional hazards models. A 5-stage classification was based upon levels of viral load and CD4+ cell count. The 5-year cumulative probabilities for AIDS and infectious disease ranged from 0% and 0%, respectively, in the first stage (less than 500 copies/mL; CD4+ cell count, 0.50×10^9/L) to 81.2% and 76.1%, respectively for the fifth stage (10,000 or more copies/mL; CD4+ cell count, 0.20×10^9/L). The 5-group staging model provided strong discrimination for both AIDS and infectious disease death in this population of minority IDUs. After controlling for the 5-stage CD4+ cell count and viral load variable, race, current drug use, and number of clinical symptoms were not statistically significantly associated with AIDS or infectious disease death.

Conclusion.—The prognostic value of viral load and CD4+ cell counts is as strong in African-American IUDs as in white homosexual men and patients with hemophilia. Combining both markers provides a simple method of prognostically staging the disease and deciding when to start therapy.

▶ This study makes a convincing case that the combination of plasma viral load and CD4+ counts makes an effective prognostic indicator. On the face of it, it also makes sense that better quality information about prognosis *should* be useful for physicians and patients in making therapeutic decisions. It is important to point out, though, that this study did not address whether patients studied in this way do any better *clinically* than patients followed up in some other way (e.g., 1 of the 2 tests only, or neither). Clinicians following the status of patients with HIV infection are usually awash in information; but we still have a lot of work to do in determining which information really makes a difference in our patients' lives.

A.O. Berg, M.D., M.P.H.

Urinary Tract Infection

Screening Dipstick Urinalysis: A Time to Change
Kaplan RE, Springate JE, Feld LG (State Univ of New York, Buffalo; Children's Hosp, Buffalo, NY)
Pediatrics 100:919–921, 1997   4–16

Introduction.—It has long been considered essential to have screening interval urinalyses in a pediatric population. The American Academy of Pediatrics recommends that a urinalysis be conducted 4 times: in infancy, early childhood, late childhood, and adolescence. Based on data from multiple studies, the usefulness of screening urinalyses in asymptomatic pediatric patients has come into question. Cost-benefit analysis is extremely important in the present health care environment.

Methods.—A calculation was made to determine the minimal cost, using a private practitioner in an urban or suburban group pediatric practice. By using current charges for supplies, tests, and an initial evaluation by a pediatric nephrologist, costs were determined. Information from published studies was also examined.

Results.—An initial abnormal urinalysis was found in 9% of patients (179 of 2,000). A persistent abnormality was found in 1.5% of the patients who were retested. In the hypothetical cohort of 2,000 asymptomatic pediatric patients, the calculated rate of a false-positive/transient abnormality was 84%. There was a cost range of $5,022 to $6,475 for the outpatient evaluation of 2,000 asymptomatic pediatric patients by dipstick urinalyses. To screen all 2,000 patients initially with a dipstick urinalysis, the cost was $1,290 or 65 cents per patient. To evaluate the 20 patients with persistent abnormality on repeat dipstick urinalysis, the cost was

$3,732 to $5,185, or $129 to $179 per patient. For 4 multiple screening urinalyses, currently recommended, the cost is $20,088 to $25,900. These costs do not include any renal imaging or function studies.

Conclusions.—In asymptomatic pediatric patients, multiple screening dipstick urinalyses are costly and should be discontinued. At school-entry age, between 5 and 6 years of age, all asymptomatic children should have a single screening dipstick urinalysis on a first-morning voided specimen.

▶ Do you routinely perform screening dipstick urinalysis in the office? I was surprised at the American Academy of Pediatrics recommendations to perform this test routinely 4 times, at scheduled intervals. This is a test that used to be regularly done during the sports preparticipation examinations but has long since been discarded as costly and unnecessary. I concur with the authors' recommendation to stop routine screening. I do not follow their logic about a "middle ground" leading to their recommendation to test at 5 or 6 years of age. No evidence is presented to support this recommendation. The title of the article should perhaps be "Screening Dipstick Urinalysis: A Time to Stop."

W.W. Dexter, M.D.

A Simple and Efficient Urine Sampling Method for Bacteriological Examination in Elderly Women

Michielsen WJS, Geurs FJC, Verschraegen GLC, et al (Univ Hosp, De Pintelaan, Belgium)
Age Ageing 26:493–495, 1997   4–17

Introduction.—Diagnosis of urinary tract infection (UTI) depends on a representative urine sample, and midstream collection has been the routine method of sampling in women. Elderly women, however, are often catheterized because midstream collection may be difficult. An alternative to catheterization, which causes discomfort, is time-consuming, and may induce infection, is to collect urine in a sterile container. Urine collected in this way was compared with urine obtained by suprapubic aspiration, the "gold standard."

Methods.—Urine samples requested by the treating physician were obtained from 58 patients with an average age of 81. The vulval region was cleansed with water, and a sterile container was placed in the toilet or in the bedpan during voiding. Samples were also obtained by suprapubic puncture of the bladder under US guidance, a safe and relatively painless procedure. All samples were examined for pyuria and bacteriuria. By applying the Kass criteria and assessing the presence of leucocyturia, UTI could be differentiated from asymptomatic bacteriuria and contamination.

Results.—Urinary tract infection was diagnosed in 13 suprapubic specimens and in 17 voided samples, not a significant difference. All 13 cases that were positive after suprapubic aspiration were positive after collection in a sterile container. Four samples were false-positive when compared to the "gold-standard," but 1 of the 4 patients did appear to have UTI.

Conclusion.—The sampling technique that involves collecting urine in a sterile container after cleaning the vulva with water identified all cases of UTI confirmed by suprapubic aspiration. This method can reduce the need for bladder catheterization in elderly women who have difficulty in providing a midstream sample.

▶ I debated whether to include this study, as the sample size was quite small and the methodology was weak (no blinding). However, I am always intrigued by studies that challenge the way we practice, particularly when applying Occams Razor (the simplest way is often the best). In the 1997 YEAR BOOK OF FAMILY PRACTICE,[1] a simple noninvasive method of collecting infants' urine for evaluation was evaluated. Catheterization, while routine, is costly (staff, time, money), uncomfortable (at best), and can cause harm (at most) in our elderly patients as well. I look forward to seeing this technique validated.

W.W. Dexter, M.D.

Reference

1. 1997 YEAR BOOK OF FAMILY PRACTICE, p 268.

Miscellaneous

Evaluation of the Computer Program GIDEON for the Diagnosis of Fever in Patients Admitted to a Medical Service
Ross JJ, Shapiro DS (Boston Univ)
Clin Infect Dis 26:766–767, 1998   4–18

Introduction.—The computer program GIDEON (Global and Infectious *Disease* and *Epidemiology Network*) has an extensive infectious disease database that uses Bayes' theorem. In a prospective study, diagnoses generated by GIDEON were compared with those of medical house officers in the assessment of febrile inpatients.

Methods.—Eligible patients were 18 or older, admitted to inpatient medical service and had a fever of 38°C or higher within 48 hours of admission. During the study period (September 1996 to January 1997), 96 patients met inclusion criteria and 86 were able to be analyzed. Forty-eight patients were immunocompetent, and 38 were immunosuppressed. The clinicians' and GIDEON's diagnoses were compared with the discharge diagnoses.

Results and Discussion.—Admitting house officers listed the correct diagnosis first in 78 (87%) cases; in 28 cases (33%), GIDEON listed the correct diagnosis before the house officers and listed the correct diagnoses in its top 5 possible diagnoses in 36% of cases. In this comparison, GIDEON had been provided with all positive findings, whatever their relevance. When irrelevant findings were excluded, GIDEON generated a correct diagnosis as the first choice in 60% of cases, and its top 5 diagnoses included the correct diagnoses in 69% of cases. The diagnostic superiority of the house officers, however, remained significant, particularly in the case of immunocompetent patients when GIDEON was provided with all data. GIDEON may be useful in patients with fever and complex diagnoses, but house officers were superior in all other situations.

▶ Computer phobic? Recurring nightmares about "HAL," the omnipotent computer from the movie *2001*? Take heart—the machines have not made us docs obsolete yet. (Well, at least not the house officers.) I notice that the authors did not stack up GIDEON against attending physicians. This small, and largely entertaining, study certainly lends weight to the old saw "garbage in, garbage out," as GIDEON did better when "irrelevant" findings were excluded. To me, therein lies one of the beauties in primary care—there really are no irrelevancies when you address the whole patient. I am all in favor of putting computers to use to improve the quality of care that we provide our patients. But here is the rub: I am not sure we can ever create a machine that will care. In the end, HAL didn't.

W.W. Dexter, M.D.

Perspectives on Switching Oral Acyclovir From Prescription to Over-the-Counter Status: Report of a Consensus Panel
Sande MA, Armstrong D, Corey L, et al (Univ of Utah, Salt Lake City; Cornell Univ, New York; Univ of Washington, Seattle; et al)
Clin Infect Dis 26:659–663, 1998

4–19

Background.—A consensus panel recently considered the proposal of switching the status of oral acyclovir from prescription to over-the-counter (OTC) for the 5-day episodic treatment of genital herpes. The findings of this ad hoc panel were reported.

Report of Consensus Panel.—The panel agreed that self-diagnosis and misdiagnosis, misuse, and adverse drug reactions were potential problems with the OTC use of acyclovir. Although acyclovir decreases the asymptomatic shedding of herpes simplex virus type 2, the decrease in transmission of virus potentially resulting from increased acyclovir use was thought to be of benefit overall, albeit of unknown extent. Acyclovir availability would probably be enhanced. Opinion differed as to whether the widespread availability of acyclovir, whether prescription or OTC, may facilitate the development of viral resistance. However, all members of the panel agreed that granting OTC status may set a bad precedent for switching from prescription to OTC use of other systemically administered anti-infective drugs. Such a precedent may result in an acceleration of multidrug-resistant bacteria. The panel concurred that acyclovir status should not be switched to OTC.

▶ As a house officer when diphenhydramine became an OTC drug, I was struck by the number of diphenhydramine overdoses we began to see in the emergency department. Acyclovir would not seem to have this abuse potential. It is very effective, safe, and the side effects are generally minimal. Concern over the development of resistance to the drug is likewise minimal, as noted by the authors. I was thrilled when this drug became available as a generic, because the cost has been a major barrier to more widespread use. The authors' state that their recommendation not to change acyclovir's status is based on concern over establishing a "precedent," citing the inevitable development of resistance. Perhaps a cautious approach is the best one, although, as they note, resistance has not been proved to develop in immunocompetent patients. I am generally skeptical of changing prescription drugs to OTC status. Given the acknowledged benefit and very low risk of adverse outcomes with acyclovir, including resistance, I am not at all sure I agree with this line of reasoning or the panel's recommendations.

W.W. Dexter, M.D.

Multicenter Study of the Efficacy and Safety of Oral Ciprofloxacin in the Treatment of Chronic Suppurative Otitis Media in Adults

Gehanno P, and the French Study Group (Hôpital Bichat, Paris)
Otolaryngol Head Neck Surg 117:83–90, 1997   4–20

Objective.—Chronic suppurative otitis media is often resistant to treatment and frequently recurs. Because ciprofloxacin has been shown to be effective in small numbers of adults with suppurative otitis media, its safety and efficacy in the routine treatment of a larger group of patients were evaluated in a prospective, open, noncomparative, multicenter study.

Methods.—During the 3-month study, oral ciprofloxacin (500 mg twice daily) was administered for 10 days to 164 adults with symptomatic suppurative otitis media for an average of 158 months. Patients were examined at days 0, 11, and 40. The most commonly identified organism were *Staphylococcus aureus, Pseudomonas aeruginosa,* and *Proteus mirabilis.*

Results.—At the end of treatment, otorrhea had been eradicated in 104 of 155 evaluable patients (67.1%) and persisted in 33 patients (21.3%). One hundred one patients were cured and 3 improved. At day 40, 110 of 118 patients (93.2%) had no recurrence. One hundred patients had bacterial eradication, and 8 had superinfections. In the 136 patients with documented infections, infection was eradicated in 100 (73.5%). At day 40 the eradication rate was 75.4% (89 of 118). The majority of the 36 adverse events reported by 24 (14.6%) patients were gastrointestinal, and 32 were probably drug-related. Four patients were withdrawn from the study because of adverse events.

Conclusion.—Ciprofloxacin is safe and effective for treatment of chronic suppurative otitis media in adults.

▶ Sometimes when I read the methodologies of studies, I am reminded of the scene in *The Wizard of Oz* when, as the wizard is exposed, he exhorts the group to "pay no attention to the man behind the curtain," hoping that they will simply believe in his wizardry. This study was open, without controls, and noncomparative. Should we believe? Well, I will not go that far. However, given the refractory nature of this problem to treatment and the relative safety of the quinolones, I am convinced enough to recommend a trial (or 2) of ciprofloxacin for suppurative otitis media.

W.W. Dexter, M.D.

Directly Observed Therapy for Treatment Completion of Pulmonary Tuberculosis: Consensus Statement of the Public Health Tuberculosis Guidelines Panel
Chaulk CP, for the Public Health Tuberculosis Guidelines Panel (Annie E. Casey Found, Baltimore, MD)
JAMA 279:943–948, 1998　　　　　　　　　　　　　　　　　　　4–21

Background.—Because pulmonary tuberculosis is a highly infectious disease that has re-emerged in recent years, it is of utmost importance that diagnosed cases are effectively cured. One of the major obstacles to cure is a lack of patient completion of the recommended 6 months of drug therapy within 12 months. One method to ensure therapy completion is directly observed therapy (DOT). Through a survey of literature on the treatment of tuberculosis using DOT, the Council on Linkages Between Academia and Public Health Practice searched for the following key words: treatment adherence, treatment completion, supervised therapy, case management, and compliance. The council then made recommendations for the effective management of tuberculosis.

Method.—The council found 497 articles published from 1966 to 1996. Then, using a list of criteria, they narrowed these down to 27 studies. Each study was reviewed by at least 2 panel members. The outcomes for various degrees of supervised therapy were noted and used toward council's recommendation.

Results.—Directly observed therapy combined with multiple enablers and enhancers produced treatment rates in excess of the 90% figure suggested by the Centers for Disease Control and Prevention. Other methods using less direct supervision did not reach the 90% recommended completion rate. Although data on cost effectiveness were limited, DOT seemed to be more cost effective than self-administered therapy.

Conclusion.—The panel recommends tuberculosis therapy centered around patients and based on DOT.

▶ This is a brief report on a consensus panel regarding the treatment of pulmonary tuberculosis. By a thorough review of the English language medical literature on tuberculosis and the combined expertise of the consensus panel, the council concluded that DOT be recommended for pulmonary tuberculosis treatment centers. They also concluded that only by this direct observation of the client's medication usage would it be possible to exceed the 90% compliance recommended by the Centers for Disease Control and Prevention.

The public's right to protect itself from individuals with infectious disease is a compelling argument for requiring treatment of patients with pulmonary tuberculosis. Most states have statutes requiring treatment and can go so far as to incarcerate a client who refuses treatment. Individuals with pulmonary tuberculosis are frequently not the most compliant patients. It seems to be common sense that if we are going to be comfortable with outpatient treatment of these individuals, we must be proactive in making sure that they take their medication.

R.C. Davidson, M.D., M.P.H.

Time to Clinical Stability in Patients Hospitalized With Community-Acquired Pneumonia: Implications for Practice Guidelines

Halm EA, Fine MJ, Marrie TJ, et al (Mount Sinai School of Medicine, New York; Univ of Pittsbugh, Pa; Dalhousie Univ, Halifax, Nova Scotia, Canada, et al)
JAMA 279:1452–1457, 1998

Objective.—Whereas community-acquired pneumonia is one of the most common medical conditions for which patients are hospitalized, the reasons for differences in hospital stays are unclear. The time course of resolution of vital signs, ability to eat, and mental status abnormalities; the risk of major adverse outcomes once vital sign stability has been achieved; and the potential opportunities for shortening length of stay safely were examined in a prospective, multicenter, observational cohort study.

Methods.—The Pneumonia Patient Outcomes Research Team study evaluated 686 patients (352 women), aged 18 to 101 years, with community-acquired pneumonia, at 3 university and 1 community teaching hospital in the United States and Canada. Outcome measures were admission to an ICU, coronary care unit, or telemetry monitoring unit.

Results.—Co-morbid illness was present in 75% of patients, and 29% were classified as moderate- or high-risk. The infecting organism was identified in only 27% of patients. The median time to stabilization of heart rate to 100 beats/min or less was 2 days and to stabilization of systolic blood pressure to 90 mm Hg or more was 2 days. The median time to stabilization of respiratory rate to 24 breaths/min or less, oxygen saturation to 90% or more, and temperature to 37.2°C or less was 3 days. The time to overall stability ranged from 3 to 7 days, depending on whether the most lenient or strictest criteria were used. Patients with more severe pneumonia took longer to achieve clinical stability. After reaching clinical stability, 4% relapsed for systolic blood pressure, 12% for heart rate, 17% for respiratory rate, 9% for oxygen saturation, 1% for ability to eat, and 2% for mental status. Recurrent fever of more than 37.2°C occurred in 26% of patients. Coronary care unit, telemetry monitoring unit, or ICU admission was required in 1% or less of patients. Most patients stayed in the hospital more than 1 day after being stabilized. The median time from stability to discontinued parenteral antibiotics was 3 days.

Conclusion.—Whereas the mean time to stability after hospitalization was 3 days, most patients were hospitalized for several days beyond that point without incident, suggesting that the hospital stay can be safely shortened.

▶ You might keep this interesting study handy for use with your hospital utilization review program. The authors studied 686 adults hospitalized with community-acquired pneumonia. They were able to show that certain risk factors predicted a longer hospital stay before adequate stability could be attained for discharge to home care. There are no particular surprises in this study, but it might be of use if you are being pressed to discharge someone before you think the patient is sufficiently clinically stable to go home.

R.C. Davidson, M.D., M.P.H.

The Influence of Antibiotics and Other Factors on Reconsultation for Acute Lower Respiratory Tract Illness in Primary Care
Holmes WF, MacFarlane JT, MacFarlane RM, et al (Univ of Nottingham, England; Nottingham City Hosp, England)
Br J Gen Pract 47:815–818, 1997

Introduction.—Lower respiratory tract illness is a common, incompletely understood symptom complex. Infections are often suspected rather than proven, and organisms are rarely identified. Few studies have measured repeat general practitioner consultations, and placebo-controlled studies of antibiotics have shown little or no benefit in treating respiratory symptoms. Factors influencing reconsultation were explored in the month after the initial management of lower respiratory tract illness in general practice.

Methods.—There were 518 patients, ages 16 years and older, with an acute lower respiratory tract illness, in which cough was the predominant symptom, and 58 general practitioners in this prospective study. Recordings were taken of the patients' presenting symptoms and signs, underlying disease, antibiotic prescriptions, and the influence of nonmedical factors on management and description of the illness. Consultations in the month after the index consultation were also recorded to detect reconsultation and the number of consultations, for any reason, taken during the 2 years before the index consultation.

Results.—Antibiotics were prescribed for 76% of patients. Reconsultations for similar symptoms occurred for 30% of patients within the next 28 days. Thirty-three percent of these patients were not given antibiotics and 29% were given antibiotics. Of patients who had seen their practitioners 15 or more times in the previous 2 years, 41% reconsulted, compared with 13% of those patients who made fewer than 5 visits. In patients with a history of underlying disease, reconsultation was more common (38.6% vs. 24.3%), as it also was in patients who reported dyspnea (41.5% vs. 24.3%).

Conclusion.—In acute lower respiratory tract illness, reconsultation is common. A heightened consulting habit before the index consultation, the presence of previous ill health, and dyspnea are associated with reconsultation. Prescribing antibiotics does not appear to influence reconsultation.

▶ The use of antibiotics in patients seen with lower respiratory tract illnesses is quite common. These authors hypothesize that one of the reasons for the high use of antibiotics is the belief that such treatment will reduce return visits by these patients. The authors prospectively studied 500 patients with lower tract respiratory illnesses. Seventy-six percent of these patients were prescribed antibiotics. The authors could find no difference in revisit rates between patients given antibiotics and those not given antibiotics. Revisit rates had a clear correlation with other health problems, as well as with prior visit rates. It seems that people who have chronic illnesses or who frequently visit the doctor for other reasons are more likely to return for a revisit with lower respiratory tract illnesses.

R.C. Davidson, M.D., M.P.H.

Cycles of Malaria Associated With El Niño in Venezuela
Bouma MJ, Dye C (London School of Hygiene and Tropical Medicine)
JAMA 278:1772–1774, 1997   4–24

Introduction.—Periodic epidemics of malaria in the tropics and subtropics have a tendency to occur in areas where the El Niño Southern Oscillation (ENSO) affects the weather. An ENSO is an unstable periodic climate system that originates in the Pacific Ocean and lasts an average of 4–5 years. This event creates rainfall and temperature fluctuations in certain geographic areas worldwide, including the north coast of South America. Historic and recent data from Venezuela were used to evaluate ENSO's potential for epidemic forecasting in this area of South America.

Methods.—Data on national malaria morbidity from 1975–1995 and mortality from 1910–1935 from the coastal zone and interior of Venezuela were retrospectively reviewed in relation to El Niño events and rainfall. These data were reviewed to assess any correlation between malaria morbidity and mortality and sea surface temperatures in the Eastern Tropical Pacific, a parameter of ENSO.

Results.—Malaria mortality and morbidity rose significantly by an average of 36.5% in years after recognized El Niño events. There was a moderate correlation between Pacific tropical sea surface temperatures during an El Niño event and malaria 1 year later. Malaria was more strongly associated with drought in the year before outbreak than to rainfall during epidemic years.

Conclusion.—Historic and recent data from Venezuela show that malaria rises by about one third in the year after an El Niño event. Alterations in malaria risk may be predicted from Pacific sea surface temperatures in the previous year. Thus, the occurrence of an El Niño event can be used to predict malaria epidemics in Venezuela.

▶ Blame it on El Niño! That refrain has been echoed across the country to account for all imaginable occurrences. Do not lose sight of the fact that weather patterns and the attendant environmental changes can cause a real shift in disease patterns. Although you may not be involved in policy decisions regarding malaria prevention programs in South America, this type of information might well be useful in counseling patients who travel to those areas. Current recommendations regarding the prevention of malaria in travelers are reviewed in a *Journal of the American Medical Association* article that accompanied this article on El Niño.[1]

W.W. Dexter, M.D.

Reference

1. Lobel H, Kozarski P: Update on prevention of malaria for travelers. *JAMA* 278:1767–1771, 1997.

5 Asthma and Allergy

Overview

Randomized controlled trials: Abstracts 5-2, 5-4, and 5-7

Asthma

- Inhaled steroids and risk of hospitalization
- Salmeterol and improved quality of life
- Efficacy of house dust mite reduction
- Effect of inactivated influenza vaccine on pulmonary function
- Lack of linkage between skin sensitivity and airway response to allergens

Miscellaneous

- Food allergy in breastfed infants
- Neonatal exposure to cows' milk and atopy
- Reliability of skin testing and oral challenge to diagnosis of penicillin allergy

Asthma and Reactive Airways Disease

Inhaled Steroids and the Risk of Hospitalization for Asthma
Donahue JG, Weiss ST, Livingston JM, et al (Brigham and Women's Hosp, Boston; Harvard Med School, Boston)
JAMA 277:887–891, 1997   5–1

Purpose.—Asthma is the main cause of hospitalization in children, and is an increasingly important cause in adults as well. Current recommendations call for a multifaceted approach to asthma treatment, including early use of anti-inflammatory drugs, especially inhaled corticosteroids. However, there are few data to support the effectiveness of these recommendations in improving asthma outcomes. The effects of anti-inflammatory treatment on the risk of hospitalization for asthma were studied.

Methods.—The computerized record system of a large HMO were used to identify patients with a diagnosis of asthma. Information on asthma pharmacotherapy and resource utilization, including hospitalization for asthma, was analyzed.

Results.—Of 16,941 patients identified, 742 were hospitalized for asthma, a rate of 4.4%. After adjustment for β-agonist treatment, treatment with inhaled steroids halved the risk of hospitalization—overall relative risk 0.5, with a 95% confidence interval of 0.4–0.6. This effect of inhaled steroid use was unaffected by additional adjustment for age, race, other antiasthma drugs, or amount and type of ambulatory care. Cromolyn also reduced the risk of hospitalization—relative risk 0.8, 95% confidence interval 0.7–0.9—particularly for children. The risk of hospitalization increased along with increasing β-agonist use, even after adjustment for other variables and medications. Patients receiving the largest amounts of β-agonists derived the greatest protection from steroid treatment.

Conclusions.—Asthma patients receiving inhaled steroids are significantly less likely to require hospitalization for exacerbations of asthma. Cromolyn has a similar but lesser protective effect. The findings support recommendations for inhaled steroid use by patients who need more than occasional β-agonist treatment to control their asthma symptoms.

▶ Accepted therapy for patients with asthma includes an inhaled bronchodilator plus an inhaled steroid. These authors used a population within an HMO and studied the rate of hospitalization for asthma. They showed a significant reduction in the necessity for hospitalization among patients who were using inhaled steroids. This was particularly dramatic among patients who needed to frequently use bronchodilators. For those patients who used greater than 8 prescriptions for bronchodilators per year, the authors showed a fourfold reduction in hospitalizations with the concurrent use of inhaled steroids.

R.C. Davidson, M.D., M.P.H.

Salmeterol Improves Quality of Life in Patients With Asthma Requiring Inhaled Corticosteroids
Kemp JP, Cook DA, Incaudo GA, et al (Allergy & Asthma Med Group, San Diego, Calif; Allergy and Asthma Med Group of Diablo Valley Inc, Danville, Calif; Allergy Associates, Chico, Calif; et al)
J Allergy Clin Immunol 101:188–195, 1998   5–2

Introduction.—Salmeterol, a selective, long-acting, β₂-adrenoceptor agonist, provides sustained improvement in pulmonary function and control of asthma symptoms. The effect of this agent on quality of life, however, has not been thoroughly studied. Using the Asthma Quality-of-Life Questionnaire, investigators sought to define the effects of salmeterol on day-to-day functioning and well-being.

Methods.—The randomized, double-blind, placebo-controlled, parallel-group study included 506 patients with stable asthma who remained symptomatic even with daily use of inhaled corticosteroids. Excluded were patients younger than 12 years, who used tobacco, who required oral corticosteroid therapy, or who had other significant illness. The 14-week study period consisted of a 2-week screening period followed by 12 weeks of treatment. Patients were instructed to take 2 inhalations twice daily (total dose 42 µg) in the morning and evening and to continue albuterol on an as-needed basis.

Results.—Compared with placebo administration, 12 weeks of salmeterol therapy produced a significantly greater mean change from baseline in asthma quality-of-life scores. Global score increases were higher after salmeterol treatment than after placebo (1.08 vs. 0.61), as were scores for each of the individual domains of the questionnaire. Compared with the placebo group, patients treated with salmeterol experienced significantly greater improvements in forced expiratory volume in 1 second, morning peak expiratory flow, and asthma symptom scores, and required significantly less supplemental albuterol.

Conclusion.—Previous studies have documented the beneficial effects of salmeterol on pulmonary function and asthma symptoms. The findings of the present study confirm that salmeterol also significantly improves quality-of-life outcomes in patients whose asthma symptoms are not well controlled with inhaled corticosteroids. Salmeterol was well tolerated by these patients and presented no additional safety risks.

▶ Long-acting inhaled bronchodilator medication has provided a significant advantage in the treatment of recurrent reactive airway disease. State-of-the-art therapy for asthma now calls for inhaled steroids and inhaled bronchodilators. This interesting study looked not at the reduction of admissions or at improved pulmonary function. Rather, it used a quality-of-life indicator. The authors found a significant improvement in quality of life, with a doubling of symptom-free days, in patients taking long-acting bronchodilator inhaled medications.

A note of caution should be applied to our interpretation of this study, since the study was funded by the makers of the medication used.

R.C. Davidson, M.D., M.P.H.

The Melbourne House Dust Mite Study: Long-term Efficacy of House Dust Mite Reduction Strategies
Sporik R, Hill DJ, Thompson PJ, et al (Royal Children's Hosp, Melbourne, Australia; QEII Med Ctr, Nedlands, Australia; Univ of West Australia, Melbourne; et al)
J Allergy Clin Immunol 101:451–456, 1998   5–3

Introduction.—Improvement of children's asthma or eczema results for the majority of house dust mite-sensitized children and young adults when they move to a totally mite-free environment. Studies conducted in the homes of asthmatic patients have resulted in variable benefits. The effectiveness of an anti-mite carpet shampoo and of using mattress encasement to control the mite environment was evaluated in 85 homes.

Methods.—In 85 homes on 10 occasions over a 16-month period, the concentration of house dust mite allergen (Der p 1) was measured on the child's mattress surfaces. All mattresses were covered with a semipermeable encasement, and the carpeted bedroom floors were randomly allocated to regular applications of an "anti-mite" shampoo cleaning or a placebo after the first 3 visits.

Results.—In the carpeted bedrooms (30.7 µg Der p 1/g) and in the mattresses (59.6 µg Der p 1/g), the concentration of Der p 1 recovered was initially high. In the treatment, placebo, and parental control groups, the concentration of mite allergen fell during the initial observation period. In the groups using the anti-mite carpet shampoo or placebo carpet shampoo, and in the parental control group, no differences were seen between the Der p 1 concentrations during the 7 treatment periods. The concentrations of Der p 1 in samples from mattress encasement (4.2 µg Der p 1/g) and uncarpeted floors (4.1 µg Der p 1/g) were low, and insufficient dust for analysis was often obtained from these sites.

Conclusion.—The use of an "anti-mite" carpet shampoo did not provide any additional benefit. A useful long-term strategy for mite allergen avoidance was the absence of carpets and the use of mattress encasement. Hot washing of encasement and reducing indoor humidity may be required to keep levels consistently low where conditions are ideal for mite growth.

▶ Many patients with asthma are known to have an allergic response to house dust mites. This study was designed to look at several mechanisms attempting to reduce the mite allergen exposure in homes with children with allergy. The authors studied 3 interventions. Two of these proved to be efficacious. The removal of carpets in the bedroom and the use of mattress encasements were found to be useful long-term strategies for mite allergen reduction. However, the use of anti-mite shampoos in rugs showed no benefit.

R.C. Davidson, M.D., M.P.H.

Randomised Placebo-controlled Crossover Trial on Effect of Inactivated Influenza Vaccine on Pulmonary Function in Asthma
Nicholson KG, Nguyen-Van-Tam JS, Ahmed AH, et al (Leicester Royal Infirmary, England; Queen's Med Centre, Nottingham, England; Dept of Health, London; et al)
Lancet 351:326–331, 1998

Introduction.—Because influenza can trigger exacerbations of asthma, annual vaccination of children and adults with chronic respiratory disease is recommended. Many patients with asthma, however, are not vaccinated against influenza, in part out of concern that the vaccine itself may trigger exacerbations of asthma. Colds can also trigger exacerbations, which may be mistaken for vaccine-related adverse events. A double-blind study assessed the safety of influenza vaccine in patients with asthma.

Methods.—The 262 patients who entered the multicenter crossover study were aged 18–75. They were randomly assigned to receive 0.5 mL

IM injections of vaccine and of placebo, separated by 2 weeks and administered in random order. Patients recorded daily peak expiratory flow (PEF), respiratory symptoms, medication, medical consultations, and hospital admission for 2 weeks before the first injection and until 2 weeks after the second injection. The main outcome measure was an exacerbation of asthma (a fall in PEF of more than 20%) within 72 hours of the injection.

Results.—Complete paired data were available for 255 patients (86%) who entered the study. Eleven recorded a fall in PEF of more than 20% after vaccine and 3 after placebo; a fall of 30% was recorded by 8 patients after vaccine, but by none after placebo. Overall, mean PEF values did not differ significantly between vaccine and placebo injections. Among the 97 first-time vaccinees, there were significantly more decreases in PEF after vaccine than after placebo (9 vs. 1).

Conclusion.—In a group of patients typical of those likely to be targeted for influenza vaccine, the risk of pulmonary complications after vaccination was quite small. The risk of these complications appears to be outweighed by the benefits of vaccination. Further trials with a wider population of patients with asthma, including children, should be conducted to confirm these findings.

▶ Current recommendations for influenza vaccination in adults include the diagnosis of asthma. However, it is not uncommon for asthma patients to be resistant to using influenza vaccine because in past years they have "gotten worse." This study used a crossover placebo methodology to study 262 adult patients with known asthma. The authors did find that adults with symptoms of colds had worse pulmonary function following influenza vaccine than they had following placebo injection. However, for those patients who did not have symptoms of colds, there was no difference. The authors conclude that the known benefits of influenza vaccine outweigh the possibility for short-term worsening of respiratory functions.

I think it is important to encourage our adult patients with asthma to take influenza vaccine. If asked, I will tell them that some patients might have a short-term worsening of symptoms. However, the protection from influenza outweighs the potential for short-term symptom exacerbation.

R.C. Davidson, M.D., M.P.H.

Skin Sensitivity to Allergen Does Not Accurately Predict Airway Response to Allergen
Bowton DL, Fasano MB, Bass DA (Wake Forest Univ, Winston-Salem, NC)
Ann Allergy Asthma Immunol 80:207–211, 1998   5–5

Introduction.—Because the airway response to allergens is similar to that of clinical asthma, allergen challenge of the asthmatic airway is widely used in the study of allergic asthma. This method is time consuming, however, for the challenge must be initiated at extremely low concentrations of allergen. To determine whether skin-test titration could be used to select initial allergen concentration, the relationship between skin test and inhaled reactivity was studied in patients with allergic asthma.

Methods.—The 22 patients underwent prick skin-test titrations and inhaled allergen challenges. The prick skin-test titrations were performed using serially diluted lyophilized antigen extracts reconstituted in normal saline from 1:100,000–1:10. A standardized tidal breathing technique was employed during methacholine bronchoprovocation. The inhaled allergen challenge was performed in the morning, using the allergen of the skin-test titration, and initiated with an allergen concentration 50% of that which caused a 2-mm wheal over saline control on skin-test titration.

Results.—Skin-test titration thresholds ranged from 1:10–1:100,000, whereas inhaled concentrations reached ranged from 1.10–1:2000. No correlation was observed between the skin-test titration and the inhaled challenge titration. Similarly, there was no correlation between the final inhaled antigen concentration and the magnitude of the early asthmatic response. Patients whose skin-testing dilutions were 1:10,000 or less, however, did appear to exhibit a relationship between skin sensitivity and inhalation response.

Conclusion.—Although a correlation between cutaneous and airways reactivity to a given allergen is present in some patients with atopy and asthma, this correlation is absent or inconsistent in other patients. Skin-test titration results are not likely to be helpful when patients have marked cutaneous sensitivity.

▶ It is a common occurrence with my patients with allergic asthma for us to have a lengthy discussion about the pros and cons of undergoing skin testing to identify their allergens. In my experience, it is so common to find multiple allergens and to have little to do about avoidance that I am not a strong proponent for such testing.

This interesting study looked at 22 known allergic asthmatic patients. The authors challenged these patients with the very antigens to which they had shown skin-test sensitivity. The authors found no correlation between skin-test threshold and the inhaled concentration required to produce a reduction in forced expiratory volume. They concluded that while a correlation between skin-test threshold and inhaled reactivity is present in some patients with allergic asthma, the relationship is inconsistent. If the relationship between skin-test sensitivity and the actual production of bronchospasm by the antigen is inconsistent, why do the test at all?

R.C. Davidson, M.D., M.P.H.

Miscellaneous

Multiple Food Allergy: A Possible Diagnosis in Breastfed Infants

de Boissieu D, Matarazzo P, Rocchiccioli F, et al (Hôpital Saint Vincent de Paul, Paris)
Acta Paediatr 86:1042–1046, 1997

Background.—Food antigens can pass from mother to infant in breast milk. Multiple food allergy as a possible diagnosis in breastfed infants was described.

Methods.—Six infants thought to have food allergy during breastfeeding were assessed. Prick tests, total IgE, radioallergosorbent tests, and intestinal permeability measures during fasting and provocation with mother's milk were administered. The mothers were placed on an elimination diet, beginning with the removal of cow's milk protein (CMP), followed by all foods suspected on the clinical history or a positive prick test in the child, followed by oral challenges in the mother's diet with the corresponding food.

Findings.—The removal of CMP from the mothers' diet was never sufficient. In 4 women, an additional diet excluding 2 to 3 foods was effective in alleviating the symptoms. In all women, oral provocations with those foods were positive. Two mothers declined a diet that excluded more than 4 foods. Symptoms in their infants cleared using an extensively hydrolysed formula. Challenges with mother's milk caused immediate reactions. Intestinal permeability was changed during provocation tests with mother's milk sampled before the maternal diet.

Conclusions.—Food allergy during breast feeding may be caused by multiple foods. The inefficacy of eliminating CMP only in the mother's diet does not exclude food sensitization.

▶ Most breastfeeding mothers are well aware that what they eat may affect their infants' behavior, both physically and mentally. However, I do not believe most physicians appreciate the relationship. Colic in breastfed infants may be caused by the amount of cow's milk protein ingested by the mother, a finding that has been known for many years. This article takes the relationship further by describing 6 cases in which infant symptoms were related to more than one food product ingested by the mother. The table shows that cow's milk protein may interact with eggs, fish, or other products to give colic, other GI symptoms, or rashes in the infants. Being alert to these possibilities, and having successful interventions, may go a long way to salvaging a breastfeeding mother–infant relationship.

J.E. Scherger, M.D., M.P.H.

Randomised Controlled Trial of Brief Neonatal Exposure to Cows' Milk on the Development of Atopy
de Jong MH, Scharp-van der Linden VTM, Aalberse RC, et al (Univ of Amsterdam)
Arch Dis Child 79:126–130, 1998

Introduction.—The relationship of exposure to cow's milk and development of atopy at a later age has not been studied by properly designed investigations. The effect of brief and early exposure to cow's milk protein on the development of atopic disease in infants and young children was assessed in a double-blind, placebo-controlled, randomized trial.

Methods.—After birth, 1,533 newborns from Dutch midwifery practices whose mothers intended to breast feed were randomized during the first 3 days of life to receive either a supplemental standard whey protein dominant cow's milk formula or a placebo formula free from cow's milk protein. Newborns aged 1 year were tested for positive radioallergosorbent (RAST) and were followed-up until aged 2 years for clinical atopic disease.

Results.—Atopic disease was detected in the first year of life in 10.0% of infants in the cow's milk group vs. 9.3% of infants in the placebo group. Positive readings of RAST tests were observed in 9.4% of infants in the cow's milk group and 7.9% of infants in the placebo group at 1 year. An analysis by family risk of atopy revealed a doubled incidence of obvious atopic disease in high-risk children; no effect was observed from intervention (Fig 3).

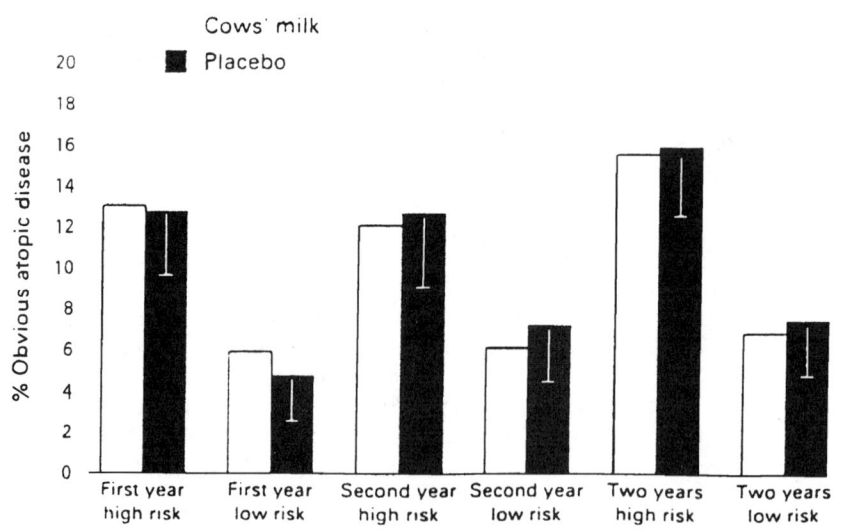

FIGURE 3.—Percentage obvious atopic disease and 95% confidence intervals in the first 2 years of life, stratified for family risk of atopy. *White bars*, cow's milk; *black bars*, placebo. (Courtesy of de Jong MH, Scharp-van der Linden VTM, Aalberse RC: Randomised controlled trial of brief neonatal exposure to cows' milk on the development of atopy. *Arch Dis Child* 79:126–130, 1998.)

Conclusion.—Breast-fed infants who received cow's milk supplementation in the first 3 days of life had the same risk of a clinical or serological expression of atopic disease as those who received placebo. These results conflict with reports by other clinicians.

▶ As a strong advocate of breastfeeding, I want to be able to discuss this topic in a balanced fashion with my patients. This article dispels one of the oft-stated rationales for not using supplements. Despite being funded by the supplement manufacturer, this was a well-controlled study looking at the notion that early exposure to cow's milk proteins leads to allergy to these proteins. On the basis of these data, development of allergies to cow's milk protein is not a valid reason to limit early supplementation. However, I am firm in my belief that there are other more compelling reasons not to supplement early; that is, this practice is negatively associated with length of breastfeeding.[1]

W.W. Dexter, M.D.

Reference

1. 1998 YEAR BOOK OF FAMILY PRACTICE, p 61.

Diagnosis of Penicillin, Amoxicillin, and Cephalosporin Allergy: Reliability of Examination Assessed by Skin Testing and Oral Challenge

Pichichero ME, Pichichero DM (Univ of Rochester, NY)
J Pediatr 132:137–143, 1998
5–8

Background.—Patients considered to have an allergy to certain antibiotics may be treated with alternative agents that are more costly and have increased toxicity. Routine elective skin testing in children is recommended as a means of identifying those who are truly at risk for an allergic reaction to penicillin, amoxicillin, and cephalosporin. A skin-testing program was conducted in a group of children and adolescents to evaluate the specificity of pediatrician-diagnosed allergic reactions to these drugs.

Methods.—The 247 study participants all were thought by their pediatrician to have experienced an adverse reaction to 1 or more of the antibiotics. It was recommended that these patients no longer be treated with any antibiotic in the β-lactam class. Skin testing was performed according to the suspected drug allergy, followed by an oral challenge, repeat testing, and prospective follow-up if no reactions were noted.

Results.—Patients ranged in age from 6 months to 18 years. In most cases, urticaria or a polymorphous rash had led to the suspicion of an adverse antibiotic reaction. Eighty-four (34%) had an IgE-type reaction on skin testing or oral challenge. Twenty-seven (32%) suspected penicillin reactions, 53 (34%) suspected amoxicillin reactions, and 13 (50%) suspected cephalosporin reactions were shown to be IgE mediated. Twenty patients with non–IgE-type clinical adverse reactions had positive skin tests. No patient experienced severe oral reactions after negative skin testing. Three (1.8%) of 163 patients who received multiple treatment courses with β-lactam antibiotics during a mean follow-up of 5.4 years had mild adverse IgE reactions.

Conclusion.—Based upon patient examination at the time of an apparent allergic reaction, pediatricians accurately predicted IgE sensitivity in 84 (34%) children and adolescents. In the remaining 66% of patients, however, the rate of possible allergy was overestimated. Elective penicillin, amoxicillin, and cephalosporin skin testing and oral challenge can accurately identify patients not at risk.

▶ It is all too common in the treatment of children to find a history of antibiotic sensitivity precluding the use of our common antibiotics. However, when we query the parents or medical record, it is not always clear whether this is a true sensitivity to the antibiotic. This very interesting study looked at 247 children and adolescents who had been reported to have an allergy to penicillin, amoxicillin, and/or an oral cephalosporin. These children were all skin tested, and those children negative by skin test were further evaluated by an oral challenge of the suspect drug. The authors found that 66% of the children who had been labeled "allergic" to one of the suspect drugs showed no evidence of such allergy on this objective testing. Even those patients who had a physician-observed suspected allergic reaction showed high percentages of no objective allergic manifestations of an IgE-mediated response.

When we have pediatric patients with suspected antibiotic allergies, we should consider skin testing them during a period when they are well and not in immediate need of an antibiotic. By this method, we might reduce the number of children precluded from using these common antibiotics.

R.C. Davidson, M.D., M.P.H.

6 Gastroenterology

Overview

Randomized controlled trials: Abstracts 6-2, 6-3, 6-8, 6-9, 6-11, and 6-12

Upper Gastrointestinal Problems

- 793 esophagogastroduodenoscopies performed by a family physician
- Two comparisons of omeprazole with misoprostol and ranitidine for ulcers associated with NSAIDs
- Screening for Barrett's esophagus
- Omeprazole in diagnosis of gastroesophageal reflux disease

Lower Gastrointestinal Problems

- Two articles on biofeedback for fecal incontinence and constipation
- Gastrointestinal symptoms and olestra

Miscellaneous

- Budesonide and mesalamine for Crohn's disease
- Risk of symptomatic gallstones related to exercise in men
- Comparison of enteral and parenteral nutrition in acute pancreatitis
- Ursodeoxycholic acid and varices in patients with biliary cirrhosis
- Prognosis in end-stage liver disease
- CT of the appendix and use of hospital resources

Upper Gastrointestinal Problems

Esophagogastroduodenoscopy Performed by a Family Physician: A Case Series of 793 Procedures
Pierzchajlo RPJ, Ackermann RJ, Vogel RL, et al (Tifon, Ga; Mercer Univ, Macon, Ga)
J Fam Pract 46:41–46, 1998   6–1

Introduction.—Flexible sigmoidoscopy is performed by up to 29% to 57% of U.S. family physicians and 42% of general internists. Primary care physicians perform esophagogastroduodenoscopy (EGD) substantially less often than flexible sigmoidoscopy. Up to 1% of some U.S. populations have endoscopy each year. Access to this technology can be problematic, particularly in rural areas. A large series of EGDs performed by a family physician in a solo rural practice is reviewed.

Methods.—Medical records were retrospectively reviewed for data regarding demographics, indications for EGD, endoscopic and pathologic findings, and complications for all EGDs performed by the family physician over 7 years.

Results.—Six hundred two patients underwent 793 EGDs. Mean age of 421 women and 181 men was 51.8 years. The second portion of the duodenum was intubated in 99% of EGDs. The most frequent indications for EGD were 60.5%, abdominal pain; 23.0%, gastrointestinal bleeding; 11.6%, dysphagia; and 10.7%, heartburn. Of 451 biopsies obtained in 385 procedures, 38% were taken from the distal esophagus and 38% were taken from the gastric antrum. The most frequent endoscopic diagnoses were 54%, gastritis; 25%, esophagitis; and 15%, normal findings. Two malignancies were found: 1 gastric lymphoma and 1 carcinoma metastatic to the stomach. There was 1 minor complication: 1 patient had an immediate urticarial rash after administration of intravenous meperidine.

Conclusion.—This is the largest reported series of EGDs by a single primary care physician. The complication rate compares favorably with the largest series in gastrointestinal literature. The physician in this series gained all of his endoscopic skills after residency.

▶ This article really caught my attention. Many of us perform flexible sigmoidoscopies, few perform esophagogastroduodenoscopies. I included this case series report simply in the hope that this might also pique your interest, and, perhaps, to motivate you, as it has me, to investigate the possibility of acquiring this skill. This is a service that family doctors can perform, and, as the author of this study has, perform expertly and safely in a busy practice setting.

W.W. Dexter, M.D.

Omeprazole Compared With Misoprostol for Ulcers Associated With Nonsteroidal Antiinflammatory Drugs

Hawkey CJ, for the Omeprazole Versus Misoprostol for NSAID-Induced Ulcer Management (OMNIUM) Study Group (Univ Hosp, Nottingham, England; Peninsula Specialist Centre, Kippa Ring, Australia; Univ Med School, Lublin, Poland; et al)
N Engl J Med 338:727–734, 1998   6–2

Background.—Although misoprostol is effective in the treatment of ulcers associated with regular nonsteroidal anti-inflammatory drug (NSAID) use, it often causes diarrhea and abdominal pain. The efficacy of omeprazole was compared with that of misoprostol in the healing and prevention of NSAID-related ulcers.

Methods.—Nine hundred thirty-five patients were enrolled in the double-blind, randomized trial. All required continuous NSAID treatment and

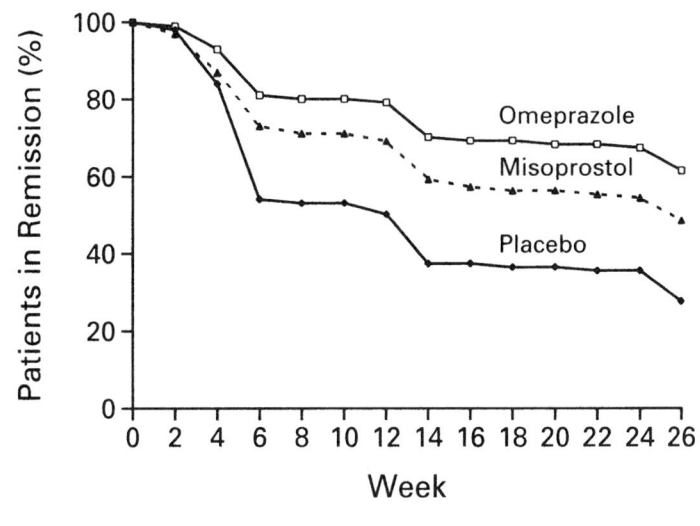

FIGURE 2.—Kaplan-Meier estimates of the rates of remission among patients treated with 20 mg of omeprazole daily, 200 μg of misoprostol twice daily, or placebo for up to 26 weeks. $P < 0.001$ for the comparison of omeprazole with placebo by the log-rank test, and $P = 0.001$ for the comparison of omeprazole with misoprostol by the log-rank test. (Courtesy of Hawkey CJ, for the Omeprazole Versus Misoprostol for NSAID-Induced Ulcer Management (OMNIUM) Study Group: Omeprazole compared with misoprostol for ulcers associated with nonsteroidal antiinflammatory drugs. N Engl J Med 338:727–734. Copyright 1998, Massachusetts Medical Society. Reprinted by permission of *The New England Journal of Medicine*. All rights reserved.)

had ulcers or more than 10 erosions in the stomach and/or duodenum. The patients took 20 mg or 40 mg of omeprazole orally in the morning, or 200 μg of misoprostol orally 4 times a day. Treatment was given for 4 or 8 weeks, depending on healing. By random assignment, 732 patients responding to treatment were given maintenance therapy with 20 mg of omeprazole daily, 200 μg of misoprostol twice daily, or placebo for 6 months.

Findings.—At 8 weeks, treatment was successful in 76% of patients receiving 20 mg of omeprazole, 75% receiving 40 mg of omeprazole, and 71% receiving misoprostol. Gastric-ulcer healing rates associated with 20 mg of omeprazole were significantly greater than with misoprostol. Healing rates among patients with duodenal ulcers were greater with omeprazole (either dose) than misoprostol. Healing rates among patients with erosions alone were greater with misoprostol. During maintenance therapy, more patients remained in remission with omeprazole than misoprostol, and with either active agent than with placebo. Patients receiving misoprostol had more adverse events in the healing phase than patients given either dose of omeprazole (Fig 2).

Conclusions.—Omeprazole and misoprostol yielded similar overall rates of successful treatment of ulcers, erosions, and symptoms associated with NSAID use. Maintenance therapy with omeprazole was more effective than with misprostol. However, omeprazole was better tolerated.

A Comparison of Omeprazole With Ranitidine for Ulcers Associated With Nonsteroidal Antiinflammatory Drugs

Yeomans ND, for the Acid Suppression Trial: Ranitidine versus Omeprazole for NSAID-Associated Ulcer Treatment (ASTRONAUT) Study Group (Univ of Melbourne, Australia; Semmelweis Univ, Budapest, Hungary; Borsod County Teaching Hosp, Miskolc, Hungary; et al)
N Engl J Med 338:719–726, 1998   6–3

Background.—Suppressing acid secretion is believed to decrease the risk of nonsteroidal anti-inflammatory drug (NSAID)–related ulcers. The best way to achieve this, however, is not known.

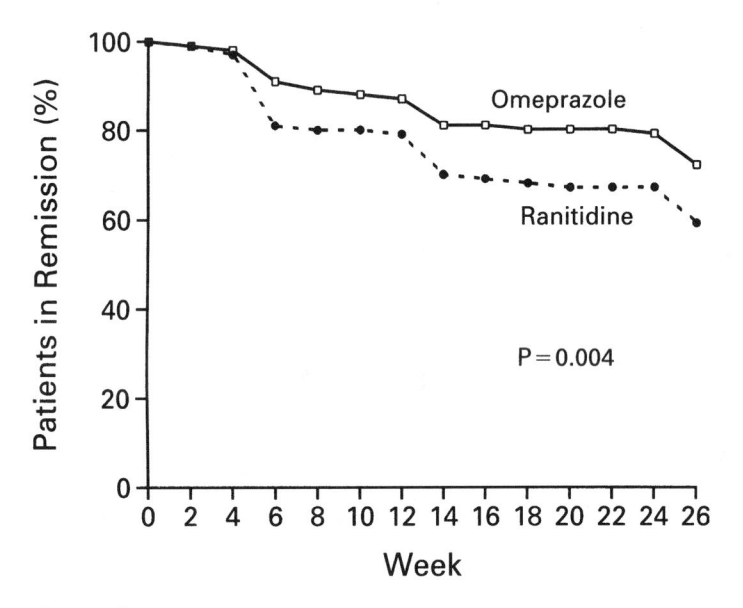

No. at Risk of Relapse

Omeprazole	210	205	177	145
Ranitidine	215	205	160	114

FIGURE 2.—Estimated rates of remission among patients treated with 20 mg of omeprazole daily or 150 mg of ranitidine twice daily for up to 26 weeks. $P = 0.004$ by the log-rank test for the difference between groups. (Courtesy of Yeomans ND, for the Acid Suppression Trial: Ranitidine versus Omeprazole for NSAID-Associated Ulcer Treatment (ASTRONAUT) Study Group: A comparison of omeprazole with ranitidine for ulcers associated with nonsteroidal antiinflammatory drugs. *N Engl J Med* 338:719–726. Copyright 1998, Massachusetts Medical Society. Reprinted by permission of *The New England Journal of Medicine.* All rights reserved.)

Methods.—Five hundred forty-one patients needing continuous NSAID treatment with ulcers or more than 10 erosions in the stomach or duodenum were studied. By random assignment, patients received omeprazole, 20 mg or 40 mg orally per day, or ranitidine, 150 mg orally twice daily, for 4 or 8 weeks depending on treatment success. Four hundred thirty-two patients in whom treatment was successful were assigned randomly to maintenance therapy with 20 mg of omeprazole per day or 150 mg of ranitidine twice a day for 6 months.

Findings.—At 8 weeks, treatment was successful in 80% of patients in the 20-mg omeprazole group, 79% in the 40-mg omeprazole group, and 63% in the ranitidine group. Healing rates for all types of lesions were greater with omeprazole than ranitidine. During maintenance treatment, the estimated proportions of patients in remission at 6 months in the omeprazole and ranitidine groups were 72% and 59%, respectively. The groups had similar rates of adverse events during both phases. The agents were tolerated well (Fig 2).

Conclusions.—Omeprazole, 20 mg daily, is superior to ranitidine in healing and preventing gastroduodenal ulcers and erosions in patients taking NSAIDs daily. Omeprazole also proved better at controlling dyspeptic symptoms.

▶ In the past few years, I have significantly reduced the number of NSAID prescriptions I have written. In many cases, the risks, particularly adverse gastrointestinal effects, have simply outweighed the benefits. Despite a history of gastrointestinal toxicity, however, many patients continue to use NSAIDs with or without my prescription. In treating these patients, I have employed all 3 strategies outlined in these 2 studies (Abstracts 6–2 and 6–3) from *The New England Journal of Medicine*, as well as testing for and treating *Helicobacter pylori* as a possible confounder. Not well-addressed in either study is the issue of *H. pylori*. Interestingly, evidence is presented by the authors that suggests *H. pylori* infection might actually be beneficial in NSAID-induced gastropathy. Overall, these well-designed studies (both supported by the manufacturer of omeprazole) provide solid evidence on which to base your decision on which approach to take when treating and prescribing prophylaxis for NSAID-induced upper gastrointestinal disease. Omeprazole is the clear winner.

W.W. Dexter, M.D.

Ten Years' Experience of Screening Patients With Barrett's Oesophagus in a University Teaching Hospital

Macdonald CE, Wicks AC, Playford RJ (Leicester Gen Hosp, England)
Gut 41:303–307, 1997   6–4

Introduction.—There is a strong link between gastroesophageal reflux disease and Barrett's metaplasia, yet the natural history of Barrett's esophagus is not well understood. Symptom severity is not a good indicator of macroscopic damage, thus symptomatology should not be used to select patients at increased risk of Barrett's metaplasia. Findings of annual screenings in 409 patients with Barrett's metaplasia were reported.

Methods.—Medical records of all patients with the suggestion of Barrett's esophagus were reviewed for data regarding age, sex, evidence of any previous endoscopy performed elsewhere, and any additional illnesses. Patients were considered to have Barrett's esophagus if there was an area of biopsy-confirmed columnar metaplasia extending over a region of 3 cm or greater. The benefit of performing annual screening in patients with Barrett's esophagus was explored.

Results.—Of 29,374 upper gastrointestinal endoscopies performed from 1984 to 1994, Barrett's esophagus was detected for the first time in 409 patients (1.4%). The sex distribution of these findings was about equal; most patients were aged 50 years or older. Thirty-five percent of patients were considered appropriate for annual screening. Throughout screening, the length of the esophagus did not vary over time. Of 379 patients in whom yearly endoscopies were performed for screening purposes, carcinoma was detected in only 1 patient as a result of annual screening. Carcinoma was discovered as a result of progressive dysphagia in 2 additional patients. All 3 of these patients had "long segment" regions of Barrett's metaplasia longer than 8 cm, with a stricture that was observed on initial endoscopy.

Conclusion.—Annual screening of all patients with Barrett's metaplasia detected on initial endoscopic examination has a poor yield. Resources need to be focused on patients who have findings of ulceration or stricture in addition to Barrett's metaplasia.

Omeprazole as a Diagnostic Tool in Gastroesophageal Reflux Disease
Schenk BE, Kuipers EJ, Klinkenberg-Knol EC, et al (Free Univ Hosp, Amsterdam; 't Lange Land Hosp, Zoetermeer, The Netherlands; Bronovo Hosp Den Haag, The Netherlands)
Am J Gastroenterol 92:1997–2000, 1997   6–5

Introduction.—A reliable and simple method for detecting gastroesophageal reflux disease (GERD) is needed. Symptoms of GERD can be alleviated within 2–4 weeks by the profound inhibition of gastric acid secretion with 20–40 mg of omeprazole. It is not likely that retrosternal complaints of non-GERD origin will respond to this therapy. The diagnostic value of empirical treatment of GERD with omeprazole was assessed in patients with symptoms suggestive of GERD.

Methods.—Upper gastrointestinal endoscopy and 24-hour esophageal pH monitoring were performed in 85 patients with symptoms suggestive of GERD, especially heartburn, regurgitation, or dysphagia. Patients with reflux esophagitis grade 0 or 1 were randomized in double-blind fashion to either 40 mg omeprazole or placebo daily. The effect of treatment was assessed after 1–2 weeks by a symptom questionnaire scored on a 4-grade Likert scale and by symptomatic response outcome. These reports were compared with findings of 24-hour pH-metry.

Results.—Of 85 eligible patients, 54 had no signs of esophagitis at endoscopy and 31 had esophagitis grade 1. The pH registration revealed pathologic gastroesophageal reflux in 47 patients (55%). Forty-one and 44 patients, respectively, were randomized to treatment with omeprazole or placebo. There was a significant association between pH registration and response to omeprazole, but not to placebo. Using pH-metry as the gold standard, the positive and negative predictive values of pH monitoring were 68% and 63%, respectively. Similar sensitivity was observed when pH-metry was compared with the presence of esophagitis.

Conclusion.—Symptom response to 40 mg of omeprazole for 14 days in patients with symptoms indicative of GERD is a simple and inexpensive method for diagnosing GERD. The sensitivity and specificity of this approach were comparable to that of 24-hour pH monitoring.

▶ Confirming diagnosis and screening for Barrett's esophagus have been 2 important reasons for having patients with GERD undergo esophagogastroduodenoscopy (EGD). These 2 articles (Abstracts 6–4 and 6–5) put this practice in a different light. The first, by Macdonald, Wicks, and Playford, reports on a very large series of endoscopies over a lengthy period with a very low incidence of Barrett's esophagus. Frankly, I was astounded at the number of EGD's performed by the 3 authors: about 900 per year per author! Basically, their methodology was simply to report the results of their own endoscopic findings. Even so, I think their conclusions regarding screening patients with Barrett's are reasonable. For me, the bigger concern raised by their data regards the widespread use of EGD for diagnosis. I draw no conclusions for or against; I am just intrigued by their data.

The second article also speaks to this issue. Schenk et al. present data that, in a fairly robust manner, support what probably is already a common practice: an empiric trial of omeprazole for presumed GERD. If such a trial is successful, an EGD is probably not warranted, certainly not to screen for Barrett's. A caveat: Note that the dose of omeprazole used was 40 mg once daily. The authors report other studies using anywhere from 20 to 80 mg. I favor 40 mg, either once daily or in 2 divided doses.

W.W. Dexter, M.D.

Lower Gastrointestinal Problems

Biofeedback Is Effective Therapy for Fecal Incontinence and Constipation
Ko CY, Tong J, Lehman RE, et al (Univ of California, Los Angeles; Univ of California, San Francisco)
Arch Surg 132:829–834, 1997   6–6

Background.—Results of surgery for fecal incontinence and constipation in elderly patients are poor. Because patients with urinary incontinence are often treated with biofeedback, it is thought that patients with fecal incontinence or constipation could benefit from this process as well.

The patients in this study used biofeedback with great success to retrain their pelvic floor.

Methods.—Biofeedback was used to treat either fecal incontinence or constipation. The 25 patients with fecal incontinence (21 women and 4 men, median age, 63 years) had neurogenic fecal incontinence (prolonged pudendal nerve terminal motor latency), mild to moderate sphincter injuries that the patient wanted to treat nonsurgically, or a failed anal sphincter reconstruction. The 17 patients with constipation (12 women and 5 men, median age, 50 years) had either pelvic floor dysfunction or could not expel a catheter balloon inflated to 60 mL.

Findings.—The 25 patients with incontinence used 2 to 13 biofeedback sessions (average, 6.5), and symptoms improved in 23 (92%) of the patients even though manometric pressures did not change. The number of patients who could sustain a 5-second contraction increased from 7 (28%) at the first biofeedback session to 12 (48%) at the last session. Likewise, more patients had a contraction range greater than 10 mV at the last visit than at the first visit (48% vs. 28%). Biofeedback significantly reduced the number of incontinent episodes, from 5.06/day to 0.77/day. Two patients with fecal incontinence experienced no improvement and had either bilateral complete pudendal neuropathy or did not follow the biofeedback program.

The 17 patients with constipation used 2 to 9 biofeedback sessions (average, 4), and symptoms improved in 13 (76%) of the patients even though, again, manometric pressures did not change. Four patients experienced no improvement and either had persistent colonic transit delay, did not follow the biofeedback program, or simply had no response to biofeedback.

Conclusions.—Biofeedback was useful in improving fecal incontinence and chronic constipation in these patients. Patient selection should begin with anorectal manometry with balloon expulsion tests and/or defecography for assessing incontinence and with transrectal ultrasonography and pudendal nerve terminal motor latency tests for assessing constipation. Patients who had the most success with biofeedback included those with only mild to moderate sphincter injuries, no or only unilateral neuropathy, and residual incontinence after previous surgical repair. The patients with bilateral complete neuropathy and fecal incontinence did not respond to biofeedback, nor did the patients with constipation and colonic inertia.

Results of Biofeedback in Constipated Patients: A Prospective Study
Karlbom U, Hállden M, Eeg-Olofsson KE, et al (Univ Hosp, Uppsala, Sweden)
Dis Colon Rectum 40:1149–1155, 1997   6–7

Introduction.—The paradoxical puborectalis contraction is probably linked to behavioral and psychological factors rather than neurologic causes. Biofeedback has been used to strengthen the pelvic floor muscles in patients with fecal incontinence. It has also been used in patients with a paradoxical sphincter contraction. Results of biofeedback treatment were prospectively evaluated in 28 patients with constipation and any degree of paradoxical sphincter contraction.

Methods.—Four patients had neurologic disease. The cause or contributing reason for constipation in the remaining patients was idiopathic. Median age range of 5 males and 23 females was 20 to 72 years. Symptom duration varied from 1 to 30 years (median, 9 years). Twenty-two patients relied on laxatives and 14 used combinations of bulking agents, motor-stimulators, and/or enemas. Six patients were managed with manually assisted defecation. A thin hook needle electromyography was placed in the external sphincter or puborectalis. Patients participated in 8 sessions with electromyography-based audiovisual feedback. Patients were asked to complete a validated bowel function questionnaire from which a symptom index was produced.

Results.—Of the 28 patients, nine (32.1%) patients with no improvement from biofeedback after 3 months of treatment had other treatments. Nineteen (67.9%) patients continued biofeedback and were followed for a median of 14 months (range, 12 to 34 months). Twelve patients (42.9%) reported improved rectal emptying. A good result was correlated with increased stool frequency, improved symptom index, and decreased laxative use. Long symptom duration, high pretreatment symptom index, and laxative use were associated with a poor outcome. Participants in the improved group tended to have less perineal descent and a prominent puborectalis impression on defectography.

Conclusion.—Biofeedback was effective for about 1 year in about 43% of patients with muscular activity during straining. Biofeedback may be used in the initial treatment of constipation in patients with paradoxical puborectalis contraction.

▶ Biofeedback has proved a useful tool in a variety of conditions from asthma to patellofemoral syndrome. Here are 2 studies (Abstracts 6–6 and 6–7) that would support at least a trial of biofeedback in your patients with constipation. Applying somewhat different methodology, including selection criteria, diagnostic and biofeedback techniques, these studies both report reasonable (not great) success. A counterpoint is provided in a similar study by Rieger et al,[1] which concluded that biofeedback is not to be recommended. This problem is noxious and embarrassing for our patients. Biofeedback certainly meets the criteria of *primum non nocere*; it is simple, noninvasive, and might be effective. Although I am not convinced that this would be my lead therapy in cases of acute constipation, I would certainly consider a trial for more chronic cases.

W.W. Dexter, M.D.

Reference

1. Rieger N, Wattchow D, Sarre R, et al: Prospective study of biofeedback for treatment of constipation. *Dis Colon Rectum* 40:1143–1148, 1997.

Gastrointestinal Symptoms Following Consumption of Olestra or Regular Triglyceride Potato Chips: A Controlled Comparison

Cheskin LJ, Miday R, Zorich N, et al (Johns Hopkins Univ, Baltimore, Md; Procter & Gamble, Cincinnati, Ohio)
JAMA 279:150-152, 1998

Objective.—There have been anecdotal reports of gastrointestinal complaints after consuming snack foods containing olestra, a nonabsorbable, energy-free fat substitute. The incidence of gastrointestinal complaints was assessed in a placebo-controlled, randomized, double-blind, parallel study allowing a large number of participants unlimited access to chips during a 2-hour sitting.

Methods.—A beverage and an unlabeled, white 369-g bag of potato chips prepared with olestra or regular triglycerides (TGs) were given to 1,123 volunteers who came to see a movie at a multiplex cinema. The volunteers were instructed to eat a meal 1-2 hours before arriving. Bags were weighed afterward to determine consumption. Telephone interviews were conducted approximately 40 hours to 10 days later to collect data on any adverse gastrointestinal reactions.

Results.—There were 1,092 evaluable volunteers, 563 in the olestra group and 529 in the TG group. The median consumption of TG chips was higher than that of olestra chips. The palatability of the TG chips was rated higher than that of olestra chips. The chips had similar satiety scores. There was no difference between the olestra and TG groups with respect to the number or type of gastrointestinal complaints (89 vs. 93). Consumption and symptom rate were not correlated.

Conclusions.—After 1 sitting and unlimited consumption of olestra or TG chips, there was no difference in number or type of gastrointestinal symptoms experienced.

▶ This study certainly makes the ones I "volunteered" for in medical school look pretty lame. Free movies and all the chips you care to eat—sure beats the gingivitis study I was recruited for, but I won't go there! Dr. Cheskin and his colleagues demonstrated that, at least for potato chips, olestra seems to be well tolerated. A happy result for Procter & Gamble—forgive me if I am a bit skeptical given the obvious bias of the sponsor. Nevertheless, as far as it goes, the science is reasonably sound. Although I would prefer to see what, if any, adverse effects occur with regular intake of this product, one of the principal concerns about olestra use, adverse gastrointestinal side effects, seems to be put to rest. Will olestra and like products prove to be a safe food product? Will it help reduce fat intake and, subsequently, reduce atherosclerotic disease risk as some other foods so touted (oatmeal for instance)? I am not sure, but for now, as a confessed "closet" chip consumer, I will feel a bit less guilty at lunch.

W.W. Dexter, M.D.

Miscellaneous

A Comparison of Budesonide and Mesalamine for Active Crohn's Disease
Thomsen OØ, for the International Budesonide–Mesalamine Study Group (Univ of Copenhagen; Hôpital Claude Huriez, Lille, France; John Radcliffe Hosp, Oxford, England; et al)
N Engl J Med 339:370–374, 1998   6–9

Introduction.—A chronic inflammatory disorder of the bowel whose cause is unknown, Crohn's disease is often treated with glucocorticoids such as prednisolone and prednisone. These drugs, however, can cause moon face, hirsutism, and acne. A highly potent topical anti-inflammatory agent with lower systemic activity than conventional glucocorticoids is budesonide. It was found to be significantly more effective than placebo in inducing remission of active Crohn's disease affecting the ileum and ascending colon. In patients with mild to moderately active Crohn's disease, slow-release formulations of mesalamine that facilitate delivery of the drug to the small intestine are often used as first-line treatment, although results in controlled studies were conflicting.

Methods.—There were 182 patients with Crohn's disease who were randomly assigned to receive 9 mg of budesonide (93 patients) daily or 2 g of mesalamine twice daily (89 patients) for 16 weeks in a double-blind, multicenter trial. The patients had scores of 200 to 400 on the Crohn's Disease Activity Index, with higher scores indicating greater disease activity.

Results.—In the budesonide group the rate of remission after 8 weeks of treatment was 69%, and in the mesalamine group the rate of remission was 45%. After 16 weeks of treatment, the rate of remission for the budesonide group was 62%, and for the mesalamine group it was 36%. In the budesonide group, 77 patients completed the 16 weeks of treatment, whereas in the mesalamine group, 50 patients completed 16 weeks of treatment. In the 2 group, the numbers of patients with adverse events were similar, but fewer severe adverse events occurred in the group assigned to the budesonide group. In 67% of the budesonide-treated patients, the morning plasma cortisol value was normal, whereas 83% of the mesalamine-treated patients had normal morning plasma cortisol values. Normal increases in cortisol in response to cosyntropin occurred in 90% of the budesonide group and in 100% of the mesalamine group.

Conclusion.—A controlled-ileal-release formulation of budesonide was more effective in inducing remission than a slow-release formulation of mesalamine in patients with active Crohn's disease affecting the ileum, the ascending colon, or both.

▶ Inflammatory bowel disease, especially Crohn's disease, can be difficult to treat effectively. Although this study was supported by the manufacturers of the drug being studied (ileal release budesonide), the results appear quite sturdy. This preparation is effective and well tolerated. Whether you actively manage these patients in your practice or refer them, here is an effective tool to help treat your patients with moderately active Crohn's disease.

W.W. Dexter, M.D.

The Relation of Physical Activity to Risk for Symptomatic Gallstone Disease in Men

Leitzmann MF, Giovannucci EL, Rimm EB, et al (Harvard School of Public Health, Boston; Harvard Med School, Boston; Brigham and Women's Hosp, Boston)

Ann Intern Med 128:417–425, 1998   6–10

Background.—Gallstone disease is a major source of morbidity in the United States. The effect of physical activity on gallstone disease has not been well studied. The effect of physical activity on the risk of development of symptomatic gallstone disease was examined in a large cohort of male health professionals in the United States.

Study Design.—The Health Professionals Follow-up Study is a longitudinal study involving 51,529 American male health professionals who were between the ages of 40 and 75 years in 1986. Participants complete a detailed health questionnaire every 2 years. For this analysis, the sample was composed of 45,813 men who had never had gallstone disease and were followed from 1986 to 1994. Physical activity was scored as metabolic equivalents, with activities requiring more than 6 metabolic equivalents per hour considered vigorous. A weekly physical inactivity score based on hours spent watching television was calculated separately. Men under the age of 65 years were compared with older men.

Results.—During the 324,263 person-years of this study, there were 828 documented cases of symptomatic gallstones, of which 661 required cholecystectomy. After adjustment for multiple confounding variables, increased physical activity was inversely related to the risk for symptomatic gallstone disease. This association was stronger for men under the age of 65 years. Sedentary behavior was positively related to risk for symptomatic gallstone disease. Men who watched television more than 40 hours per week had a significantly higher risk for symptomatic gallstone disease than those who watched less than 6 hours per week. Increasing exercise to 30 minutes of endurance training 5 times a week could prevent 34% of cases of symptomatic gallstone disease in men.

Conclusion.—Physical activity may be important in the prevention of symptomatic gallstone disease in men. These results can be generalized to American men over the age of 40 years and may not apply to other at-risk populations. Further research is needed to expand these findings to other groups, especially women, who are at higher risk for gallstones.

▶ Here is one more reason to encourage your patients—and engage yourself—in regular exercise. Or at least to get off the couch: Increased TV time increases gallstone risk. (Can you believe that there is a subgroup of health professionals who watch more than 40 hours of television per week?) One big hole in this study is the fact that gallstones are far more common in women than men, and the Health Professionals Follow-up Study includes men only. Thus, exercise may not provide similar risk reduction for women, although I suspect it would. The authors cite conflicting studies on this point. This ongoing study is generating some very interesting epidemiologic data. Although data are all self-report and done by retrospective questionnaire, the scope lends credence to the findings.

W.W. Dexter, M.D.

Enteral Nutrition Is Superior to Parenteral Nutrition in Severe Acute Pancreatitis: Results of a Randomized Prospective Trial
Kalfarentzos F, Kehagias J, Mead N, et al (Univ of Patras, Greece)
Br J Surg 84:1665–1669, 1997
6–11

Background.—Early aggressive nutritional support is essential in severe acute pancreatitis. The standard method of providing exogenous nutrients to these patients has been total parenteral nutrition (TPN). The usefulness, tolerance, clinical outcome, and cost of TPN were compared with enteral feeding (EF) for nutritional support of patients with severe acute pancreatitis in a prospective, randomized clinical trial.

Methods.—Between July 1990 and December 1995, 326 patients with acute pancreatitis participated in this study. All patients were intensively monitored for 72 hours and given fluid replacement and respiratory support as needed. Patients were randomized to EF through a nasoenteric feeding tube with a peptide-based formula (18 patients) or standard TPN through a subclavian catheter (20 patients). Patient records were reviewed for complications, ICU stay, hospital stay, ventilator days, number of days of nutritional support, antibiotics, and average cost.

Results.—Enteral feedings was well tolerated by patients with severe acute pancreatitis and were as efficacious as TPN. The EF patients had fewer complications and had a lower risk of sepsis development, compared with the TPN patients. The cost of TPN support was 3 times higher than the cost of EF support for these patients.

Conclusion.—Enteral support was safe, well-tolerated, and effective and was associated with fewer complications and fewer infections than TPN. The results of this prospective, randomized trial suggest that EF should be the preferred method of nutritional support for patients with severe acute pancreatitis.

▶ "Nothing by mouth" has been a standard order written for patients with acute pancreatitis. This study challenges this dogma while supporting a lesson I learned during my surgical rotations as a medical student: If the gut works, use it. This was a small study of patients who were quite ill. Enteral feedings proved less costly, were effective and safe, and led to few complications.

This population probably does not represent the typical pancreatitis patient a family physician might manage. One wonders if this approach would work as well for patients with less severe disease. Note that the patients in this study all received nothing by mouth during the first 3 days of treatment, about the length of time it takes to "quiet down" someone with moderate disease.

Thus, I am not ready to change my practice just yet. I would like to see a larger study that also looks at more moderate disease and earlier feeding. For severe disease, these results are very intriguing, and early EF is worth discussing with your consultants as you manage these patients.

W.W. Dexter, M.D.

Ursodeoxycholic Acid Delays the Onset of Esophageal Varices in Primary Biliary Cirrhosis
Lindor KD, Jorgensen RA, Therneau TM, et al (Mayo Clinic, Rochester, Minn)
Mayo Clin Proc 72:1137–1140, 1997   6–12

Introduction.—Earlier trials have shown that ursodeoxycholic acid (UDCA) treatment in patients with primary biliary cirrhosis (PBC) provides biochemical improvement, delays time until treatment failure, and prolongs time until liver transplantation or death. The effect of UDCA on the development of varices has not been determined, therefore the effect of UDCA therapy on the development of esophageal varices was prospectively assessed in 180 patients with PBC.

Methods.—Patients were randomized to up to 4 years of treatment with either UDCA, 13–15 mg/kg daily, or placebo. All patients underwent endoscopy every 2 years or as clinically necessary. All patients in the placebo group were offered UDCA at completion of the 4-year assessment period. The risk of the development of endoscopically confirmed varices was calculated.

TABLE 3.—Time to Development of Esophageal Varices in Study Patients With Primary Biliary Cirrhosis, Stratified by Type of Treatment

| | | With esophageal varices | | | | |
| | | UDCA | | | Placebo | |
Time	%	95% CI	No. of patients	%	95% CI	No. of patients
Baseline	0	...	70	0	...	69
Year 2	11	3-19	60	22	10-33	54
Year 4	16	3-27	25	58	29-75	24

Note: Patients were censored from the study at last esophagogastroduodenoscopy.
Abbreviations: CI, confidence interval; UDCA, ursodeoxycholic acid.
(Courtesy of Lindor KD, Jorgensen RA, Therneau TM, et al: Ursodeoxycholic acid delays the onset of esophageal varices in primary biliary cirrhosis. *Mayo Clin Proc* 72:1137–1140, 1997.)

Results.—At trial entry, esophagogastroduodenoscopy revealed that of 180 patients, 139 had no esophageal varices and 41 had varices. At completion of the 4-year treatment, the risk of new development of endoscopically confirmed varices was significantly less for the UDCA group than for the placebo group (16% vs. 58%) (Table 3). Treatment with UDCA was correlated with a significantly lower risk of varices development in patients with PBC.

Conclusion.—Treatment with UDCA reduces the risk of the development of esophageal varices in patients with PBC. These findings support the growing evidence that UDCA is an effective therapy for patients with this disease.

▶ The last line of the article is really the bottom line: "The results of the current study further support the growing evidence that UDCA is an effective treatment for patients with PBC." The reduction in varices in this placebo-controlled trial is just one of a number of positive results from this medication. Interestingly, the incidence of variceal bleeding actually increased. The explanation, that UDCA treatment increases time to transplant, allowing more time to have a bleed, is certainly plausible. In any case, I included this article as a reminder that UDCA is effective therapy for PBC.

W.W. Dexter, M.D.

A Prognostic Model for Patients With End-Stage Liver Disease
Cooper GS, Bellamy P, Dawson NV, et al (Case Western Reserve Univ, Cleveland, Ohio; Univ of California, Los Angeles; Marshfield Clinic, Wis; et al)
Gastroenterology 113:1278–1288, 1997   6–13

Introduction.—Survival of patients with end-stage liver disease is difficult to predict. A 2-stage, prospective cohort investigation was undertaken at 5 teaching hospitals to develop and analyze a model for prediction of death in patients with end-stage liver disease. Phase I and phase II patients were enrolled from June 1989 to June 1991 and January 1992 to January 1994, respectively.

Methods.—Data from 538 patients hospitalized with end-stage liver disease and 2 or more signs of decompensation were abstracted from medical charts from trial day 3 regarding the following: hospital discharge, each hospitalization during the next 6 months at the same facility, demographics, cause of liver disease, reason for admission, co-morbid illnesses, physical findings, laboratory indices of liver function, the Glasgow coma score, and severity of illness.

Results.—The cumulative incidence of death at 30 days and 6 months were 30% and 50%, respectively. The time to death in 295 patients in phase I was independently associated with 5 factors examined on day 3: renal insufficiency, cognitive dysfunction, ventilatory insufficiency, age 65 years or older, and prothrombin time of 16 seconds or more (Table 3). These risk factors were used to stratify the 243 patients in phase II into

TABLE 3.—Independent Predictors of Survival Time: Results of Cox Proportional Hazards Analysis Among 295 Patients in Phase I

Variable*	Relative hazard (95% CI)†	Points
Renal insufficiency		
Creatinine 1–2 mg/dL	1.65 (1.32–2.07)	1
Creatinine >2 mg/dL	2.73 (2.17–3.43)	2
Cognitive dysfunction		
Glasgow coma score 10–14	1.66 (1.28–2.16)	1
Glasgow coma score <10	2.76 (2.13–3.59)	2
Age ≥65 yr	1.71 (1.17–2.51)	1
Prothrombin time ≥16 s	1.60 (1.13–2.26)	1
Mechanical ventilation or hypoxemia (pO_2 < 60)	2.19 (1.49–3.21)	1

*All variables were measured on study day 3.

†In the multivariate model, the relative hazards for serum creatinine, Glasgow coma score, and hypoxemia/mechanical ventilation were different from 1 ($P < 0.001$). The relative hazard for age was different from 1 ($P = 0.006$); the relative hazard for prothrombin time was different from 1 ($P = 0.009$).

Abbreviations: CI, confidence interval; pO_2, partial pressure of oxygen.

(Courtesy of Cooper GS, Bellamy P, Dawson NV, et al: A prognostic model for patients with end-stage liver disease. Gastroenterology 113:1278–1288, 1997.)

low-, middle-, and high-risk groups. The cumulative incidences of death in the model created from phase I disease at 30 days were 12%, 40%, and 74%, respectively, for low-, middle-, and high-risk groups (Fig 2). Integration of this prognostic model with physicians' predictions improved estimates of the probability of death. Transplantation after trial entry was independently correlated with enhanced survival; intensity of other acute therapies was not correlated with enhanced survival.

Conclusion.—The risk of death in patients with end-stage liver disease could be calculated using 5 independent risk factors. These data provide a quantitative basis for supplementing physicians' prognostic estimates.

▶ Over the past year, I have been involved as a preceptor in the care of several patients with end-stage liver disease. Having had this study available would have been most useful. Decisions regarding transplantation, quality of life, and end of life entered into almost every office visit and, certainly, each hospitalization. Desiring, but often lacking, prognostic information, the patient, family, and physician struggle with these decisions. The information presented here will not guide treatment recommendations per se, but it will certainly inform the discussion with the patient and family.

W.W. Dexter, M.D.

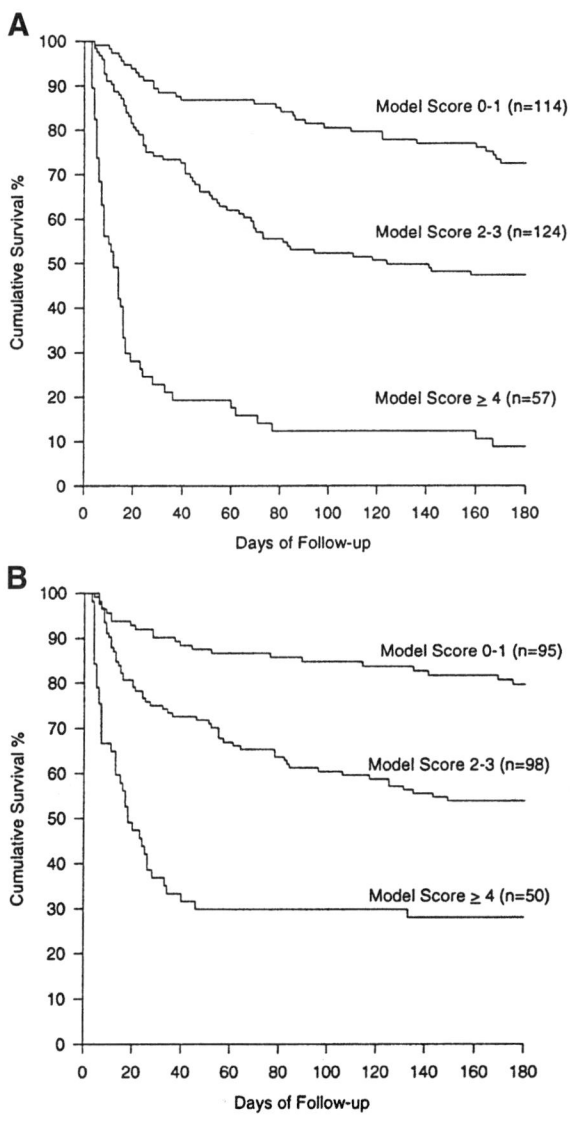

FIGURE 2.—The association of point score assigned by the multivariate model with survival in (**A**) phase I and (**B**) phase II. In each phase, survival differed between patients with different point scores (*P* less than 0.0001 in phase I and phase II by the log rank test). (Courtesy of Cooper GS, Bellamy P, Dawson NV: A prognostic model for patients with end-stage liver disease. *Gastroenterology* 113:1278–1288, 1997.)

Effect of Computed Tomography of the Appendix on Treatment of Patients and Use of Hospital Resources

Rao PM, Rhea JT, Novelline RA, et al (Massachusetts Gen Hosp, Boston)
N Engl J Med 338:141–146, 1998

Objective.—Approximately half the patients hospitalized for suspected appendicitis ultimately receive a diagnosis for another condition. About 20% of appendicitis cases are missed, and 15% to 40% of patients undergo appendectomies unnecessarily. The accuracy of CT in diagnosing or ruling out appendicitis was evaluated.

Methods.—Computed tomography was performed on 100 consecutive patients (43 males), aged 6 to 75 years, admitted for suspected appendicitis. The CT results were compared with surgical findings, and by clinical follow-up at 2 months in 41 patients. Treatment plans before CT were compared with actual treatment after CT. Utilization of hospital resources was analyzed retrospectively.

Results.—At surgery for appendicitis or other conditions, 53 patients had appendicitis and 47 did not. The CT results were positive in 53 patients, negative in 45, false positive in 1, and false negative in 1, for sensitivity, specificity, positive predictive value, negative predictive value, and overall accuracy rates of 98%. The CT results changed treatment strategies for 59 patients, including prevention of unnecessary appendectomy in 13, admission for observation in 18, admission for observation prior to appendectomy in 21, and admission for observation prior to diagnosis by CT of other medical conditions in 11. Prevention of unnecessary appendectomy in 13 patients resulted in a savings of $47,281 in surgical and allied costs and in a savings of 50 hospitalization days ($20,250). After deducting the cost of 100 CT scans ($22,800), the resulting savings per patient was $447.

Conclusion.—Routine CT scans of patients with suspected appendicitis decrease unnecessary surgery and reduce the use of hospital resources, resulting in a $447 per patient savings.

▶ Just when we think the clinical diagnosis of acute appendicitis is well established, along comes definitive proof that routine CT scanning is indicated. Most of us were taught to accept up to 50% normal appendices at operation for clinically suspected appendicitis. That was fine for being careful not to miss cases but may not be well liked by all of those patients receiving "unnecessary surgery." Routine CT scanning offers the promise of more accurate diagnosis and a reduction in unnecessary surgery.

J.E. Scherger, M.D., M.P.H.

7 Skin Conditions

Overview

Randomized controlled trials: Abstracts 7–2 and 7–4

Sun Exposure
- Sunscreens in the prevention of actinic damage and skin cancer
- Vitamins C and E in protecting against sunburn
- Pathophysiology of damage induced by ultraviolet light

Therapeutics
- Anti-inflammatory activity of antifungals
- The cytochrome P-450 system and dermatologic therapies
- Treating palmar hyperhidrosis with botulinum toxin
- Treatment of severe vulvar lichen sclerosus
- Potent steroid found in Chinese herbal topical cream

Miscellaneous
- Differences among physicians in prescribing for cutaneous fungal infections
- Atopic dermatitis and food hypersensitivity
- Incidence of invasive cancer following basal cell cancer
- Photoaging and topical tretinoin

Sun Exposure

The Case for Sunscreens: A Review of Their Use in Preventing Actinic Damage and Neoplasia
Naylor MF, Farmer KC (Univ of Oklahoma, Oklahoma City)
Arch Dermatol 133:1146–1154, 1997   7–1

Objective.—Recently controversy has arisen over the use of sunscreens. The use of sunscreens for the prevention of photodamage and carcinogenesis was reviewed.

Ultraviolet Damage and Sunscreens.—Ultraviolet (UV) radiation can cause direct tissue and cellular damage and also local and systemic immunosuppression that can lead to carcinogenesis via DNA damage.

Sunscreen Controversy.—Sunscreens can lead to cutaneous reactions and potentially to vitamin D deficiency by decreasing its synthesis. 2-Ethylhexyl *p*-methoxycinnamate (2–EHMC) has shown weak mutagenicity in the Ames test, which is known to have a high false positive rate. Compounds such as retinoic acid can promote tumor growth in mice. Because mutagenic substances would have to penetrate the multilayered epidermis before significant damage could occur, evidence indicates that the protective effects of sunscreens outweigh their potential risks. There is little evidence to suggest that immunosuppression resulting from sunscreen use is a significant problem, although research continues. Evidence indicates that there is an increased risk of melanoma associated with exposure to UV-B and short UV-A wavelengths, but for ethical reasons, controlled human studies of sunscreen use for protection against melanoma have not been conducted. Because melanoma incidence and mortality have declined in Australia with increased use of sunscreen, it would appear that sunscreen use does not cause melanoma. Sunscreens are usually not applied thickly enough to maximize their high sun protection factor (SPF) content.

Conclusions.—Sunscreens are the most flexible and practical tool for protecting against sunlight-induced skin cancers.

▶ Recently, in both the lay and professional press, there have been questions raised about the efficacy of sunscreens in the prevention of skin cancers, in particular, melanoma. As the authors of this review correctly point out, a controlled human trial to investigate this would be unethical. Thus, our recommendations to use sunscreens must be based principally on epidemiologic studies, some of which offer conflicting evidence. While the conclusions reached by the authors are not surprising, I do feel they have constructed a solid theoretical and practical case from the available evidence supporting sunscreen use. We need to continue to educate our patients about melanoma risks. I will continue to recommend high SPF sunscreen to my patients and family.

W.W. Dexter, M.D.

Protective Effect Against Sunburn of Combined Systemic Ascorbic Acid (Vitamin C) and d-α-Tocopherol (Vitamin E)
Eberlein-König B, Placzek M, Przybilla B (Dermatologische Klinik und Poliklinik der Ludwig-Maximilians-Universität München, Munich)
J Am Acad Dermatol 38:45–48, 1998 7–2

Objective.—Ultraviolet (UV)-induced skin damage is caused by free radical oxygen species. Use of antioxidants may decrease the damage. The effect of oral ascorbic acid (vitamin C) and d-α-tocopherol (vitamin E) on sunburn was investigated in a double-blind, placebo-controlled study.

Methods.—Either 2 g of ascorbic acid plus 1,000 IU of vitamin E or placebo was administered for 8 days to 20 healthy white volunteers (4 women), aged 23 to 46 years. At baseline and 8 days later, 12 areas on the lower back of each volunteer were exposed to increasing UVB doses, sufficient to elicit sunburn (minimal erythema dose). The cutaneous blood flow at each site was measured with a laser Doppler flowmeter and compared with measurements at adjacent, nonirradiated sites.

Results.—Whereas the minimal erythema dose increased significantly from 80 to 96.5 mJ/cm^2 in the treated group compared with baseline, minimal erythema dose values decreased significantly from 80 to 68.5 mJ/cm^2 in the placebo group. Ultraviolet-activated molecules induce membrane lipid peroxidation, which vitamin E inhibits. Vitamin C responds synergistically by regenerating vitamin E in a reaction similar to those that occur with unsaturated lipids in micelles or in phosphatidyl liposomes. The effect of combined vitamin C and E use is small when compared with the protection conferred by sunscreens with protection factors of 20 or larger.

Conclusion.—A combination of oral vitamins C and E reduces the damage caused by UVB irradiation and may decrease the risk of long-term skin damage. The increase in sunburn in the placebo group at second exposure may be the result of a "priming" effect.

▶ This study from Germany shows that a combination of 2 g of vitamin C and 1,000 IU of vitamin E taken together orally reduces sunburn. The overall effect is rather small (SPF 1.4), and should not be seen as an alternative to using sunscreen or wearing protective clothing. It appears that the 2 antioxidant vitamins taken together are substantially more effective than either taken alone. The significance of these findings is not yet clear, and family physicians should not be advised to recommend this therapy as definitive protection from sunburn and sun-damaged skin. However, some people are repeatedly and continuously exposed to sunlight (e.g., lifeguards), and taking these 2 vitamins may have some protective effect.

J.E. Scherger, M.D., M.P.H.

Pathophysiology of Premature Skin Aging Induced by Ultraviolet Light
Fisher GJ, Wang ZQ, Datta SC, et al (Univ of Michigan, Ann Arbor)
N Engl J Med 337:1419–1428, 1997   7–3

Objective.—Characteristics of photoaged skin include wrinkles, pigmentary alterations, and loss of skin tone. Histologic and ultrastructural studies of photoaged skin have shown major changes in the collagenous extracellular matrix of connective tissue. The matrix-degrading metalloproteinases were investigated as possible mediators of collagen damage in photoaging.

Methods.—The study included 59 white research subjects (age range, 21–58 years). All had light-to-moderate skin pigmentation and no current or previous skin disease. Buttock skin was irradiated by fluorescent ultraviolet lights, and specimens of irradiated and nonirradiated skin were obtained. The effects of tretinoin or vehicle—applied to the skin under occlusion for 48 hours before irradiation—were studied as well. In situ hybridization, immunohistologic, and in situ zymographic studies were performed to assess the expression of matrix metalloproteinases. Radioimmunoassay of soluble cross-linked telopeptides was done to measure irradiation-induced degradation of skin collagen, and Western blotting was used to assess the protein level of tissue inhibitor of matrix metalloproteinases type 1.

Results.—After just 1 exposure to ultraviolet radiation, there were significant increases in expression of 3 matrix metalloproteinases in the skin connective tissue and outer skin layers compared with nonirradiated skin. These were collagenase, a 92-kd gelatinase, and stromelysin. Irradiated skin showed a 58% increase in degradation of endogenous type I collagen fibrils. After 4 exposures to ultraviolet irradiation, collagenase and gelatinase activity remained at peak levels for 7 days. Tretinoin pretreatment was associated with a 70% to 80% inhibition of induction of matrix metalloproteinase proteins and activity in both connective tissue and outer skin layers. A tissue inhibitor of matrix metalloproteinases-1, which regulates the enzyme, was also induced by ultraviolet irradiation. Tretinoin had no effect on the induction of this inhibitor.

Conclusions.—Ultraviolet irradiation causes sustained increases in matrix metalloproteinases that degrade skin collagen. These metalloproteinases may play an important role in photoaging. Topical tretinoin inhibits the induction of matrix metalloproteinases in response to irradiation but does not affect their endogenous inhibitor.

▶ This is an experimental study providing partial information regarding the mechanism of skin damage induced by ultraviolet light. The study also suggests a partial role for topical tretinoin in inhibiting this damage. I included this article (1) to provide more description about the important problem of skin damage caused by ultraviolet light from the sun and (2) to show that medical treatment is only a partial solution. Burning of the skin with ultraviolet light should be avoided whenever possible and is a new health education recommendation that must be reinforced repeatedly by family physicians.

J.E. Scherger, M.D., M.P.H.

Therapeutics

Anti-inflammatory Activity of Antifungal Preparations
Rosen T, Schell BJ, Orengo I (Baylor College of Medicine, Houston)
Int J Dermatol 36:788–792, 1997   7–4

Objective.—Because steroid/antifungal treatments can lead to adverse effects, primarily because of the steroid component, an antifungal drug with anti-inflammatory properties would be useful. The anti-inflammatory properties of several antifungal drugs were determined and compared in a randomized, double-blind, controlled study using the erythema response to ultraviolet (UV) light.

Methods.—The non–sun-exposed skin of the ventral forearm of 20 healthy white volunteers (3 men), aged 25 to 53 years, was irradiated at 8 sites, using a 150-W xenon short-arc solar simulator with UVB. Each

TABLE 1.—Erythema Scores After 2 Minimum Erythema Doses of Ultraviolet B Irradiation

Variable	Minimum	Maximum	Mean	Std Deviation	Std Error
Ciclopirox	0.0	4.0	2.15	1.26	0.28
Naftifine	0.0	4.0	2.40	0.94	0.21
Terbinafine	0.0	5.0	2.50	1.14	0.25
Ketoconazole	0.0	5.0	2.95	1.09	0.24
Oxiconazole	2.0	5.0	3.45	0.68	0.15
Econazole	3.0	4.0	3.60	0.50	0.11
Hydrocortisone	2.0	5.0	3.85	0.87	0.19
Control	3.0	5.0	4.30	3.51	0.12

Note: Scores are based on a 0 (no erythema) to 5 (severe erythema) scale.
(Courtesy of Rosen T, Schell BJ, Orengo I: Anti-inflammatory activity of antifungal preparations. *Int J Dermatol* 36:788–792, 1997. Used with permission of Blackwell Science Ltd.)

individual's minimum erythema dose was determined. One day after exposure, skin portals were evaluated for erythema. Study creams (2.5% hydrocortisone, 1% terbinafine, 1% ciclopirox olamine, 1% naftifine hydrochloride, 2% ketoconazole, 1% oxiconazole nitrate, and 1% econazole nitrate) were applied to different skin portals on each arm twice daily for 2 days, with 1 portal left untreated as the control. On day 3, the skin was cleaned and irradiated again at twice the individual's minimum erythema dose. Creams were applied (except to the control portal) immediately and at 12 hours (except to the control portal). Skin portals were evaluated 24 hours after irradiation and graded on a 1 to 5 color scale (Table 1).

Results.—Ciclopirox, naftifine, and terbinafine were significantly superior to econazole, oxiconazole, hydrocortisone, and control. Ketoconazole was intermediate in effectiveness and significantly better than econazole, hydrocortisone, and control.

Conclusion.—Antifungal preparations such as ciclopirox, naftifine, and terbinafine possess anti-inflammatory activity.

▶ The inflammatory component of fungal infections of the skin has only recently been recognized. Treating the inflammation along with an effective antifungal drug clears the lesions more rapidly. Hence, many physicians have chosen combined steroid/antifungal topical preparations. This study shows that many antifungal medications have substantial anti-inflammatory activity. As the table indicates, this anti-inflammatory activity may be greater than that of 2.5% hydrocortisone! No more use of those expensive combinations.

J.E. Scherger, M.D., M.P.H.

Cytochrome P-450 3A: Interactions With Dermatologic Therapies
Singer MI, Shapiro LE, Shear NH, et al (Univ of Toronto)
J Am Acad Dermatol 37:765–771, 1997

7–5

Purpose.—Drug interactions involving the cytochrome P-450 mixed function oxidase system have emerged as an important cause of toxicity and reduced treatment efficacy. The cytochrome P-450 3A3/4 isoenzymes are involved in many of the clinically significant drug interactions. Understanding the principles of these interactions could help to avoid potentially serious interactions involving both new and familiar drugs. Interactions involving the cytochrome P-450 3A (CYP3A) subfamily of isoenzymes are reviewed.

CYP3A Drug Interactions.—The CYP3A isoenzymes are a major metabolizing isoform for many commonly prescribed dermatologic drugs, particularly the CYP3A3 and CYP3A4 isoforms. Drug interactions involving CYP3A may occur through either enzyme inhibition or induction. Inhibition of CYP3A can lead to increased plasma drug concentration, increased drug response, and thus toxicity. Beginning with the first or second dose, CYP3A inhibition may be maximal by the time drug steady-state concentration is achieved. Some drugs are "accomplices" that cause another drug to become dangerous or less effective; others are "bullets" or "blanks" that cause toxicity or decreased efficacy, respectively. Some inhibitory interactions occur through complex formation with the heme moiety of cytochrome P-450 isoenzyme, such as cimetidine, ketoconazole, and macrolide antibiotics. Others, such as chloramphenicol or spironolactone, cause cytochrome-inactivating suicidal reactive intermediate metabolites. Numerous other mechanisms are operative as well, including simple cytochrome P-450 binding site competition between 2 drugs metabolized by the same enzyme. Substrates metabolized by CYP3A3/4 isoenzymes include cyclosporine, tacrolimus, cisapride, terfenadine, astemizole, and nifedipine, while inhibitors of these enzymes include imidazole-triazole antifungals, oral contraceptives, cimetidine, and macrolide antibiotics. Peripheral edema may occur from an interaction between nifedipine and itraconazole. It may be possible to predict such adverse interactions using in vitro testing.

Other interactions can occur as a result of induction of CYP3A. Such drugs include rifampin, the most potent inducer of P-4503A; dexamethasone, anticonvulsants; and griseofulvin. Rifampin may induce CYP3A3/4 that metabolizes estrogens, causing oral contraceptive failure. Porphyritic crises may result from persistent cytochrome P-450 induction by anticonvulsants and/or alcohol. Accomplice drugs can also bioactivate a CYP3A substrate to active, potentially toxic metabolites. Metabolic activation of cyclophosphamide leads to the formation of acrolein, which is a cause of bladder toxicity. Drugs that induce CYP3A may increase conversion of a prodrug to its active metabolites, thus leading to increased pharmacologic effect and increased toxicity.

Summary.—The CYP3A3/4 isoenzymes mediate a number of diverse and potentially serious drug interactions. These interactions may result from inhibition or induction of CYP3A. Knowing the principles of these interactions, and their recently discovered molecular mechanisms, may have a major influence on patient outcome.

▶ Family physicians must become familiar with this mechanism of drug interaction and aware of the groups of drugs influenced by this enzyme system. While dermatologic medications are among the most commonly involved, many other drugs are also included. This type of biochemical understanding of drug interactions is likely to become more common, including genetic testing for identifying patients at risk.

J.E. Scherger, M.D., M.P.H.

Botulinum Toxin Therapy for Palmar Hyperhidrosis
Shelley WB, Talanin NY, Shelley ED (Med College of Ohio, Toledo)
J Am Acad Dermatol 38:227–229, 1998   7–6

Background.—Severe palmar hyperhidrosis is a chronic disease that can cause serious social, psychological, and occupational problems. Conservative treatment is not always effective. A permanent treatment is endoscopic transthoracic sympathectomy, but this can cause pneumothorax and complications from general anesthesia. Botulinum toxin therapy has been used successfully for localized hyperhidrosis. It blocks the release of acetylcholine from presynaptic membranes, thereby inhibiting sweat production. It can help various conditions, such as blepharospasm, strabismus, focal dystonia, spasmodic dysphonia, and achalasia.

Methods.—The short-term and long-term effectiveness of botulinum toxin therapy was determined in 4 female patients with severe palmar hyperhidrosis. The patients were between 14 and 34 years of age and had had palmar hyperhidrosis since childhood. Patients were given regional nerve blocks of the median and ulnar nerves, then 50 injections, 2 mouse units each, of botulinum toxin in each palm. Follow-up was 12 months.

Results.—Significantly reduced sweat production in the treated areas of the palms was noted after botulinum toxin injection. In 1 patient, anhidrosis lasted for 12 months. In the other 3 patients, anhidrosis lasted for 7 months and 4 months. One patient had mild weakness of the thumb that resolved in 3 weeks. There were no other side effects.

Discussion.—These results show that superficial botulinum toxin injections are effective treatment for palmar hyperhidrosis. The treatment is comparatively safe and relieved sweating from 4 to 12 months. Subepidermal rather than subcutaneous injections were given to deliver the botulinum toxin as close as possible to the sweat glands. Nerve blocks made the injections significantly less painful for patients.

▶ Who would think that the toxin of botulism would find widespread use in medicine? There is very little that we can offer patients with hyperhidrosis, and this treatment may seem somewhat drastic. I am impressed by the growing list of conditions for which this treatment may be used. I suspect that we may be hearing more about this novel form of therapy.

J.E. Scherger, M.D., M.P.H.

Clobetasol Dipropionate 0.05% Versus Testosterone Propionate 2% Topical Application for Severe Vulvar Lichen Sclerosus
Bornstein J, Heifetz S, Kellner Y, et al (Carmel Med Ctr, Haifa, Israel)
Am J Obstet Gynecol 178:80–84, 1998

Objective.—The various topical and systemic drugs that have been used to treat lichen sclerosus have not produced satisfactory results. Testosterone propionate 2% has been the treatment of choice because of concern that corticosteroids will exacerbate the atrophy already seen. The corticosteroid clobetasol does not cause atrophy. The topical treatment by testosterone propionate 2% and clobetasol 0.05% for lichen sclerosus was compared for short- and long-term applications.

Methods.—Between 1988 and 1993, 20 women treated with testosterone propionate 2% and 20 treated with clobetasol 0.05% for lichen sclerosus were followed up for at least 1 year. Patients were evaluated at 3 months and 1 year, and responses and degree of atrophy were recorded.

Results.—Patients were postmenopausal women whose average age was 64 years. At 3 months, subjective outcomes were similar, whereas gynecologic examination indicated that the clobetasol group was significantly more improved than the testosterone group. At 12 months, 90% of the clobetasol group and 10% of the testosterone group had a response (Table 3). Significantly more testosterone patients than clobetasol patients discontinued treatment because of lack of response. Six patients in the testosterone group and 1 patient in the clobetasol group had side effects. Significantly more women in the clobetasol group than in the testosterone group were satisfied with their treatment (18 vs. 7).

Conclusions.—Clobetasol is significantly more effective than testosterone for the treatment of lichen sclerosus and results in fewer side effects.

▶ This article convinces me to switch from testosterone to clobetasol for treating vulvar lichen sclerosus. I used testosterone because of my fear that the steroids would lead to more skin atrophy. The difference in outcome at

TABLE 3.—Treatment Outcome at 12-Month Follow-up

	Complete Response No.	Complete Response %	Incomplete Response No.	Incomplete Response %	No Response No.	No Response %	Total No.
Subjective (symptoms)*							
Clobetasol	10	50	8	40	2	10	20
Testosterone	5	25	3	15	12	60	20
Objective (signs)†							
Clobetasol	10	50	8	40	2	10	20
Testosterone	5	25	3	15	12	60	20

*$P \leq 0.02$.
†$P \leq 0.02$.
(Courtesy of Bornstein J, Heifetz S, Kellner Y, et al: Clobetasol dipropionate 0.05% versus testosterone propionate 2% topical application for severe vulvar lichen sclerosus. Am J Obstet Gynecol 178:80–84, 1998.)

1 year between testosterone and clobetasol was remarkable, and the patient adherence rates corresponded. The patients had severe conditions and were referred, which may not be typical for what is seen in the family physician office. As the authors do not note whether the subjects were randomized, or whether the assessments were blinded, the amount of difference may be overstated.

M.A. Bowman, M.D., M.P.A.

Potent Topical Steroid in a Chinese Herbal Cream
Wood B, Wishart J (Auckland Hosp, New Zealand)
N Z Med J 110:420–421, 1997

Objective.—With the growing popularity of "alternative medicine," there is concern over the possible contents of some of the preparations used in treatment. Some of these products may have inherent toxicities, which may be difficult to identify without correct labeling. A very potent topical steroid marketed as a Chinese herbal remedy is reported.

Case Report.—Woman, 53, consulted a dermatologist because of psoriasis. She had been using a topical cream recommended by a Chinese health center. Her psoriasis improved considerably but she could not afford the medication any longer. Liquid chromatography was performed on a sample of the cream, showing that it contained a high concentration of clobetasol propionate. The authors notified the Health Department, which took appropriate action.

Discussion.—A "Chinese herbal cream" that proved to contain the potent steroid clobetasol propionate is reported. Potentially hazardous drugs are being sold at unauthorized outlets by untrained personnel to patients seeking "alternative" remedies. The clinician should be aware that such illegal products may be available to patients.

▶ This remarkable brief report is included to remind us that not all herbal presentations are as innocent as herbal tea. This report from New Zealand describes a Chinese herbal cream that contained a potent topical steroid. We must be alert for the possibility of serious drugs included in alternative therapies and not recommend products we do not know about.

J.E. Scherger, M.D., M.P.H.

Miscellaneous

Nondermatologists Are More Likely Than Dermatologists to Prescribe Antifungal/Corticosteroid Products: An Analysis of Office Visits for Cutaneous Fungal Infections, 1990–1994

Smith ES, Fleischer AB Jr, Feldman SR (Wake Forest Univ, Winston-Salem, NC)
J Am Acad Dermatol 39:43–47, 1998
7–9

Introduction.—Dermatologists are more accurate than nondermatologists in diagnosing cutaneous disease; how this affects outcome is not known. Compared with dermatologists, nondermatologists tend to prescribe more combination corticosteroid/anti-infective products for all skin diseases. Office-based physician visits for fungal skin infections were retrospectively analyzed to determine whether nondermatologists are more likely than dermatologists to prescribe combination products for treatment of common fungal skin infections.

Methods.—Databases from 1990 to 1994 of the National Ambulatory Medical Care Survey (NAMCS) were reviewed for frequency of primary, secondary, and tertiary drugs used to treat a primary diagnosis of fungal skin infections by office-based providers. Drug costs were estimated.

Results.—Of 4.1 million office-based visits for cutaneous fungal disease, 82% were to nondermatologists. Combination drugs or agents were used by 34.1% of nondermatologists and by 4.8% of dermatologists, a significant difference (Table 1). If nondermatologists prescribed combination agents at the same rate as dermatologists, an estimated $24.9 million would be saved if clotrimazole were used instead of clotrimazole/betamethasone dipropionate; $10.3 million would be saved using ketoconazole instead of the combination drug.

TABLE 1.—Drug Mentions for Combination and Single Antifungal Drugs for Primary Diagnoses of Common Fungal Infections by Physician Specialty (1990-1994)

Physician Specialty	Single Agent No.†	%	Combination Agent* No.	%
Family/General practice	1547	71	640	29
Medicine	31	49	329	51
Pediatrics	597	83	121	17
Other specialties	64	45	78	55
Dermatology	699	95	35	5
Total of all nondermatology	2263	66	1170	34

*Combination antifungal and corticosteroid medication.
Abbreviation: No., drug mentions in thousands.
(Courtesy of Smith ES, Fleischer AB Jr, Feldman SR: Nondermatologists are more likely than dermatologists to prescribe antifungal/corticosteroid products: An analysis of office visits for cutaneous fungal infections, 1990–1994. *J Am Acad Dermatol* 39:43–47, 1998.)

Conclusion.—Nondermatologists are more likely to prescribe a less cost-effective regimen for treating cutaneous fungal disease. The NAMCS database provides information on a cross-section of visits; it does not follow-up patients. Further investigation is needed to accurately determine cost-effectiveness over time.

▶ Fungal skin infections are a common problem. The conclusion reached in the study is, I think, valid. Unfortunately, for whatever reason, primary care physicians, as a group, are not optimally treating this entity. The authors try to stretch this finding into an argument for dermatologists being the first line for almost all skin care in managed care settings. That, to me, is quite a stretch. Nevertheless, there is a good take-home message here. Fungal skin infections should be treated with single, not combination, agents.

W.W. Dexter, M.D.

Atopic Dermatitis and Food Hypersensitivity Reactions
Burks AW, James JM, Hiegel A, et al (Univ of Arkansas, Little Rock; Arkansas Children's Hosp Research Inst, Little Rock)
J Pediatr 132:132–136, 1998   7–10

Background.—Food hypersensitivity can play a role in atopic dermatitis (AD) in some children. Identification and elimination from the diet can result in improvement in AD. The prevalence of food hypersensitivity in AD and the accuracy of skin prick screening tests for food allergens in patients with AD were assessed in a double-blind, placebo-controlled study.

Study Design.—Patients with AD attending the Arkansas Children's Hospital Pediatric Allergy Clinic participated in this study. A medical history and physical examination were obtained at the start of the study. Patients had allergy skin prick tests with at least 12 food antigens. The average diameter of erythema and wheal reactions were recorded. Based on the results of the skin prick tests, patients were asked to eliminate the suspected foods for 2–3 weeks. Double-blind, placebo-controlled food challenges were performed at the hospital after this period. The type, onset, severity, and duration of reaction were recorded.

Findings.—The study group consisted of 165 participants aged 4 months to 21.9 years. Of this study group, 98 had at least 1 positive skin prick test reaction. Food challenges were performed on the basis of the skin prick tests. A positive food challenge was observed in 64 of these 98 study group members. Milk, egg, peanut, soy, wheat, cod or catfish, and cashew together accounted for 89% of all positive food challenges. Using a skin prick screening test for these 7 foods, 99% of patients with AD with food allergies could be identified.

Conclusions.—This double-blind, placebo-controlled study of food allergies in children with AD confirms that many of these children have food allergies. Skin prick tests are effective in identifying those children with AD who have food allergies. Screening for food allergy should include milk, eggs, peanuts, wheat, soybean, fish, and tree nuts. As sensitivity changes over time, repeat challenges should be included in follow-up studies.

▶ The most useful part of this article is highlighting the 7 foods that cause the great majority of food allergies. These are milk, eggs, peanuts, soy, wheat, cod and catfish, and cashews. The authors are confident that screening skin prick tests are useful in identifying patients with food allergies. I need more evidence before I share this confidence. However, knowledge of these 7 most common foods allows the family physician to use an elimination diet approach. It is also important to remember that many patients with AD have this disease because of food hypersensitivity.

J.E. Scherger, M.D., M.P.H.

Incidence of Invasive Cancers Following Basal Cell Skin Cancer
Levi F, La Vecchia C, Te V-C, et al (Centre Hospitalier Universitaire Vaudois, Lausanne, Switzerland; Registre Neuchâtelois des Tumeurs, Neuchâtel, Switzerland; Università degli Studi Milano, Italy)
Am J Epidemiol 147:722–726, 1998   7–11

Introduction.—Basal cell carcinoma (BCC) usually occurs in older patients and has a favorable prognosis. A number of studies, however, report an excess incidence of other cancers in individuals who have had BCC. To determine the risk of invasive cancers after a diagnosis of BCC of the skin, a group of patients were followed for up to 20 years.

Methods.—Incident cases of BCC listed in the cancer registries of the Swiss cantons of Vaud and Neuchâtel between 1974 and 1994 were actively followed through December 1994 for the occurrence of subsequent invasive neoplasms. A total of 11,878 histologically confirmed BCCs of the skin had been diagnosed during the study period. Patients ranged in age from 15 to 100 years (median age, 68 years).

Results.—Overall, 1,543 metachronous cancers were observed in patients previously diagnosed with BCC. The number of cancers that would be expected was 1,397.9, corresponding to a standardized incidence ratio (SIR) of 1.1. When subsequent skin cancers were excluded, there were 975 second primary cancers observed vs. an expected 1,059.0, for an SIR of 0.9. Certain cancers did show significant excesses: cancer of the lip (SIR = 2.2), squamous cell skin cancer (SIR = 4.5), melanoma of the skin (SIR = 2.5), and non-Hodgkin's lymphoma (SIR = 1.9). The SIR for lung cancer was 0.9. The SIRs remained elevated 5 or more years after BCC diagnosis, particularly for squamous cell cancer and melanoma of the skin. At 19 years, the cumulative incidence of squamous cell skin cancer in patients with previous BCC was 13%.

Conclusion.—With a few exceptions, patients diagnosed with BCC do not have a generalized excess risk of nonskin cancers. But because of their excess rate of other skin cancers, such patients should continue to be monitored for suspicious skin lesions.

▶ Basal cell skin cancers are considered of minor importance because, with rare exception, they do not metastasize and threaten life. This study from Switzerland indicates that the population diagnosed with basal cell skin cancers have a much higher incidence of other more serious skin cancers than might be expected. A good practical suggestion is made that patients who have been identified with basal cell skin cancer should be regularly and thoroughly evaluated for other skin cancers.

J.E. Scherger, M.D., M.P.H.

Photoaging and Topical Tretinoin: Therapy, Pathogenesis, and Prevention
Kang S, Fisher GJ, Voorhees JJ (Univ of Michigan, Ann Arbor)
Arch Dermatol 133:1280–1284, 1997   7–12

Objective.—Subjects with repeated exposure to ultraviolet (UV) radiation from the sun during a period of many years show premature skin aging. The characteristics of photoaged skin are similar to those of aging, including wrinkles, mottled pigmentation, dryness and roughness, and loss of skin tone. Topical tretinoin has been shown to improve photoaged skin, generating great attention among the public, the media, and the medical community. The effectiveness of tretinoin has led to new knowledge that may explain wrinkle effacement. The authors review current understanding of photoaging, particularly wrinkle formation.

Photoaging and Tretinoin.—The first sign of improvement in photoaged skin treated with tretinoin is improvement in fine wrinkles. Because this effect is unlikely to result from epidermal alterations, the dermal component is apparently the therapeutic target. This is consistent with the findings in animal models of photoaging. Studies have shown that tretinoin increases collagen levels in photoaged human skin. Because of its unique molecular structure, collagen is resistant to nonspecific proteolytic attack in the insoluble extracellular matrix. Photoaging decreases collagen, and retinoic acid restores it. Thus, the wrinkling associated with photoaging may involve reduction and disorganization of fibrillar collagen. This suggests that UV irradiation leads to collagen loss, probably through enhanced collagen degradation. The authors' studies of the UV effects mediating photoaging suggest that even UV exposure insufficient to cause sunburn can still lead to degeneration of skin collagen. Treatment with tretinoin significantly reduces UV-B–mediated induction of matrix metalloproteinases, a group of enzymes responsible for collagen degradation. Whatever the mechanism of this effect, it suggests that topical tretinoin use may prevent photoaging.

Discussion.—Recent research strongly suggests that deficiency of superficial dermal collagen is the cause of skin photoaging. Based on this research, the authors propose a mechanism whereby a lifetime of UV radiation exposure could lead to reduced collagen and photoaging. Understanding this mechanism raises the possibility of treating and even preventing skin photoaging with the use of tretinoin.

▶ This comprehensive review comes from the authors who originally described the benefits of topical tretinoin in treating photoaging skin. Of course, no matter how much is learned about the pathophysiology of photoaging, prevention using protective clothing will always be worth more than a pound of curative cream.

J.E. Scherger, M.D., M.P.H.

8 Urological Conditions

Overview

Randomized controlled trials: Abstracts 8–1, 8–6, 8–7, 8–8, and 8–9

Prostate Disease

- Finasteride and the need for surgical treatment of men with benign prostatic hyperplasia
- Treatment of chronic prostatitis with α-blockers and antibiotics
- Informed consent and preferences of elderly men for prostate-specific antigen testing
- The effects of screening on early detection of prostate cancer
- Serendipity and screening for prostate cancer

Circumcision

- Two articles on four anesthetic techniques for routine circumcision

Miscellaneous

- Pelvic floor electrical stimulation and stress incontinence
- Sildenafil and erectile dysfunction

Prostate Disease

The Effect of Finasteride on the Risk of Acute Urinary Retention and the Need for Surgical Treatment Among Men With Benign Prostatic Hyperplasia
McConnell JD, for the Finasteride Long-Term Efficacy and Safety Study Group (Univ of Texas, Dallas; Univ of Wisconsin, Madison; The Johns Hopkins Med Institutions, Baltimore, Md; et al)
N Engl J Med 338:557–563, 1998   8–1

Introduction.—Finasteride is reported to improve urinary symptoms in men with benign prostatic hyperplasia (BPH). It is not known to what extent the benefit is sustained or whether finasteride decreases the incidence of related events, particularly the need for surgery and the development of acute urinary retention. The long-term effects of finasteride on the symptoms of BPH and on the incidence of important outcomes related to taking the drug were assessed in 3,040 men with moderate to severe BPH in a 4-year, double-blind, randomized, placebo-controlled trial.

Methods.—Patients were randomized to receive either finasteride, 5 mg daily, or placebo for 4 years. Patients were observed every 4 months for symptom scores (scale of 1–34) and side effects and for measurement of urinary flow rate. Serum prostate-specific antigen was measured every 4

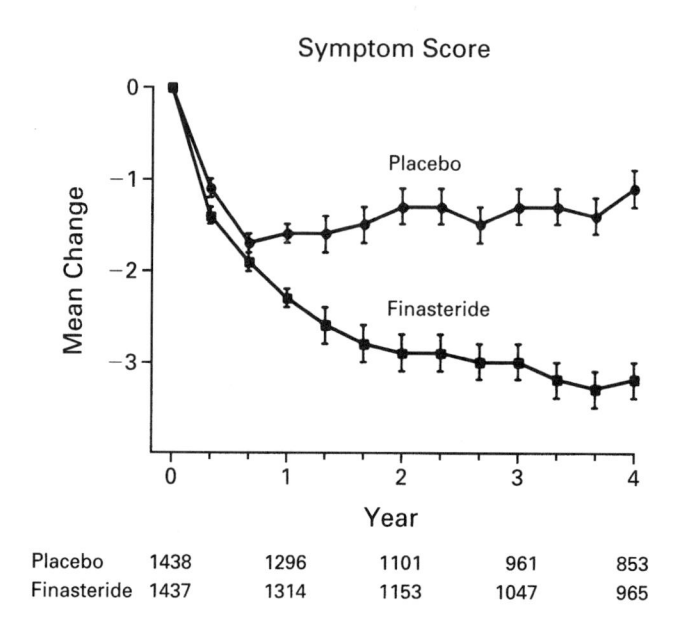

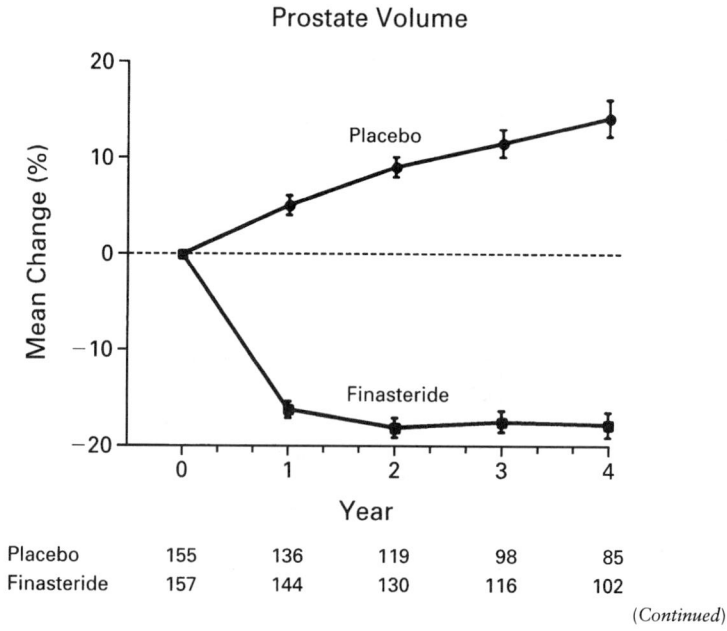

Symptom Score

Placebo	1438	1296	1101	961	853
Finasteride	1437	1314	1153	1047	965

Prostate Volume

Placebo	155	136	119	98	85
Finasteride	157	144	130	116	102

(*Continued*)

FIGURE 3 (cont.)

Maximal Urinary Flow Rate

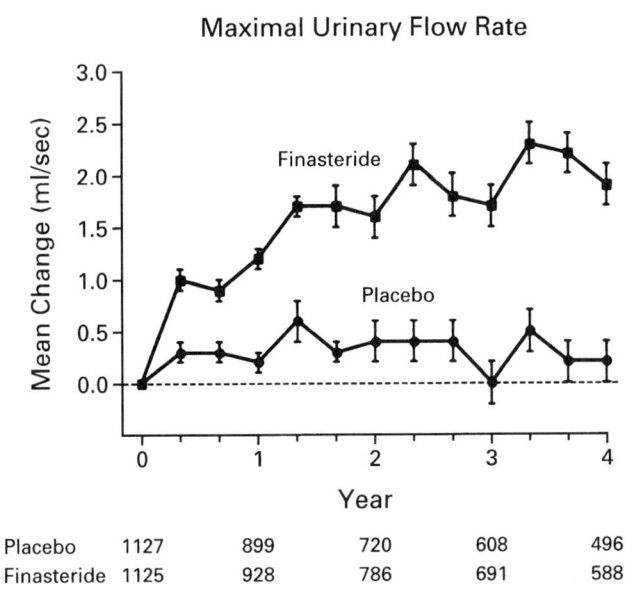

[Graph showing Mean Change (ml/sec) vs Year (0 to 4) for Finasteride and Placebo groups, with Finasteride rising to approximately 2.0 ml/sec and Placebo remaining near 0.3–0.5 ml/sec.]

	0	1	2	3	4
Placebo	1127	899	720	608	496
Finasteride	1125	928	786	691	588

FIGURE 3.—The effect of finasteride or placebo on symptom scores (on the quasi-AUA symptom scale), prostate volume, and maximal urinary flow rate over time. Values are mean (±SE) changes from baseline. The numbers below the panels show the numbers of patients with valid data who remained in the study. *Abbreviations: AUA*, American Urological Association; *SE*, standard error. (Reprinted by permission of *The New England Journal of Medicine* from McConnell JD, for the Finasteride Long-Term Efficacy and Safety Study Group: The effect of finasteride on the risk of acute urinary retention and the need for surgical treatment among men with benign prostatic hyperplasia. *N Engl J Med* 338:557–563. Copyright 1998, Massachusetts Medical Society. All rights reserved.)

months for 1 year and every 8 months thereafter. Patients underwent a yearly physical examination and magnetic resonance imaging of the prostate. Prostate volume was measured in a subgroup of men.

Results.—Complete data were available for 2,760 men. During the 4-year assessment period, 152 of 1,503 men in the placebo group (10%) and 69 of 1,513 men in the finasteride group (5%) had surgery for BPH. Seven percent of the men in the placebo group had acute urinary retention, compared with 3% in the finasteride group. Mean decreases in symptom scores were significantly greater in the finasteride group than in the placebo group (3.3 vs. 1.3). Finasteride significantly improved urinary flow rate and reduced prostate volume (Fig 3).

Conclusion.—Treatment with finasteride for 4 years decreases symptoms and prostate volume, increases urinary flow, and lowers the probability of surgery and acute urinary retention in men with symptoms of urinary obstruction and prostatic enlargement.

▶ These are solid, believable results from a large, long-term, well-controlled study. Finasteride has been shown to be quite useful in controlling symptoms of BPH, a finding echoed in this study (see Fig 3). The treatment of

BPH was reviewed extensively in the 1997 YEAR BOOK OF FAMILY PRACTICE (pp 163–173). Medical treatment with finasteride, as well as doxazosin, terazosin, and a newer agent, tamsulosin, was shown to be effective in reducing symptoms of BPH as well as prostate size. From the results in this study, it now appears that finasteride can play an important role in preventing complications of progressive BPH, which is not so benign if it results in acute urinary retention. Do these findings suggest we should be prescribing finasteride for all our patients with BPH to avoid the possibility of urinary retention and the potential need for surgery? Not at all, although in the final analysis, this might prove to be a cost-effective strategy. For your patients who fit the study group characteristics, this is evidence on which to base your practice of medicine.

W.W. Dexter, M.D.

α-Blockers for the Treatment of Chronic Prostatitis in Combination With Antibiotics
Barbalias GA, Nikiforidis G, Liatsikos EN (Univ of Patras, Greece)
J Urol 159:883–887, 1998   8–2

Introduction.—Patients with nonprostatodynia, abacterial prostatitis (group 1, 134 patients), prostatodynia (group 2, 72), and chronic bacterial prostatitis (group 3, 64) took part in a study designed to evaluate the immediate and long-term effects of α-blockers and antibiotics in the treatment of chronic prostatitis. Researchers hypothesized that the painful male urethral syndrome that characteristically responds to α-blockade may be the first step in a chain of events than can end in an adverse effect on the prostate.

Methods.—Patients evaluated for enrollment had clinical complaints of the painful male urethral syndrome and chronic prostatitis. All patients in groups 1 and 2 were administered α-blockers. These patients had a mean maximal urethral closure pressure of 110 cm H_2O. Half of the group 3 patients also received α-blockers. Therapy was usually started at a low dose, then titrated weekly until the optimal dose was achieved for each patient. This dose level was continued for an additional 8 months. No patient received more than 5 mg of terazosin or 7.5 mg of alfuzosin daily. All patients with positive segmental prostatic cultures (group 3) and half of those with abacterial prostatitis and greater than 10 white blood cells per high-power field in the expressed prostatic secretion (group 1) received antibiotics. Mean follow-up was 22 months.

Results.—Treatment with α-blockade significantly reduced the recurrence rate of bacterial prostatitis and provided relief of symptoms for many months. Among patients with abacterial prostatitis, the rate of symptom occurrence was lower for those who received only α-blockers than those treated with a combination of α-blockers and antibiotics.

Conclusion.—Patients with abacterial and bacterial prostatitis, as well as those with prostatodynia, can benefit from α-blockers. In this series, α-blockade enhanced clinical improvement among patients with abacterial and bacterial prostatitis and reduced recurrences. The use of α-blockade reduces intraluminal urethral pressure, obviating urethral hypertonia and interrupting the cycle that leads to chronic prostatitis.

▶ α-Blockers, both the older nonselective agents and the newer selective $α_{1A}$-agents, are proving to be very useful drugs in treating male genitourinary disease. This ranges from symptomatic improvement in benign prostatic hypertrophy to the prevention of complications such as bladder outlet obstruction.[1-3] Here is another potential use for α-blockers. Despite the problems with this study such as small numbers, single site, and no blinding, I tend to believe the results, particularly given α-blockers' efficacy in similar and related problems. Thus, while I will certainly be interested in seeing a multicenter, double-blinded, placebo-controlled trial, I will begin using these agents on my patients with chronic prostatic symptoms as well as lower urinary tract symptoms described by the authors as the painful urethral syndrome.

W.W. Dexter, M.D.

References

1. Kirby RS: Doxazosin in benign prostatic hyperplasia: Effects on blood pressure and urinary flow in normotensive and hypertensive men. *Urology* 46:182–186, 1995. (1997 YEAR BOOK OF FAMILY PRACTICE, p 164.)
2. Lepor H, Williford WO, Barry MJ, et al: The efficacy of terazosin, finasteride, or both in benign prostatic hyperplasia. *N Engl J Med* 335:533–539, 1996. (1997 YEAR BOOK OF FAMILY PRACTICE, p 169.)
3. Chapple CR, Wyndaele JJ, Nordling J, et al: Tamsulosin, the first prostate-selective $α_{1A}$-adrenoceptor antagonist: A meta-analysis of two randomized placebo-controlled, multicentre studies in patients with benign prostatic obstruction (symptomatic BPH). *Eur Urol* 29:155–167, 1996. (1997 YEAR BOOK OF FAMILY PRACTICE, p 171.)

Preferences of Elderly Men for Prostate-Specific Antigen Screening and the Impact of Informed Consent
Wolf AMD, Schorling JB (Univ of Virginia, Charlottesville)
J Gerontol 53A:M195-M200, 1998   8–3

Introduction.—Screening for prostate cancer with prostate-specific antigen (PSA) can detect cancer at an earlier stage compared with digital rectal examination alone; yet screening with PSA has not been shown to improve patient outcomes. The question of whether to use PSA screening in elderly patients is particularly difficult, for the potential harm of intervention may outweigh benefits in those aged 70 years and older. A group of elderly men took part in a study designed to assess their preferences for such screening.

Methods.—Study participants were men aged 65 years or older who were in a randomized controlled trial on the effect of information on patients' interest in PSA screening. Of the 205 men involved in the trial, 104 had no history of prostate cancer and had not previously undergone PSA screening. Randomization was to a scripted overview of PSA screening or to a brief control message. Those in the former group received information about known risk factors for prostate cancer, implications of an abnormal PSA result, and the uncertain benefits and common complications of early prostate cancer treatment. The 2 groups were compared for their attitudes about PSA screening.

Results.—Men who received the informational message were significantly less interested in PSA screening than were men who were given the control message. Informed men viewed screening to be of significantly less benefit than did uninformed men. Both groups, however, showed a correlation between perceived efficacy of screening and interest in having PSA screening. Among the uninformed men, but not the informed men, perceived seriousness of prostate cancer predicted interest in screening. Marital status did not predict screening interest among the uninformed men, whereas informed men who were married had less interest in screening than did informed men who were single, divorced, or widowed.

Conclusion.—It is important to provide elderly patients with information about the benefits and burdens of PSA screening. Interest in screening was significantly decreased when elderly men received such information. Men who did not receive information about the potential effects of screening were likely to be influenced by the perceived seriousness of prostate cancer.

▶ This is an important study with implications beyond screening for prostate cancer. The underlying issue is that of patient preferences, a topic too long ignored by researchers and practitioners alike. This study tells us that informed patients will make different decisions than will uninformed patients and that the added information could lead to a decision not to have a test done, even when the test is widely promoted and readily available. A large HMO in our area has implemented a similar educational program and has seen even more dramatic decreases in the ordering of PSA tests. I think we will see more empirical evidence that high-quality information must be available to patients when a health care decision is made and that patients will use the information to make decisions that meet their needs ("utilities" in the jargon) rather than match their physicians' preferences.

A.O. Berg, M.D., M.P.H.

Prostate Carcinoma Incidence and Patient Mortality: The Effects of Screening and Early Detection
Brawley OW (Natl Cancer Inst, Bethesda, Md)
Cancer 80:1857–1863, 1997   8–4

Introduction.—New screening and diagnostic technologies have led to a dramatic increase in the rate of diagnosis of prostate carcinoma in the

United States. There is concern that a significant number of men will be treated unnecessarily and experience morbidity and complications. Data collected from the Surveillance, Epidemiology, and End Results (SEER) Program of the National Cancer Institute, were used to describe national and regional trends in prostate carcinoma incidence and the impact that screening has had in the United States.

Methods.—The SEER Program is a population-based cancer database containing information on all cancers diagnosed among nearly all residents of 9 defined areas in the United States. Data from the SEER Program and demographic data of the U.S. census are used to make projections of cancer incidence and mortality.

Results.—During 1973 to 1994, incidence rates of prostate carcinoma increased for both black and white men, and the increase in mortality rates slowed in both races. Both incidence and mortality rates, however, were significantly higher among blacks. There was a decline in distant disease at diagnosis and an increase in local and regional disease. All of these changes are attributed to increased numbers of men undergoing screening and early detection, but they are also consistent with lead-time bias, length bias, and a decline in mortality. Incidence rates of prostate carcinoma varied considerably among the 9 SEER regions. Mortality rates declined in recent years, but the decline was small compared with the rise in incidence rates. In Connecticut, for example, a state with less screening than the other areas, the mortality rate declined from 25.3 to 23 per 100,000 white men.

Discussion.—Although prostate carcinoma can be diagnosed, it is difficult to distinguish those who need treatment from those who do not. It is estimated that one third of men who receive a diagnosis fall into the category of those for whom cure is necessary but not possible. Although the benefits of screening and early detection are theoretically possible, treatment prompted by screening results has clearly caused harm.

▶ The findings in this study will not surprise those who have been skeptical about the benefits of screening for prostate cancer. It does not provide a definitive answer but is consistent with the possibility that screening often detects cancers that would be better left alone. What is truly surprising is that this paper appears under the heading of a communication from the American Cancer Society, an organization that has strongly advocated screening in the past. The organization's policy toward screening has been tempered recently. Skeptics of screening long ago conceded that there is currently insufficient evidence to make a strong recommendation one way or the other for asymptomatic men; it is nice to see the traditional proponents moving in the same direction.

A.O. Berg, M.D., M.P.H.

Early Detection of Prostate Cancer: Serendipity Strikes Again
Collins MM, Ransohoff DF, Barry MJ (Massachusetts Gen Hosp, Boston; Univ of North Carolina, Chapel Hill)
JAMA 278:1516–1519, 1997   8–5

Objective.—Prostate cancers may be detected by accident. Whether serendipity plays a role in cancer screening was examined by reviewing articles on prostate cancer screening for serendipitous results.

Definition of Detection by Serendipity.—Serendipitous discovery of prostate cancer during digital rectal examinations (DREs) would occur if a random biopsy in an area other than the suspicious one revealed prostate cancer. Serendipitous discovery of prostate cancer in prostate-specific antigen (PSA) screening would occur if a random biopsy of a nonpalpable tumor too small to cause elevated PSA levels revealed prostate cancer.

Magnitude of Prostate Cancer Detection by Serendipity.—Serendipity accounted for approximately 25% of prostate cancers detected during DREs and approximately 25% of prostate cancers detected during PSA screening. Serendipity may be responsible for the detection of prostate cancer in 30% to 100% of tumors less than 1.0 cm^3.

Conclusion.—Prostate cancers detected by serendipity may contribute to overestimating the value of DRE and PSA screening. Whether serendipitous detection of smaller prostate cancers makes a significant difference in outcome depends on their importance. If they are indolent, their detection may encourage overly aggressive treatment. If they are fast-growing, not enough are being found.

▶ Serendipity doesn't sound like it should properly be the province of scientific medical care, but these authors raise an interesting argument, suggesting that it's there whether we recognize it or not. The clinical take-home in this article is that 36% to 100% of small (less than 1 cm) prostate cancers detected at biopsy after a PSA test may be discovered more or less accidentally. The reason that this is potentially important is that it is precisely these small tumors that might best be left alone. Intervening with surgery or radiation might not be in the patient's best interest.

A.O. Berg, M.D., M.P.H.

Circumcision

Efficacy of EMLA Cream Prior to Dorsal Penile Nerve Block for Circumcision in Children
Serour F, Mandelberg A, Zabeeda D, et al (Edith Wolfson Med Ctr, Holon, Israel)
Acta Anaesthesiol Scand 42:260–263, 1998   8–6

Objective.—EMLA cream is a topical anesthetic that has been proven effective for cutaneous procedures in children. The efficacy of EMLA cream before dorsal penile nerve block for circumcision was evaluated in a prospective, double-blinded, placebo-controlled, randomized study.

Methods.—Ambulatory circumcision was performed in 42 boys, aged 7–17 years, with application of EMLA cream (group A, n = 21) or placebo cream (group B, n = 21) to the pubic area before needle penetration and infiltration of local anesthesia. Pain intensity and global discomfort were graded from 1 to 4 by patients using a visual analog scale.

Results.—There was no significant difference in application times between groups A and B (61–108 minutes vs. 64–103 minutes). There were no major complications in either group. There were 2 patients with edema in group A and 3 in group B, and 4 patients had hematomas in group A and 6 in group B. There were no group A patients who reported pain at skin penetration, whereas 2 patients in group B reported slight pain and 19 reported moderate pain. Three group A patients reported slight pain at infiltration and 18 reported moderate pain. One group B patient reported slight pain at infiltration and 20 reported moderate pain.

Conclusions.—EMLA cream was effective as a topical anesthetic during needle penetration but had no effect on the pain of infiltration.

▶ EMLA cream has become popular even though it is much less effective than dorsal penile nerve block and takes much longer to work. There must be some incentive to using a cream over injecting a needle into a newborn's skin. However, the cream is of limited benefit, and subdermal injections quickly provide excellent local anesthesia and prevent the pain of circumcision.

J.E. Scherger, M.D., M.P.H.

Comparison of Ring Block, Dorsal Penile Nerve Block, and Topical Anesthesia for Neonatal Circumcision: A Randomized Controlled Trial
Lander J, Brady-Fryer B, Metcalfe JB, et al (Univ of Alberta, Edmonton, Canada)
JAMA 278:2157–2162, 1997

Background.—Because of beliefs about the safety and efficacy of current anesthetics, many newborns are circumcised without the benefit of anesthesia. Ring block, dorsal penile nerve block, a topical eutectic mixture of local anesthetics (EMLA), and topical placebo were compared during neonatal circumcision.

Methods.—Fifty-two healthy, full-term boys aged 1 to 3 days were enrolled in the randomized, controlled trial. The main outcome measures were heart rate, cry, and methemoglobin level.

Findings.—Untreated newborns showed homogeneous responses consisting of sustained increases in heart rate and high-pitched cry during and after circumcision. Two boys in this group became ill after the procedure, experiencing choking and apnea. Crying and heart rates were significantly reduced in the 3 active treatment groups during and after circumcision.

The ring block was equally effective throughout all stages of the circumcision. The dorsal penile nerve block and EMLA were ineffective during foreskin separation and incision. Methemoglobin levels were greatest in the boys given EMLA, although none of the infants needed treatment.

Conclusion.—An anesthetic should be administered to infants before circumcision is performed. In this series, the ring block was the most effective anesthetic for neonatal circumcision, and EMLA was the least effective.

▶ It is appalling how many circumcisions are still going on in the United States without anesthesia. We now have multiple techniques, and this article describing a randomized controlled trial shows that the injection methods are safe and more effective than placebo. Interestingly, a lead article in the *New England Journal of Medicine* promoted the topical anesthetic method.[1] The injection methods, such as a ring block or dorsal penile nerve block, are very easy to administer and may be readily taught right in the nursery. Those of us performing circumcisions should make a special effort to have all of the providers on the medical staff give anesthesia to infants undergoing this procedure.

J.E. Scherger, M.D., M.P.H.

Reference

1. Taddio A, Stevens B, Craig K, et al: Efficacy and safety of lidocaine-prilocaine cream for pain during circumcision. N Engl J Med 336:1197–1201, 1997.

Miscellaneous

Pelvic Floor Electrical Stimulation in the Treatment of Stress Incontinence: An Investigational Study and a Placebo Controlled Double-blind Trial

Yamanishi T, Yasuda K, Sakakibara R, et al (Chiba Univ, Japan)
J Urol 158:2127–2131, 1997
8–8

Introduction.—Success rates of treating genuine stress incontinence with electrical stimulation range from 6% to 90%. This treatment is used infrequently because of the widespread lack of information about physiologic and technical principles. A small electrical stimulation device was used in an investigational study and a placebo-controlled, double-blind trial to determine the usefulness of electrical stimulation in 44 patients with stress incontinence.

Methods.—Forty-four patients (mean age, 63 years) were included in the study. Six men and 38 women (9 patients in the investigational study, 35 patients in the double-blind investigation) with stress plus mild urge incontinence were assessed. A vaginal electrode was placed in females and an anal electrode was placed in males. Urethral pressure was measured in the investigational trial before, during, and after 15 minutes of stimulation in the investigational study. Patients in the double-blind trial were randomized to either an electrical stimulation device or a dummy device group. Efficacy was judged from a subjective patient report, records from a frequency/volume chart, results of a 1-hour pad test, and from urodynamic parameters after 4 weeks of treatment.

Results.—Maximum urethral closure pressure before, during, and after stimulation was 44.4, 64.5, and 46.8 cm H_2O, respectively. The increase during stimulation was significant. In the double-blind trial, patient impressions were good in 60% and 8% of the active device and dummy device groups, respectively. Significant improvement was noted for the pad test in the active vs. dummy device group. There was a 45% and 7.7% cure rate in the active and dummy device groups, respectively. Significantly more patients were cured or improved in the frequency of leakage and pad tests in the active device vs. dummy device group.

Conclusion.—Pelvic floor electrical stimulation is safe and useful as an alternative to surgery for stress urinary incontinence.

▶ Surgical correction for stress incontinence, while effective, is an option many patients are reluctant to choose for, perhaps, the obvious reasons of risk, discomfort, cost, or fear. Exercise and medications provide some relief but are often not adequate. The results noted in this study were echoed in a recent study by Brubaker et al., which looked at 121 women with detrusor instability.[1] Electrical stimulation is a simple technique and is apparently well tolerated. Given the somewhat invasive nature of the device, however, I wonder whether these results would hold up in an office-based trial. Nevertheless, treatment with electrical stimulation would seem to be an attractive alternative short of surgery. Discuss this with your local urogynecologic specialist. This seems a reasonable approach to recommend to your patients.

W.W. Dexter, M.D.

Reference

1. Brubaker L, Benson JT, Bent A, et al: Transvaginal electrical stimulation for female urinary incontinence. *Am J Obstet Gynecol* 177:536–540, 1997.

Oral Sildenafil in the Treatment of Erectile Dysfunction
Goldstein I, for the Sildenafil Study Group (Boston Univ; Univ of California, San Francisco; Univ of Southern California, Los Angeles; et al)
N Engl J Med 338:1397–1404, 1998
8–9

Introduction.—Sildenafil (Viagra), a selective and potent inhibitor of cyclic guanosine monophosphate in the corpus cavernosum, restores the natural erectile response to sexual stimulation in men with erectile dysfunction. The oral therapy offers advantages over previously available treatments that required injections, prostheses, or surgery. Two sequential studies evaluated the efficacy and safety of sildenafil in men with erectile dysfunction of organic, psychogenic, or mixed causes.

Methods.—The 2 studies included a total of 861 men aged 18 years or older with a clinical diagnosis of erectile dysfunction of at least 6 months' duration. In a study of dose response, efficacy, and safety, 532 men were randomly assigned to receive 25, 50, or 100 mg of sildenafil or placebo for 24 weeks. Tablets were to be taken approximately 1 hour before planned sexual activity but not more than once daily. Men were advised not to consume more than 2 alcoholic drinks within 1 hour of sexual activity. The 12-week dose-escalation study included 329 different men, randomly assigned to receive placebo or 50 mg of sildenafil 1 hour before sexual activity. Participants were able to double or reduce the dose by 50% according to therapeutic response and adverse effects. The men were questioned about their frequency of penetration and maintenance of erections after penetration.

Results.—The dose-response study showed an association between improved erectile function with increasing doses of oral sildenafil. On the question about achieving erections, men who received 100 mg of the drug increased their mean score by 100% (to 4.0 after treatment vs. 2.0 at baseline, from a possible score of 5.0). In the dose-escalation study, 69% of attempts at sexual intercourse during the last 4 weeks of the study were successful in the sildenafil group. The success rate in the placebo group at this time was only 22%. The mean number of successful attempts at sexual intercourse was 5.9 per month in the sildenafil group vs. 1.5 per month in the placebo group. In the dose-response study, 10% of men in the sildenafil group and 17% in the placebo group stopped treatment because of adverse effects; corresponding figures for the dose-escalation study were 6% and 8%. The most common adverse effects, reported by 6% to 18% of men, were headache, flushing, and dyspepsia.

Discussion.—Sildenafil improved sexual function in men with erectile dysfunction, causing erection in response to sexual stimulation. The therapeutic response of the drug was similar in men with various causes of erectile dysfunction. Increasing doses, from 25 to 100 mg, improved the frequency of penetration and the maintenance of erections after penetration. Sildenafil is simple to use and generally well tolerated.

▶ Well, the results seem to be in. The patients (and doctors) are voting with their prescriptions. This drug has received an unprecedented amount of publicity and has been treated, in the advice columns of the newspapers anyway, as being both the savior of relationships as well as the downfall! It clearly seems to be an effective alternative to the various other more invasive treatments for erectile dysfunction, a number of which have been reviewed in these pages in past years. This drug seems reasonably safe but not completely so. Don't get swept up in the euphoria over this drug. There are significant side effects and potentially dangerous drug interactions, especially with nitrates, particularly in the patient group most likely to want to use this drug.

W.W. Dexter, M.D.

9 Musculoskeletal Conditions and Fibromyalgia

Overview

Randomized controlled trials: Abstracts 9–1, 9–7, 9–8, and 9–10

Back Pain

- Nortriptyline and chronic low back pain
- Back pain in children and adolescents
- Back pain during pregnancy

Fibromyalgia

- Behavioral and educational interventions for fibromyalgia
- Fibromyalgia in children and adolescents

Miscellaneous

- Functional outcomes in upper extremity disorders
- Hydroquinone in muscle cramps
- Chiropractic treatment of carpal tunnel syndrome
- Effectiveness of topical NSAIDs
- Effects of hot- and cold-pack therapies
- Clinical and MR findings in children and adolescents with knee injuries
- Prognosis in whiplash

Back Pain

A Placebo-controlled Randomized Clinical Trial of Nortriptyline for Chronic Low Back Pain

Atkinson JH, Slater MA, Williams RA, et al (San Diego VA Healthcare System, Calif; Univ of California–San Diego, La Jolla; San Diego State Univ, Calif)
Pain 76:287–296, 1998   9–1

Introduction.—Society spends more than $22 billion annually to treat chronic low back pain, a leading reason for physician visits. As analgesics for this disorder, tricyclic antidepressants are prescribed widely because they are known to inhibit transmission of pain at the level of the spinal cord and midbrain. However, because of methodological limitations in previous studies, no convincing scientific evidence supporting or refuting the use of tricyclic antidepressants to relieve back pain exists. In patients with chronic low back pain without major depression, the efficacy of nortriptyline, a standard tricyclic antidepressant, was compared with a placebo for relief of pain and improvement of function and health-related quality of life.

Methods.—Seventy-eight men were recruited from a primary care and general orthopedic setting for this study. All 78 participants had chronic low back pain, defined as pain at T-6 or below on a daily basis for 6 months or longer. They participated in a randomized, double-blind, placebo-controlled 8-week trial and received either inert placebo or nortriptyline titrated to within the therapeutic range for treating major depression at 50–150 ng/mL. The outcomes used were pain, disability, health-related quality of life, mood, and physician-rated outcome. These outcomes were rated using several scales including the Descriptor Differential Scale, the Sickness Impact Profile, the Quality of Well-Being Scale, the Beck Depression Inventory, and the Clinical Global Impression.

Results.—Participants randomized to nortriptyline had significantly greater reduction in pain intensity scores. Their pain was reduced by 22% compared with 9% for those receiving the placebo. Nortriptyline also resulted in a marginally favorable reduction in disability over placebo, but health-related quality of life, mood, and physician ratings of overall outcome did not differ significantly between treatments. The intent-to-treat analysis was supported by a subgroup analysis.

Conclusion.—The modest reduction in pain intensity experienced by participants of this trial suggests that physicians should carefully weigh the risks and benefits of using nortriptyline to treat patients with chronic back pain and depression.

▶ This was a cleanly performed randomized controlled trial of nortriptyline alone as an analgesic. Most previous studies have examined the effects of tricyclics as an adjunct to other more typical analgesics and focused on patients with pain and signs of depression. As the authors point out, the quality of evidence supporting use of tricyclics in this clinical setting is inadequate; thus, the attempt here is to isolate the effect of the tricyclics alone. The investigators documented a positive effect of nortryptyline alone, but the effect was small. I believe these findings lend weak support to the use of tricyclics in chronic low back pain. I would use them as adjuncts with other analgesics and have limited expectation for success.

A.O. Berg, M.D., M.P.H.

Back Pain in Children and Adolescents: A Retrospective Review of 648 Patients

Combs JA, Caskey PM (Shriner's Hosp for Crippled Children, Spokane, Wash)
South Med J 90:789-792, 1997

Background.—It is traditionally taught that back pain in children should be regarded as reflecting a serious problem—tumor or an infection—until proven otherwise. Observations at the authors' children's hospital suggested a change in the pattern of diagnoses among children with back pain. These changes were analyzed retrospectively.

Methods.—The review included 648 children seen for chief complaints referable to the spine during a 2.5-year period. Of these, 265 were classified as having pain and 383 as having no pain. Detailed evaluations of these 2 groups were performed, including diagnoses, studies performed, and demographic data.

Results.—The pain group included 167 girls and 98 boys, with an average age of 14 years. The no-pain group consisted of 245 girls and 138 boys, with an average age of 12 years. Back pain with no organic cause was the primary diagnosis among children in the pain group, affecting 57% of patients. The most common concurrent diagnosis in this group of patients was psychosocial problems. In the no-pain group, spinal asymmetry was the major diagnosis for 44% of patients and scoliosis for 40%. Only 1 child in the pain group had a malignancy, and none had an infection diagnosed. In the pain group, symptoms were sometimes associated with psychosocial problems such as depression, attempted suicide, and abuse; a family history of disability; or pending litigation.

Conclusions.—Patterns of back pain in children and adolescents appear to be shifting; the diagnoses in children with back pain are now similar to those in the adult population. Emotional, psychiatric, and social problems are much more common in children with back pain than in children with nonpainful back conditions. The findings underscore the importance of preventing and treating first-time occurrences of back pain in children. Psychosocial causes of back pain should be considered in children who have a negative workup for organic disease.

▶ Back pain in children and adolescents is a common problem seen by primary care physicians. However, it must be taken seriously because it may be a harbinger of significant problems.

This study was interesting, looking at 648 young patients with known spinal disorders treated at a Shriner's hospital. Even among this very select group of patients with known pathology, the authors found that 57.4% of these patients who had back pain had no known organic cause. Scoliosis was by far the most common known cause for back pain in this population. The authors also found an interesting correlation between back pain and confounding associations such as psychosocial problems in the family, disabilities in the family, or a pending lawsuit. They concluded that the range of back pain causes and its relationship to other variables are very similar in children and adolescents as that seen in adult populations.

My take-home message is that we should continue to do what we have always done—take seriously the complaint of back pain in our young patients and evaluate them thoroughly. During this evaluation, we must remember that a high percentage of them will have no known organic cause.

R.C. Davidson, M.D., M.P.H.

Follow-up of Patients With Low Back Pain During Pregnancy
Brynhildsen J, Hansson Å, Persson A, et al (Univ Hosp Linköping, Sweden)
Obstet Gynecol 91:182–186, 1998   9–3

Background.—During pregnancy, 50% to 75% of all women report low back pain. The reason for this pain is not well understood and the long-term prognosis is not known. To determine the long-term risk for low back pain among women who had disabling low back pain during pregnancy, a follow-up questionnaire was administered.

Study Design.—A previous study performed from 1983 to 1984 had identified 79 women with disabling low back pain during pregnancy in Linköping, Sweden. Of those 79 women, 62 were included in the current study. All women visiting a single antenatal clinic from 1983 to 1984 in Linköping without disabling low back pain were invited to serve as controls. A questionnaire, including age, weight, height, smoking, occupation, parity, and presence of low back pain, was sent to both groups of women in 1996.

Findings.—The questionnaire response rate was 84% in the low back pain group and 80% in the control group. The basic characteristics of these 2 groups were similar. Ten of the women in the low back pain group stated that they had avoided subsequent pregnancy because of fear of low back pain. Among those women with severe low back pain in previous pregnancies, 94% experienced this pain in subsequent pregnancies, compared to 44% in the control group. Even when they were not pregnant, the women in the low back pain group had more back pain than the control group. The location of the pain did not affect prognosis. Logistic regression analysis indicated that low back pain during pregnancy was the only independent risk factor for low back pain during a subsequent pregnancy.

Conclusions.—The risk of recurrence of severe low back pain, both during pregnancy and when not pregnant, is high among women who had disabling low back pain during a previous pregnancy. Further studies are necessary to understand the mechanism of this pain and to develop preventive therapies.

▶ Any family physician providing prenatal care knows that low back pain is very common during pregnancy. A particular low back pain that is more common in pregnancy is subluxation of the sacroiliac joint. This important article from Sweden describes the follow-up of patients with back pain after their pregnancy, and suggests that many of them have recurrent back problems. Although not conclusive, this article should alert us to watching these patients closely for the later development of back pain and consider preventive measures such as strengthening exercises and teaching good posture to avoid recurrent back problems.

J.E. Scherger, M.D., M.P.H.

Fibromyalgia

A Comparison of Behavioral and Educational Interventions for Fibromyalgia
Nicassio PM, Radojevic V, Weisman MH, et al (California School of Professional Psychology, San Diego; Univ of California–San Diego, La Jolla)
J Rheumatol 24:2000–2007, 1998   9–4

Objective.—Neither behavioral nor educational approaches have been definitively shown to be effective in reducing fibromyalgia (FM) symptoms and disability. Self-reported indices of pain severity and objective measures of pain behavior and disability were used to separate behavioral and educational elements, and the role of intervening variables in mediating improvement in clinical outcomes was evaluated.

Methods.—For 10 weeks, 48 participants in the behavioral condition were taught pain-coping skills, and 35 in the education/control condition were given information on a variety of health-related topics. Participants (88.7% women) ranged in age from 24 to 78 years and had had FM for an average of 11.1 years. Outcome measures were pain index, self-reported pain behavior, observed pain behavior, depression, disability, and myalgia score. The intervening variables of helplessness, pain coping, and social support were also assessed.

Results.—Both groups showed significant reductions in depression, self-reported pain behavior, observed pain behavior, and myalgia scores, and there was no difference between groups. The 2 groups demonstrated similar significant reductions in helplessness and passive coping. According to multiple regression analysis, helplessness and passive coping were related to improvements in several clinical outcomes for participants overall and for the behavioral condition group. Only helplessness and pain scores were significantly higher in the education/control group.

Conclusion.—Behavioral and educational approaches are effective in reducing depression, myalgia scores, and pain behaviors in patients with

FM. Reducing helplessness and improving coping skills result in improved clinical outcomes.

▶ Fibromyalgia is one of the most perplexing problems facing patients and their physicians. Little is known of the etiology of this condition and most treatment interventions are fraught with high rates of failure in the reduction of symptoms. This interesting article looks at the efficacy of behavioral and psychoeducational strategies in reducing pain and depression. The results tell a tale of good news/bad news. The authors were not able to demonstrate any reduction in pain in the behavioral or educational format. The 1 variable that seemed to have a significant impact was the feeling of helplessness. Particularly impressive was the follow-up study showing a significant reduction in pain scores for those patients who had had a great decrease in the feeling of helplessness.

It's hard to place much stock in these findings. I don't think they would convince many managed care companies to approve funding for these therapies. However, so many of these patients are desperate for any type of help that referral for behavioral counseling and an education program seems prudent.

R.C. Davidson, M.D., M.P.H.

Fibromyalgia Syndrome in Children and Adolescents: Clinical Features at Presentation and Status at Follow-up
Siegel DM, Janeway D, Baum J (Univ of Rochester, NY)
Pediatrics 101:377–382, 1998

Introduction.—The precise etiology of fibromyalgia syndrome (FS), a painful, noninflammatory disorder that affects many more women than men, has not been identified. The disorder also occurs in children, and its presentation there appears to differ in several important aspects from that described in adults. A retrospective, descriptive study was conducted to further characterize FS as it appears in the pediatric population.

Methods.—The study setting was a university-affiliated pediatric rheumatology clinic that serves as a regional subspecialty referral service. Patients were identified by a review of medical records from 1989 to 1995. All had the diagnosis of FS, confirmed by a pediatric rheumatologist, as well as characteristic findings of diffuse pain, tender points, and poor sleep. A structured telephone interview was conducted to determine current status and response to treatment.

Results.—Forty-five children with a mean age of 13.3 years were identified in the review. Forty-one were girls and 42 were white. Thirty-three patients were available for a telephone interview at a mean of 2.6 years from initial diagnosis. Of the 15 symptoms that might be associated with FS, these children reported a mean of 8. Nearly all (more than 90%) experienced diffuse pain and disturbed sleep. Less frequent, but still common, were headaches (71%), generalized fatigue (62%), and morning

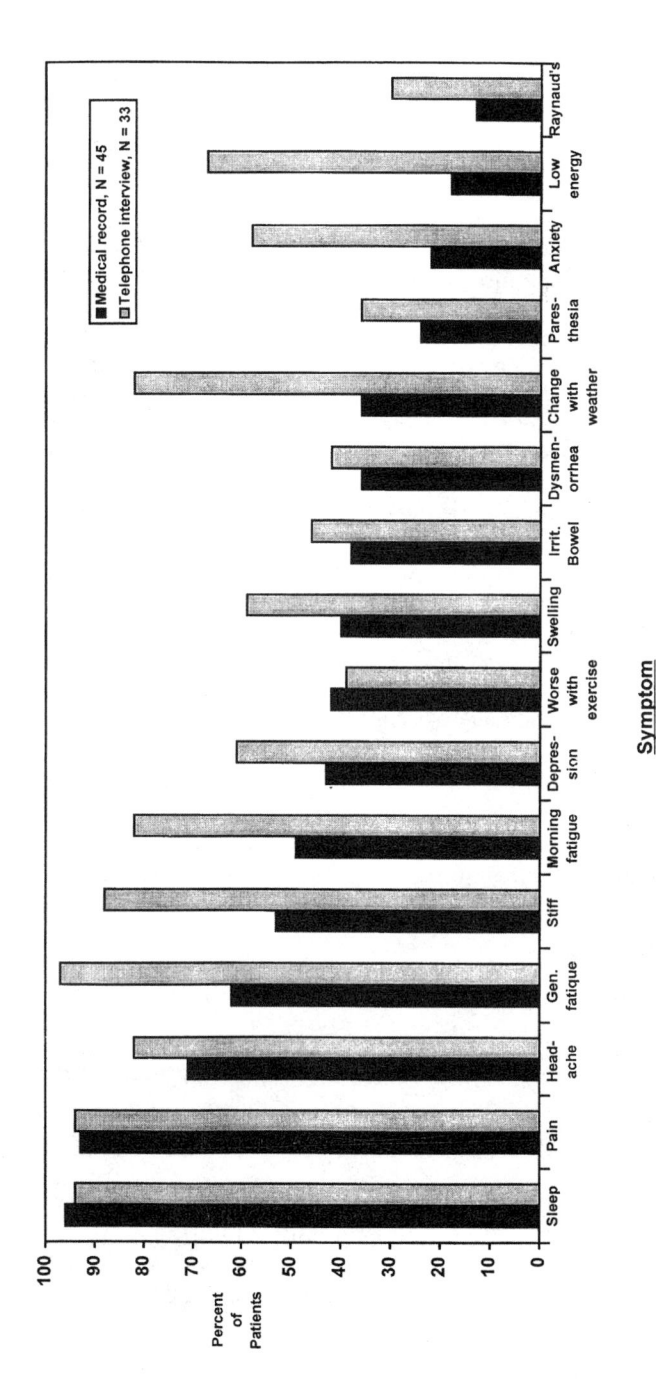

FIGURE.—Initial (medical record) and cumulative (telephone interview) symptoms in children and adolescents with FS. *Abbreviation:* FS, fibromyalgia syndrome. (Courtesy of Siegel DM, Janeway D, Baum J: Fibromyalgia syndrome in children and adolescents: Clinical features at presentation and status at follow-up. *Pediatrics* 101:377–382, 1998. Reproduced with permission from *Pediatrics*.)

stiffness (53%). Whereas a diagnosis of FS in adults requires a minimum of 11 (of 18) tender points, these children had a cumulative mean of 9.7 tender points. Most of the patients reported improvement at follow-up (Figure). Drugs frequently prescribed were cyclobenzaprine, nortriptyline, and amitriptyline.

Conclusion.—Fibromyalgia syndrome is not a rare or unusual diagnosis in children. As in adults, diffuse pain is an almost universal complaint, but sleep disturbance is as important to the establishment of a diagnosis. Children also tend to have fewer tender points than adults. The prognosis for children with FS is quite good.

▶ Fibromyalgia syndrome is a vexing problem for the patient and the physician. It is a noninflammatory disorder characterized by diffuse pain and specific tender spots. Although much more common in adults, it also occurs in children. This article reports a descriptive study from a pediatric rheumatology clinic, documenting the frequency of symptoms in children diagnosed with FS. Although there are some differences between children and adults in rank order of frequency, the overall pattern of symptoms seems quite similar. Sleep disturbances, pain, headache, general fatigue, and stiffness seem to be present in more than 50% of the children.

I think this is a helpful descriptive study. However, its population had severe disease and had been referred to a university pediatric rheumatology clinic. The symptoms in this population might be very different from the symptoms family physicians see in their offices. My purpose in including this article, however, is to increase our collective awareness of the possibility of FS in children and adolescents.

R.C. Davidson, M.D., M.P.H.

Miscellaneous

Measuring Functional Outcomes in Work-related Upper Extremity Disorders: Development and Validation of the Upper Extremity Function Scale
Pransky G, Feuerstein M, Himmelstein J, et al (Univ of Massachusetts, Worcester; Univ of Health Sciences, Bethesda, Md; Harvard Med School, Boston; et al)
J Occup Environ Med 39:1195–1202, 1997   9–6

Introduction.—Upper extremity disorders (UEDs), especially those that are work related, have been the subject of many recent studies. There is little evidence, however, to support the effectiveness of a particular intervention on functional outcome. Researchers report development of the Upper Extremity Function Scale (UEFS) to measure the impact of UEDs on the ability to perform physical tasks. The UEFS was evaluated for its reliability, discriminant validity, sensitivity to relevant clinical changes, and possible floor-and-ceiling effects.

Methods.—Eight items were selected for inclusion in the UEFS, using input from physicians, occupational therapists, and UED patients (Table

TABLE 1.—Upper Extremity Function Scale Questionnaire

	No Problem								Major Problem (Can't do it at all)	
A. Sleeping	1	2	3	4	5	6	7	8	9	10
B. Writing	1	2	3	4	5	6	7	8	9	10
C. Opening jars	1	2	3	4	5	6	7	8	9	10
D. Picking up small objects with fingers	1	2	3	4	5	6	7	8	9	10
E. Driving a car more than 30 minutes	1	2	3	4	5	6	7	8	9	10
F. Opening a door	1	2	3	4	5	6	7	8	9	10
G. Carrying milk jug from the refrigerator	1	2	3	4	5	6	7	8	9	10
H. Washing dishes	1	2	3	4	5	6	7	8	9	10

(Courtesy of Pransky G. Feuerstein M, Himmelstein J, et al: Measuring functional outcomes in work-related upper extremity disorders: Development and validation of the Upper Extremity Function Scale *J Occup Environ Med* 39:1195–1202, 1997.)

1). The instrument was tested in a group of 108 patients with work-related UEDs and 165 patients with carpal tunnel syndrome (CTS). Patients were asked to rate, on a scale of 1 (no problem) to 10 (major problem, unable to perform) their level of difficulty in performing each of the activities (sleeping, writing, opening jars, picking up small objects, driving a car for more than 30 minutes, opening a door, carrying a milk jug, and washing dishes).

Results.—Women made up 66% of the UED group and 67% of the CTS group. Over half in each group had been symptomatic for more than 1 year. Over one third of UED patients and 20% of CTS patients had undergone previous surgery for their condition. Compared with measures of symptom severity and clinical findings, the UEFS exhibited good internal consistency, a relative absence of floor effects, and excellent convergent and discriminant validity. In patients with CTS, the UEFS was more responsive to significant improvements over time than were clinical measures such as grip-and-pinch strength.

Conclusion.—The self-administered questionnaire reported here shows the feasibility of this method for measuring physical function in work-related UEDs. The UEFS performed well in terms of acceptability, validity, responsiveness to change, and adequate reliability.

▶ Pain and the limitations imposed by painful conditions are difficult to assess. We all have different "pain thresholds" and react to pain in different ways. Some of the most difficult, and most important, recommendations we make to our injured patients is how and when to return to work and to play. This is certainly the case in the management of cumulative trauma disorders of the upper extremity. The authors point out that some objective clinical measures, such as strength, may not correlate well with functional ability to return to activity. This has been well known in the sports medicine world when assessing athletes' ability to return to play—functional and field tests are more reliable indicators. However, this can be a cumbersome approach in the office. The author's presentation of a quick, self-administered tool to assess function really caught my eye. This appears to be a reliable tool, created by practitioners. I have some concerns. For instance, the study relied only on Phalen's test (often not done correctly and easily misinterpreted) as a measure in CTS. Also, the study focused only on chronic pain patients in a referral center. I definitely think that more work needs to be done. Nevertheless, this instrument provides a tool with which to monitor the effects of treatment in your cumulative trauma disorder patients. I am going to give it a try.

W.W. Dexter, M.D.

Randomised Controlled Trial of Hydroquinine in Muscle Cramps
Jansen PHP, Veenhuizen KCW, Wesseling AIM, et al (Ziekenhuis Gelderse Vallei, Ede, The Netherlands; Catholic Univ of Nijmegen, The Netherlands; ASTA Medica BV, Diemen, The Netherlands)
Lancet 349:528–532, 1997

Background.—Quinone and hydroquinone are often prescribed for muscle cramps. However, the results of studies of these agents' efficacy have been mixed.

Methods.—One hundred twelve patients with 3 or more muscle cramps per week were enrolled in a randomized, double-blind, placebo-controlled, parallel-group trial. Patients received 300 mg of hydroquinone hydrobromide dihydrate or placebo daily for 2 weeks.

Findings.—In both groups, the total number of muscle cramps and of cramp days declined during the treatment period, compared with the preceding 2-week period. However, the active treatment group had a median of 8 fewer cramps and 3 fewer cramp days, compared with only 3 and 1, respectively, in the placebo group. Sixty-five percent of the participants in the hydroquinone group had a 50% or greater decrease in the number of muscle cramps. Hydroquinone did not decrease the severity or duration of cramps after cramp onset. A sustained effect was noted after therapy was stopped. The adverse effects associated with hydroquinone were mild.

Conclusion.—This dose of hydroquinone is safe and effective in the short term for preventing frequent ordinary muscle cramps. The therapeutic effect of this agent continued beyond the treatment period.

▶ Leg cramps—particularly nocturnal leg cramps—are a common symptom of adults seeking primary care physician help. Assuming that the physical examination and history do not show any more serious pathology, quinine is frequently used as a therapy to reduce leg cramps. These authors from the Netherlands found a significant reduction in cramps in patients who used quinone. This seems to correlate well with most primary care physicians' findings that it does not always help but it often does.

Let us not forget nonpharmacologic interventions. In my own experience, nightly stretching of the Achilles tendon before going to bed is a safe and effective mechanism for helping to reduce nocturnal leg cramps.

R.C. Davidson, M.D., M.P.H.

Comparative Efficacy of Conservative Medical and Chiropractic Treatments for Carpal Tunnel Syndrome: A Randomized Clinical Trial
Davis PT, Hulbert JR, Kassak KM, et al (Northwestern College of Chiropractic, Bloomington, Minn; American Univ, Beirut, Lebanon)
J Manipulative Physiol Ther 21:317–326, 1998　　　　　　　　　　9–8

Introduction.—A variety of conservative and surgical interventions are used in the treatment of carpal tunnel syndrome (CTS). The American Academy of Neurology has recently recommended a conservative, nonsurgical approach as the primary treatment. A randomized trial compared the efficacy of conservative medical care with chiropractic care in the treatment of CTS.

Methods.—Men and women aged 21 to 45 years with self-reported symptoms of CTS were recruited using notices in local newspapers and on local radio. Excluded were those with a currently prescribed treatment for CTS or previous wrist surgery. Ninety-one of 96 eligible individuals with symptoms had CTS confirmed by clinical examination and nerve conduction studies. The 2-group, randomized, single-blind trial consisted of 9 weeks of treatment followed by an interview 1 month later. Those who received medical treatment took ibuprofen (800 mg 3 times a day for 1 week, 800 mg twice a day for 1 week, and 800 mg as needed to a maximum daily dose of 2,400 mg for 7 weeks) and wore wrist supports at night. Chiropractic treatment consisted of manipulation of the soft tissues and bony joints of the upper extremities and spine, US over the carpal tunnel, and wrist supports at night.

Results.—Outcome was determined by the patients' self-reported assessments of their physical and mental distress, focusing on hand discomfort and function. Objective assessment involved vibrometric thresholds of finger sensation. Both medical and chiropractic treatment groups exhibited significant improvements in perceived comfort and function, nerve conduction, and finger sensation. Differences between the 2 groups were not significant.

Conclusion.—Patients with CTS associated with median nerve demyelination, but not axonal degeneration, benefit equally from the common components of conservative medical or chiropractic therapy. No attempt was made to examine the relative cost of medical vs. chiropractic interventions.

▶ This might be a first for the YEAR BOOK OF FAMILY PRACTICE: a randomized, controlled trial extracted from a chiropractic journal. I was favorably impressed by the rigor of the methods. I was also favorably impressed that they published "negative" results. Mainstream biomedical journals are presumed to have a "publication bias" in that the results of studies showing a positive effect are more likely to be published than studies (like this one) that show no differences between treatments. I hope that more research into the clinical value of manipulative and physical treatments is conducted and that more of it is of this high quality. This study provides excellent evidence that manipulative therapies offer no clinical advantage over traditional medical treatment. The authors should be commended for their scientific integrity.

A.O. Berg, M.D., M.P.H.

Quantitive Systematic Review of Topically Applied Non-steroidal Anti-inflammatory Drugs
Moore RA, Tramèr MR, Carroll D, et al (Univ of Oxford, England)
BMJ 316:333–338, 1998   9–9

Background.—Although topical pain medications containing nonsteroidal anti-inflammatory drugs are big business, many physicians view such preparations as ineffective. A large, systematic literature review was undertaken to examine available evidence of the safety and efficacy of topical nonsteroidal anti-inflammatory drugs.

Methods.—MEDLINE, Excerpta Medica Database, and the Oxford Pain Relief Database were searched for reports of randomized, controlled trials of topical nonsteroidal anti-inflammatory drugs in which pain was an outcome. Additional reports were identified from retrieved report reference lists and from contacting companies that manufacture topical nonsteroidal anti-inflammatory products in the United Kingdom. A total of 86 trials involving 10,160 patients were identified.

Conclusions.—The results of this large, quantitative literature review indicate that topical nonsteroidal treatments are significantly more effective than placebo for relief of both acute and chronic pain. In particular, ketoprofen, felbinac, ibuprofen, and piroxicam were all significantly more effective than placebo, while indomethacin and benzydamine were no more effective than placebo. Both local and systemic adverse effects were rare. Further research should focus on identifying those patients who would benefit from using topical rather than oral nonsteroidal anti-inflammatory medication.

▶ I am frequently asked whether any of the topical medications for pain really work. One needs only to peruse the shelves of the local pharmacy to realize that it is a large industry and that many people perceive some type of benefit from these creams. Many of the preparations work as a rubefacient. These include menthol or some other ingredient to increase the blood flow to the area and give a feeling of warmth. Other preparations add a topical pain medication, frequently salicylate or some other nonsteroidal anti-inflammatory drug.

This article is an interesting mega-analysis of the published literature on 86 trials studying the pain-relieving effect of topically applied nonsteroidal anti-inflammatory drugs. The authors found a quite strong concurrence among the studies that these topical medications are effective in relieving pain in both acute and chronic conditions. This was true whether or not there was a rubefacient effect in the cream. These studies did not measure whether the topical medication was actually absorbed or if there was any anti-inflammatory effect locally from the application. However, there is fairly strong evidence that people do get pain relief from the use of these medications.

R.C. Davidson, M.D., M.P.H.

Cold- and Hot-pack Contrast Therapy: Subcutaneous and Intramuscular Temperature Change
Myrer JW, Measom G, Durrant E, et al (Brigham Young Univ, Provo, Utah)
J Athletic Train 32:238–241, 1997   9–10

Background.—Contrast therapy, the repeated alternation of thermotherapy and cryotherapy, is a common treatment for soft-tissue injury. However, no scientifically validated parameters have been established. On the assumption that the physiologic effects of contrast therapy are caused by significant fluctuations in soft-tissue temperature, the temperature changes in vivo in subcutaneous and IM tissue were investigated in 16 healthy volunteers.

Methods.—The study group consisted of 16 healthy college students. Subcutaneous and muscle tissue temperatures were measured by microprobes. The control treatment group had an ice pack placed over the triceps surae muscle group for 20 minutes. The contrast group received 5 minutes of a standard hydrocollator pack, followed by an ice pack for 5 minutes. These 2 treatments were alternated for a total of 20 minutes. Intramuscular and subcutaneous temperatures were recorded every 30 seconds during treatment and for 30 minutes after treatment. Then the 2 groups crossed over to the other treatment regimen. A multivariate analysis of variance was performed to determine whether significant changes in temperature occurred during these treatments.

Results.—During contrast therapy, muscular temperature did not change significantly over the 20-minute treatment period. Subcutaneous temperature fluctuated from 8°C to 14°C during each 5-minute treatment interval. During 20 minutes of ice pack treatment, muscle temperature decreased 7°C and subcutaneous temperature decreased 17°C.

Conclusions.—These results demonstrate that alternating cold- and hot-pack contrast therapy has little effect on muscle temperature. If beneficial effects depend on significant fluctuations in IM tissue temperature, then use of contrast therapy for soft-tissue injury should be reconsidered.

▶ It is interesting that as we delve further into evidence-based medicine, we continually need to question our assumptions for even simple "commonsense" types of therapies. This article, although clearly not a definitive study, asks such a question. These faculty members from a school of physical education designed this study to objectively measure temperature changes in muscle tissue during the frequently used contrast therapy. Their findings show that with this alternating contrast therapy, very little temperature fluctuation in muscle tissue could be measured. There was a greater temperature variation in subcutaneous tissue. When the authors used cold therapy for only 20-minute periods, demonstrable reductions in temperature in muscle tissue could be measured.

As I read this article, I thought back to the hundreds of times I have ordered physical therapy with alternating heat and cold for weekend injuries. This article suggests that if there is any therapeutic effect from this alternating contrast therapy, it is probably placebo in nature.

R.C. Davidson, M.D., M.P.H.

Correlation of Arthroscopic and Clinical Examinations With Magnetic Resonance Imaging Findings of Injured Knees in Children and Adolescents

Stanitski CL (Children's Hosp of Michigan, Detroit)
Am J Sports Med 26:2–6, 1998   9–11

Background.—Magnetic resonance imaging has become a widely used technique for diagnosis of knee disorders. However, few studies have correlated the results of MRI with the clinical and arthroscopic findings, and there is very little information regarding these relationships in children. The clinical, MRI, and arthroscopic findings in a series of children and adolescents with knee injuries were correlated.

Methods.—The study included 28 patients (average age, 14 years) who underwent MRI followed by arthroscopic surgery of the knee. The clinical and MRI diagnoses were evaluated against the arthroscopic findings, which were considered the standard for comparison. The analysis included meniscal, anterior cruciate ligament (ACL), and articular surface injuries.

Results.—There was total disagreement between the clinical and MRI findings in 75% of patients. In contrast, in 78.5% of patients, there was complete agreement between the clinical and arthroscopic findings. The accuracy of clinical evaluation was 96% for ACL injuries, 93% for meniscal injuries, and 89% for articular surface injuries. In contrast, there was total disagreement between the MRI and arthroscopic findings in 78.5% of patients. The accuracy of MRI was 89% for ACL injuries, 37.5% for meniscal injuries, and 79% for articular surface injuries. In addition to accuracy, positive and negative predictive values, sensitivity, and specificity were all greater with clinical examination than with MRI.

Conclusion.—In the evaluation of injured knees in children and adolescents, clinical examination offers much better diagnostic information than MRI. Little information useful for patient management is provided by MRI, which has a high false negative rate. In pediatric knee injuries, MRI should be used as an adjunct when the diagnosis is in question after clinical and radiographic assessment. The radiologist performing MRI should always be made aware of the clinical findings.

▶ So much for the thinking that the MRI is a definitive gold standard in the evaluation of acute knee injuries. This remarkable study of children and adolescents suggests that the clinical evaluation of the patient may be more accurate than MRI. This study may be quoted to parents who demand an MRI for knee injuries when the clinical examination is diagnostic.

J.E. Scherger, M.D., M.P.H.

The Effect of Socio-Demographic and Crash-Related Factors on the Prognosis of Whiplash
Harder S, Veilleux M, Suissa S (McGill Univ, Montreal; Montreal Gen Hosp)
J Clin.Epidemiol 51:377–384, 1998   9–12

Objective.—It is common for individuals in motor vehicles during crashes to experience whiplash injuries. The outcome is not predictable and problems may persist for more than 6 months. The effects and relative contributions of sociodemographic and crash-related factors on prognosis were investigated in a large, population-based incident cohort of patients with whiplash.

Methods.—The recovery of a cohort of 3,014 patients with whiplash in Quebec, Canada, was followed for 6 years. The duration of recovery time was defined as the duration of compensation.

Results.—Because 204 individuals had a recurrence, the recovery of the remaining 2,810 was analyzed. The recovery rate for whiplash alone was 1.37/100 patients per day. The 1,259 patients with injuries in addition to whiplash had slower recoveries. Among whiplash-only patients, 25% recovered within 1 week; the median recovery time was 30 days, and 1.9% of patients had not recovered in a year. Among patients with injuries in addition to whiplash, 19% recovered within 1 week; the median recovery time was 31 days, and 4.1% had not recovered in a year. Among the whiplash-only group, older age, female sex, larger number of dependents, married status, not being employed full-time, being in a truck or bus, being a passenger, colliding with a moving object, and colliding head-on or sideways were associated with a significantly lower chance of recovery. The likelihood of recovery was 15% lower for passengers and 14% lower for every 10-year increase in age.

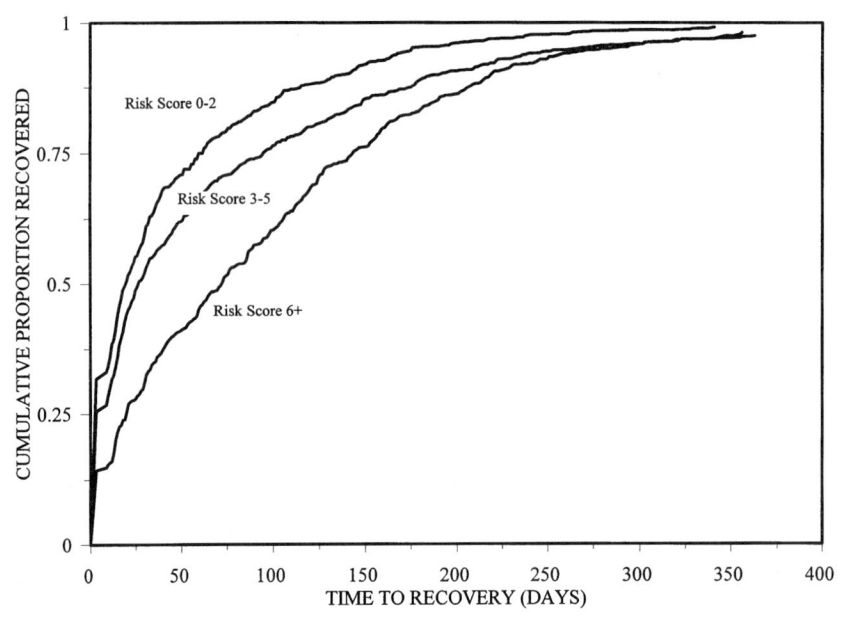

FIGURE 2.—One-year cumulative recovery curves among subjects with a whiplash injury alone according to the prediction score: 0–2 (fastest recovery profile); 3–5 (average recovery profile); and 6–11 (slowest recovery profile). The prediction score is the sum of ones or zeros, respectively, for the presence or absence of female sex, one or more dependents, not being employed full-time, crash in a bus or truck, being a passenger, collision with a moving object, collision at 90 degrees or head-on, as well as of 0, 1, 2, 3, and 4, respectively, for age less than 30 years, 30–39, 40–49, 50–59, and 60 and over. (Reprinted by permission of the publisher from Harder S, Veilleux M, Suissa S: The effect of socio-demographic and crash-related factors on the prognosis of whiplash. *J Clin Epidemiol* 51:377–384, copyright 1998 by Elsevier Science Inc.)

Among patients with injuries in addition to whiplash, older age, not being employed full-time, severity of collision, being in a truck or bus, and being a passenger were associated with a significantly lower chance of recovery. A prediction score from 0 to 11 was constructed, based on these factors, and was used to stratify patients. Patients with scores of 0 to 2 (a maximum of 2 risk factors) had the fastest recovery time, whereas patients with scores of 6 or greater had the slowest recovery time (19 and 71 days, respectively) (Fig 2).

Conclusion.—Sociodemographic and crash-related factors contribute to the duration of recovery from whiplash injury in a motor vehicle crash. These factors are easily measured and can be used to identify patients with a poor prognosis.

▶ Whiplash injury, especially after a motor vehicle accident, is a common problem for the primary care physician. This is a very interesting longitudinal study of over 3,000 patients in Canada who sustained whiplash injuries from motor vehicle accidents. There are no surprises in these data. Persons injured in truck or bus accidents took a longer time to recover than those injured in automobile accidents. Persons who were wearing seat belts were more likely to get whiplash injury and to take a longer time to recover. However, the authors did not study other injuries in patients not wearing seat belts.

The authors developed a prognosis score for rating variables that prolong time to recovery. For patients with a risk score greater than 6, there was a significantly longer time to recovery. The significant factors that related to a higher risk score included female gender, older age, larger number of dependents, married status, not being employed full-time, being in a truck or bus, being a passenger, collision with a moving object, and colliding head-on or sideways.

I am not sure that this study is of much use. We will continue to need thorough documentation of symptoms because many of these injuries are involved in legal issues. I do find this study interesting, however, as documentation of the intuitive findings that I have had as a primary care physician.

R.C. Davidson, M.D., M.P.H.

10 Mental Health and Psychiatry

Overview
  Randomized controlled trials: Abstracts 10–4, 10–18, and 10–21

Dementia and Alzheimer's Disease
- The Mini-Mental State Examination in diagnosing dementia
- Effects of special care units on Alzheimer's disease functional outcome
- Cost-effectiveness of tacrine for Alzheimer's disease
- Ginkgo biloba for dementia

Drug and Alcohol Use
- Single question for problem drinking
- Two articles on alcohol consumption and mortality
- Naltrexone in alcohol dependence

Marital Distress and Domestic Violence
- Validating the concept of abuse
- Guidelines for managing abuse
- Screening men for partner violence
- Couple and family interventions for marital distress and mental health problems

Mental Health Services and Insurance
- Costs of unlimited mental health coverage in managed care
- Insurance status and recognition of psychosocial problems

Miscellaneous
- Can money buy happiness?
- Psychosocial correlates of workplace harassment
- Suicide after natural disasters
- Nondirective therapy and routine care for emotional problems
- Restraint reductions and psychoactive drug use
- Creativity and mental illness
- Paroxetine and social phobia

- Munchausen by proxy
- Sabotaging one's own medical care

Dementia and Alzheimer's Disease

Limitations of the Mini-Mental State Examination in Diagnosing Dementia in General Practice
Wind AW, Schellevis FG (Vrije Universiteit Amsterdam)
Int J Geriatr Psychiatry 12:101–108, 1997   10–1

Objective.—As society ages, dementia becomes an increasing health care problem. Whether cognitive tests are useful in diagnosing dementia is controversial. The value of the Mini-Mental State Examination (MMSE), advocated by the Dutch College of General Practitioners, was validated by comparing the diagnostic value of a set of items in the MMSE to that of the total MMSE score in a suspect population.

Methods.—Cross-sectional data were collected on 533 community-based elderly individuals (214 men) aged 65–84 years in Amsterdam, judged by their 36 physicians to be suffering from minimal to severe dementia. The Geriatric Mental State Schedule (GMS) was administered to all patients, and the AGECAT algorithm was applied to weight symptoms. The MMSE was administered to all patients. Total scores and 2 sets of categories were evaluated for validity. The first set consisted of 3 categories: normal (27–30), suspect (22–26), and poor (21 or less) cognitive functioning; and the second set consisted of 2 categories: normal (24–30) and deviant (23 or less). The most accurate combination of items for predicting dementia was determined using stepwise logistic regression analysis, and the predictive ability of the total MMSE score for diagnosing dementia was calculated using logistic regression analysis.

Results.—General practitioners judged 319 patients with minimal dementia, 106 with mild dementia, and 36 with severe dementia. The average MMSE score for all patients was 24.2, 149 scored 23 or less, and 114 scored 21 or less. Organic syndrome was diagnosed in 114 patients by the GMS/AGECAT. Individual items did not discriminate well between those with and without dementia. Patients with suspect scores (22–26) and those with poor scores (21 or less) were 6.5 and 91.1 times more likely to have dementia as a patient with a normal score (27–30) (Table 2). The best predictive combination included date, day of the week, patient's address, and current prime minister (sensitivity, 64.9%; specificity, 96.4%). This combination was as accurate as the entire MMSE in distinguishing between dementia and nondementia (sensitivity, 64.7%; specificity, 93.3%).

Conclusion.—Whereas the 4-component combination of date, day of the week, patient's address, and current prime minister was as accurate as the total MMSE score in differentiating between dementia and nondementia in a selected group of elderly individuals, the value of MMSE in

TABLE 2.—Relationship Between the Diagnosis of Dementia and a Set of Items, Two Sets of MMSE Score Categories (Composed of Three and Two Categories, Respectively), Adjusted for Age, Sex, and Education

Items	Categories	Odds Ratio	(95% CI)
Set of items			
Date (d/m/y)	0 m/l–3 m*	5.4	(2.6–11.0)
Day of the week	Correct/incorrect	5.5	(2.2–13.7)
Address, excl. postal code	Correct/incorrect	15.7	(5.6–44.2)
Current prime minister	Correct/incorrect	9.5	(4.9–18.6)
MMSE scores divided into 3 categories	27–30	1.0	
	22–26	6.5	(2.6–16.4)
	≤ 21	91.1	(35.6–233.1)
MMSE scores divided into 2 categories	24–30	1.0	
	≤ 23	21.2	(12.2–36.7)

Note: Population composed of individuals suspected by their general practitioners to be possibly suffering from dementia. N = 533.
*Geriatric Mental State Schedule/AGECAT-based diagnosis of organic syndrome: 3 or more = suffering from dementia (N = 114) vs. 2 or less = not suffering from dementia (N = 419, reference population).
Abbreviation: m, mistakes.
(Reprinted by permission of John Wiley & Sons Ltd., from Wind AW, Schellevis FG: Limitations of the Mini-Mental State Examination in diagnosing dementia in general practice. *Int J Geriatr Psychiatry* 12:101–108, 1997. Copyright 1997 by John Wiley & Sons Ltd.)

diagnosing dementia in the general population is limited. Cognitive test scores are only 1 aspect of the patient's overall clinical condition.

▶ The MMSE has achieved status as a sort of gold standard in screening patients for likely dementia. The good news is that a 4-item subset was as discriminating as the whole thing in this group of patients. The great thing about this is that the cumulative risk of the 4 items is multiplicative (see Table 1). In other words, age and sex being equal, a patient with incorrect answers on date and day of the week is 30 times more likely (5.4 × 5.5) to have dementia than a patient who answered all 4 questions correctly. This approach holds promise for being a quicker and an at-least-as-accurate screen as doing the whole MMSE.

A.O. Berg, M.D., M.P.H.

Effects of Residence in Alzheimer Disease Special Care Units on Functional Outcomes
Phillips CD, Sloane PD, Hawes C, et al (Menorah Park Ctr for the Aging, Beachwood, Ohio; Univ of North Carolina, Chapel Hill; Research Triangle Inst, Research Triangle Park, NC)
JAMA 278:1340–1344, 1997

Objective.—Although Alzheimer's disease special care units (SCU) are becoming more common, their effect on patient outcome has not been investigated. Results of the first large-scale evaluation of the effects of SCUs on resident outcomes were reviewed.

Methods.—Activities of daily living function, continence, and weight for 77,337 residents in more than 800 nursing homes in 4 states, including 1,228 residents in 48 SCUs, were assessed quarterly in a cohort study over a 1-year period. Decline in locomotion, transferring, toileting, eating, dressing, activities of daily living, bowel continence, urinary incontinence, and weight were outcome measures.

Results.—When SCU residents, residents in traditional units in facilities with SCUs, and residents in facilities without SCUs were compared, there were no statistically significant differences in any of the 9 variables.

Conclusion.—Residents with Alzheimer's disease in SCUs did not have a better outcome than did residents in traditional nursing homes.

▶ These data provide nearly population-based data on the actual use-effectiveness of SCUs for patients with Alzheimer's disease. These results diverge from earlier smaller studies, some of which documented improvements in patients residing in SCUs. The numbers studied here were enormous—nearly 250,000 assessments on more than 75,000 residents. I believe the data are persuasive that SCUs do not retard functional decline, at least for large populations of average patients residing in average settings. The principal remaining question is whether SCUs provide other important benefits, perhaps related to quality of life or social outcomes, not studied in this research. If indeed the designation "special care" predicts nothing special in functional outcomes, families who are considering placing members in SCUs should be sure that they understand what is being provided, what outcomes are expected, and at what cost.

A.O. Berg, M.D., M.P.H.

Treatment of Alzheimer Disease With Tacrine: A Cost-Analysis Model
Wimo A, Karlsson G, Nordberg A, et al (Umeå Univ, Sweden; Stockholm School of Economics; Karolinska Inst, Stockholm; et al)
Alzheimer Dis Assoc Disord 11:191–200, 1997   10–3

Introduction.—It has been hypothesized that the cognitive decline characteristic of Alzheimer's disease results from low levels of acetylcholine. Thus, drugs that increase the cholinergic activity in the brain, such as the acetylcholinesterase inhibitor tacrine, may have positive effects on cognitive function. A cost-analysis model was developed to determine the economic effects of tacrine treatment for patients with Alzheimer's disease.

Methods.—In this Swedish study, tacrine treatment was compared with no treatment for patients with Alzheimer's disease. Also examined were the costs of starting tacrine treatment in the early stages of disease vs. a later stage. In the sensitivity analysis, the main alternative and the alternative outcomes were based on tacrine's effect on cognitive function expressed as the Mini-Mental State Examination (MMSE) score. Extra costs of tacrine treatment were based on the costs of different doses, laboratory tests, extra visits to physicians, and diagnostic procedures. A model of survival was constructed in which the placement of patients with Alzheimer's disease in care organizations was assumed to be influenced by the use of tacrine.

Results.—When benefits were calculated for the entire Alzheimer disease population in Sweden, the benefit of tacrine treatment was a cost reduction of 1.3%. The annual benefit per patient was estimated to be approximately U.S. $320 (1993). An early start of treatment (MMSE score = 24 points) resulted in lower costs than a later score, even though most such patients are at home rather than in institutional care. Benefits of tacrine improve to 4.1% if the treatment and its effects are assumed to continue to death. Savings are 4.6% if nursing home care is postponed by 1 year.

Discussion.—This model found tacrine treatment would have modest beneficial effects on the cost of Alzheimer's disease in Sweden. The 17% cost reduction reported in a 1994 U.S. study assumed a greater reduction in institutional care, a more rapid decline in the MMSE score, and a shorter survival period. Tacrine may facilitate the trend of deinstitutionalization, which is already under way in Sweden.

▶ This is a welcome study following on the findings of a few years ago that tacrine has a modest effect on the course of Alzheimer's disease: what is the treatment's cost? The fact that this study was conducted using Swedish data compromises generalizability to the United States; but, on the other hand, the strength of the model is its population base, unobtainable in this country. The bottom line is a modest—indeed a very modest—effect at a very modest cost. An even more useful study would be a full cost-effectiveness analysis, in which the costs per quality-adjusted year of life saved would be calculated. That would allow us to more directly compare the cost-effectiveness of tacrine treatment with other competing interventions.

A.O. Berg, M.D., M.P.H.

A Placebo-controlled, Double-blind, Randomized Trial of an Extract of Ginkgo Biloba for Dementia
Le Bars PL, for the North American EGb Study Group (New York Inst for Med Research, Tarrytown; et al)
JAMA 278:1327–1332, 1997   10–4

Introduction.—An extract of ginkgo biloba, EGb 761, has been used in Europe to treat cognitive disorders and was recently approved in Germany for the treatment of dementia. The mechanism of action of this plant extract seems to be related to its antioxidant properties. A multicenter trial was conducted at 6 research centers in the United States to examine the safety and efficacy of EGb in Alzheimer's disease (AD) and multi-infarct dementia (MID).

Methods.—The 327 patients enrolled in the double-blind, placebo-controlled study had mild to moderately severe dementia and no other significant medical conditions. After a 14-day placebo run-in period, the subjects were randomized to treatment with EGb (120 mg/day) or placebo. Safety assessments were performed at 4-, 12-, 26-, and 52-week visits and assessments of primary outcome measures at 12, 26, and 52 weeks. Change was evaluated in the areas of cognitive impairment, daily living, and social behavior, using the Alzheimer's Disease Assessment Scale–Cognitive subscale (ADAS-Cog), Geriatric Evaluation by Relative's Rating Instrument (GERRI), and Clinical Global Impression of Change (CGIC).

Results.—The study group had 251 patients with AD and 76 with MID; 309 were included in intent-to-treat (ITT) analysis (236 with AD and 73 with MID) and 202 provided evaluable data for the 52-week end point analysis. In the ITT group, a greater proportion of those treated with EGb achieved at least a 4-point improvement on the ADAS-Cog (27% vs. 14%) and were considered improved on the GERRI (37% vs. 23%). Their CGIC score was unchanged. Approximately 30% of patients in each treatment group reported at least 1 adverse event. Only about half of these events were related to the study drug, however, and most were considered mild to moderate. Three patients were withdrawn from the trial because of adverse events: 2 treated with EGb and 1 receiving placebo.

Conclusion.—Treatment with the extract of ginkgo biloba, EGb, was shown to be superior to placebo in stabilizing or improving cognitive performance and social functioning in patients with mild to moderately severe dementia. Improvement was demonstrated objectively by the ADAS-Cog and was of sufficient magnitude to be recognized by caregivers who completed the GERRI.

▶ This article is a real showstopper: a high-quality, randomized controlled trial of an herbal remedy published in a front-rank U.S. medical journal showing a positive effect of treatment—and on dementia yet. The benefits were statistically significant and were noticeable by caregivers. In my view, in addition to identifying a possibly useful treatment for dementia, the study shows that one should keep an open mind regarding nonconventional therapy. Nonconventional interventions that appear to be useful in descriptive studies, have a favorable safety profile, and are available at reasonable cost are worth studying.

A.O. Berg, M.D., M.P.H.

Drug and Alcohol Use

Screening for Problem Drinking: Does a Single Question Work?
Taj N, Devera-Sales A, Vinson DC (Univ of Missouri-Columbia)
J Fam Pract 46:328–335, 1998 10–5

Introduction.—Problem drinking is a major cause of morbidity and mortality. Alcohol consumption may be significantly reduced by brief physician interventions with at-risk drinkers; yet, according to the 1991 National Health Interview Survey of Health Promotion and Disease Prevention, only 39% of respondents who visited a physician in the previous 2 years indicated that they were asked by their physician about alcohol use. A systematic approach to screening may increase the rate at which primary care physicians discuss health behaviors with their patients. It was explored whether a single screening question could effectively identify problem drinkers, including *at-risk drinkers*, defined as those who drink more than safe limits but without major recurrent consequences, and those with an *alcohol-use disorder*, defined as alcohol abuse or dependence.

Methods.—An initial 3-question screen was presented to 1,435 patients. The screen included the question, "On any single occasion during the past 3 months, have you had more than 5 drinks containing alcohol?" The question was placed between other questions about seat belt and tobacco use. Of the 1,368 patients who answered the questions, a sample of 101 patients who answered yes and 99 who answered no were given the Alcohol Use Disorders Identification Test in writing. Two gold standard interview instruments were also given: alcohol questions in the Composite International Diagnostic Interview, with alcohol-use disorders defined by the *Diagnostic and Statistical Manual of Mental Disorders*, ed 4, (DSM-IV) criteria; and a calendar-based review of drinking. *Problem drinking* was defined as either at-risk drinking in the previous month or an alcohol-use disorder in the past 12 months.

Results.—A positive predictive value of 74% resulted with the single question. The negative predictive value was 88% for problem drinking, with a specificity of 93% and a sensitivity of 62%. The question's utility in detecting both at-risk drinking and current alcohol-use disorders was similar. All 29 patients who had both were correctly identified.

Conclusion.—At-risk drinking and current alcohol-use disorders can be detected by means of a single question with clinically useful positive and negative predictive values.

▶ Here's the latest in the long-standing quest for the absolute minimum intervention to detect problem drinking. Is it possible that a *single* question is good enough? Well, Table 3 in this article is astonishing. Sensitivity, specificity, positive predictive value, and negative predictive value are in a range that would be acceptable for any number of other commonly used screening tests. It would be premature to discard other screening tools, such as the CAGE and the Michigan Alcoholism Screening Test, that can be answered in written questionnaire format before the patient even sees the physician (thus being quicker than asking even 1 question in the clinical interview). But as a backup in a busy practice with the patient who may not have time for a health maintenance questionnaire, this single question looks like a good bet to me.

A.O. Berg, M.D., M.P.H.

Alcohol Consumption and Mortality Among Middle-aged and Elderly U.S. Adults
Thun MJ, Peto R, Lopez AD, et al (American Cancer Society, Atlanta, Ga; Univ of Oxford, England; World Health Organization, Geneva)
N Engl J Med 337:1705–1714, 1997   10–6

Background.—The consumption of alcohol is known to have both adverse and beneficial effects on health. The balance between these separate effects of alcohol was prospectively studied in a large population of American adults.

Study Design.—The Cancer Prevention Study II is a large prospective study of mortality among almost 1.2 million American adults. The current study included 490,000 of these participants, aged 30 years and older, who completed a 4-page questionnaire on mortality factors, including both alcohol and tobacco use. The participants were more likely than the U.S. population to be white, married, middle class, and college educated. The study was begun in 1982, and the participants were followed up for 9 years. Cause-specific death rates and all-cause death rates were compared across categories of baseline alcohol consumption.

Findings.—Alcohol consumption was associated with cirrhosis; alcoholism; cancers of the mouth, esophagus, pharynx, larynx, and liver; breast cancer in women; and injuries in men. Mortality from breast cancer was 30% higher among women who reported consumption of at least 1 drink per day than among nondrinkers. The rate of death from cardiovascular disease was 30% to 40% lower among men and women reporting consumption of at least 1 drink per day, than among nondrinkers (Fig 1). Overall death rates were lowest for those reporting consumption of about 1 drink per day. All-cause mortality increased with increasing alcohol consumption, especially among adults younger than 60 years with lower risks of cardiovascular disease. Consumption of alcohol was associated with a small reduction in mortality risk among middle-aged Americans, whereas smoking approximately doubled this risk (Fig 2).

Conclusions.—Moderate alcohol consumption—1–2 drinks per day—was associated with lower all-cause mortality than was nondrinking. The age, background, and health risks of participants had an effect on the balance of adverse and beneficial effects of alcohol consumption. Any benefit from alcohol consumption was far lower than the increased risk of mortality produced by smoking. The social policy implications of these findings are beyond the scope of this study.

▶ Alcohol consumption is a frequent topic at our health maintenance visits. This study should reassure those who have preached moderation not abstinence. I am thoroughly impressed by the sheer volume of this study—nearly half a million participants. This certainly gives the results some credence. However, I wonder whether specific conclusions can be drawn from this study as there are factors not studied because of its size. The authors did control for smoking (Fig 2)—no surprise there. Also note that for other

Chapter 10–Mental Health and Psychiatry / **201**

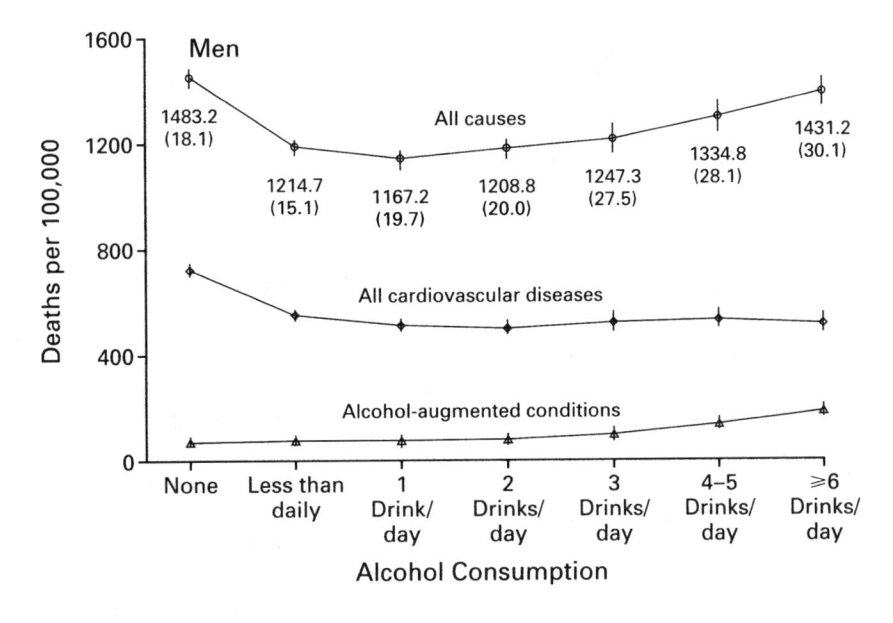

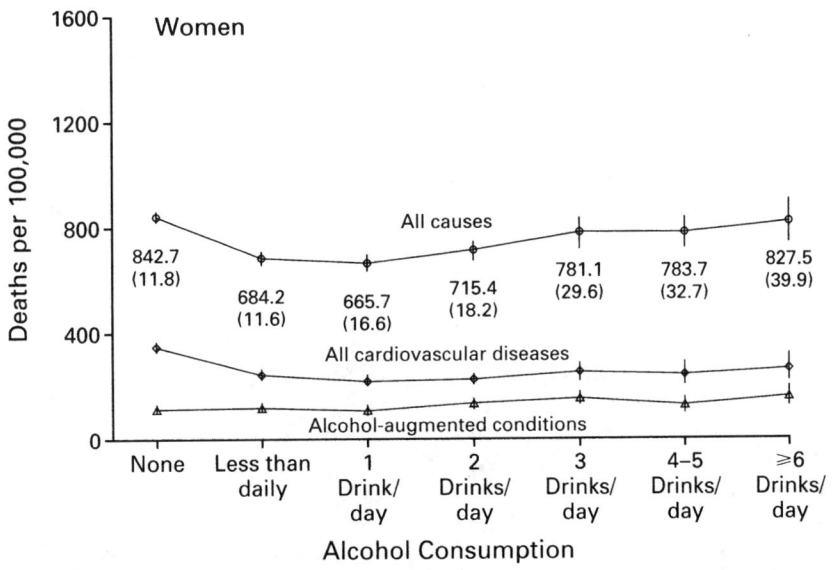

FIGURE 1.—Rates of death from all causes, all cardiovascular diseases, and alcohol-augmented conditions from 1982 to 1991, according to baseline alcohol consumption. Alcohol-augmented conditions are cirrhosis and alcoholism, alcohol-related cancers, breast cancer in women, and injuries and other external causes. "Less than daily" alcohol consumption was defined as drinking 3 or more times per week, but less than 1 drink per day. The numbers in parentheses are the standard errors of the rates of death from all causes. (Courtesy of Thun MJ, Peto R, Lopez AD, et al: Alcohol consumption and mortality among middle-aged and elderly U.S. adults. *N Engl J Med* 337:1705–1714. Copyright 1997, Massachusetts Medical Society. Reprinted by permission of *The New England Journal of Medicine*. All rights reserved.)

Men

Nondrinkers
- Nonsmokers: 26
- Smokers: 46

Drinkers
- Nonsmokers: 22
- Smokers: 43

Probability (%)

Women

Nondrinkers
- Nonsmokers: 17
- Smokers: 30

Drinkers
- Nonsmokers: 14
- Smokers: 28

Probability (%)

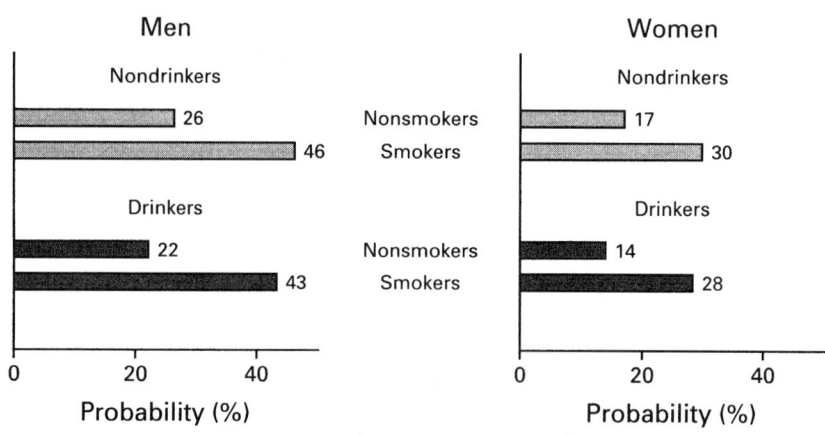

FIGURE 2.—Estimated probability of death from any cause in the general U.S. population from 35 to 69 years of age for 4 combinations of alcohol consumption and smoking. The probabilities projected for the general U.S. population are based on relative risks calculated in this study, combined with prevalence and mortality data for the U.S. population in 1990. They reflect the smoking of approximately 1 pack of cigarettes per day by smokers and consumption of approximately 1–2 drinks per day by those reported drinking alcohol in 1982. (Courtesy of Thun MJ, Peto R, Lopez AD, et al: Alcohol consumption and mortality among middle-aged and elderly U.S. adults. *N Engl J Med* 337:1705–1714. Copyright 1997, Massachusetts Medical Society. Reproduced by permission of *The New England Journal of Medicine*. All rights reserved.)

entities (e.g., breast cancer), the risk for disease may increase with modest alcohol intake, and the potential social/family costs are not mentioned. My other concern is that the population studied (white, educated, married, middle class) is not representative of the U.S. population. Nevertheless, moderate drinking, for many of our patients, would seem to be a relatively safe (not necessarily prudent) dietary habit that, based on the study findings, need not be discouraged. For another look at this topic, see the next article (Abstract 10–7).

W.W. Dexter, M.D.

Association of Alcohol Consumption to Mortality in Middle-aged U.S. and Russian Men and Women

Deev A, Shestov D, Abernathy J, et al (Natl Ctr for Preventive Medicine of the Russian Federation, Moscow; Russian Academy of Med Sciences, St Petersburg, Russia; Univ of North Carolina, Chapel Hill)
Ann Epidemiol 8:147–153, 1998   10–7

Introduction.—Although alcohol use increases the risk of mortality from certain diseases and types of accidents, many recent studies report benefits from moderate use of alcohol. In both men and women, moderate alcohol consumption appears to have a protective effect for cardiovascular disease (CVD). The relationships of alcohol consumption to total and CVD mortality were assessed in U.S. and Russian men and women.

TABLE 3.—Age-adjusted Mortality Rates for All Causes and CVD Deaths by Drinking Category, U.S. and Russian Men Aged 40–59 and Women Aged 40–69

Drinking Category	U.S. All Causes	U.S. CVD	Russia All Causes	Russia CVD
Men				
Non-drinker	17.3	11.5	29.0	18.8
Level 1	16.8	10.1	23.2	13.6
Level 2	13.7	6.8	24.3	14.4
Level 3	12.7	5.9	24.0	11.9
Level 4	15.1	8.7	33.6	18.1
Women				
Non-drinker	16.7	8.4	16.6	8.1
Level 1	13.1	5.0	12.4	5.7
Level 2	13.3	5.6	9.2	4.3
Level 3	12.7	5.0	25.7	13.4

Abbreviation: CVD, cardiovascular disease.
(Courtesy of Deev A, Shestov D, Abernathy J, et al: Association of alcohol consumption to mortality in middle-aged U.S. and Russian men and women. *Ann Epidemiol* 8:147–153. Copyright 1998 by Elsevier Science Inc. Reprinted by permission.)

Methods.—The U.S.-Russian Lipid Research Clinics Prevalence Study was conducted between 1972 and 1982. In both countries, men aged 40–59 years and women aged 40–69 years were screened and followed up for mortality for 13 years. Alcohol consumption by study participants was based on a 7-day recall of drinks of beer, wine, mixed drinks, and liquors. Given the amount consumed in the previous week, participants were classified as nondrinkers or into 4 levels of alcohol consumption.

Results.—In the United States, most men (72%) and women (53%) had at least 1 drink last week; 11% of men and 21% of women were classified as nondrinkers. Russian men showed a similar pattern, but only 27% of Russian women reported consuming at least 1 drink in the previous week. More than half (55%) of Russian women were level 1 drinkers, defined as at least 1 drink during the previous year but none last week. For both U.S. and Russian men, age-adjusted mortality rates for all causes of death and for CVD were highest for nondrinkers and lowest for level 3 drinkers (has more than 12 g but less than or equal to 24 g last week). An exception was all-cause mortality in Russian men (Table 3), where the rate for level 1 drinkers was slightly lower than for level 4 drinkers (more than 24 g last week). Adjustment for other risk factors showed that mortality rates remained higher for nondrinkers in U.S. men and women, but no difference in mortality rates was present between drinkers and nondrinkers in Russia. An exception to Russian findings was in women who were level 2 drinkers (less than or equal to 6 g last week).

Conclusions.—Alcohol consumption has a protective effective on all-cause and CVD mortality in men and women in the United States, but this protective effect was not observed in Russian men and women. The difference may be explained by higher rates of mortality and hypertension in Russia or by variations in drinking patterns.

▶ Here is another take on alcohol consumption and its relationship to mortality. This study, while smaller than that of Thun et al. (Abstract 10–6), reports similar results. Moderate consumption of alcohol (the definition in this study varied significantly from that used by Thun et al.) seems to reduce all-cause and CVD mortality—but only in the United States. Left unexplained is the lack of effect in Russia. Even so, there is no increase in mortality in the Russian population study. The final word? Probably not. I would prefer to see data that allow more precise counseling of patients, i.e., risk of specific diseases such as breast cancer (increased risk) or macular degeneration (decreased risk).[1] In the meantime, moderation is still the watchword.

W.W. Dexter, M.D.

Reference

1. Obisesan TO, Hirsch R, Kosoko O, et al: Moderate wine consumption is associated with decreased odds of developing age-related macular degeneration in NHANES-1. *J Am Geriatr Soc* 46:1–7, 1998.

A Preliminary Investigation of the Management of Alcohol Dependence With Naltrexone by Primary Care Providers
O'Connor PG, Farren CK, Rounsaville BJ, et al (Yale Univ, New Haven, Conn)
Am J Med 103:477–482, 1997
10–8

Introduction.—Patients identified in the primary care setting as having problem drinking and alcohol dependence are typically referred to specialized alcohol treatment programs. Those with problem drinking who continue to have primary care–based treatment often participate in minimal or brief interventions. Naltrexone, a new form of pharmacotherapy for alcohol dependence, was evaluated as an adjunct to a counseling strategy used by primary care providers.

Methods.—Twenty-nine alcohol-dependent individuals were enrolled in the study. All were managed within a primary care model located at a university-affiliated substance research program. None had major comorbidity or were at high risk for complicated withdrawal. Participants were required to have current alcohol dependence by the *Diagnostic and Statistical Manual of Mental Disorders*, ed 3, revised criteria, and abstinence for 5 days before study entry. On day 1, patients received 25 mg of naltrexone followed by 50 mg/day on subsequent days. An initial 45-minute counseling session was used to review substance abuse history, develop a treatment plan, refer to Alcoholics Anonymous, and set goals for later follow-up sessions. Seven brief follow-up visits were scheduled for the 10-week study.

Results.—Most patients were employed white men. Twenty-one (72%) of those enrolled completed treatment. The percent of days abstinent increased significantly (from 36.6% to 88.8%), as did the percent days abstinent from heavy drinking (from 48.7% to 97.3%); the mean number of drinks per occasion significantly fell from 9.2 to 2.5. Mean serum γ-glutamyl transferase level decreased compared to baseline from 67.1 U/L to 45.3 U/L. Providers reported that 33% of the patients had improved "very much" and 24% "moderately." Participant ratings were "much better" for 29% and "somewhat better" for 19%. Seventeen of the 21 patients who completed the study continued treatment with their primary care provider and 4 were referred to other treatment.

Conclusion.—Counseling by primary care providers, combined with naltrexone treatment, proved to be both feasible and effective for alcohol-dependent individuals. Overall, 45% of the 29 patients who enrolled remained abstinent and 35% relapsed to heavy drinking.

▶ This is the only trial I've seen testing naltrexone in a primary care setting. I include it because of its novelty, even though its small size, nonreproducible recruitment strategy (advertisements, referrals, volunteers), and management by a general internist make it hard to generalize to typical family practice settings. Still, everything so far about this approach in the literature is promising. One hopes that more research in typical settings will bring it into the mainstream of family practice.

A.O. Berg, M.D., M.P.H.

Marital Distress and Domestic Violence

Validating the Concept of Abuse: Women's Perceptions of Defining Behaviors and the Effects of Emotional Abuse on Health Indicators
Wagner PJ, Mongan PF (Med College of Georgia, Augusta)
Arch Fam Med 7:25–29, 1998   10–9

Introduction.—High rates of violence against women are consistently shown by research; yet health care professionals often react to reports of family violence with disbelief. Up to 54% of women visiting an emergency department have reported a lifetime prevalence of exposure to violence. Providers do not consistently query their female patients about their exposure to violence. There may be a lack of agreement between patients and providers on the definition of abuse. Women's definitions of abusive behavior were examined. The construct of emotional abuse was validated by assessing its association with health status, symptoms, and use of medical services.

Methods.—Four hundred seven women over the age of 18 were interviewed, and their medical records were reviewed. One half of the women were from a rural setting and one half were from an urban setting; 64% were black. To identify the women's perceptions of abusive behaviors, modified directions to the Conflict Tactics Scale were used. Self-report was used to determine a personal history of abuse. The Medical Outcomes Study Short-Form Health Survey-36 was used to measure health status.

Medical records were used to determine the use of medical services. Symptom experience was measured with the Symptom Inventory.

Results.—More behaviors were seen by women as abusive than are typically identified by the Conflict Tactics Scale. Abusive behaviors were identified more often by abused women than by nonabused women. Women who reported emotional abuse with no concurrent physical or sexual abuse had significant health status differences when compared to nonabused women on 7 of the 8 dimensions of the Short-Form Health Survey health status scales, including physical role functioning, emotional role functioning, sexual functioning, bodily pain, mental health, vitality, and general health perceptions. There were also differences on 25% of the measured symptoms, including difficulty in sleeping, in losing weight, excessive perspiration, feeling tired, muscular tension, poor health in general, feeling hot or cold regardless of weather, arm or leg aches or pains, shakiness, and swelling of arms, hands, legs, or feet. More medical visits were found among the emotionally abused groups than among the nonabused group.

Conclusion.—Many behaviors are considered by women to be abusive. More behaviors are perceived to be abusive by abused women than by nonabused women. In patient health behavior, emotional abuse can be viewed as a critical variable, given that significant health status differences are shown between emotionally abused and nonabused women.

▶ I now commonly (almost routinely) ask about violence. This article suggests that inquiries about interpersonal abuse should include emotional abuse, since it is associated with lower health status across multiple domains. As compared with physical violence, it is not uncommon to witness verbal abuse either in the office or during telephone conversations with a patient. In these cases, tactful inquiries or comments may be helpful, with later follow-up. Less clear to me is the meaning of the study's finding that abused women define more actions as abusive than do nonabused women. Perhaps it is of little meaning since the differences were not large. Perhaps it is because abused women have had so many more occurrences or concurrent abusive actions that more actions feel abusive. In either case, feeling emotionally abused lowers the woman's level of subjective health.

M.A. Bowman, M.D., M.P.A.

Guidelines for Managing Domestic Abuse When Male and Female Partners Are Patients of the Same Physician
Ferris LE, for the Delphi Panel and for the Consulting Group (Univ of Toronto; Sunnybrook Health Science Centre, North York, Ont, Canada; Inst for Clinical Evaluative Sciences, North York; et al)
JAMA 278:851–857, 1997   10–10

Objective.—It may be difficult for a physician to deal with domestic abuse when both partners are patients. Guidelines may help physicians to make ethical decisions in this situation. Clinical guidelines for management of physical wife abuse when both male and female partners are patients of the same physician were developed and refined.

Methods.—An 11-member multidisciplinary consulting group representing medicine, consumers, police, psychology, social work, and nursing identified 144 clinical scenarios. A 15-member expert panel, made up of individuals from family practice, gynecology, emergency medicine, medical ethics, nursing, psychology, law, and social work, ranked the scenarios in terms of best practice using a modified Delphi technique involving 4 iterations. Focus groups, made up of abused women and previously abusive men, and the consulting group commented on the panel's results. Guidelines were approved by the panel and the consulting group and comments from the focus groups were included.

Recommended Guidelines.—Physicians should have up-to-date information about the health effects, costs, etiology, psychology, and social repercussions of domestic violence. It is not unethical for a physician to deal with domestic violence when both perpetrator and victim are patients. Both patients are entitled to confidentiality. Both should be treated independently. Physicians should discuss domestic abuse with the woman's partner only with her consent. Joint counseling is not recommended, particularly if the physician is not adequately trained or both patients are not willing.

Conclusion.—Physicians need to be aware of domestic abuse and its ramifications and be prepared to manage it even when both partners are patients in the same practice. The recommended guidelines address the issues involved.

▶ Having both male and female partners in a domestic abuse situation is more common for family physicians than any other type of physician. We also tend to have the unique circumstance of seeing these patients over years, and knowing many other family members, which may allow us to detect more abuse and provide support. We are often in the position of knowing or suspecting abuse, and must decide our appropriate actions. This article represents 1 group's opinion with the help of a Delphi Panel and Consulting Group on how we should function. In general, I think their opinions and presentations are good, but not sufficiently detailed as to help a physician with individual circumstances. These situations can be very difficult, but our roles in detecting abuse and supporting patients should be encouraged.

M.A. Bowman, M.D., M.P.A.

Screening Men for Partner Violence in a Primary Care Setting: A New Strategy for Detecting Domestic Violence

Oriel KA, Fleming MF (Univ of Wisconsin, Madison)
J Fam Pract 46:493–498, 1998

Introduction.—Over the last decade, domestic violence has been recognized as a major public health issue. Removing an abused woman from the home is not always practical, because up to 34% of women may be physically assaulted by a male partner during their lifetime. In the medical literature, prevention and intervention strategies for men are inadequately addressed. It has been recommended that physicians screen men for violent behavior by asking them what they do when they argue with their partners. Abusers may be troubled by their own violent behavior and may feel relief when asked to discuss the problem. A study was undertaken to determine whether men would answer questions about partner violence in a health care setting.

Methods.—Three hundred seventy-five men were screened by means of an anonymous written survey. Of these men, 237 met the inclusion criteria. To measure aggressive and violent behavior, the Conflict Tactics Scale was used. Minor violence was defined as throwing, pushing, or slapping. Severe violence was defined as kicking, beating, or threatening to use or using a knife or gun. Demographic variables and health behaviors were also assessed.

Results.—Thirty-two men (13.5%) disclosed physical violence toward their partners in the previous 12 months. Severe violence was reported by 10 men (4.2%). Minor violence was reported by all of the men who reported severe violence. Violent behavior was more likely to be reported by men with increased alcohol consumption, depression, or a history of abuse as children. A probability of violence of 41% was found if all 3 variables were present. If none of the risk factors were present, the baseline probability of violence was 7%.

Conclusion.—It is suggested that primary care physicians screen male patients for aggressive behavior toward their intimate partners. Men who are depressed, who are heavy users of alcohol, or who were childhood victims of abuse are most likely to be abusers themselves, and physicians should be aware of this possibility among these groups.

▶ The absolute number of male patients who reported violent partnerships seems in line with information we hear from women. However, this article has made me think differently about what I do in the office. I have asked men about partner violence, but not on a regular basis. This article suggests that I should ask more often. I am impressed by how many men were willing to answer the survey questions; I wonder if they would answer the same if asked directly by the physician. In general, if the response is positive for violence, we will need to be prepared with individual therapists or therapy programs willing to work with individuals involved in violent relationships.

Should we consider asking only those with risk factors inasmuch as the rate was low in those with no risk factors?

M.A. Bowman, M.D., M.P.A.

Empirically Supported Couple and Family Interventions for Marital Distress and Adult Mental Health Problems

Baucom DH, Shoham V, Mueser KT, et al (Univ of North Carolina, Chapel Hill; Univ of Arizona, Tucson; Dartmouth Univ, Hanover)
J Consult Clin Psychol 66:53–88, 1998

10–12

Background.—During the past 3 decades, many different forms of couple- and family-based therapies for the treatment of adult mental health problems have been studied. Empirical data on the efficacy, clinical significance, and effectiveness of various couple and family interventions for marital distress and individual adult disorders were reviewed.

Couples Therapy for Relationship Distress.—Several different forms of therapy for marital distress have been studied. The best studied of these is behavioral marital therapy, which is efficacious and specific. Also efficacious and possibly specific is emotion-focused therapy. Research findings suggest that other forms of therapy—including insight-oriented marital therapy, cognitive-behavioral marital therapy, cognitive therapy for couples, and couples' systemic therapy—may be efficacious as well. All of these interventions have proven superior to a waiting list treatment condition. There is some evidence to suggest that insight-oriented therapy may offer better long-term results. Helping couples to understand the issues and needs behind their destructive interactions appears to be an important component of long-term maintenance of gains. There is no way to tell which marital intervention will be most appropriate for a specific couple; some couples remain distressed despite treatment, regardless of what intervention they receive.

Couples-Based Interventions for Individual Disorders.—Couple- and family-level treatments for adult individual disorders may be partner- or family-assisted interventions, disorder-specific partner or family interventions, or general couples or family therapy. Involving the partner or family in treatment for obsessive-compulsive disorder is at least as effective as individual therapy. Family involvement may be particularly important when the patient needs home reinforcement to follow through with treatment. Partner involvement in interventions for agoraphobia may lead to enhanced benefit. Such interventions may be beneficial even if there is no overt relationship distress at baseline. Interventions for depression have targeted the general relationship as a means of eliminating depressive symptoms. Such interventions have included behavioral marital therapy and conjoint interpersonal psychotherapy. One study found behavioral marital therapy superior to no treatment; the efficacy of marital vs. individual psychotherapy remains unclear. Marital therapy may be preferred over individual psychotherapy for couples with marital discord and a depressed wife.

Four possibly efficacious and specific psychosocial treatments for female sexual dysfunction have been identified, but none for men. Efficacy may be underestimated for the less recently studied treatments. Including the spouse in treatment appears to produce better results than treating the woman alone. A direct focus on sexual interactions appears to be important; it is unclear whether communication or the sexual problem should be addressed first. Involving partners in the treatment of alcoholism has enhanced treatment outcomes. Although the data on effectiveness are sparse, they are highly promising. There is evidence that marital status and marital adjustment may provide useful information for predicting response to treatment for alcoholism. Many studies have shown that family programs are efficacious for schizophrenia; however, most families do not have access to such programs. More work is needed to implement family intervention programs for use by a broad range of clinicians.

Discussion.—There is evidence that several types of couple- and family-based interventions are beneficial for the treatment of marital distress and individual disorders. The research findings are limited, however, particularly in terms of cultural generalizability. With increasing understanding of marital therapy and its theoretical bases, it is hoped that guidelines for involving spouses and other family members in treatment will continue to evolve.

▶ This lengthy article contains a wealth of information that is difficult to summarize. In general, couple- or family-focused interventions have been found to be helpful for many adult mental health problems (marital distress, obsessive-compulsive disorder, female sexual disorder, may be depression, alcohol abuse, and schizophrenia). However, most of the studies did not involve minority individuals or couples, or those with more than 1 disorder (such as alcohol abuse *and* sexual dysfunction), as pointed out by the authors. This reinforces that partners and families are important to individual functioning, which is well known to family physicians.

M.A. Bowman, M.D., M.P.A.

Mental Health Services and Insurance

How Expensive Is Unlimited Mental Health Care Coverage Under Managed Care?
Sturm R (RAND, Santa Monica, Calif)
JAMA 278:1533–1537, 1997

Purpose.—Under the Mental Health Parity Act of 1996, employers are required to increase the limits for mental health coverage to equal those for medical care but are not required to offer either type of coverage. Little is known about the impact of such policies; it will depend on how employers perceive the cost consequences. Older data on the costs of mental health coverage do not consider trends in the health care market or in treatment patterns—including the trend toward outpatient care; thus, they may overestimate the costs of the new legislation. The cost consequences of unlimited mental health coverage in the managed care era were studied.

Methods.—The study analyzed 1995 and 1996 claims data on 24 new managed care plans, all of which provided unlimited mental health coverage with minimal co-payments. The costs of removing various coverage limits for mental health care were analyzed, including limits not affected by the Mental Health Parity Act but possibly by newer state laws. The probability of care, intensity of care, and total costs were analyzed in terms of service type and type of enrollee. The findings were compared with the assumptions made in recent policy debates.

Results.—The debate over the Mental Health Parity Act overestimated the actual costs of managed care by fourfold to eightfold. Factors leading to lower costs in the plans analyzed included reduced hospitalization rates, the shift toward outpatient care, and reduced payments per service. At the same time, 7.0% of enrollees had accessed the mental health specialty care compared with 6.5% in previous fee-for-service plans and 5.0% with free care in the RAND Health Insurance Experiment. Eliminating a $25,000 annual limit on mental health care would raise insurance rates by only about $1 per year per enrollee. The greatest beneficiaries of mental health parity would be families with seriously mentally ill children.

Conclusions.—The debate over the Mental Health Parity Act was limited by incorrect assumptions and old data and overestimated the impact of removing limits on mental health coverage. This study demonstrates that the cost impact under managed care will actually be quite small. Children will be the greatest beneficiaries of the new legislation, which is a fact that has not received adequate attention.

▶ Family physicians will not be surprised by what is expressed in this article. We know that patients with mental health problems often receive very extensive (and expensive) health care unless their mental health problems are addressed. Managed care health plans seem frightened by the costs of mental health care and set up structures to avoid delivering these necessary services. This important article describes how foolish this policy is and provides a strong voice for the up-front and generous coverage of mental health care. It is important to remember that the majority of mental health care is provided by primary care physicians, who should be recognized and reimbursed for this service.

J.E. Scherger, M.D., M.P.H.

Insurance Status and Recognition of Psychosocial Problems: A Report From the Pediatric Research in Office Settings and the Ambulatory Sentinel Practice Networks

Kelleher KJ, Childs GE, Wasserman RC, et al (Univ of Pittsburgh, Pa; Pediatric Research in Office Settings, Elk Grove Village, Ill; Ambulatory Sentinel Practice Network, Denver)
Arch Pediatr Adolesc Med 151:1109–1115, 1997
10–14

Introduction.—There are several reports regarding the association between insurance status and discrepancies in health care provision. The effect of insurance status on clinician recognition of psychosocial problems for pediatric primary care visits was evaluated.

Methods.—Children aged 4–15 years made 10,250 consecutive visits for nonemergent care to 172 primary care clinicians. Clinician recognition of psychosocial problems was evaluated in children with parent-reported behavior problems. Clinician reports of psychosocial problems were compared with parent reports of the Pediatric Symptoms Checklist (PSC). Insurance status was recorded.

Results.—Agreement was high between clinicians and PSC for children with negative PSC scores. Clinicians recognized only 54% of positive PSC scores identified by parent report. Rates of recognition were not associated with insurance status. Increased recognition of psychosocial problems was associated with provider familiarity with patients, provider discipline, and patient demographics.

Conclusions.—Insurance status did not affect rates of recognition of childhood psychosocial problems by clinicians. Psychosocial problems of children and adolescents were most likely to be recognized when clinicians identified them as their own patients and when patients were older, male, or non–African-American.

▶ In this period of patients changing health plans and doctors, usually for financial reasons, articles stressing the importance of continuity of care provide vital information. Many involved in the business of health care do not appreciate the value of a long-term doctor-patient relationship. I loved the editor's note attached to this article, "Familiarity breeds content."

J.E. Scherger, M.D., M.P.H.

Miscellaneous

Can Money Buy Happiness? Depressive Symptoms in an Affluent Older Population

West CG, Reed DM, Gildengorin GL (Buck Ctr for Research in Aging, Novato, Calif)
J Am Geriatr Soc 46:49–57, 1998
10–15

Introduction.—In cross-sectional and prospective studies, depressive symptoms in older people have been associated with lower income. The relationship between income level and poor health outcomes may be associated with differences in behavioral risk factors, access to medical care, and social and physical environment. Important correlates of depressive symptomatology in older adults are concurrent medical and health problems, physical disability, and social support. The relationship between income and depressive symptoms was explored in a population-based cohort of affluent community-dwelling older adults.

Methods.—The cohort included 1,948 randomly selected, noninstitutionalized residents 55 years and older from an affluent county. The participants completed a questionnaire and a physical performance test. A *high level of depressive symptoms* was defined as a score of greater than or equal to 16 in the Center for Epidemiologic Studies–Depression scale.

Results.—There was a lower prevalence of high levels of depressive symptoms in this affluent population than in most other population-based samples. Lower levels of depressive symptoms were significantly associated with increasing income levels; however, the nature of the relationship appeared quadratic rather than linear. When measures of health conditions, physical disability, and social support were included in the model, the magnitude of the association between depressive symptoms and income decreased and was not statistically significant in multivariate regression analyses that included potential confounding risk factors.

Conclusion.—Poor health, physical disability, and social isolation are the major factors responsible for the observed inverse relationship between income and symptoms of depression in both affluent and economically disadvantaged older populations.

▶ This gets the award for the year's catchiest title; and, fortunately, the study delivers at least some of what the title promises. One of the strengths of the study is that it was population-based, so the findings are likely to apply elsewhere. The observed inverse relationship between income and depression in older studies washed out here because the researchers used more sophisticated statistical methods that I believe more accurately model reality. So, the short answer to the question posed in the title is no. The prevalence of depression was also lower than expected in this population of elders with typical numbers of chronic medical conditions. The conclusion that physical health, functional status, and emotional health are more important than affluence is an important finding.

A.O. Berg, M.D., M.P.H.

Psychosocial Correlates of Harassment, Threats and Fear of Violence in the Workplace
Cole LL, Grubb PL, Sauter SL, et al (Natl Inst for Occupational Safety and Health, Cincinnati, Ohio; Northwestern Natl Life, Minneapolis)
Scand J Work Environ Health 23:450–457, 1997   10–16

Introduction.—The National Institute for Occupational Safety and Health reports that homicide is the second leading cause of workplace death. During the period from 1980 to 1989, approximately 7,600 murders occurred in the workplace. Data from a telephone survey commissioned by Northwestern National Life Insurance were used to examine prevalence rates and risk factors for forms of nonfatal workplace violence, which may be experienced by 25% of full-time American workers.

Methods.—Study participants were 600 workers aged 19 or older who had worked for a single employer 35 hours or more a week during at least 8 of the 12 previous months. All were selected through a national random sample of telephone numbers and contacted by phone. Respondent profiles indicated that the sample was reasonably representative of full-time civilian employees in the United States. The survey included questions on work climate variables, job uncertainty factors, respondent and workplace demographics, and professional or career status variables.

Results.—Harassment on the job during the last 12 months was reported by 19% of respondents; 13% reported threats in the past 5 years. Sixty-two (10%) had feared becoming a victim of workplace violence in the last 12 months, and 82 reported physical attacks on other persons. A variety of factors appeared to place workers at risk of nonfatal occupational violence. Work climate variables, such as work group harmony and supervisor and co-worker support, were predictive of threats, harassment, and fear of becoming a victim of violence. Structural aspects of the job, such as work schedule and money handling, were predictive of threats and becoming a victim of violence.

Conclusion.—Both psychosocial factors and structural aspects of the job have an impact on nonfatal occupational violence. Stressors (reduced co-worker and supervisory support, layoff worries) are related to violence outcome, and structural variables, such as work schedule, recent layoffs, and money handling, are predictive of fear of violence, harassment, and physical attacks. Violence prevention strategies need to consider the design of work systems and workplace culture.

▶ Talking with our patients about violence at home has been (or should be) a routine part of our health and prevention screening. Lately, it seems, there has been a spate of violent deadly instances in the workplace. I was astounded by the National Institute for Occupational Safety and Health statistics on homicide deaths in the workplace. While the sample size seemed small for a survey of this scope, the population studied seemed representative of the workforce. I wonder if, in fact, the data actually underestimates the problem because there was a high rate of nonparticipation in the survey as a result of language barriers or refusal. Dr. Berg, in the 1997 YEAR BOOK OF FAMILY PRACTICE, reviewed an article that outlined the significant amount and effects of violence in our schools.[1] I suggest that not only should we be aware of this problem in our conversations with our patients, but that we also should actively solicit a history of violence and look for risk factors. Often, these issues become a game of "you don't ask and they won't tell." Ask. Ask about violence at home, at school, and in the workplace. Be comfortable with the questions, and anticipate the answers. As physicians, we may not be able to alter the reality of violence in society, but we are in a position to help those whose lives are being affected.

W.W. Dexter, M.D.

Reference

1. Everett SA, Price JH: Students' perceptions of violence in the public schools: The MetLife Survey. *J Adolesc Health* 17:345–352, 1995. (1997 YEAR BOOK OF FAMILY PRACTICE, p 301.)

Suicide After Natural Disasters
Krug EG, Kresnow M-J, Peddicord JP, et al (Natl Ctr for Injury Prevention and Control, Ctrs for Disease Control and Prevention, Atlanta, Ga)
N Engl J Med 338:373–378, 1998   10–17

Introduction.—Millions of individuals around the world are affected every year by natural and man-made disaster. Injury is experienced by about 1.5 million households in the United States as a result of floods, tornadoes, hurricanes, or earthquakes. For up to 5 years after a disaster, increased respiratory, gastrointestinal, and cardiovascular symptoms have been reported. Posttraumatic stress disorder, insomnia, depression, and problems, such as substance abuse and domestic violence, have also been reported. The psychological sequelae, which can result from the death or injury of family members, loss of property, financial assets, or employment, or from the disruption of the social fabric of community life, can also persist. There may be a relationship between suicide rates and disasters. In sites where single natural disasters occurred, the suicide rates were examined.

Methods.—There were 377 counties selected that had each been affected by a single natural disaster during a 4-year period from a list of all the events declared by the U.S. government to be federal disasters. Data on suicides during the 36 months before and the 48 months after the disaster were collected and aligned around the month of the disaster. According to the type of disaster, pooled rates were calculated. In the affected counties and in the entire United States, comparisons were made between the suicide rates before and those after disasters.

Results.—In the 4 years after floods, suicide rates increased by 13.8%, from 12.1 to 13.8 per 100,000. There was an increase of 31% in the 2 years after hurricanes from 12 to 15.7 per 100,000. There was a 62.9%

increase in the first year after earthquakes, from 19.2 to 31.3 per 100,000. There was no statistical significance in the 4-year increase of 19.7% after earthquakes. There were stable rates for the entire United States that were computed in a similar manner. Both sexes and all age groups accounted for the increases in suicide rates. After tornadoes or severe storms, the suicide rates did not change significantly.

Conclusion.—After severe earthquakes, floods, and hurricanes, suicide rates increase, and the need for mental health support after severe disasters is confirmed. Strategies of prevention can include providing social support and facilitating aid to victims.

▶ As a resident of the Pacific Northwest where we await "the big one" (earthquake, that is), I was dismayed to see that suicide risks went up the most after earthquakes, compared to floods and hurricanes. Every year I read stories of family physicians practicing in the aftermath of natural disasters, so I know this issue is out there even though still rare for any individual family physician. The advice of these authors to pay attention to mental health support after natural disasters is well founded, reinforcing what the average family physician would likely be doing anyway.

A.O. Berg, M.D., M.P.H.

Randomised Controlled Assessment of Non-directive Psychotherapy Versus Routine General-Practitioner Care
Friedli K, King MB, Lloyd M, et al (Royal Free Hosp, London)
Lancet 350:1662–1665, 1997   10–18

Objective.—Although brief psychotherapy, formal sessions in which patients try to define their problems and achieve their own solutions, has become increasingly more popular in England during the last 20 years, its clinical efficacy and cost-effectiveness have not been established. Brief psychotherapy was compared with routine general practitioner care for patients with emotional difficulties to evaluate clinical efficacy and patients' satisfaction.

Methods.—Between August 1993 and October 1994, 136 patients aged 18 years or older with emotional difficulties were recruited from 14 general practices in north London. Patients were randomly assigned to brief psychotherapy (nondirective rogerian model) in the intervention group (n = 70, 77% female) or routine general practice care in the control group (n = 66, 85% female). Patient satisfaction was assessed at 3 and 9 months. Psychological outcome was measured using the Beck Depression Inventory, the brief symptom inventory, and the computerized revised clinical interview schedule. Results were compared using analysis of covariance.

Results.—Depression was reported by 52% of patients and anxiety by 22%. Symptoms were most frequently the result of relationship and family difficulties according to patients. Patients in the psychotherapy group attended an average of 7.7 sessions. Fourteen did not complete the course suggested by the therapist, and 4 never saw a therapist. All patients improved significantly over the course of the study. Ten patients in the psychotherapy group and 12 control patients were prescribed antidepressants between baseline and 3-month follow-up. Patients were more satisfied with the therapist at 3 and 9 months than with the general practitioner, although there were no differences between groups with respect to coping ability.

Conclusion.—Both intervention and control patients improved significantly over time. At the last assessment, intervention patients were more satisfied with their therapists than control patients were with their physicians, but they showed no differences in coping skills.

▶ I have always admired the ability of British general practitioners to conduct useful research in real practice settings. This study lacks precision in the initial diagnosis and management plan, but U.S. family physicians will be won over by its common-sense approach. The clinical take-home is also reassuring in its validation of usual care. I have no difficulty accepting these results as likely true for a large number of patients with mild emotional problems seen in typical practice. The study does not address, of course, the patient with more severe mental health problems.

A.O. Berg, M.D., M.P.H.

Effects of a Restraint Reduction Intervention and OBRA '87 Regulations on Psychoactive Drug Use in Nursing Homes
Siegler EL, Capezuti E, Maislin G, et al (New York Univ, Brooklyn; Univ of Pennsylvania, Philadelphia)
J Am Geriatr Soc 45:791–796, 1997

Background.—In nursing homes, behavioral problems historically have been treated with physical and "chemical" restraints, such as psychoactive medications. A previous study in 3 Philadelphia nursing homes showed that staff education and expert consultation can lead to a significant decline in the number of restraints used. Whether a reduction in the use of physical restraints had an effect on the use of psychoactive medications was investigated.

Methods.—Three nursing homes were studied (446 residents in 16 wards)—a control site, a site that received staff education about restraint use, and a site that received education coupled with expert consultation. Data on the use of neuroleptics, benzodiazepines, and antidepressants were evaluated to see whether drug use changed over time. Evaluations were based on measurements taken after the Omnibus Budget Reconciliation Act (OBRA) mandates of 1987 (T1), immediately after the educational intervention (T2), and 3 (T3) and 6 (T4) months after the intervention.

Findings.—Neuroleptic medications were used at T1 in 19%, 14%, and 18% of the control, education, and education plus consultation sites, respectively. After 6 months (T4), only the control site had a significant decrease in neuroleptic drug use (11%, 16%, and 19% for the 3 sites, respectively). Benzodiazepine use, however, declined significantly from T1 to T4 in all 3 sites (from 33% to 27% in the control site, from 37% to 27% in the education site, and from 22% to 18% in the education plus consultation site). Antidepressant use varied greatly and nonlinearly, but in general, it was low. In each ward, the use of neuroleptic drugs and physical restraints seemed to either decrease or increase together.

Conclusions.—Using fewer restraints did not cause an increase in the use of psychoactive drugs. In fact, in many wards, the use of benzodiazepines and physical restraints decreased in tandem. Although the effects of the OBRA 1987 mandate were not uniform (especially with regard to antidepressant use), each of the 3 sites did show reductions in the use of physical and/or chemical restraints over time.

▶ A few years ago there was wide concern about the potential combined impact of reducing restraints and reducing psychoactive drug use at the same time in nursing homes. This well-designed, controlled trial (not randomized, though) shows that the concerns were not well founded. Psychoactive drug use (especially benzodiazepines) can be kept in check even when restraints are reduced. I found it most interesting that the "control" home was actually the most successful in reducing neuroleptic use according to the OBRA guidelines.

A.O. Berg, M.D., M.P.H.

Creativity and Mental Illness: Is There a Link?
Waddell C (McMaster Univ, Hamilton, Ont, Canada)
Can J Psychiatry 43:166–172, 1998   10–20

Background.—Creativity has been linked to mental illness. This review assessed studies of creativity and mental illness to evaluate the scientific evidence for this association.

Study Design.—A MEDLINE literature search for English-language studies and reviews from this century that examined creativity and mental illness in the same individuals was performed. These were reviewed and critically evaluated by currently accepted scientific standards.

Findings.—The literature search revealed 29 empirical studies of mental illness and creativity. Of these studies, 15 negated and 9 supported an association between creativity and mental illness. All studies were case-series or case-control in design. Fourteen early studies did not use standardized definitions of mental illness. The 15 later studies did, but only 4 measured creativity; none selected participants randomly, only 3 used prospective designs, and only 2 rated subjects blindly. Six did not use living subjects. Thirty-four reviews of creativity and mental illness were found in the literature search; none met current standards for literature reviews. There were no meta-analyses. No studies measured community samples for comparison. Confounding variables were rarely dealt with.

Conclusion.—This review evaluated the scientific evidence for an association between creativity and mental illness. The evidence was not sufficient to establish such a linkage. Despite the paucity of evidence, much enthusiasm for this association was displayed in the studies examined. Definitive studies in this area have not yet been performed. Such studies would be larger, would be prospective, and would include randomly selected living participants with matched controls and blinded assessment. Creativity and mental illness should be defined and measured with standardized instruments. Evidence from several different studies, using randomized and prospective methodologies and demonstrating a strong association between creativity and mental illness, is required before such a relationship can be suggested.

▶ This is my 1 indulgence for the 1999 YEAR BOOK: updating a topic that I have been following for many years. This report is the first attempt at a systematic review using evidence-based methods and is easily the most complete and rigorous review of the topic in the literature. The poor quality of research documented here is not likely to be remedied; the subject will never lend itself to high-quality cohort studies, much less randomized controlled trials. (What a thought!)

For those interested in the subject, obtaining a copy of the entire article is a must. The short, philosophical discussion at the end of the paper is an exceptionally clear and concise summary of the issues. I agree with one of the author's concluding comments: "...the eloquence of creative or gifted people who comment on their own mental health problems attracts attention and compels us to spuriously connect their creativity with their problems."

A.O. Berg, M.D., M.P.H.

Paroxetine Treatment of Generalized Social Phobia (Social Anxiety Disorder): A Randomized Controlled Trial
Stein MB, Liebowitz MR, Lydiard RB, et al (Univ of California at San Diego, La Jolla; Columbia Univ, New York; Med Univ of South Carolina, Charleston; et al)
JAMA 280:708–713, 1998   10–21

Background.—Social anxiety disorder is a severe, often disabling form of social anxiety affecting about 5% of the general population. Monoamine oxidase inhibitors or benzodiazepines appear to be effective treatments, but neither of these treatments is used widely. The efficacy of paroxetine, a selective serotonin reuptake inhibitor, was compared with that of placebo in adults with generalized social phobia.

Methods.—Thirteen U.S. centers and 1 Canadian center enrolled a total of 187 patients in the 12-week, randomized, double-blind trial. All patients met criteria for generalized social phobia. Patients were assigned to treatment with paroxetine at an initial dose of 20 mg, with weekly increases of 10 mg/day permitted after week 2 of treatment, or to placebo.

Findings.—Fifty-five percent of paroxetine recipients and 23.9% of placebo recipients were much improved or very much improved by the end of treatment. Mean total scores on the Liebowitz Social Anxiety Scale were reduced by 39.1% and 17.4%, respectively.

Conclusions.—Paroxetine is effective in the treatment of generalized social phobia. Short-term treatment produces clinically meaningful reductions in symptoms and disability. Future research should focus on whether extended treatment or the addition of specific educational-cognitive-behavioral methods can further improve outcomes.

▶ This article describes a nicely conducted study with clinically useful results. Social phobia is more common than most of us recognize, with a lifetime prevalence of around 13%. Treatment with paroxetine was effective in a little over half of these patients, and had more than double the success of placebo. One might expect that other selective serotonin reuptake inhibitors would work as well, but I am sure we will not have long to wait before every manufacturer conducts a similar study of its own product. This article does not address long-term efficacy or adverse effects, but extensive long-term experience with selective serotonin reuptake inhibitors for other conditions is reassuring.

A.O. Berg, M.D., M.P.H.

Procedures, Placement, and Risks of Further Abuse After Munchausen Syndrome by Proxy, Non-accidental Poisoning, and Non-accidental Suffocation
Davis P, McClure RJ, Rolfe K, et al (Univ of Wales, Cardiff; St James's Univ Hosp, Leeds, England)
Arch Dis Child 78:217–221, 1998   10–22

Background.—In Munchausen syndrome by proxy, an adult caregiver causes harm to a child so that medical attention can be obtained. Such children are often seen repeatedly by health care providers. Poisoning and suffocation are common mechanisms of injury. The outcomes, management, and prevention of Munchausen syndrome by proxy, nonaccidental poisoning, and nonaccidental suffocation were reported.

Methods and Findings.—One hundred nineteen children younger than 14 years were included in the review. Follow-up ranged from 12 to 44 months. No previous diagnosis of Munchausen syndrome by proxy was found to be the result of other organic disease. Forty-six children were discharged home with no signs or symptoms at follow-up. Victims of suffocation, poisoning, and direct harm and children younger than 5 years were less likely to go home. At follow-up, 24% of the children still showed symptoms or signs of abuse. One hundred eight children were on a child protection register initially, and 35 were on the register at follow-up. Twenty-nine percent of the adult victimizers had been prosecuted, and most had been convicted. Seventeen percent of the children with milder abuse who were allowed to go home were abused again. Data collected on siblings suggested that further abuse, potentially fatal, occurred in 50% of the families in which a child had been suffocated, and in 40% in which a child had been poisoned.

Conclusions.—Munchausen syndrome by proxy, nonaccidental poisoning, and nonaccidental suffocation involve severe abuse, associated with high rates of death, injury, family disruption, repeated abuse, and harm to siblings. Follow-up by a child protection expert is warranted for children who are victimized by such abuse.

▶ This article is from the United Kingdom, but I think that in spite of cultural, social, and legal differences, there are some findings that are probably generalizable and worth remembering. In no case was a genuine medical disorder later found as the cause of what had been identified as Munchausen syndrome by proxy, which means medical providers tend to be certain before applying the label, but also that we are probably underdiagnosing the syndrome. A substantial number of children allowed to return home after "mild" Munchausen syndrome by proxy were abused again (17%), many (24%) had ongoing symptoms or problems from the abuse, and many siblings were abused. In the groups with suffocation or nonaccidental poisoning, the rate of other sibling abuse, some fatal, was very high. Of note, the abuse of siblings was not necessarily of the same type as in the study case. These are difficult cases, and judges may be unsure of when it is right to deny parental rights, but these families are generally highly disturbed and children in them are at very high risk for bad outcomes.

M.A. Bowman, M.D., M.P.A.

Sabotaging One's Own Medical Care: Prevalence in a Primary Care Setting
Sansone RA, Wiederman MW, Sansone LA, et al (Univ of Oklahoma, Tulsa; Ball State Univ, Muncie, Ind; Med Care Associates of Tulsa, Okla)
Arch Fam Med 6:583–586, 1997
10–23

Objective.—Little has been written about patients who sabotage their own medical care. A series of self-sabotaging behaviors from factitious disorder (the pathologic and intentful creation of false symptoms) to medication noncompliance and its associated nonpathologic factors were identified and explored.

Methods.—Nineteen sabotaging behaviors were identified on a survey filled out by 411 nonemergent outpatients (63 men) aged 18–81 years seen at the Family Medicine Clinic, University of Oklahoma College of Medicine, Tulsa. Demographically, 41.6% were married, 33.1% were single, 18.2% were divorced, 6.3% were widowed, and 3% indicated no marital status. The highest educational level attained was not a high school graduate (21.9%), high school graduate (42.1%), some college (25.5%), a bachelor's degree (7.3%), postgraduate education (2.7%), and no education status listed (0.5%).

Results.—At least 1 respondent endorsed each of the 19 behaviors. The most commonly checked behaviors, "not taken a prescribed medication intentionally" (25.1%) and "not gone for medical treatment despite knowing you needed it" (37.2%), were excluded. Significantly more men (4.8%) than women (0.6%) reported not following a physician's or a nurse's instructions to prolong an illness. The prevalence of the remaining items was determined. At least 1 additional sabotaging behavior was reported by 27 (6.6%) of the respondents, 23 of whom indicated 1 (63%) or 2 (22.2%) other sabotaging behaviors. The remaining 4 patients reported an additional 4–12 sabotaging behaviors. Significantly more women (26.4%) than men (17.5%) reported not taking prescription medication.

Conclusion.—In this study, 6.6% of the patients actively sabotaged their medical care.

▶ Physician, beware! In addition to the everyday noncompliance, patients sabotage their medical care in more overt and covert ways daily. I was shocked by the numbers, because I can only think of a few patients who I have recognized as actively sabotaging their care. When have I missed this? What can I do about it when I recognize it? Is it our job to find such things as insurance fraud or abuse of job privileges? I wonder how many of those purposefully self-injuring patients have psychiatric illnesses.

M.A. Bowman, M.D., M.P.A.

11 Preventive Medicine

Overview

Randomized controlled trials: Abstracts 11–4, 11–10, 11–11, 11–16, and 11–17

Fitness and Physical Activity
- Two articles on fitness and functional status in older adults
- An evolutionary perspective on physical activity
- Written prescriptions for exercise
- Aerobic demands in lawn mowing
- Walking and mortality in older men

Smoking
- Smoking and the progression of atherosclerosis
- Environmental smoke and heart disease risk
- Maternal smoking and expenditures for childhood respiratory illness
- Telephone support and transdermal nicotine for smoking cessation
- Buproprion and smoking cessation
- Preemption in tobacco control
- Mailed smoking advice for young men with asbestos exposure

Antioxidants
- Antioxidants and heart disease prevention
- Pathophysiology of antioxidants on arterial endothelium
- Vitamin E and nitrate tolerance in men with ischemic heart disease

Garlic
- Garlic and serum lipids
- Garlic and aortic elasticity

Fitness and Physical Activity

Physical Fitness and Functional Limitations In Community-Dwelling Older Adults

Morey MC, Pieper CF, Cornoni-Huntley J (Duke Med Ctr, Durham, NC; Univ of North Carolina, Chapel Hill)
Med Sci Sports Exerc 30:715–723, 1998

Introduction.—Most geriatric models of disability use disease as its underlying cause. Morphological factors, muscular performance, and motor ability are fitness components that are correlated with favorable outcomes that potentially decrease or delay the onset of physical disability. The relationship between functional limitations and cardiorespiratory, morphological, and strength components of fitness were assessed in a series of older adults. This is the first known trial to characterize a broad set of individual fitness components as they relate to functional limitations and the first to assess directly measured cardiovascular fitness within the context of existing disability models.

Methods.—The mean age of a convenience sample of 161 community-dwelling older adults was 72.5 years (range, 65 to 90 years) at baseline. For 5 years, participants were followed up for cervical range of motion, cervical rotation, functional axial rotation-pointer, shoulder flexion, ankle dorsiflexion strength, hip abduction strength, disease index, and symptom index. During that time, a series of 5 tests of functional limitations, pathology, psychosocial variables, cardiovascular fitness, and anthropometric measures were also given.

Results.—The cardiorespiratory, morphological, and strength fitness components were significantly correlated with functional limitations after controlling for age, race, sex, education, and depressive symptoms. The only fitness component directly related to pathology was the cardiorespiratory.

Conclusion.—Individual fitness components are directly associated with functional limitations; associations that are independent of pathology. Exercise interventions for older adults should be tailored to underlying impairments within each fitness component to fully optimize potential gains in physical functioning.

▶ Amen. Declining function often equates to declining quality of life. Despite the limitations of the study (size and sample), these results make sense. In my office, I often preach the fitness gospel. I now have some solid evidence on which to base my faith. Perhaps this article will convince the nonbelievers out there. Perhaps even the third-party payers.

W.W. Dexter, M.D.

Physical Activity, Energy Expenditure and Fitness: An Evolutionary Perspective
Cordain L, Gotshall RW, Eaton SB, et al (Colorado State Univ, Fort Collins; Emory Univ, Atlanta, Ga; Marshall Univ, Huntington, WVa)
Int J Sports Med 19:328–335, 1998 — 11-2

Introduction.—For all mammals except *Homo sapiens*, food procurement depends upon energy expenditure. In the affluent nations of today, food energy has become more affordable and accessible, and an energy surplus exists. An evolutionary perspective of physical activity, energy expenditure, and fitness, based on an extensive literature review using MEDLINE, Sport Discus, and Colorado Alliance Research Libraries and bibliographies of original articles, is discussed.

Human Evolution.—The genetic composition of contemporary humans has changed little over the last 40 millennia. The relationship among energy intake, energy expenditure, and specific motor activity remains equivalent to that of Stone Age people who lived in a foraging environment. The amount of obligatory physical exertion necessary for hunting, gathering, carrying, digging, and escape from predators has been lessened with agriculture and industrialization. The result is an energy surplus, increased body weight, and distorted body composition with an overabundance of adipose tissue relative to bone and muscle.

Energy Expenditure.—Resting metabolic rate (RMR) and total energy expenditure (TEE) expressed per kilogram of body weight probably remained consistent for 3.5 million years until contemporary *H. sapiens* became affluent and sedentary. Typical Westerners have TEE/kg per day values that barely equal the RMR/kg per day of recent hunter-gatherers and that estimated for preagricultural humans. The RMR/kg per day decrease observed in modern humans probably reflects altered body composition (more fat, less muscle) as a direct result of sedentary living. The TEE/kg per day of 20th century contemporary humans is probably about 65% that of late Paleolithic Stone Age people.

Aerobic Fitness.—Hunter-gatherers and other traditional populations have aerobic fitness levels that range from good to excellent when plotted against fitness norms of Americans. The limited physical activity of modern affluent humans has resulted in mediocre aerobic fitness.

Guidelines for Fitness and Health.—The American College of Sports Medicine (ACSM) guidelines recommend participating in physical activity 3 to 5 days per week at 50% to 85% of maximum intensity continuously for 20 to 60 minutes to improve athletic performance and overall health. For health promotion, the ACSM recommends 30 minutes of physical activity for most days of the week. If ACSM recommendations for health promotion can be considered the minimum, what level is needed for optimizing health benefits? If the answer lies in that of our ancestors, the physical activity energy expenditure would be the equivalent of walking 406 kilometers (252 miles) per month, in addition to current physical activities.

Conclusion.—In the evolutionary perspective, it is the sedentary existence of today's affluent nations that is the extreme—not the lifestyle that prevailed before industrialization. The ACSM guidelines for health promotion are 44% of those of hunter-gatherers for the level of energy expended by physical activity. These guidelines are almost certainly far below those of our preagricultural ancestors, and very likely beneath the level for which our genetically determined physiology and biochemistry have been programmed through evolution.

▶ Have some fun with this one. All this time I have thought that (1) we should really be quadripeds given all the back pain I treat; and (2) we are too heavy simply from eating too much and watching too much TV. No hard science here, just a very interesting evolutionary perspective on why we should still be hunter-gatherers. Will we eventually evolve (or engineer?) a "sedentary" gene allowing us to burn calories more efficiently while we sit? Works for me, but then I am a Darwinian.

W.W. Dexter, M.D.

Physical Activity and Health Promotion for Older Adults in Public Housing
Buchner DM, Nicola RM, Martin ML, et al (Univ of Washington, Seattle)
Am J Prev Med 13(Suppl 2):57–62, 1997   11–3

Introduction.—Special objectives are established for older, low-income, and minority adults by Healthy People 2000. For these adults, health promotion and disease prevention are important to addressing national objectives. However, few studies have been conducted on older residents of public housing, and it is not clear whether such programs for older residents should emphasize preventive care or lifestyle modification. It would be useful to determine which health-promotion and disease-prevention programs residents would participate in. A study was undertaken to identify the needs of health promotion and disease prevention of older public housing residents and to determine whether there was a need for lifestyle modification or for preventive care.

Methods.—In a needs assessment survey, the needs of 199 older public housing residents were compared with the needs of 2,289 community older HMO enrollees. Residents were also interviewed about major life concerns and interest in health-promotion and disease-prevention activities and in interventions to reduce barriers and observe residents' interest in on-site exercise classes.

Results.—It was found that the majority of residents could benefit from physical activity programs, inasmuch as 75% spent less than 60 minutes per week of exercise; 21% of residents could benefit from smoking cessation programs; and 4% could benefit from alcohol counseling. There was a greater need among residents than among HMO enrollees for physical activity promotion. Similar use of preventive care services was reported by the 2 groups. Interest in physical activity programs was demonstrated by residents, even though they seldom identified physical inactivity as a major concern. An exercise class offered at the older residents' facility resulted in 41% of residents participating regularly or irregularly. Residents successfully lobbied city government to sustain the class when it was scheduled to be discontinued.

Conclusion.—A major goal of health-promotion and disease-prevention programs for older residents of public housing should be promotion of physical activity.

▶ The premise of this study struck me as a really terrific idea. As the authors point out, the lower-income elderly are at particular risk of and from inactivity. I was also intrigued by the finding that far more individuals could benefit from physical activity programs than from smoking cessation. Although a small nonrandom survey of public housing in 1 city is probably not sufficient evidence to change public policy nationwide, I would bet that the basic tenet is true. In the past 5 years or so, there has been an explosion of research regarding physical activity in the elderly. The benefits are many, and the risks are few. I would like to see these data replicated across a wider population and geographic area. In the meantime, it is enough to at least begin discussion with your patients and local policy makers.

W.W. Dexter, M.D.

The Green Prescription Study: A Randomized Controlled Trial of Written Exercise Advice Provided by General Practitioners
Swinburn BA, Walter LG, Arroll B, et al (Univ of Auckland, New Zealand; Univ of Otago, New Zealand)
Am J Public Health 88:288–291, 1998   11–4

Background.—General practitioners have used several strategies in an attempt to promote physical activity among their patients. Whether written advice, in addition to verbal advice, is more effective than verbal advice alone in increasing physical activity levels among sedentary persons was determined.

Methods.—Four hundred ninety-one sedentary patients were given verbal advice by their general practitioner to increase their level of physical activity. The patients were then assigned randomly to an exercise prescription group or a control group. Thirty-five participants were lost to follow-up.

Findings.—The number of patients engaging in any recreational physical activity increased substantially at 6 weeks. An intention-to-treat analysis indicated that significantly more patients in the exercise prescription group increased their activity level than did patients in the control group.

Conclusion.—General practitioners can play an important role in effecting lifestyle changes among their patients. Writing down goal-oriented prescriptions for increasing physical activity is more effective than verbal advice alone in effecting such a change.

▶ Patients were identified by their physicians as willing and able to increase their exercise. A randomized group had the recommendations for exercise written down, such that the group for whom they were written had the physician spend slightly more time with them. The physicians estimated that they spent an average of 5 minutes discussing exercise.

Using intention-to-treat analysis, 2 of the 5 measures showed a statistically significant difference, with the group given the written prescription increasing their exercise in the ensuing 6 weeks more than those given verbal advice alone. The take-home message is that writing down the goal-oriented exercise recommendations may make a small but clinically significant difference in the outcome. I suspect the same could be said for many other types of advice we give.

M.A. Bowman, M.D., M.P.A.

Aerobic and Myocardial Demands of Lawn Mowing in Patients With Coronary Artery Disease
Haskin-Popp C, Nazareno D, Wegner J, et al (William Beaumont Hosp, Royal Oak, Mich)
Am J Cardiol 81:1243–1245, 1998

Background.—Lawn mowing is a common activity, but there has been little research on the aerobic and myocardial demands of grass cutting for patients with coronary artery disease (CAD). The ECG, cardiorespiratory, hemodynamic, and perceptual responses to manual and automated lawn mowing were evaluated and compared to maximal treadmill testing in a group of CAD patients.

Methods.—The study group consisted of 10 men with CAD who had low-risk clinical status, little to no functional aerobic impairment, physician approval, no orthopedic limitations, and completion of a treadmill test to volitional fatigue without cardiac symptoms. Participants cut two 4-cm-high × 25-m-long tracts of grass using manual and automated cutting in random order with a 15-minute rest between. During the 10-minute mowing sessions, heart rate, oxygen consumption, blood pressure, and perceived exertion were assessed.

Results.—Each participant completed the grass cutting without cardiac signs or symptoms. The highest heart rates for each participant during manual lawn mowing ranged from 71% to 109% and from 51% to 85% of the peak heart rate of exercise treadmill testing during automated lawn mowing. $\dot{V}O_2$ during manual lawn mowing averaged 20.3 mL/kg/min or 5.8 metabolic equivalents (METs) and 15.4 mL/kg/min or 4.4 METs during automated lawn cutting.

Conclusions.—The energy cost of lawn mowing is 4 METs for automated and 6 METs for manual grass cutting. Heart rate and blood pressure during manual lawn mowing may approach or exceed that attained during maximal treadmill exercise testing. These excessive cardiac demands may be hidden by the moderate aerobic demands and perceived low effort of grass cutting.

▶ The title of this article piqued my interest among the many articles that we review for inclusion in the YEAR BOOK OF FAMILY PRACTICE. It probably caught my eye because I was facing a good-sized lawn to mow the following weekend. Numerous studies have shown the risk to patients with CAD of working in extreme cold, such as shoveling snow. Little has been documented regarding the risks of mowing lawns. It was troublesome to me to read in this study that mowing a lawn with a manual lawn mower met or exceeded the oxygen consumption demands of an exercise treadmill test. I'm not sure how many of our patients still use manual lawn mowers, but I suspect a fair number. I certainly don't want to discourage our patients from exercise. However, in our patients with known CAD, we should counsel them regarding the risks of weekend exercise, such as mowing the lawn. Most of us understand this when we think of winter exercise activities. I think we need to add lawn mowing as a risk exercise for patients with known CAD.

R.C. Davidson, M.D., M.P.H.

Effects of Walking on Mortality Among Nonsmoking Retired Men
Hakim AA, Petrovitch H, Burchfiel CM, et al (Univ of Virginia, Charlottesville; Univ of Minnesota, Minneapolis; Univ of Hawaii; Honolulu; et al)
N Engl J Med 338:94–99, 1998   11–6

Background.—The possible benefits of low-intensity activity in prolonging life among older men are unclear. The relationship between walking and mortality in a cohort of retired men who were nonsmokers and physically able to participate daily in low-intensity activities was investigated.

Methods.—Seven hundred seven men, aged 61–81 years, enrolled in the Honolulu Heart Program, were studied. Distances walked were recorded at a baseline examination, between 1980 and 1982. Mortality data were collected during 12 years of follow-up.

Findings.—Two hundred eight deaths occurred during follow-up. After adjusting for age, mortality among men walking less than 1 mile per day was almost twice that of those walking more than 2 miles per day. These rates were 40.5% and 23.8%, respectively. The cumulative incidence of death after 12 years among the most active walkers occurred in less than 7 years among the least active walkers. Distance walked was inversely associated with mortality after adjustment for overall measures of activity and other risk factors (Fig 1).

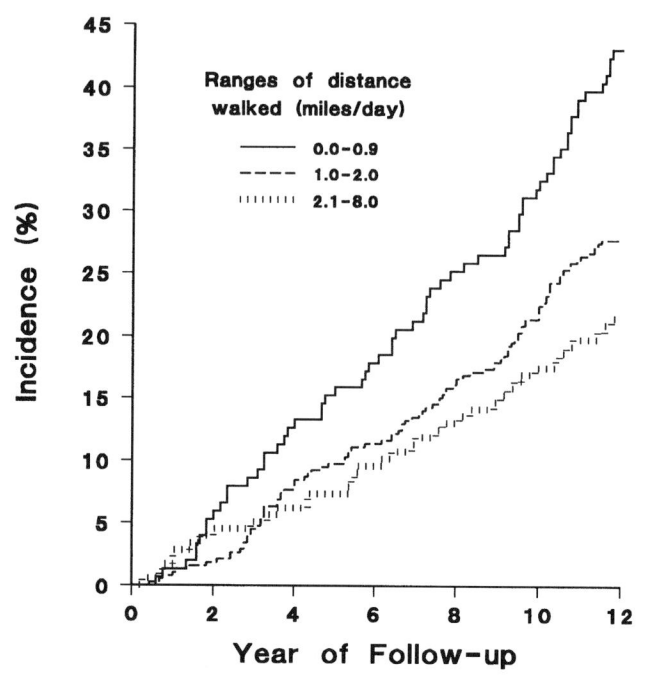

FIGURE 1.—Cumulative mortality according to year of follow-up and distance walked per day. To convert distances to kilometers, multiply by 1.609. (Courtesy of Hakim AA, Petrovitch H, Burchfiel CM, et al: Effects of walking on mortality among nonsmoking retired men. *N Engl J Med* 338:94–99. Copyright 1998, Massachusetts Medical Society. Reprinted by permission of *The New England Journal of Medicine*. All rights reserved.)

Conclusions.—Regular walking is associated with a reduced overall mortality among older, physically capable men. Thus, encouraging elderly individuals to walk may increase their survival.

▶ The message from this research study is critically important to anyone taking care of older individuals. It is a well-designed prospective study of men involved in a longitudinal surveillance program in Hawaii. The authors studied the relationship between the average distance walked in miles per day and overall mortality. As you might expect, they found a significant reduction in overall mortality in men who walked a greater distance on average each day. This is especially valuable in that no equipment or exercise program memberships were required. The one thing I wish the authors would have added to this study is some measure of quality of life. I have a strong suspicion that those who walk on a daily basis also have a significantly better quality of life.

There are 3 problems that I find with this study. The first is that it looked at men only. The U.S. research community continues to be criticized, and I believe rightfully so, in studies which look only at men's health. The second problem is that it is a group of a certain ethnic subculture (Japanese men). I cannot think of any factor in Japanese men that would make them more prone to have a benefit from walking than men from other cultures. However, it's unfortunate that it was limited to this subculture. The third problem is that the study took place entirely in Hawaii. It seems intuitive to me that men would have an easier time walking in Hawaii than they would in Duluth, Minn, in winter. I wonder whether regular walking at 10° below zero would actually reduce overall mortality.

R.C. Davidson, M.D., M.P.H.

Smoking

Cigarette Smoking and Progression of Atherosclerosis: The Atherosclerosis Risk in Communities (ARIC) Study
Howard G, for the ARIC Investigators (Wake Forest Univ, Winston-Salem, NC; The Johns Hopkins Univ, Baltimore, Md; Univ of Minnesota, Minneapolis; et al)
JAMA 279:119–124, 1998   11–7

Background.—Cigarette smoking is known to be a strong risk factor for incident heart disease and stroke. However, the association of active and passive smoking with the progression of atherosclerosis has not been determined.

Methods.—A population-based cohort of middle-aged individuals from 4 U.S. communities was studied in this longitudinal assessment of the relationship between smoking exposure determined at the initial visit and changes in atherosclerosis 3 years later. A total of 10,914 individuals enrolled in the Atherosclerosis Risk in Communities (ARIC) study between 1987 and 1989 were included.

Findings.—Exposure to cigarette smoke was correlated with progression of atherosclerosis. Compared with individuals who never smoked, current smokers had a 50% increase in progression of atherosclerosis, after adjustment for demographic factors, cardiovascular risk factors, and lifestyle variables. Past smoking was associated with a 25% increase. Compared with individuals not exposed to environmental tobacco smoke (ETS), those exposed to ETS had a 20% increase. The effects of smoking on atherosclerosis progression was greater for individuals with diabetes and hypertension. Although more pack-years of exposure was correlated independently with faster progression, after adjustment for number of pack-years, the progression rates of current and past smokers did not differ.

Conclusions.—Both active smoking and ETS exposure are correlated with the progression of atherosclerosis. Smoking is especially detrimental to atherosclerosis progression among patients with diabetes and hypertension. Some adverse effects of smoking may be cumulative and irreversible.

▶ Our previous chairman of surgery here at the U.C. Davis School of Medicine is a renown cardiovascular surgeon. While giving a Grand Rounds presentation on carotid atherosclerotic disease, he made the statement that in his 25 years of operating on carotid arteries, he has yet to have 1 patient who did not have a significant smoking history. He concluded that this is a disease of smokers.

This is a large, well-controlled study of 4 communities in the United States with 11,000 participants. As expected, they found a significant relationship between current smoking and risk of atherosclerotic disease. They also found a relationship between exposure to environmental tobacco products and the risk of disease. They found a higher risk among previous smokers, suggesting that there are some irreversible changes from previous smoking exposure.

There are no surprises in this study. I included it because it is such a powerful study from its size and design, and its message is so important.

R.C. Davidson, M.D., M.P.H.

Environmental Tobacco Smoke Exposure and Ischaemic Heart Disease: An Evaluation of the Evidence
Law MR, Morris JK, Wald NJ (Royal London School of Medicine)
BMJ 315:973–980, 1997
11–8

Objective.—The risk of ischemic heart disease has been found to be 30% greater in nonsmokers who live with smokers. This finding appears to be excessive. The possible explanations for this reported large association were examined.

Methods.—A meta-analysis was performed on all 19 published studies of exposure of nonsmokers to environmental tobacco smoke. A dose-response relationship between smoking and ischemic heart disease from 5 cohort studies of men recruited during the 1950s was analyzed, and the amount of excess risk of ischemic heart disease that is reversible many years after stopping smoking was determined in the 5 cohort studies. The increase in the risk of ischemic heart disease attributable to a decrease of 1 standard deviation in consumption of fruit, vegetables, and antioxidant vitamins was analyzed; the risk of ischemic heart disease according to platelet aggregation was analyzed; and the increased risk of ischemic heart disease was calculated for a 1–standard deviation increase in platelet aggregation.

Results.—The relative risk of ischemic heart disease in nonsmokers exposed to environmental tobacco smoke was 1.30 at age 65 years, compared with the risk of ischemic heart disease associated with smoking 1 cigarette a day (1.39) or 20 cigarettes a day (1.78). Because nonsmokers living with smokers eat less fruits and vegetables than nonsmokers living with nonsmokers, the former nonsmokers are at a 6% higher risk of ischemic heart disease, increasing the risk of environmental tobacco smoke to 23%. An increase in platelet aggregation of 1 standard deviation increases the relative risk of increased ischemic heart disease to 1.33.

Conclusion.—Exposure to environmental tobacco smoke increases a nonsmoker's risk of ischemic heart disease nonlinearly by approximately 25%.

▶ This meta-analysis covers 19 published research studies on the risk of ischemic heart disease in lifelong nonsmokers who are exposed to environmental smoke. With the power of the meta-analysis behind them, the authors can unequivocally state that exposure to other people's smoke is an important risk factor for ischemic heart disease.

R.C. Davidson, M.D., M.P.H.

Maternal Smoking and Medical Expenditures for Childhood Respiratory Illness
Stoddard JJ, Gray B (Univ of Wisconsin, Madison)
Am J Public Health 87:205–209, 1997   11–9

Background.—Exposure to environmental tobacco smoke contributes to childhood respiratory illnesses. The cost of medical treatment of such illnesses is high. The association between environmental tobacco smoke exposure because of maternal smoking and health care expenditures for respiratory illnesses among U.S. children was examined.

Study Design.—The National Medical Expenditure Survey is a population-based nationwide survey designed to estimate health care usage and expenditure by the civilian, noninstitutionalized U.S. population. In this study, analysis was restricted to the sample of 2,624 children younger than the age of 5 years. The dependent variable was expenditures for medical services in which a respiratory illness was the coded diagnosis. The independent variable was self-reported maternal smoking status. All results were statistically weighted to reflect 1987 population estimates.

Results.—Multivariate analysis that controlled for several sociodemographic factors associated with heath care usage was performed and revealed that respiratory-related health care expenditures were significantly higher for young children whose mothers smoked than for young children of nonsmoking mothers. The truncated regression estimate of the cost of maternal smoking was $120 per year for children younger than 5 years and $175 per year for children younger than 2 years. These results indicate that passive smoking was associated with $661 million in additional medical expenditures in 1987. This represents 19% of the total expenditures for childhood respiratory conditions.

Conclusions.—Environmental tobacco smoke exposure from maternal smoking is associated with significantly increased medical expenditures for respiratory illnesses in young children. These costs contribute significantly to the overall cost of medical care to society. Therefore, it would be prudent for health care organizations to provide smoking cessation and prevention programs targeted to young women. The figures presented in this paper may be useful in tobacco-related illness litigation.

▶ The United States seems to have finally woken up to the huge costs that smoking produces in our health industry. We continue to see debates regarding a settlement between the tobacco companies and various states and other class action groups. Sometimes the figures used in the settlement seem astronomical. However, I'm convinced that we have underestimated the true costs of smoking.

This interesting study looked at the cost of increased health services for the children of families who smoke. It is not surprising that they found a significantly increased number of respiratory illnesses requiring intervention by health care providers, and they also noted its inherent cost.

We must continue to work vigilantly to reduce smoking as an acceptable social behavior in the United States.

R.C. Davidson, M.D., M.P.H.

Telephone Support as an Adjunct to Transdermal Nicotine in Smoking Cessation
Lando HA, Rolnick S, Klevan D, et al (Univ of Minnesota, Minneapolis)
Am J Public Health 87:1670–1674, 1997   11–10

Background.—The reported efficacy of transdermal nicotine patches has been promising. The value of telephone support as an adjunct to nicotine patch therapy in a managed care–based, single-session group smoking cessation program was investigated.

Methods.—By random assignment, 509 subjects participated in a group session without telephone support, in a session plus access to a toll-free help line, or in a session with a telephone help line plus active telephone outreach.

Findings.—No outcome differences were noted among groups. Overall abstinence rates at 6 months and 1 year were 22% and 21%, respectively. Less than 1% of the eligible subjects used the telephone help line. A mean 3.8 of a possible 4 calls were completed in the telephone outreach condition.

Conclusions.—Abstinence outcomes obtained in this program were similar to those achieved with more extensive counseling. However, telephone support did not appear to improve results beyond the initial physician-led group orientation session.

▶ Smoking cessation is the most important public health intervention that can be practiced in the office. While sincerely advising a patient to quit smoking is the most important initial intervention, a follow-up program including transdermal nicotine plays a major role to increase the rate of smoking cessation. This study shows that a toll-free help line for patients was rarely used and did not play a key role in smoking cessation. However, a physician-led group orientation session for the use of medication and a program for quitting smoking are helpful. Those patients who are highly motivated to quit will follow the program, and those who are not are likely to relapse.

J.E. Scherger, M.D., M.P.H.

A Comparison of Sustained-release Bupropion and Placebo for Smoking Cessation

Hurt RD, Sachs DPL, Glover ED, et al (Mayo Clinic and Mayo Found, Rochester, Minn; Palo Alto Ctr for Pulmonary Disease Prevention, Calif; West Virginia Univ, Morgantown; et al)
N Engl J Med 337:1195–1202, 1997   11–11

Introduction.—Because nicotine appears to act as an antidepressant in some smokers, antidepressant medications may be of value as nicotine-replacement therapy for smoking cessation. Results of clinical trials, however, have been mixed. A double-blind, placebo-controlled trial was designed to evaluate the efficacy and safety of a sustained-release form of bupropion as an aid to smoking cessation.

Methods.—Volunteers for the trial were recruited from 3 centers. Of the 742 evaluated individuals, 615 met study criteria. Those eligible for the study had smoked an average of 15 cigarettes a day for the past year, wanted to stop smoking, and were in generally good health. Smokers with a history of major depression were included, but not those with current depression. Randomization was to placebo or bupropion at doses of 100, 150, or 300 mg/day for 7 weeks. The target quitting date was 1 week after the start of treatment. Participants received brief counseling weekly during treatment and several times during follow-up. Self-reports of smoking cessation were confirmed by a carbon monoxide level in expired air of 10 parts per million.

Results.—After 7 weeks of treatment, rates of smoking cessation were 19.0% in the placebo group, 28.8% in the 100-mg group, 38.6% in the 150-mg group, and 44.2% in the 300-mg group (Table 2). Rates of cessation had fallen to 12.4%, 19.6%, 22.9%, and 23.1%, respectively, at 1 year. Only the 300- and 150-mg groups had significantly better cessation rates than the placebo group. For the 103 participants who were continuously abstinent during the treatment phase, mean weight gain after 7 weeks was negatively associated with dose (2.9 kg in the placebo group, 2.3 kg in the 100- and 150-mg groups, and 1.5 kg in the 300-mg group). Mean weight gain at 6 months (5.5 kg, 6.6 kg, 4.4 kg, and 4.5 kg, respectively) in the 59 individuals who were continuously abstinent during this period was not significantly associated with dose. Treatment had no effect on depression, as measured by Beck Depression Inventory scores. Adverse events occurred at similar rates in the 4 groups and caused 37 participants to stop treatment prematurely.

Conclusion.—Although many study participants were smoking at 1-year follow-up, bupropion proved to be an effective treatment for smoking cessation. The 300-mg dose (150 mg twice a day) is recommended as the most effective dose and is associated with lower weight gain during the treatment phase.

▶ Any improvement on interventions to help patients stop smoking is welcome. The authors of this study properly (conservatively) point out that

TABLE 2.—Point Prevalence Smoking-Cessation Rates Confirmed by Carbon Monoxide Measurement

Time after Target Quitting Date	Percentage of Subjects Not Smoking				P Value*			
	Placebo (N=153)	100 mg of Bupropion (N=153)	150 mg of Bupropion (N=153)	300 mg of Bupropion (N=156)	Overall	Placebo vs. 100-mg Dose	Placebo vs. 150-mg Dose	Placebo vs. 300-mg Dose
6 wk†	19.0	28.8	38.6	44.2	< 0.001	0.04	< 0.001	< 0.001
3 mo	14.4	24.2	26.1	29.5	0.01	0.03	0.01	< 0.001
6 mo	15.7	24.2	27.5	26.9	0.06	0.06	0.01	0.02
12 mo	12.4	19.6	22.9	23.1	0.06	0.09	0.02	0.01

Note: Point prevalence was estimated weekly.
*The P values given are from analyses that did not include site as a covariate; therefore, they can be obtained directly from the given cessation rates. In logistic regression analyses that included site as a covariate, the same differences were found to be statistically significant. The overall P value is for the simultaneous comparison of all 4 groups treated categorically. When dose was treated as a continuous variable, a significant dose effect was detected at all times ($P < 0.001$ at week 6, $P = 0.003$ at 3 months, $P = 0.02$ at 12 months). The pairwise dose comparisons presented were identified a priori, and the corresponding P values are unadjusted.
†Week 6 was the final week of study medication.
(Reprinted by permission of *The New England Journal of Medicine*, from Hurt RD, Sachs DPL, Glover ED, et al: A comparison of sustained-release bupropion and placebo for smoking cessation. N Engl J Med 337:1195–1202, Copyright 1997, Massachusetts Medical Society. All rights reserved.)

more than three quarters of all patients were smoking at 1 year, but the quit rate with 150–300 mg of buproprion was still almost twice the quit rate for placebo (12% vs. 23%—Table 2). The magnitude of this effect is roughly equivalent to the benefit from using a nicotine patch or gum, so there's no breakthrough here. Also, it is important to note that a combination of buproprion and patches or gum has not been tested. The most encouraging new finding is the control of weight gain after quitting. So, add this to your armamentarium; here's one more thing to try.

A.O. Berg, M.D., M.P.H.

Preemption in Tobacco Control: Review of an Emerging Public Health Problem
Siegel M, Carol J, Jordan J, et al (Boston Univ; Americans for Nonsmokers' Rights, Berkeley, Calif; American Cancer Society ASSIST Project, Atlanta, Ga; et al)
JAMA 278:858–863, 1997   11–12

Introduction.—In response to an increasing number of local ordinances against smoking in public places and selling tobacco to minors, the tobacco industry has used its influence to promote state legislation that preempts local regulations. Laws that restrict local authority to regulate tobacco products have been enacted in 29 states. Various data sources were reviewed to determine the nature, extent, and public health significance of preemption in tobacco control.

Methods.—Sources of data included local tobacco control ordinances, state laws regulating tobacco, state tobacco preemption bills introduced in 1996, and materials on the subject provided by state tobacco control coalition leaders. A MEDLINE search, using the key word "preemption" was also conducted. A number of observers analyzed state laws and preemption bills for content.

Results.—By the end of 1995, approximately 1,006 communities had enacted a local tobacco control ordinance. Such ordinances provided protection from secondhand smoke to 60% of the population in California and 50% in Massachusetts. The tobacco industry responded by advancing preemptive legislation in 29 states; such bills were enacted in 2 states during 1996. In California alone, the tobacco industry spent $18.9 million in 1994 in an attempt to repeal all local control ordinances and eliminate local authority to enact new ordinances. The industry has a strong influence at state and national levels, but is less able to influence local elected officials.

Discussion.—Local government regulation is the most appropriate and effective strategy to confront threats to the health of a community. If tobacco control comes under the sole jurisdiction of the state, it is extremely unlikely that effective tobacco control will be enacted. Thus, preemption of local tobacco regulation will have serious, adverse health consequences. An important public health priority should be regaining the ability to develop community-based tobacco control policy interventions.

▶ This article makes a very convincing case for the motives underlying the apparently baffling behavior on the part of tobacco companies to enact state laws restricting tobacco use. The findings are alarming, revealing a strategy used quietly and successfully over the last decade by the tobacco companies. The study should be read and understood by any physician locally active in the fight to restrict tobacco sales and use.

A.O. Berg, M.D., M.P.H.

Effectiveness of Postal Smoking Cessation Advice: A Randomized Controlled Trial in Young Men With Reduced FEV₁ and Asbestos Exposure
Humerfelt S, Eide GE, Kvåle G, et al (Univ of Bergen, Norway)
Eur Respir J 11:284–290, 1998   11–13

Introduction.—Smoking cessation is known to have beneficial effects on morbidity and mortality from obstructive lung disease. Very few community-based intervention trials using randomization, control groups, and biochemical validation have been conducted with minimal smoking interventions, such as written or verbal advice, in individuals at risk for ob-

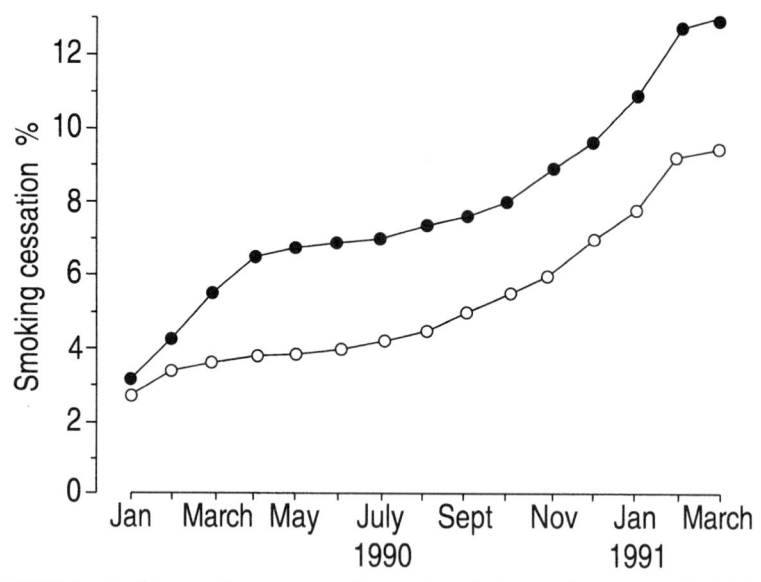

FIGURE 1.—Smoking cessation among participants from the intervention group *(solid circles)* and from the control group *(open circles)* by self-reported month of quitting, given retrospectively by March 1991 (n = 2,282). The advice to quit smoking was posted on January 15, 1990. Information was missing about 9 and 7 participants, respectively. (Courtesy of Humerfelt S, Eide GE, Kvåle G, et al: Effectiveness of postal smoking cessation advice: A randomly controlled trial in young men with reduced FEV₁ and asbestos exposure. *Eur Respir J* 11:284–290, 1998.)

structive lung disease. The effectiveness of smoking cessation advice from a respiratory physician was evaluated in men at high risk for lung cancer and obstructive lung disease.

Methods.—There were 2,619 men who were smokers between the ages of 30 and 45 years who responded to a cross-sectional community survey, in which they provided information about their smoking habits and occupational asbestos exposure. Measurements of reduced forced expiratory volume in 1 second were taken with a dry-wedge bellow spirometer. Half of the smokers received a mailed personal letter from a respiratory physician with person-specific health advice to quit smoking and a pamphlet on smoking cessation, and the remaining smokers did not receive any information. Information on smoking habits was re-examined using a postal questionnaire 12 months after the intervention.

Results.—Among the 2,282 respondents, there was a 13.7% rate of reported cessation in smoking, compared to a 9.9% rate in the control group (Fig 1). There was a 5.6% 1-year sustained quit rate, representing no smoking at all during the last year, for the intervention group, and a 3.5% rate for the controls. Self-reported nonsmoking was confirmed with measurements of carbon monoxide in expired air (with 10 parts or less per million).

Conclusion.—The 1-year sustained success rate was improved by 60% in identified high-risk smokers when this simple postal smoking cessation advice based on person-specific risk factors was given by a respiratory physician.

▶ I included this article to remind us that physician advice regarding smoking cessation does make a difference. This was a very interesting prospective study of a group of men with a high risk for respiratory problems because of reduced pulmonary function and/or asbestos exposure. Half of those men identified were contacted by a personal letter from a physician giving specific advice on how to quit smoking. The other men acted as controls and did not receive any intervention. The study showed a significant increase in smoking cessation in the intervention group.

Even though the overall success rate was low (12% in the intervention group), it still was worth the effort to increase the number of patients who successfully stopped smoking from 8% to 12%.

R.C. Davidson, M.D., M.P.H.

Antioxidants

Is There a Role for Antioxidant Vitamins in the Prevention of Cardiovascular Disease? An Update on Epidemiological and Clinical Trials Data
Lonn EM, Yusuf S (McMaster Univ, Hamilton, Ont, Canada)
Can J Cardiol 13:957–965, 1997   11–14

Introduction.—Preventive strategies to reduce the incidence of cardiovascular disease (CVD) have been the focus of substantial research in recent years. The effects of antioxidants, including the naturally occurring vitamin E, vitamin C, and beta-carotene, are of particular interest. A review of epidemiologic studies and randomized clinical trials was conducted to determine the role of these antioxidants in CVD prevention.

Methods.—Studies were identified through a search of MEDLINE and the Science Citation Index, and through manual searches on the role of antioxidant vitamins in CVD management. Only prospective epidemiologic studies and double-blind, controlled, randomized clinical trials including 100 or more participants were eligible for review. Relative risk reductions were evaluated for the clinical trials and relative risk for the epidemiologic studies. Because of significant differences in overall study design, study populations, dosages, and durations of follow-up, a formal meta-analysis was not performed.

Results.—Five prospective observational studies of vitamin E, 10 of vitamin C, and 9 of beta-carotene followed participants for periods ranging from 4 to 20 years. These investigations suggest that an increased intake of the antioxidant vitamins, particularly vitamin E, is associated with a reduction in cardiovascular risk. The 14 large randomized trials, some ongoing and others with follow-up ranging from 510 days to 12 years, were inconclusive about the roles that vitamin E and vitamin C play in cardiovascular protection, and showed no effect and a potential for harm associated with the use of beta-carotene.

Conclusion.—An analysis of prospective epidemiologic studies and randomized clinical trials found no clear evidence for the benefits of vitamin E, vitamin C, or beta-carotene supplementation in the prevention of CVD. There is some evidence, which needs to be confirmed in clinical trials, that vitamin E is of value, but beta-carotene supplementation should be avoided.

▶ This well-done review of the epidemiologic and clinical trials data on antioxidant vitamins brings a note of caution to all of us. The authors did a review of the world's literature. They included only those studies with more than 100 participants in a double-blinded, controlled, randomized clinical trial. The authors concluded that there is significant evidence that vitamin E intake does reduce overall cardiovascular risk. They were not convinced that vitamin C has any protective effect, and they actually found a negative effect with beta-carotene.

In this era of evidence-based medicine, it is important to maintain the gold standard of well-controlled, large double-blinded placebo studies before we jump on the bandwagon of a new treatment. However, because there seems to be little risk from taking antioxidant vitamins, and because at least with vitamin E there is a statistically proven benefit, I still feel that it is efficacious to recommend antioxidant vitamins to appropriate patients for coronary artery risk reduction.

R.C. Davidson, M.D., M.P.H.

Effect of Antioxidant Vitamins on the Transient Impairment of Endothelium-dependent Brachial Artery Vasoactivity Following a Single High-fat Meal

Plotnick GD, Corretti MC, Vogel RA (Univ of Maryland, Baltimore)
JAMA 278:1682–1686, 1997
11–15

Background.—A high-fat diet promotes atherosclerosis through elevation of serum cholesterol. It may also directly impair endothelial function, caused by transient accumulation of triglyceride-rich lipoproteins. Intake of antioxidant vitamins reduces coronary heart disease risk. This study examined the effects of a high-fat meal, with or without antioxidant pretreatment, on endothelial function in healthy subjects.

Methods.—The randomized trial included 20 healthy volunteers, all with normal total and low-density lipoprotein levels. There were 13 women and 7 men, aged 24–54 years. The subjects were randomized to receive a high-fat meal, providing 3,766 J of energy and 50 g of fat; a low-fat meal, providing 3,766 J of energy but 0 g of fat; a high-fat meal with oral vitamins C and E, 1 g and 800 IU, respectively; or a low-fat meal with vitamins. The effects of the 4 meals on flow-mediated, endothelium-dependent vasodilation were assessed noninvasively in the brachial artery using high-frequency ultrasound and blood pressure cuff–induced hyperemia. The percent diameter change in flow-mediated vasodilation was assessed before and 6 hours after each meal.

Results.—In subjects eating the high-fat meal, flow-mediated vasodilation decreased from a mean of 20% before the meal to 12% at 2 hours, 10% at 3 hours, and 8% at 4 hours. None of the other 3 groups showed a significant change in flow-mediated vasodilation after their assigned meal. After both the high- and low-fat meals, the change in flow-mediated vasodilation was inversely correlated with the change in triglyceride levels 2 hours after the meal.

Conclusions.—In normal subjects, consuming a high-fat meal produces a short-term reduction in endothelial function, most likely via buildup of lipoproteins rich in triglycerides. Pretreatment with the antioxidant vitamins C and E prevents this reduction in endothelium-dependent vasoactivity. The findings help in understanding the opposing effects of fat and antioxidant intake on coronary heart disease risk, and may lead to a better mechanistic approach to antioxidant administration for disease prevention and management.

▶ When this article was published in *JAMA* in November 1997, it caused a short-term flurry of interest in both local and national media. The authors' purpose was to study the effects of the antioxidants vitamins C and E on arterial endothelial function following a high-fat meal. What the media picked up seemed to imply that it was OK to have a high-fat meal as long as you followed it with a chaser of vitamins C and E. Herein lies the danger of this study. Somehow the message got out that it's OK for a McDonald's double cheeseburger, but just carry some C and E in your pocket to take as a chaser.

One might even envision complimentary C and E tablets stuffed in the fast-food bag as a marketing ploy.

There are more and more data showing the cardioprotective and antioxidant advantages of an adequate intake of vitamins C and E. However, let's not delude ourselves into thinking that we will be able to eat whatever we want as long as we chase it with a vitamin.

R.C. Davidson, M.D., M.P.H.

Randomized, Double-blind, Placebo-controlled Study of Supplemental Vitamin E on Attenuation of the Development of Nitrate Tolerance
Watanabe H, Kakihana M, Ohtsuka S, et al (KINU Med Assoc Hosp, Mitskaido, Japan; Ibaraki Prefectural Univ, Ami, Japan; Univ of Tsukuba, Ibaraki, Japan)
Circulation 96:2545–2550, 1997 11–16

Introduction.—Patients receiving organic nitrates for the treatment of cardiovascular diseases quickly develop tolerance. One mechanism of nitrate tolerance is reduced intracellular production of cyclic guanosine monophosphate (cGMP). In vitro studies in nitrate-tolerant vessels have demonstrated an increase in superoxide levels and a reduction in activation of guanylate cyclase. The antioxidant drug vitamin E was tested for its ability to prevent nitrate tolerance.

Methods.—The study included 24 normal volunteers and 24 patients with ischemic heart disease (IHD). Both groups were randomly assigned to either vitamin E, 200 mg 3 times daily, or placebo. Their vasodilator

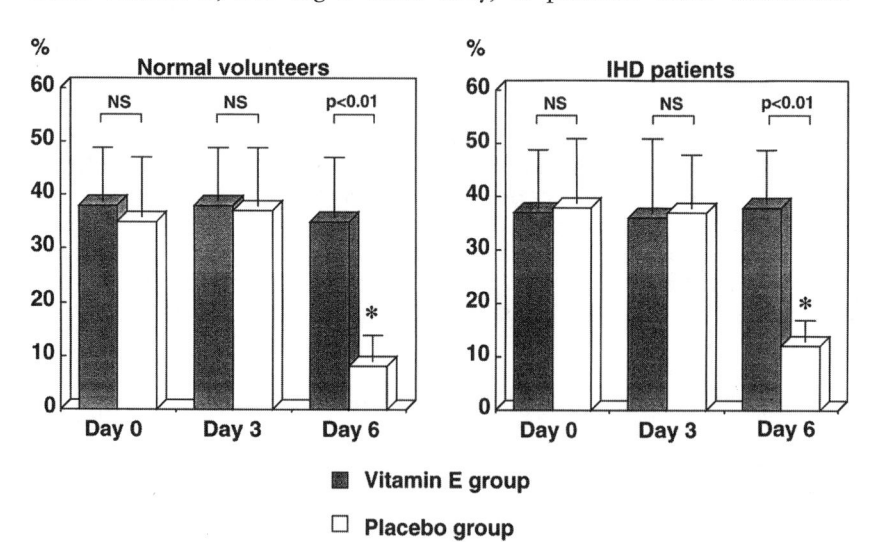

FIGURE 5.—Percent increase of platelet cyclic guanosine monophosphate level after sublingual nitroglycerin. Data are mean ± SD. *P < .05 vs day 0 and day 3. *Abbreviations:* *IHD* indicates ischemic heart disease; *NS*, not significant. (Courtesy of Watanabe H, Kakihana M, Ohtsuka S, et al: Randomized, double-blind, placebo-controlled study of supplemental vitamin E on attenuation of the development of nitrate tolerance. *Circulation* 96:2545–2550, 1997.)

response to nitroglycerin, 0.3 mg sublingually, was assessed using plethysmography to measure the change in forearm blood flow (FBF) before and 5 minutes after administration. At the same times, venous blood samples were obtained for measurement of the platelet cGMP level. These measurements were made at baseline, day 0; at day 3, after treatment with vitamin E or placebo; and at day 6, 3 days after application of a 10-mg/ 24-hr nitroglycerin tape, given with vitamin E or placebo.

Results.—The groups did not vary in their FBF and cGMP responses to sublingual nitroglycerin on day 0 or day 3 (Fig 5). However, on day 6, both values were significantly lower than at baseline, and significantly different between groups. In normal volunteers, day 6 FBF was 30% with vitamin E vs. 17% with placebo; in patients with IHD, these values were 28% vs. 17%, respectively. Day 6 values for cGMP in normal volunteers were 35% with vitamin E vs. 8% with placebo; in patients with IHD, these values were 38% vs. 12%, respectively.

Conclusions.—Combination therapy with vitamin E may be a useful means of preventing the development of nitrate tolerance in patients with IHD. This antioxidant vitamin prevents reductions in FBF and production of platelet cGMP in response to sublingual or transdermal nitroglycerin application. The authors call for more research into the potential benefits of antioxidant supplementation to prevent nitrate tolerance.

▶ As I review my selections for this year's YEAR BOOK OF FAMILY PRACTICE, I feel a little like a soapbox zealot for vitamin E. However, we are finding increasingly important and well-validated studies showing the multiple positive effects of vitamin E on cardiovascular risk factors. This particular study did not look at a reduction of risk factors, but rather a reduction in body resistance to the vasodilative effects of nitrates on patients who were given vitamin E. In patients receiving continuous nitroglycerin, those without vitamin E showed a significant reduction in response to the nitrate. The addition of vitamin E appeared to block this resistance.

Since most patients on nitrates also have coronary artery disease, it would seem logical to make sure our patients who are on long-term nitrates also are taking vitamin E.

R.C. Davidson, M.D., M.P.H.

Garlic

Effect of Garlic Oil Preparation on Serum Lipoproteins and Cholesterol Metabolism: A Randomized Controlled Trial
Berthold HK, Sudhop T, von Bergmann K (Univ of Bonn, Germany)
JAMA 279:1900–1902, 1998   11–17

Introduction.—Despite a lack of evidence of their efficacy, garlic-containing preparations have been recommended for the treatment and prevention of a number of diseases. Studies of the lipid-lowering effects of garlic have yielded contradictory results. A double-blind, randomized, placebo-controlled trial was used to analyze the hypocholesterolemic effect of garlic oil and its possible mechanism of action.

Methods.—Twenty-five patients, 14 men and 11 women, participated in the trial. The mean age of the patients was 58 years and they had moderate hypercholesterolemia. They adhered to their usual diet during the study but were prohibited from taking additional garlic or other food supplements. In a crossover design, patients took a steam-distilled garlic oil preparation (5 mg twice daily) or placebo for 12 weeks with washout periods of 4 weeks. Patients were evaluated for serum lipoprotein concentrations, cholesterol absorption, and cholesterol synthesis.

Results.—Compliance with the garlic oil preparation was excellent, and there were no serious adverse events. Body weights remained constant during the study. There were virtually no effects from the garlic drug on the measured variables of cholesterol metabolism. At the end of the study, the placebo and garlic treatment groups were similar in mean total cholesterol levels, triglyceride levels, cholesterol absorption, cholesterol synthesis, mevalonic acid excretion, and changes in the ratio of lathosterol to cholesterol in serum.

Conclusion.—The commercially available garlic preparation analyzed in this study had no effect on serum lipoprotein levels of patients with moderate hypercholesterolemia. The overall evidence for a positive effect of garlic on serum lipid levels is questionable.

▶ I had to keep my string going. Each year I have included at least 1 article on the health effects of garlic. I do identify a conflict of interest because I enjoy garlic. Some past studies have shown a slight relationship to risk reduction for coronary artery disease with use of garlic. However, this small study of 25 patients with moderate hypercholesterolemia showed no value to the use of commercial garlic oil preparations. The authors were not looking at the use of garlic in food preparation. They were studying the potential benefit of commercial garlic oil preparations that have become quite common in health food stores. Because these have no taste, there seems little value in recommending them. When asked, I will cite this study to show that there appears to be no benefit. However, I plan to continue to use plenty of garlic in my food preparation.

R.C. Davidson, M.D., M.P.H.

Protective Effect of Chronic Garlic Intake on Elastic Properties of Aorta in the Elderly
Breithaupt-Grögler K, Ling M, Boudoulas H, et al (Centre for Cardiovascular Pharmacology, Mainz, Germany; Ohio State Univ, Columbus, Ohio)
Circulation 96:2649–2655, 1997   11–18

Introduction.—Garlic appears to have a protective effect against cardiovascular diseases, but the precise mechanisms responsible for the ben-

Reservation Card for the Year Book

Yes! I would like my own copy of *Year Book of Family Practice*® at the price of **$69.00** (**$76.00** outside the U.S.) plus sales tax, postage, and handling. Please begin my subscription with the current edition according to the terms described below.* I understand that I will have 30 days to examine each annual edition.

Name _____

Address _____

City _____ State _____ ZIP _____

Method of Payment

Check (in U.S. dollars, drawn on a U.S. bank, payable to *Year Book of Family Practice*®)

❑ VISA ❑ MasterCard ❑ Discover ❑ AmEx ❑ Bill me

Card number _____ Exp. date: _____

Signature _____

Prices are subject to change without notice.   PMC-346

Subscribe to the related journal in your field!

Yes! Begin my one-year subscription to *Disease-a-Month*® (12 issues).

Name _____

Institution _____

Address _____

City _____ State _____

ZIP/PC _____ Country _____

Specialty _____
(Students/residents, please list Institution)

Method of payment

Enclose payment (check or credit card number) and we'll send an extra issue FREE!

❑ Check (in U.S. dollars, drawn on a U.S. bank, and payable to *Disease-a-Month*®)

❑ VISA ❑ MasterCard ❑ Discover

❑ AmEx ❑ Bill me Exp. date_____

Card # _____

Signature _____

*Includes Canadian GST

Subscription prices (through 9/30/99)

	USA	Canada*	Int'l
Individuals ❑	$95.00	$118.77	$111.00
Institutions ❑	147.00	174.41	163.00
Students, residents ❑	51.00	71.69	67.00

Individual/student subscriptions must be in the name of, billed to, and paid for by the individual.

Airmail rates available upon request.
Prices subject to change without notice.

J062991YB

---

*Your Year Book service guarantee:

When you subscribe to the *Year Book*, you will receive advance notice of future annual volumes about two months before publication. To receive the new edition, you need do nothing—we'll send you the new volume as soon as it is available. If you want to discontinue, the advance notice allows you time to notify us of your decision. If you are not completely satisfied, you have 30 days to return any *Year Book*.

BUSINESS REPLY MAIL
FIRST-CLASS MAIL   PERMIT NO 135   ST LOUIS MO

POSTAGE WILL BE PAID BY ADDRESSEE

SUBSCRIPTION SERVICES
MOSBY, INC.
11830 WESTLINE INDUSTRIAL DRIVE
ST. LOUIS   MO 63146-9988

NO POSTAGE
NECESSARY
IF MAILED
IN THE
UNITED STATES

BUSINESS REPLY MAIL
FIRST-CLASS MAIL   PERMIT NO 135   ST LOUIS MO

POSTAGE WILL BE PAID BY ADDRESSEE

SUBSCRIPTION SERVICES
MOSBY, INC.
11830 WESTLINE INDUSTRIAL DRIVE
ST. LOUIS   MO 63146-9988

NO POSTAGE
NECESSARY
IF MAILED
IN THE
UNITED STATES

Want to speed up the process?

To order a *Year Book* or *Advances*, you also may call 1-800-426-4545

To subscribe to a journal today, call toll-free in the U.S.:
1-800-453-4351
or fax 314-432-1158
Outside the U.S., call: 314-453-4351

Visit us at: *www.mosby.com/periodicals*

Mosby, Inc.
Subscription Services
11830 Westline Industrial Drive
St. Louis, MO   63146 U.S.A.

M Mosby

eficial effects are not known. A study was designed to test the hypothesis that regular garlic intake would delay age-related stiffening of the aorta.

Methods.—Participants were healthy, nonsmoking men and women aged 50–80 years. All had taken 300 mg or more garlic powder preparation per day for 2 or more years immediately preceding the study. Controls were matched to study participants by age, sex, and body weight, but the controls did not regularly consume garlic powder. The elastic properties of the aorta were measured using pulse wave velocity (PWV) and pressure-standardized elastic vascular resistance. Twenty-four individuals from each group were studied for the effects of wave reflection on pulse height.

Results.—The 202 research participants (101 in each group) were all Caucasians and lived in the same geographic area. Garlic users reported ingesting an average of 44.6 100-mg garlic tablets for an average of 7.1 years. The 2 groups were similar in blood pressures, heart rates, and plasma lipid levels. Compared with controls, those who had regularly taken garlic powder had significantly lower PWV and elastic vascular resistance. There was a significant correlation between PWV and both age and systolic blood pressure (SBP). Any degree of increase in age or SBP led to significantly lower PWV increases in the garlic group. Garlic intake was divided into 3 levels: 300 mg/day, 400 mg/day, and 600 mg/day. Analysis of the relations between intake level and study outcomes did not reveal a dose effect. Age and SBP were the most important determinants of PWV, and the effect of garlic on PWV was independent of confounding factors such as blood pressure and serum lipids.

Conclusion.—Age-related increases in aortic stiffness were reduced, relative to controls, in healthy participants who had taken garlic powder tablets on a regular basis for an average of 7 years. Data strongly support the hypothesis that the protective effect of garlic against cardiovascular diseases is related to garlic's ability to maintain the elastic properties of the aorta.

▶ I'm sure glad that garlic seems to be good for you, because to me it sure tastes good. The health food stores and drug store displays tout the benefits of various types of garlic. However, it remains unclear why garlic would be of value in cardiovascular risk reduction.

This study looked at the aortic stiffness in older healthy adults aged 50–80 years who were taking large amounts of garlic powder. The authors found a reduction in aortic stiffness in those taking the garlic. However, the number in this study was small (101), and the time of the study was only 2 years. I included this article, however, since I am frequently asked by my patients whether they should take garlic. I always leave the decision up to them, but now at least I will tell them that there is 1 study showing a reduction in stiffness of the arteries in people who take garlic powder.

R.C. Davidson, M.D., M.P.H.

12 Neurologic Conditions

Overview

Randomized controlled trials: Abstracts 12-3, 12-5, 12-6, 12-8, and 12-9

Stroke and Stroke Prevention

- Public perception of stroke warning signs
- Hypertension and intracerebral hemorrhage
- Stroke prevention in patients with atrial fibrillation using aspirin
- Serum uric acid as a predictor of stroke in patients with NIDDM
- HMG-CoA reductase inhibitors and stroke incidence
- Stroke outcome in stroke and general medical units

Headache

- Epidemiology of tension headache
- Homeopathic prophylaxis of migraine
- Aspirin, acetaminophen, and caffeine in migraine

Stroke

Public Perception of Stroke Warning Signs and Knowledge of Potential Risk Factors
Pancioli AM, Broderick J, Kothari R, et al (Univ of Cincinnati, Ohio)
JAMA 279:1288–1292, 1998   12–1

Introduction.—The third leading cause of death and adult disability in the United States is stroke. Decreasing the time from stroke onset to hospital arrival and improved control of stroke risk factors offer the greatest opportunities for effective treatment and prevention of stroke. Public knowledge of stroke warning signs and risk factors is necessary for rapid patient presentation and risk reduction. To assess current public knowledge of warning signs and risk factors for stroke, a population-based telephone survey was conducted.

Methods.—A total of 17,634 telephone calls made to individuals whose age, race, and sex that matched those of the population of patients with acute stroke yielded 2,642 demographically eligible individuals. Of these, 1,066 (71.2%) responded to the interview in which they were asked to report risk factors, hypertension, diabetes, previous stroke, current smoking, past smoking or warning signs, including dizziness, numbness, headaches, weakness, unspecific pain, slurred speech, vision problems, chest pain, and shortness of breath.

Results.—At least 1 of the 5 established stroke warning signs was correctly listed by 1,066 respondents (57%). At least 1 of the established stroke risk factors was correctly listed by 1,274 respondents (68%). Of 818 respondents with a history of hypertension, 469 (57%) listed hypertension as a risk factor. Of 402 respondents who were current smokers, 142 (35%) listed smoking as a risk factor. Of 255 respondents with diabetes, 32 (13%) listed diabetes as a risk factor for stroke. Respondents 75 years or older were less likely to correctly list at least 1 stroke warning sign (47%) than those younger than 75 (60%). They were also less likely to list at least 1 stroke risk factor (72% of those younger than 75 vs. 56% of those older than 75 years).

Conclusion.—To increase the public's awareness of the warning signs and risk factors for stroke, considerable education is needed. Those who are the least knowledgeable about these warning signs and risk factors are the very elderly, the population at greatest risk of stroke. There is great lack of unawareness of an increased risk of stroke among those with self-reported risk factors for stroke.

▶ No startling revelations here. I included this article as a "heads up" for office practice. The treatment of stroke, or "brain attack," has been revolutionized in the last few years. We, including physicians, nurses, hospitals, public health organizations, etc., have done a very good job of changing how we all approach "heart attack" care. Now we all need to apply this same energy toward changing our approach to brain attack. Early identification and intervention can, and does, prevent mortality and, perhaps even more important, morbidity. If you are not educating your patients, particularly those at increased risk regarding this entity, start today.

W.W. Dexter, M.D.

Three Important Subgroups of Hypertensive Persons at Greater Risk of Intracerebral Hemorrhage

Thrift AG, for the Melbourne Risk Factor Study Group (Austin and Repatriation Med Ctr, Heidelberg, Australia)
Hypertension 31:1223–1229, 1998   12–2

Objective.—Whereas hypertension is the most serious risk for intracerebral hemorrhage (ICH), risks in specific groups have not been quantified. Risks for ICH were assessed in specific subgroups of hypertensive patients in a predominantly white population with a high level of detection and treatment of hypertension.

Methods.—Between 1990 and 1993, 331 consecutive patients (200 men), aged 18–80 years, from 13 hospitals, with verified ICH and 331 age-

and sex-matched controls were interviewed to ascertain risk factors for stroke. The size and site of hemorrhage were determined.

Results.—The stroke risk was 1.95 for hypertensive patients taking antihypertensive medication and 4.98 for those who had stopped taking medication. Hypertensive smokers had a risk of stroke of 6.12, and hypertensive nonsmokers had a risk of 2.92, compared with normotensive nonsmokers. Hypertensive patients younger than 55 years had a risk of 7.68, compared with normotensive individuals. The size and location of the hemorrhage was not affected by the presence of hypertension. Hypertensive patients were at higher risk for fatal ICH, compared with normotensive individuals (odds ratio, 10.84).

Conclusion.—The risk of ICH is higher for hypertensive individuals, those younger than 55 years, smokers, and those who have discontinued antihypertensive medication.

▶ Patients with hypertension are known to be at greater risk for ICH. These authors studied multiple factors in persons with hypertension to determine what factors predicted a higher risk for ICH. They found that younger persons, current smokers, and those discontinuing antihypertensive therapy were all at greater risk. It is this third subgroup that is the most important for us to remember. When it is necessary to stop antihypertensive medication in one of our patients, we should be particularly vigorous in reducing other risk factors and counseling the patient regarding the risk of ICH.

R.C. Davidson, M.D., M.P.H.

Patients With Nonvalvular Atrial Fibrillation at Low Risk of Stroke During Treatment With Aspirin: Stroke Prevention in Atrial Fibrillation III Study
The SPAF III Writing Committee for the Stroke Prevention in Atrial Fibrillation Investigators (SPAF Statistical Coordinating Ctr, Seattle)
JAMA 279:1273–1277, 1998
12–3

Objective.—Whereas individuals with nonvalvular atrial fibrillation (AF) are at increased risk for stroke, there are no valid methods for stratifying patients at risk. A risk stratification scheme was prospectively validated by recruiting AF patients without prespecified thromboembolic risk factors, giving them aspirin, and measuring the subsequent rate of stroke and systemic embolism.

Methods.—Patients with AF (n = 892, 78% men), with an average age of 67 years, from 20 clinical sites were given 325 mg/day of aspirin and followed up at 3 and 6 months and then at 6-month intervals, with telephone call interviews in between, for an average of 2 years. Patients without any of the 4 thromboembolic risk factors (recent congestive heart failure or left ventricular fractional shortening of less than 25%, previous thromboembolism, systolic blood pressure greater than 160 mm Hg, or female sex and older than 75 years of age) were predicted to have a risk of stroke and systemic emboli of less than 3% annually. Outcome measures were strokes, systemic emboli, or transient ischemic attacks.

Results.—Patients had histories of ischemic heart disease (16%), diabetes (13%), and hypertension (46%). The yearly rate of primary events was 2.2%, with a rate of ischemic stroke of 2.0%, disabling ischemic stroke of 0.8%, and transient ischemic attack of 1.3%. Patients with hypertension had a significantly higher rate of primary events than did other participants (3.6% vs. 1.1%) and a higher rate of disabling ischemic strokes (1.4% vs. 0.5%). According to multivariate analysis, patients with hypertension had a relative risk of primary events of 3.3. Age was also a significant predictor with a relative risk increase of 1.7 for every decade. The rate of major bleeding from aspirin was 0.5% per year.

Conclusion.—Patients with AF with a low risk of stroke can be prospectively identified during aspirin therapy.

▶ The use of anticoagulation by warfarin products in a patient with chronic AF is a standard of practice in this community. This study is an attempt to identify a subpopulation with chronic AF who can be safely treated with aspirin alone. The authors concluded that patients with AF who did not have any of 4 specific risk factors for thromboembolism could be safely treated with aspirin alone. The risk factors requiring warfarin therapy included impaired left ventricular function, hypertension, prior ischemic stroke or transient ischemic attack, or being female and older than 75 years. Because there may be significant complications with anticoagulation, it can be helpful to be able to identify this low-risk population for avoidance of anticoagulation.

R.C. Davidson, M.D., M.P.H.

Serum Uric Acid Is a Strong Predictor of Stroke in Patients With Non–Insulin-Dependent Diabetes Mellitus
Lehto S, Niskanen L, Rönnemaa T, et al (Univ of Kuopio, Finland; Univ of Turku, Finland)
Stroke 29:635–639, 1998

Introduction.—Up to a fourfold greater risk of all manifestations of atherosclerotic vascular disease, including stroke, is found among those with non–insulin-dependent diabetes mellitus. Serum uric acid has been defined as a metabolically inert end product of purine metabolism and was thought to be without physiologic significance. More recently, however, it has been associated with insulin resistance. An elevated level of uric acid has furthermore been shown to be an independent predictor of coronary heart disease and total mortality for nondiabetic subjects. In a prospective population-based study that included a large number of patients with non–insulin-dependent diabetes mellitus, serum uric acid was examined as a factor for stroke.

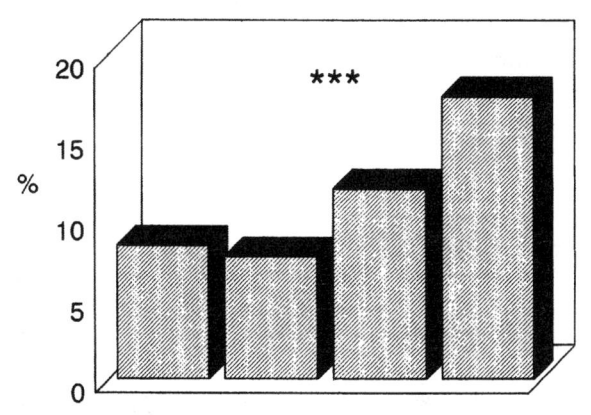

FIGURE.—Seven-year incidence (%) of stroke events (fatal or nonfatal stroke) with respect to the quartiles of serum uric acid concentration (expressed as micromoles per liter) (quartile limits: less than 243, 243–295, 296–356, and greater than 357). ***P < .001. (Courtesy of Lehto S, Niskanen L, Rönnemaa T, et al: Serum uric acid is a strong predictor of stroke in patients with non–insulin-dependent diabetes mellitus. *Stroke* 29:635–639, 1998.)

Methods.—A total of 1,017 patients (551 men and 466 women) were studied for cardiovascular risk factors. They had non–insulin-dependent diabetes mellitus and were between the ages of 45 and 64 years. They were followed up for 7 years with respect to stroke events.

Results.—Death from stroke occurred among 31 patients with non–insulin-dependent diabetes mellitus (19 women and 12 men). Fatal or nonfatal strokes occurred among 114 patients (55 men and 59 women). A significant increase was seen in the incidence of stroke by quartiles of serum uric acid levels (Figure). The risk of fatal and nonfatal stroke was significantly associated with a high uric acid level (above the median value of more than 295 µmol/L by Cox regression analysis). Even after adjustment for all cardiovascular risk factors, this association remained statistically significant.

Conclusion.—In middle-aged patients with non–insulin-dependent diabetes mellitus, hyperuricemia is a strong predictor of stroke events, independent of other cardiovascular risk factors. Further research should focus on the mechanisms by which hyperuricemia increases the risk of stroke.

▶ Uric acid has been thought to have no physiologic role in the body. However, this and other studies are questioning this presumption. Low uric acid levels have been noted in multiple sclerosis, and there is currently a trial to give uric acid to patients with severe multiple sclerosis. High levels of uric acid are associated with gout, but now several investigators suggest that they are also associated with higher levels of death and coronary heart disease. Many patients with diabetes and elevated levels of uric acid were taking diuretics, but the relationship with stroke remained after controlling for this and other factors. Could uric acid just reflect the patient's diet rather than be physiologically active? This study did not answer that question.

M.A. Bowman, M.D., M.P.A.

Effect of HMGcoA Reductase Inhibitors on Stroke: A Meta-analysis of Randomized, Controlled Trials
Bucher HC, Griffith LE, Guyatt GH (Kantonsspital Basel, Switzerland; McMaster Univ, Hamilton, Ont, Canada)
Ann Intern Med 128:89–95, 1998

Background.—Scientists have not adequately determined the correlation of hypercholesterolemia and stroke. This study examines the relationship between stroke and the administration of antilipidemic interventions.

Methods.—Researchers searched MEDLINE and EMBASE through October 1996 to find controlled, randomized studies of cholesterol-lowering interventions. Selection of studies was based on random assignment of treatment, use of control, and reporting of cases of stroke, death from coronary disease, and overall mortality. Researchers took differences in antilipidemic treatments into account and reviewed each trial for criteria, methods, and outcomes. Twenty-eight trials were used. The intervention group numbered 49,477 and the control group numbered 56,636. Researchers combined data for fatal and nonfatal strokes.

Results.—Researchers tabulated risk ratios at 0.95 (95% confidence interval, 0.86–1.05; test of heterogeneity, $P = 0.2$) for total risk, 0.76 (confidence interval, 0.062–0.92; test of heterogeneity, $P = 0.2$) for 3-hydroxy-3-methylglutaryl coenzyme A (HMG-CoA) reductase inhibitors, and 1.0 for interventions other than HMG-CoA, including fibrates, resins, and dietary interventions. Summary estimate differences between HMG-CoA reductase inhibitors and other interventions were statistically significant and clinically important. Rates of overall mortality and death from coronary heart disease were also reduced in HMG-CoA trials.

Conclusion.—According to this meta-analysis, HMG-CoA reductase inhibitors reduce the incidence of stroke by lowering cholesterol much more effectively than older drugs.

▶ By now, quite a few studies of HMG-CoA reductase inhibitors and lowering cholesterol have been published, with an interesting consistent byproduct showing reduced incidence of strokes in treated groups. Because stroke was not one of the primary end points in many of the studies, the numbers available for analysis have been less than ideal for determining biological and statistical significance of the differences observed. This is the first well-designed meta-analysis of the data from the 28 best trials, and shows the expected result: the drugs reduce stroke incidence.

The important clinical question not addressed in this meta-analysis is *how much* stroke incidence is reduced. The risk ratios give only a general idea. Here's how I would approach this question, using a number-needed-to-treat analysis. The baseline risk for nonfatal and fatal strokes, at its highest, is approximately 10 strokes per 1,000 patient-years. If the summary meta-analysis is correct, treatment with HMG-CoA reductase inhibitors lowers that risk by about 25% to 7.5 strokes per 1,000 patient-years, an absolute reduction of 2.5 strokes per 1,000 patient-years. An individual patient treated with these drugs for 20 years, then, can expect an average reduction of 0.05 events. In other words, you would need to treat 20 patients (the reciprocal of 0.05) for 20 years to prevent 1 fatal or nonfatal stroke. This number-needed-to-treat calculation places the treatment well in line with other recommended and well-accepted interventions.

A.O. Berg, M.D., M.P.H.

Stroke Units Versus General Medical Wards: Twelve- and Eighteen-Month Survival: A Randomized, Controlled Trial

Rønning OM, Guldvog B (Central Hosp of Akershus, Nordbyhagen, Norway)
Stroke 29:58–62, 1998   12–6

Objective.—Mortality at 1 year for stroke patients in stroke units (SUs) is lower than for stroke patients who are not managed in SUs. Whether lower mortality is the result of early treatment or later rehabilitation efforts is not known. The hypothesis that patients in an SU have a shorter stay and increased survival at 12- and 18-months was tested.

Methods.—Between January 1993 and February 1994, 802 patients aged 60 years or older, admitted to the Central Hospital of Akershus in Norway within 24 hours after a first or recurrent stroke, were randomly allocated to treatment in the general medical ward (GMW) (n = 438) or the SU (n = 364). Survival was assessed at 10 days and at 1, 3, 6, 12, and 18 months.

Results.—Distributions of the type of stroke were similar between groups. Survival rates were significantly higher at all time points for SU patients. Overall mortality at 10 days was 9.1% for SU patients and 16.7% for GMW patients, at 12 months was 30.8% and 37.3%, and at 18 months was 34.9% and 41.9%, respectively. Mortality at 10 days, 12 months, and 18 months for SU and GMW patients with intracerebral hemorrhage was 24.5% and 51.6%, 52.8% and 69.4%, and 56.6% and 71.0%, respectively.

Conclusion.—Stroke patients treated in SUs have a significantly higher survival rate at 12 and 18 months than stroke patients in the GMW.

▶ Population-based trials of this magnitude are always interesting. Even though this was not quite a fully randomized study, only the most critical epidemiologist would be concerned with the authors' method of patient assignment. Further, the technology of SUs is sufficiently well developed around the world that I do not have a problem accepting the Norwegian source of the data. I am entirely comfortable with the authors' conclusions. At the very least, data like these should prompt hospitals with adequate volume to seriously consider establishing SUs. But hospitals that do so should not stop there; they should evaluate outcomes to make sure that patients actually do better in the specialized facilities.

A.O. Berg, M.D., M.P.H.

Headache

Epidemiology of Tension-Type Headache
Schwartz BS, Stewart WF, Simon D, et al (The Johns Hopkins Univ, Baltimore, Md; Albert Einstein College of Medicine, New York)
JAMA 279:381–383, 1998   12–7

Objective.—Although tension headaches are common and disabling, there have been few large epidemiologic studies. The 1-year period prevalence of episodic tension-type headache (ETTH) and chronic tension-type headache (CTTH) in a population sample was estimated. Also, the demographic factors associated with 1-year period prevalence were described, and the societal impact of ETTH and CTTH were estimated.

Methods.—A telephone survey of 13,345 individuals was conducted from 1993 to 1994 in Baltimore County, Maryland, to collect demographic data and to determine the type, frequency, and severity of headache respondents experienced, together with the location, quality, associated symptoms, and disability using International Headache Society criteria.

Results.—For respondents with the most severe headaches, 25.3% had ETTH and 1.4% had CTTH. For the next most severe headaches, 19.5% had ETTH and 0.8% had CTTH. The overall prevalence of all ETTHs was 38.3%, with women having a higher prevalence than men. The highest headache prevalence occurred in the 30- to 39-year-old group for both men and women, with whites having a significantly higher prevalence than blacks for both men (40.1% vs. 22.8%) and women (46.8% vs. 30.9%). Prevalence increased with educational level, peaking in men (48.5%) and women (48.9%) with a graduate school education. Women were twice as likely to have CTTH than men (2.8% vs. 1.4%). Blacks had a lower prevalence of CTTH than whites.

Prevalence of CTTH declined significantly with an increasing educational level, particularly in women. Women were more likely than men to have both ETTH (a ratio of 2:1) and CTTH (a ratio of 1.16:1). The proportion of subjects over 50 years of age was higher for CTTH (men, 18.8%; women, 29.6%) than for ETTH (men, 16.8%; women, 19.5%). Among individuals with ETTH, 8.3% reported an average of 8.9 lost workdays and 43.6% reported reduced effectiveness days. Among individuals with CTTH, 11.8% reported an average of 27.4 lost workdays and 46.5% reported reduced effectiveness days.

Conclusion.—A high prevalence of ETTH results in a significant number of lost workdays and reduced effectiveness days. Although CTTH is more disabling, it is less prevalent and has a smaller societal impact.

▶ This excellent, large-scale study uses the rigorous International Headache Society criteria. I found most interesting the data showing that ETTHs are strongly related to socioeconomic status (as pointed out by the authors, they could almost be used as a surrogate), with prevalence increasing with higher socioeconomic status. The contrasts with migraine are also instructive (migraines are inversely related to socioeconomic status, are more common in women, and increase with age). With virtually half of some population subgroups experiencing ETTHs in a given year, obviously most individuals do not seek medical care for their headaches or we would have time for nothing else in practice. This makes that subgroup seeking medical attention especially interesting. What is it about their headaches, or (more likely) about them, that makes a visit to the physician "necessary?"

A.O. Berg, M.D., M.P.H.

Double-blind Randomized Placebo-controlled Study of Homoeopathic Prophylaxis of Migraine
Whitmarsh TE, Coleston-Shields DM, Steiner TJ (Charing Cross Hosp, London)
Cephalalgia 17:600–604, 1997   12–8

Introduction.—The acceptance of homeopathy is growing, particularly in Europe, but this system of complementary medicine remains highly controversial. A 1991 review of 107 clinical studies concluded that more good quality trials were needed to provide evidence of the efficacy of homeopathy. The value of homeopathic remedies for migraine, which are statutorily offered by the National Health Service in the United Kingdom, was examined in a randomized, double-blind, placebo-controlled trial.

Methods.—Patients were recruited from a hospital-based headache center in London. Those eligible for inclusion were aged 18–60 years, had a definite diagnosis with or without aura, had had recognizable attacks for at least the past 2 years and 2–8 attacks per month in each of the past 3 months, and had symptoms conforming to the prescribing criteria for any of 11 homeopathic remedies. After a 1-month, single-blind placebo run-in period, patients received 3 months of individualized homeopathic treatment or placebo. Patients were seen monthly and completed diary cards rating the treatment for efficacy and side effects.

Results.—Three patients dropped out, leaving 30 in each treatment group. Overall compliance was good. Although both homeopathic and placebo groups improved while on therapy, neither showed great reductions in the primary outcome measure of attack frequency (19% reduction with verum and 16% with placebo). Toward the end of the treatment period, however, the effects of placebo appeared to be decreasing and those of verum developing (Fig 1). Analyses of secondary outcome measures—including analgesic consumption, total number of headache days, and subjective rating of efficacy—added no useful information.

Discussion.—In this first trial of homeopathic prophylaxis of migraine conducted according to International Headache Society guidelines, homeopathic treatment had no clear advantages over placebo. It is possible that

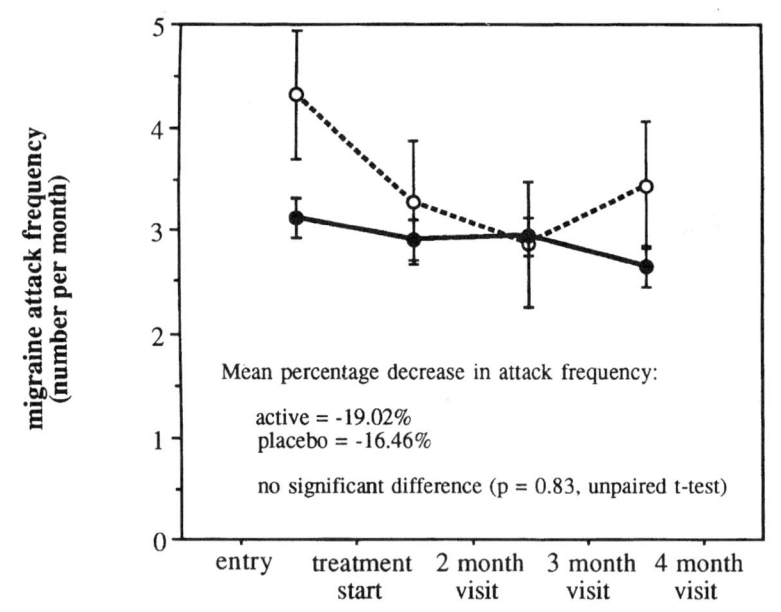

FIGURE 1.—Change in mean attack frequency per month during the trial by treatment group. *Bars* indicate standard deviations. The groups were not ideally matched at entry. There was improvement in each group which was not marked in either but appeared to be following a different course: early on placebo, delayed on verum. As follow-up ended, there were signs that the effect of placebo, but not of homeopathy, was undergoing reversal. *Solid circles* indicate active therapy; *open circles* indicate placebo. (Reprinted from Double-blind randomized placebo-controlled study of homeopathic prophylaxis of migraine by Whitmarsh TE, Coleston-Shields DM, Steiner TJ from *Cephalalgia* 17:600–604, 1997, by permission of Scandinavian University Press.)

a different dosage regimen and longer duration of treatment might have confirmed a benefit for homeopathic treatment of migraine.

▶ The growing interest in this country in "alternative" or "complementary" medicine has not been matched by a growing research base testing the efficacy and effectiveness of the interventions. This article reports on a well-designed, randomized, controlled trial of homeopathic treatment for migraine, showing no overall effect (see Fig 1).

Note that there were actually 11 separate homeopathic treatments administered among the 63 patients. In the conventional research paradigm, this would be a fatal flaw, because too few patients were studied in each subgroup. The authors argue persuasively, though, that at this early stage of research into alternative therapies, it is appropriate to combine the groups, in effect studying the efficacy of homeopathy as a whole rather than individual homeopathic interventions.

A "price" is paid for this strategy, however, in the limited conclusions that one can draw. The study shows that there was no overall benefit, but one cannot conclude that all 11 treatments are ineffective. It is possible that 1 or more of the therapies is effective in some as-yet-unstudied part of the population. One last observation: The opening paragraph casually comments that homeopathic inpatient and outpatient facilities are part of the British National Health Service! Is this what we have to look forward to in the United States?

A.O. Berg, M.D., M.P.H.

Efficacy and Safety of Acetaminophen, Aspirin, and Caffeine in Alleviating Migraine Headache Pain: Three Double-blind, Randomized, Placebo-controlled Trials
Lipton RB, Stewart WF, Ryan RE Jr, et al (Albert Einstein College of Medicine, Bronx, NY; The Johns Hopkins School of Public Health, Baltimore, Md; St Louis Univ, Mo et al)
Arch Neurol 55:210–217, 1998

Background.—Migraine affects an estimated 23 million Americans, producing a wide spectrum of pain and disability. More than 90% of those experiencing migraine treat their headaches with nonprescription medications, although only prescription medications are approved for this indication in the United States. A combination of acetaminophen, aspirin, and caffeine is approved for treating migraine headaches in other countries. If effective, this drug combination could provide cost savings and safety advantages over the currently approved prescription medications. This report describes the results of 3 independent studies evaluating the efficacy of the nonprescription drug combination of acetaminophen, aspirin, and caffeine for the relief of migraine headache pain.

Methods.—The 3 studies were conducted between August 1995 and June 1996 using a uniform double-blind, randomized, parallel-group, placebo-controlled design. The studies differed only in methods of patient recruitment. Two of the studies were multicenter. Two of the studies relied on both conventional and random-digit dialing methods for panel recruitment. All participants met International Headache Society diagnostic criteria for migraine, were at least 18 years of age, were in good general health, and had had migraines at least every 2 months but not more than 6 times monthly. Headaches were at least moderately intense but were not incapacitating. Patients were trained to complete a study diary. Then they were randomly assigned to either a single dose of combined acetaminophen, aspirin, and caffeine or placebo to treat the pain of 1 acute self-recognized migraine. The primary effectiveness assessments were pain intensity difference from baseline and percentage of patients with reduced pain after 2 hours. Patients rated pain, disability, nausea, vomiting, photophobia, and phonophobia at baseline and at 0.5, 1, 2, 3, 4, and 6 hours after medication.

Results.—Of the 1,357 patients included in these 3 studies, 1,250 took their medication. The efficacy-evaluable patient group differed from the intention-to-treat patient group by 27 patients. There were significantly greater reductions in migraine pain intensity from 1 through 6 hours after medication in the treatment group vs. the placebo group in all 3 studies.

Pain intensity was minimal after 2 hours in 59% of the 602 treated patients vs. 33% of the 618 in the placebo group. Pain intensity was minimal after 6 hours in 79% of the treated vs. 52% of the placebo subjects. Other migraine symptoms were also significantly improved in the treatment group compared to the placebo group.

Conclusion.—The results of these 3 large clinical trials show that the nonprescription combination of acetaminophen, aspirin, and caffeine is effective for treating the pain, disability, and associated symptoms of migraine headache. There were no serious adverse effects of the medication. This nonprescription combination appears to be a safe and cost-effective treatment alternative for patients with migraine headaches.

▶ Lest there be any ambiguity, the over-the-counter combination tested here was identical to Excedrin Extra Strength, which contains 250 mg each of aspirin and acetaminophen and 65 mg of caffeine. The study was paid for by the manufacturer, Bristol-Myers Squibb Co. The 3 studies reported here shared excellent study design, and the results are impressive.

The standard way of reporting results should have been the intention-to-treat (ITT) analysis, but the authors chose to report the "efficacy evaluable" (EE) group, i.e., those who actually took the medication. They state that the ITT results were the same and that the numbers lost in the EE group were small; still it would have been better to report the results using the ITT approach because it would have blunted criticism of the findings.

In this country, the debate in treating patients with migraine focuses on prescription drugs, even though a minority of patients with migraines uses them. In other countries, specific formulations like this one are the norm. Physicians will eventually want to see studies in which over-the-counter drugs are pitted directly against prescription drugs, so that advice for patients who seek care can be informed by comparative efficacy information. Although this study is imperfect, I think it appropriately moves the debate toward careful evaluation of treatment options with nonprescription drugs that leave therapeutic decisions in the hands of patients themselves.

A.O. Berg, M.D., M.P.H.

13 Eye, Ear, Nose, and Throat Conditions

Overview

Randomized controlled trials: Abstracts 13-3 and 13-4
- Glaucoma and quality of life
- Radiology of the sinuses in normal men
- Homeopathic treatment of vertigo
- Oral pseudoephedrine vs. topical oxymetazoline for air travel–associated barotrauma
- Sport nasal strips and airflow

Quality of Life Among Patients With Glaucoma in Sweden
Wändell PE, Lundström M, Brorsson B, et al (Karolinksa Inst, Stockholm; Hosp of Blekinge, Karlskrona, Sweden; Swedish Council on Technology Assessment in Health Care, Stockholm)
Acta Ophthalmol Scand 75:584–588, 1997   13–1

Background.—Ocular disease can have a major effect on health-related quality of life (HRQOL). In patients with glaucoma, different factors may influence HRQOL. The impact of glaucoma severity, treatment, and co-existing diseases on HRQOL was investigated.

Methods.—Two hundred seventy patients from 2 ophthalmology departments in different parts of Sweden were included in the cross-sectional survey study. The Swedish HRQOL Survey, a generic HRQOL instrument adapted from the Medical Outcomes Study, was administered.

Findings.—Compared with a random standard population sample, the patients with glaucoma had a lower mean score on the pain scale only. The patients' mean score on the sexual functioning scale was higher than that of the population sample. A lower HRQOL-scales score was significantly associated with reduced visual acuity and visual field as well as comorbid cardiovascular and nonvascular systemic diseases. β-Blockers with or without miotic agents did not adversely affect HRQOL.

Conclusions.—In general, patients with glaucoma have a good HRQOL, especially when their vision is intact. Topical β-blockers do not adversely affect HRQOL.

▶ This is a good example of the newer breed of studies that attempt to determine how disease states and their treatments affect overall quality of life. As this type of research proliferates, I expect to see some surprises. Every now and then we are likely to find high levels of quality of life in patients whom we would expect to be miserable and low levels of quality of life in patients whom we would expect to be perfectly happy. The findings in this study strike me as more in the former category showing that patients with a chronic disease are doing quite well, contradicting the usual presumption of "dis-ease" in chronic conditions. I expect that we will see more of this kind of work, reminding us to pay attention to how patients say they are doing and functioning, rather than relying only on objectively measured intermediate and physiologic outcomes.

A.O. Berg, M.D., M.P.H.

Radiological Findings in the Maxillary Sinuses of Symptomless Young Men
Savolainen S, Eskelin M, Jousimies-Somer H, et al (Natl Public Health Inst, Helsinki; Kuopio Univ, Finland)
Acta Otolaryngol (Stockh) 529:153–157, 1997   13–2

Background.—Acute maxillary sinusitis (AMS) is a not infrequent complication of the common cold. As AMS can be difficult to diagnose, radiographs are often used to detect abnormalities of the sinus. To interpret these findings correctly, physicians need knowledge of the findings in healthy research subjects as a prerequisite. To provide baseline radiologic data for the maxillary sinuses, investigators analyzed radiographic findings in a large group of symptomless young men.

Study Design.—The study group consisted of 404 conscripts, aged 17–29 years, who were admitted to the Ear, Nose and Throat Department of the Central Military Hospital because of severe acoustic trauma between 1985 and 1989. All participants underwent ear, nose, and throat examinations. None of the study participants had symptoms suggestive of respiratory tract infections. Maxillary sinuses were examined radiologically by occipitomental projection (Waters' projection). Samples from the posterior nasal cavities were collected in 100 participants for bacteriologic culture. Between 1986 and 1989, 265 participants underwent examination for allergies.

Findings.—Abnormalities were detected in 13.3% of the sinuses from 404 symptomless study participants. The most common abnormalities detected were mucosal thickening of greater than 6 mm in 12.3%, cysts or polyps in 7.2%, and completely opacified sinuses in 3.3%. Normal radiographic findings were more common in the summer, and mucosal thickening was more common in the winter. Findings of normal flora or of pathogenic bacteria were equally common in those with normal and abnormal radiographs, except that mucosal cysts were more commonly associated with pathogens. Sinus lavage revealed fluid retention indicative of subclinical sinusitis in 1% to 2% of the participants. Allergies were not associated with mucosal abnormalities in this study group.

Conclusions.—Radiographic abnormalities classified as pathologic were detected in the maxillary sinuses of more than 20% of symptomless young men, although sinus lavage detected subclinical sinusitis in only 1% to 2%. Allergies were not associated with pathologic sinus changes.

▶ The diagnosis of chronic sinusitis is difficult. Most primary care physicians rely heavily on a history of sinusitis and the symptoms seen in the patient. If standard therapies don't seem to be working, it is common to seek radiologic imaging of the sinuses and possible referral to an ear, nose, and throat specialist.

This was an interesting study of young men who had radiologic examinations of the sinus area because of complaints not related to sinusitis. The authors found that 20% of these young men had significant abnormalities in the sinuses by x-ray examination.

In this community, we have veered away from standard radiographs of the sinus area for diagnosis of chronic sinusitis because of its lack of specificity. More commonly, we use CT views of the sinus area. This certainly delineates the soft tissue better than standard radiographs. However, even with the advances of CT scans, we cannot diagnose chronic sinusitis simply from a film. It has to be a constellation of the history, a physical examination, and the response to therapies. It appears that there are an awful lot of asymptomatic adults with chronic mucosal thickening and mucosal cysts in their sinuses.

R.C. Davidson, M.D., M.P.H.

Homeopathic vs Conventional Treatment of Vertigo: A Randomized Double-blind Controlled Clinical Study
Weiser M, Strösser W, Klein P (Biologische Heilmittel Heel GmbH, Baden-Baden, Germany; Datenservice Eva Höning GmbH, Rohrbach, Germany)
Arch Otolaryngol Head Neck Surg 124:879–885, 1998   13–3

Introduction.—Dizziness has been found as the ninth most common symptom at initial evaluation in the outpatient setting, according to 1 study. Vertigo may be caused by lesions in the CNS or by disturbances of the vestibular nerve and vestibular cochlear system. Nausea, emesis, sweating, collapse, and tinnitus are symptoms of vertigo, as are disturbances of equilibrium, systematic imbalance, or instability. An effective medication is necessary to reduce the frequency, intensity, and duration of vertigo attacks. A homeopathic preparation containing ambra grisea D6, anamirta cocculus D4, conium maculatum D3, and petroleum rectificatum

D8 was compared with betahistine hydrochloride, a standard treatment for vertigo.

Methods.—One hundred nineteen patients with vertigo of various origins participated in the randomized, double-blind, controlled clinical trial. The main outcome measures were frequency, duration and intensity of vertigo attacks.

Results.—A clinically relevant reduction in the mean frequency, duration, and intensity of vertigo attacks was found with both homeopathic and conventional treatments. In both treatment groups, vertigo-specific complaints were significantly and similarly reduced. Clinical relevance was established in the improvement of the quality of life and the reduction of vertigo attacks. The homeopathic remedy and betahistine were statistically established to have therapeutic equivalence.

Conclusion.—The therapeutic equivalence between the homeopathic remedy and betahistine was found to be statistically significant in the main efficacy variable. The frequency, duration, and intensity of vertigo attacks during a 6-week treatment period were reduced by both treatments. In both treatment groups, vertigo-specific complaints were also significantly reduced.

▶ This study of homeopathic treatment comes from the industrialized world's homeopathic center, Germany. Success of the conventional and homeopathic treatments was the same, with adequate statistical power to detect a difference if there had been one. The most important limitation to this study is the lack of a placebo control, especially relevant in this case because these were first episodes of vertigo that might be expected to resolve spontaneously. The findings in Figure 1 of the original article are consistent with either explanation. Still, carefully crafted studies, like this one, of an alternative intervention put the ball back into the court of conventional medicine: Where is the proof that our treatment is any better?

A.O. Berg, M.D., M.P.H.

A Double-blind Comparison Between Oral Pseudoephedrine and Topical Oxymetazoline in the Prevention of Barotrauma During Air Travel
Jones JS, Sheffield W, White LJ, et al (Butterworth Hosp, Grand Rapids, Mich; Akron Gen Med Ctr, Ohio)
Am J Emerg Med 16:262–264, 1998   13–4

Objective.—Recovery from otic barotrauma can take as long as 4 weeks. For prevention of middle ear barotrauma during air travel, some sources recommend prophylactic use of oral or topical nasal decongestants. The efficacy of oral pseudoephedrine vs. topical oxymetazoline for the prophylaxis of aerotitis media during air travel was tested in a randomized, double-blind clinical trial.

Methods.—Either 120 mg of pseudoephedrine, 0.05% oxymetazoline hydrochloride, or a placebo (capsule or nasal spray) was administered 30 minutes before flying to 150 adult volunteers with a history of recurrent ear discomfort during air travel. After arrival at their destination, the volunteers filled out a questionnaire about any otologic symptoms they experienced during the flight. Results were compared between groups.

Results.—There were 124 subjects who completed the study—41 taking pseudoephedrine, 42 taking oxymetazoline, and 41 taking placebo. Symptoms of ear discomfort were significantly more common among placebo users than among pseudoephedrine users (71% vs 34%). Fewer oxymetazoline users (64%) than placebo users (71%) had ear discomfort, but the difference was not significant. Fifteen percent of pseudoephedrine users reported dry mouth and drowsiness. Nasal irritation was reported by 14% of oxymetazoline users.

Conclusion.—Administration of pseudoephedrine 30 minutes before flight time significantly reduces ear discomfort in individuals with recurrent ear pain during air travel.

▶ This is an interesting small study of a common problem. The authors compared oral pseudoephedrine with a nasal decongestant and with placebo. They found a significant reduction in symptoms in patients pretreated with pseudoephedrine, but they found no reduction with a nasal decongestant. The authors recommend treatment with 120 mg of pseudoephedrine at least 30 minutes before flying for patients who have known ear-related symptoms. This sounds like a reasonable option.

R.C. Davidson, M.D., M.P.H.

Do Sports Nasal Strips Improve Nasal Airflow? A Preliminary Report
Fergie N, Bingham BJG (Victoria Infirmary, Glasgow, Scotland)
J Otolaryngol 27:113–114, 1998   13–5

Introduction.—There were 160 million nasal strips sold in the United States in 1995. The nasal strips are attached across the nasal bridge to the upper lateral cartilages by adhesive, and they pull the cartilages apart, dilating the nasal valve area and reducing the airway resistance. As demonstrated in terms of pulmonary function tests, nasal breathing is beneficial, and nasal strips may allow more effective nasal breathing over a wider level of activity. The effect of commercially available external nasal splints on nasal inspiratory flow rates was assessed.

Methods.—Eight healthy volunteers, aged 18–50 years, used a transparent oronasal mask. Their peak inspiratory flow per nasum was measured from functional residual capacity to total lung capacity. They were tested with and without splints at rest, and with and without splints immediately after intense exercise.

Results.—At rest, the participants' peak inspiratory flow increased as a total from 13 (100%) to 15.49 (119%) with the addition of a splint. With exercise, the peak inspiratory flow increased as a total from 13.02 (100%) to 21.61 (166%) with the addition of a splint.

Conclusion.—While wearing the nasal strips, all participants felt a definite subjective improvement in ease of nasal breathing. Peak nasal inspiratory flow is increased with nasal strips, particularly with exercise. It is still unknown whether this increase improves athletic performance.

▶ Being a northern Californian, I enjoy following the San Francisco 49ers. When perennial all-star wide receiver Jerry Rice began using a nasal strip and claiming increased breathing capability, it became an overnight sensation for athletes of all kinds to use these nasal strips. Perhaps he knew what he was talking about. This preliminary study showed an increase of between 13% and 15% peak inspiratory flow at rest with the use of these nasal strips. With exercise, the peak inspiratory flow increased from 13% to 21%. My guess is we will continue to see many athletes using these nasal strips.

R.C. Davidson, M.D., M.P.H.

14 Children's Health

Overview

Randomized controlled trials: Abstracts 14–10 and 14–12

Immunization
- Post-licensure varicella vaccine effectiveness in a day care outbreak
- Varicella serology in children with uncertain history of chickenpox
- Physician reaction to universal varicella vaccination recommendation
- Two articles on vaccine response in premature infants

Infectious Diseases
- Risk of bacteremia in post-*Haemophilus influenza* type b era
- Amoxicillin/clavulanate and chronic adenotonsillar hypertrophy
- Acute otitis media and bronchiolitis
- *H. pylori* and abdominal symptoms in preschoolers
- Albuterol in bronchiolitis
- A diagnostic marker for early onset neonatal infection
- Early feeding in gastroenteritis
- Perinatal transmission of human papillomavirus in infants

Sudden Infant Death Syndrome
- Effect on SIDS of abandoning prone sleeping
- Counseling parents to reduce risk
- Caffeine during pregnancy and SIDS risk
- Weather temperature and SIDS risk

Injury
- Predictors of injury mortality
- Injuries due to trampolines

Preparticipation Examinations
- Preparticipation cardiovascular screening
- Mayo Clinic experience with preparticipation screening
- Screening for hypertrophic cardiomyopathy

Miscellaneous

- Preschool screening using the sentence repetition test
- Variation in bone age in healthy children
- Renal function following ibuprofen use
- Hepatotoxicity associated with acetaminophen
- Clinical and radiologic findings in adenoidal obstruction
- Evaluating gynecomastia in adolescent boys
- Effects of a condom availability program in high school
- Hyperactive boys grown up

Immunization

Postlicensure Effectiveness of Varicella Vaccine During an Outbreak in a Child Care Center

Izurieta HS, Strebel PM, Blake PA (Georgia Dept of Human Resources, Atlanta)
JAMA 278:1495–1499, 1997

Objective.—Varicella virus vaccine must be stored at −15°C and given within 30 minutes of reconstitution. Under field conditions, vaccine effectiveness can be compromised. The epidemiologic factors of a 1996 outbreak of varicella among children in a child care center, severity and impact of disease among vaccinated and unvaccinated children, effectiveness of varicella vaccine, and risk factors for vaccine failure were investigated in a retrospective cohort study.

Methods.—Children enrolled in the day care center and not having varicella before January 1, 1996 were eligible for the study. Parents filled out a self-administered questionnaire on disease status, severity and impact of disease, and risk factors for varicella and for vaccine failure. Pediatricians and teachers were interviewed. Vaccine effectiveness was based on the attack rate in vaccinated vs. attack rate in unvaccinated children.

Results.—In the 15-week outbreak, 81 of 148 children got varicella. Nine of 66 vaccinated children and 72 of 82 unvaccinated children got varicella. Attack rates by age group were similar among vaccinated and unvaccinated children. The median duration of disease was 4.5 days in vaccinated children and 7.0 days in unvaccinated children. The 9 vaccinated children had mild cases. Unvaccinated children had significantly more severe disease with 19 mild cases, 43 moderate cases, and 10 severe cases. Vaccine effectiveness was 86% against all forms of varicella and 100% against moderate and severe disease. Vaccinated children with asthma or other respiratory diseases were 7.1 times more likely to have varicella than were vaccinated children without respiratory diseases.

Conclusion.—Varicella vaccine was 86% effective in preventing all forms of varicella and 100% effective in preventing moderate and severe forms of the disease. Other respiratory diseases, such as asthma, are a risk factor for varicella.

▶ This study reports reassuring data proving the real-world use-effectiveness of varicella vaccine. There are 2 clues that the study was conducted in quite an unusual day care center: they had a 100% response rate to their questionnaire, and 92% of the parents had at least a college degree. Although the usual footnotes about a selected population in an unusual setting apply, it is hard for me to imagine credible arguments that similar results wouldn't be obtainable in more typical settings. What was tested here was the effectiveness of vaccine administered by typical physicians, not characteristics of the setting in which the exposure occurred, so I am comfortable with the authors' conclusions. Despite the relative fragility of varicella vaccine, use by nonpublic health physicians produces excellent results.

A.O. Berg, M.D., M.P.H.

Varicella Serology Among School Age Children With a Negative or Uncertain History of Chickenpox
Lieu TA, Black SB, Takahashi H, et al (Kaiser Permanente, Oakland, Calif; Permanente Med Group, Berkeley, Calif; Univ of California, San Francisco)
Pediatr Infect Dis J 17:120–125, 1998   14–2

Introduction.—Now that varicella vaccination is available, physicians have the clinical dilemma of whether to vaccinate presumptively children aged 7 to 12 years whose history is uncertain or to recommend varicella serology. Although young adults with a negative or uncertain history of chickenpox usually have positive serology, the varicella prevalence among children 7 to 12 is not known.

Methods.—A cross-sectional study of children whose clinicians had ordered varicella serotesting sought to describe the seroprevalence among 7- to 12-year-olds with a negative or uncertain history of chickenpox, to determine parental preferences for serotesting vs. presumptive vaccination and to examine the cost effectiveness of these 2 options. The HMO guidelines specified that varicella serology be obtained when history was uncertain. Parents were interviewed about their preferences after the serotest was performed but before results were known.

Results.—Seroprevalence was low (9%) among 7-year-olds whose parents said they had definitely not had chickenpox but quite high (68%) among 11-year-olds whose parents were unsure of their status. Almost half (48%) of the children whose parents expressed uncertainty about their chickenpox history proved seropositive. Most children whose parents thought they probably or definitely had chickenpox were seropositive (74% and 89%, respectively). Exposure to a household member with known chickenpox was associated with a 65% seropositive rate. Most (73%) parents whose children experienced serotesting said they would prefer this method to presumptive vaccination. Varicella serology was the cost-effective option for children aged 9 to 12 with uncertain histories of chickenpox. The HMO had a relatively low cost of serotesting.

Conclusion.—Varicella serotesting of children with negative or uncertain histories of chickenpox yields a wide variety of results, depending on age and clinical history. Among 7- to 12-year olds, seropositivity increases with age. Parents often favor serotesting over presumptive vaccination, a cost-effective method when low-cost serotesting is available. In some settings, however, the vaccine costs far less than serotesting.

▶ Acceptance of the varicella vaccine is growing. Deciding whether to have older children vaccinated is a dilemma for parents as well as their providers. Since it is often difficult to know for certain if a child has had chickenpox (though I can assure you the Dexter children have had it!), serotesting is often performed. This is one clinical decision that is usefully informed by considering cost implications. This study helps illuminate this issue while not allowing conclusive recommendations. Find out what serotesting costs are at your lab (at this writing, $56 in ours) and what vaccination costs are ($51 in ours) to inform your office policies.

W.W. Dexter, M.D.

Reactions of Pediatricians to the Recommendation for Universal Varicella Vaccination
Newman RD, Taylor JA (Univ of Washington, Seattle)
Arch Pediatr Adolesc Med 152:792–796, 1998   14–3

Introduction.—Live attenuated varicella vaccine was licensed for use in children 12 months of age and older by the Food and Drug Administration. The recommendation of its use for this population has been endorsed by the American Academy of Pediatrics and the Centers for Disease Control and Prevention. This vaccine has been shown to be theoretically cost-effective, saving more than $5 for each dollar spent on immunization, and it reduces the morbidity and mortality associated with varicella infection. Nevertheless, the medical community has not unanimously endorsed routine immunization against varicella. A survey of pediatricians was conducted to determine the rate of adherence to the varicella immunization recommendation, to understand sources of concern, and to evaluate factors that might influence adherence.

Methods.—A survey was sent to 574 pediatricians in the state of Washington, and the response rate was 76%. They were asked about demographic characteristics, attitudes about varicella vaccine, and previous experiences with the disease that were associated with self-reported adherence to universal varicella immunization recommendations.

Results.—Of those who completed the survey, 42% reported following a policy of universal varicella immunization. The recommendation was associated with pediatrician attitudes of agreement regarding the effectiveness of varicella vaccine in reducing rare but serious complications of the disease and in decreasing parental time lost from work. Those who universally recommended the vaccine disagreed with statements concerning the lack of the need for varicella immunization because complications are rare, that it is not required for school entry, or that it is not medically cost-effective. Adherence to the recommendations was also associated with experience with varicella encephalitis. Those who were less likely to report recommending universal vaccination were pediatricians who were concerned that varicella vaccine might not provide lifelong immunity.

Conclusion.—Universal varicella vaccination was recommended by fewer than 50% of the responding pediatricians. Personal experiences, perceptions about the potential seriousness of varicella, and beliefs about the societal and medical cost-effectiveness of varicella vaccine appear to influence adherence to the recommendation.

▶ Do you routinely recommend the varicella vaccine to your patients? Do you at least offer or discuss it? Well, it seems that our pediatric colleagues are reluctant to embrace this, too. The two most prominent concerns I have heard voiced are (1) that chickenpox is a benign, self-limited illness (not necessarily true) and (2) that immunity may wane, leaving young adults, in whom varicella can be a severe illness, susceptible (we could, of course, revaccinate). Clearly, there needs to be more education done on this for both patients and physicians. What are *your* barriers to using this vaccine?

W.W. Dexter, M.D.

Three-Year Follow-up of Vaccine Response in Extremely Preterm Infants
Khalak R, Pichichero ME, D'Angio CT (Strong Children's Research Ctr, Rochester, NY; Univ of Rochester, NY)
Pediatrics 101:597–603, 1998
14–4

Introduction.—With certain exceptions, the American Academy of Pediatrics recommends that premature infants be immunized at their chronological age after birth, rather than gestational age. Some studies, however, suggest that protective levels achieved in extremely preterm infants are lower after the primary immunization series than those in full-term infants and premature infants of older gestational age. Sixteen former extremely premature and 17 former full-term infants were compared for antibody titer measurements at 3–4 years of age.

Methods.—The former extremely premature infants were delivered at less than 29 weeks' gestation and weighed less than 1,000 g at birth. Both groups of infants had received the primary series and first booster vaccines for diphtheria, pertussis, tetanus, polio, and *Haemophilus influenzae* type b. Twelve preterm and 14 full-term children also completed the hepatitis B vaccine series. The primary outcome variable studied was the geometric mean titer (GMT) of antibody to each antigen.

Results.—Findings of serum analysis at 3–4 years of age showed that former preterm and full-term children had similar GMT values of antibodies to tetanus, diphtheria, and pertussis. The mean GMT value of *Haemophilus* polyribosylribitol phosphate (PRP) was lower in preterm

(0.99 µg/mL) than in full-term children (3.06 µg/mL). Fewer preterm children (50%) than full-term children (88%) had PRP antibody levels of greater than 1.0 µg/mL; anti-PRP titers of greater than 0.15 µg/mL were found in 100% of preterm and 88% of full-term children. The 2 groups had similar GMT values of neutralizing antibodies to polio serotypes 1 and 2, with nearly all children achieving greater than protective levels. Fewer preterm children, however, had protective titer values of polio serotype 3 (75% vs. 100% for full-term children). Similar percentages of preterm and full-term children (75% and 71%) vaccinated against hepatitis were protected.

Conclusions.—For most immunizing antigens, extremely preterm children immunized at chronological age demonstrated antibody responses similar to those for full-term children. Normal immunologic responses persisted at 3–4 years of age. Responses of the preterm children were less robust to polio serotype 3 and *Haemophilus* PRP.

▶ We are all seeing more and more preterm and extremely preterm infants. Are we all following the immunization recommendations made by the American Academy of Pediatrics? This study provides excellent evidence to reinforce our current practice of immunization based on chronological age after preterm birth, or to persuade us to begin to follow these guidelines.

W.W. Dexter, M.D.

Immune Responses of Prematurely Born Infants to Hepatitis B Vaccination: Results Through Three Years of Age

Kesler K, Nasenbeny J, Wainwright R, et al (Providence Alaska Med Ctr, Anchorage)
Pediatr Infect Dis J 17:116–119, 1998

Introduction.—Hepatitis B vaccination of the newborn is a cost-effective practice that may have a greater impact on childhood health than other commonly administered vaccinations. A study of premature infants was designed to determine the long-term immunogenicity in premature infants.

Methods.—Alaskan native infants were chosen for the study because of their high incidence of hepatitis B virus infection. The 69 infants included had all been delivered at less than 37 weeks. Immunizations were given just before discharge, 1 month later, and 6 months after the first. Venous blood samples obtained 1 to 3 months after (early titer) and 2.5 to 3 years after (late titer) the third immunizations were tested for antibody to hepatitis B surface antigen. A comparison group consisted of 108 infants born at full term.

Results.—Paired serum samples were available for 37 of the preterm infants. Compared with term infants, those born before term had lower early and late blood sample antibody to hepatitis B surface antigen titers. The differences between early titer preterm and term (23.1 vs. 56.8 mIU/

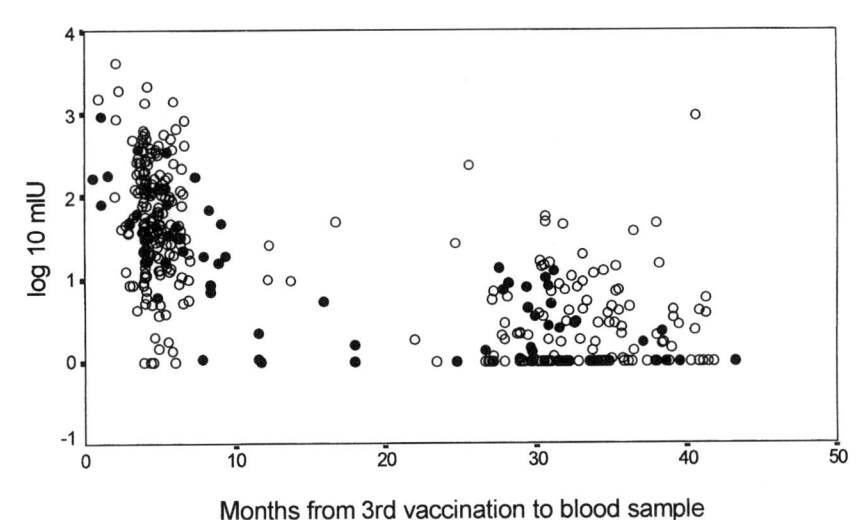

![Figure 1 scatter plot: log 10 mIU vs Months from 3rd vaccination to blood sample]

Months from 3rd vaccination to blood sample

FIGURE 1.—Logarithm 10 of anti-HBs by interval from third dose of hepatitis B vaccine to date of blood sample (undetectable levels are reported as zero). ●, preterm infants; ○, term infants. (Courtesy of Kesler K, Nasenbeny J, Wainwright R, et al: Immune responses of prematurely born infants to hepatitis B vaccination: Results through three years of age. *Pediatr Infect Dis J* 17:116–119, 1998.)

mL) and late titer preterm and term (0.7 vs. 1.32 mIU/mL) were not statistically significant, however. Both groups had a significant drop in titer over time (Fig 1) and a significant decrease in the percent of infants with titers equal to or greater than 10 mIU/mL. A decreased antibody titer was associated with prematurity and with a longer interval between the third vaccination and the blood sample. No infant showed evidence of hepatitis B infection.

Conclusion.—Although preterm and term infants who have received hepatitis B vaccination show a similar decline in antibody titers in the 3 years, the decline is generally greater in preterm infants. There appeared to be no association between birth weight and antibody titer among the premature infants.

▶ Here's a heads up, folks. Vaccination of the newborn for hepatitis B, including preterm infants, is, hopefully, now standard in your practice. These data, while a little sketchy, indicate that the standard 3-shot series may not be sufficient for infants, particularly infants born prematurely. No guidance on who or when to test, or when or if to give boosters yet. So, stay tuned.

W.W. Dexter, M.D.

Infectious Diseases

Risk of Bacteremia for Febrile Young Children in the Post-*Haemophilus influenzae* Type b Era

Lee GM, Harper MB (Children's Hosp, Boston)
Arch Pediatr Adolesc Med 152:624–628, 1998

Introduction.—It is difficult to distinguish children with bacteremia from those with self-limiting viral illnesses. A child with occult bacteremia is clinically similar to the well-appearing febrile child. The risk of bacteremia was assessed in a prospective cohort of well-appearing febrile children aged 3 to 36 months after introduction of the *Haemophilus influenzae* type b conjugate vaccine. The predictive ability of objective criteria in identifying children with occult pneumococcal bacteremia from those at risk were assessed.

Methods.—All children seen from 1993 to 1996 aged 3 to 36 months with a temperature of 39.0°C or higher with no identified source of infection (except otitis media) were considered at risk. Databases and medical records were reviewed for data regarding demographics, chief complaint, temperature at initial evaluation, disposition, diagnoses, white blood cell count, differential, blood culture results, recent antibiotic therapy, and immunizations within the previous 48 hours.

Results.—Of 199,868 patient visits to the emergency department, 11,911 (6%) children were determined to be at risk for occult bacteremia. Blood cultures were collected from 79% of this cohort. There were 149 (1.57%) blood cultures with pathogenic organisms. The best predictors for occult pneumococcal bacteremia were white blood cell count and absolute neutrophil count. A white blood cell count cutoff value of 15 cells × 10^9/L (sensitivity, 86%; specificity, 77%; and positive predictive value, 5.1%) would result in the treatment of about 19 children with no bacteremia for each child with bacteremia.

Conclusion.—There was a 1.6% prevalence of occult bacteremia in children aged 3 to 36 months with temperatures of 39.0°C or higher with no obvious source of infection. A complete blood cell count and blood culture are useful in the clinical evaluation of nontoxic-appearing children aged 3 to 36 months with temperatures of 39.0°C or higher without an identifiable source of infection.

▶ This is an interesting look at bacteremia in young children. It is not surprising that there is less bacteremia overall, probably because of widespread use of the *Haemophilus influenzae* type b vaccine. Though retrospective, the sheer size of this study lends weight to the discussion regarding use of the white blood cell count (WBC) in evaluating febrile infants. The take-home for the office is that bacteremia, though uncommon, is still a problematic but important diagnosis to make, and a WBC with absolute neutrophil count remains a most useful tool in our decision-to-treat analysis in febrile children.

W.W. Dexter, M.D.

Treatment of Symptomatic Chronic Adenotonsillar Hypertrophy With Amoxicillin/Clavulanate Potassium: Short- and Long-term Results
Sclafani AP, Ginsburg J, Shah MK, et al (New York Eye & Ear Infirmary; New York Med College, Valhalla)
Pediatrics 101:675–681, 1998   14–7

Introduction.—Many children with recurrent tonsillitis (RT) and obstructive adenotonsillar hypertrophy undergo adenotonsillectomy, one of the most commonly performed surgical procedures in children. An effective nonsurgical treatment would be of value, particularly for children who are poor surgical candidates. The short- and long-term effects of treatment of symptomatic chronic adenotonsillar hypertrophy (CATH) with amoxicillin/clavulanate potassium (AMOX/CLAV) were prospectively studied.

Methods.—A review of the charts of 100 pediatric patients who underwent adenoid and/or tonsillar procedures during a 2-month period revealed that adenotonsillectomy was the most frequently performed procedure. The most common single indication for surgery was CATH (36%), and more than half of the patients who underwent surgery had evidence of symptomatic adenotonsillar hypertrophy. In the randomized, double-blind study, 86 patients entered the AMOX/CLAV arm and 81 the placebo arm. The average age of the patients was 6.5 years; 88 were boys and 79 were girls. All had obstructive symptoms attributable to CATH, but no history of recurrent adenotonsillitis. Children in the active treatment group received AMOX/CLAV, 40 mg/kg/day in 3 divided doses for 30 days. At 30-day evaluation children were referred for surgery if necessary. Those not referred were scheduled for reevaluations at 3 and 24 months post-treatment.

Results.—Compared with placebo, treatment with AMOX/CLAV significantly reduced the need for surgery in the short-term (37.5% vs. 62.7%). The reduced need for surgery persisted in the AMOX/CLAV group at both 3 months (54.5% vs. 85.7% in the placebo group) and 24 months (83.3% vs. 98.0% in the placebo group). Diarrhea and rash caused cessation of treatment in 6 patients and 3 patients, respectively, and the difference in complications between AMOX/CLAV and placebo groups was not statistically significant.

Conclusions.—Treatment with AMOX/CLAV can reduce the need for adenotonsillectomies in children with CATH. Because approximately 500,000 adenotonsillar surgeries are performed each year in the United States, even a modest long-term reduction in symptoms requiring surgery could have a significant impact. Costs savings from 15,000 surgeries not being performed are estimated at between $37.5 million to $45 million.

▶ The use (misuse) of antibiotics in upper respiratory tract infection has received much publicity in the past several years, including articles reviewed in these pages. In this tightly controlled study, the authors present a convincing argument for the longer-term use of antibiotics in CATH. While rates for tonsillectomy have dropped dramatically over the past 3 decades (I lost mine at age 6—ether anesthesia to boot!), it is, as noted, a common procedure. The potential downside of long-term antibiotics notwithstanding, it seems to me that the very real potential for avoiding surgery makes this treatment protocol worth a try before referring our patients for tonsillectomy.

W.W. Dexter, M.D.

Acute Otitis Media in Children With Bronchiolitis
Andrade MA, Hoberman A, Glustein J, et al (Univ of Pittsburgh, Pa; Children's Hosp of Pittsburgh, Pa)
Pediatrics 101:617–619, 1998   14–8

Introduction.—Acute otitis media (AOM) is reported to occur in approximately two thirds of children with respiratory syncytial virus (RSV) infection, and is also frequently encountered in children with bronchiolitis. The prevalence and etiology of AOM in children with bronchiolitis were examined prospectively to determine whether AOM in such patients is caused entirely or mainly by RSV. Were this the case, routine antimicrobial treatment would not be appropriate.

Methods.—Children eligible for the study were aged 2–24 months and had received a diagnosis of bronchiolitis. Those determined to have AOM at entry had nasal washings obtained for RSV enzyme-linked immunosorbent assay (ELISA). Middle-ear aspirates collected at tympanocentesis were examined by Gram-stained smear, bacterial culture, and reverse transcriptase–polymerase chain reaction (PCR) to detect the presence of

TABLE 2.—Bacterial Pathogens Isolated From 33 Middle-ear Aspirates (25 Patients)

Organisms	No. (%)
Streptococcus pneumoniae	13 (39)
Haemophilus influenzae	8 (24)
Moraxella catarrhalis	6 (18)
Streptococcus pneumoniae + *Moraxella catarrhalis*	2 (6)
Staphylococcus aureus	2 (6)
No growth	2 (6)
Total	33 (100)

(Courtesy of Andrade MA, Hoberman A, Glustein J, et al: Acute otitis media in children with bronchiolitis. *Pediatrics* 101:617–619. Copyright 1998 by the American Academy of Pediatrics. Reproduced by permission of *Pediatrics*.)

RSV. Children without AOM were reevaluated at 48–72 hours, 8–10 days, and 18–22 days.

Results.—Forty-two children with a mean age of 6.75 months were studied. Mean duration of rhinorrhea was 4.0 days. Evidence of AOM was present in 21 children (50%) at study entry and developed in 5 during the first 10 days after entry. At final follow-up, 26 patients (62%) had AOM (unilateral in 18 and bilateral in 8), and 10 additional patients had otitis media with effusion (OME); only 6 patients maintained a normal middle-ear status throughout the study period. Tympanocentesis, performed in 25 children (33 ears), yielded at least 1 bacterial pathogen from each patient (Table 2). Seventeen of 24 patients with AOM had RSV identified by ELISA in nasal washings and/or by PCR in middle-ear aspirates.

Conclusions.—No previous report has described the prevalence or etiology of AOM in infants and young children with bronchiolitis. Most of the patients in this series either had AOM at entry or showed evidence of AOM soon after entry. The usual middle-ear bacterial pathogens were identified in all patients with AOM who underwent tympanocentesis. Thus RSV is rarely the sole cause of AOM in infants and children with bronchiolitis, and antibiotic treatment may be indicated.

▶ Acute otitis media is often seen in the youngsters who are seen in our offices and emergency departments with bronchiolitis. Hats off to Andrade and colleagues for investigating whether this is caused by bacterial pathogens. These data certainly support my (usual) decision to treat with antibiotics. However, whether these patients actually benefit from antibiotics remains unanswered. Respiratory syncytial virus was isolated from a large percentage of the middle-ear aspirates. It may be that once the RSV clears, antibiotics would not be needed. For now, until someone studies efficacy and outcome of antibiotics for AOM in the face of RSV, I will continue to treat this entity with antibiotics.

W.W. Dexter, M.D.

Helicobacter pylori **and Abdominal Symptoms: A Population-based Study Among Preschool Children in Southern Germany**
Bode G, Rothenbacher D, Brenner H, et al (Univ of Ulm, Germany)
Pediatrics 101:634–637, 1998   14–9

Introduction.—There appears to be a clear correlation between *Helicobacter pylori* bacterial load and the severity of inflammation in adults and children with gastritis and peptic ulcer disease. It has been difficult, however, to establish a causal relationship between *H. pylori* gastritis and abdominal symptoms. The relation of *H. pylori* infection with gastrointestinal symptoms in children was examined in a cross-sectional study.

Methods.—The study group was drawn from a group of preschool children living in Ulm, Germany. Infection status was determined by means of the ^{13}C-urea breath test, performed during a screening evaluation

TABLE 3.—Frequency of Symptoms in Children With (+) and in Children Without (−) *H. pylori* Infection

Symptom	H. pylori Status	Never	Rarely	Sometimes	Often	P Value*
Abdominal pain	+	57.6	19.5	17.8	5.1	
	−	39.7	30.5	23.4	6.5	.311
	Overall	42.1	29.0	22.6	6.3	
Vomiting	+	78.6	14.5	4.3	2.6	
	−	62.8	29.0	7.4	0.8	.066
	Overall	64.9	27.0	7.0	1.0	
Diarrhea	+	77.6	14.7	6.9	0.9	
	−	50.8	33.2	14.7	1.2	.015
	Overall	54.4	30.7	13.7	1.2	

*Pooled P value of Mantel-Haenszel χ^2 for association of infection status with abdominal symptoms (adjusted for nationality).
(Courtesy of Bode G, Rothenbacher D, Brenner H, et al: *Helicobacter pylori* and abdominal symptoms: A population-based study among preschool children in southern Germany. *Pediatrics* 101:634–637. Copyright 1998, by the American Academy of Pediatrics. Reproduced by permission of *Pediatrics*.)

for school fitness. Parents completed a questionnaire on the children's medical history and history of abdominal symptoms. Of the 1,201 children eligible for the voluntary study, 945 participated.

Results.—After children with recent antibiotic treatment were excluded, the final study sample consisted of 863 children. Gender distribution was equal in the sample, and most children were 6 years of age. The abdominal symptoms score was significantly higher in children of German nationality (40.1%) than in those of Turkish (21.1%) or other nationalities (26.1%). Overall, 118 children (13.7%) were infected with *H. pylori*. The prevalence of infection was 6.1% in children of German nationality, 44.8% in the Turkish children, and 27.6% in children of other nationalities. Presence of the infection showed no positive relation to specific gastrointestinal symptoms, and fewer symptoms were found in the infected children than in the uninfected children (Table 3).

Conclusions.—Because most children with *H. pylori* infection are asymptomatic, the presence of abdominal symptoms provides no evidence of the infection. There was no association between specific gastrointestinal symptoms and *H. pylori* in children.

▶ The idea that *H. pylori* plays a central role in gastritis and peptic ulcer disease has been relatively quickly accepted into our medical dogma. There have been hundreds of studies demonstrating this relationship and investigating treatment regimens. Not so fast! This large population-based study sheds some doubt on the relationship between *H. pylori* and gastrointestinal symptoms, at least in children. Admittedly, the findings pertain only to several specific symptoms, not disease. However, these findings certainly are intriguing. It raises several questions: Is *H. pylori* the causative agent in gastritis and peptic ulcer disease (at least in kids)? Does colonization or infection in childhood lead to adult disease? If so, should we be treating children? Is there a role for screening youngsters? Studies like this raise questions about our closely held beliefs—which hopefully makes us question the rationale for our practices. A useful exercise.

W.W. Dexter, M.D.

The Use of Albuterol in Hospitalized Infants With Bronchiolitis
Dobson JV, Stephens-Groff SM, McMahon SR, et al (Maricopa Med Ctr, Phoenix, Ariz)
Pediatrics 101:361–368, 1998   14–10

Introduction.—Characterized by fever, rhinitis, tachypnea, expiratory wheezing, or increased respiratory effort, bronchiolitis is an acute inflammatory respiratory illness of children that occurs in the first 2 years of life. Peak incidence occurs in the winter to spring months. Several viral agents have been identified as the cause, including respiratory syncytial virus, parainfluenza virus, adenovirus, influenza virus, and rhinovirus. The care of hospitalized infants with bronchiolitis costs about $300 million each year. For more than 20 years, the use of nebulized albuterol and other β-adrenergic agents in the treatment of bronchiolitis has been debated. A study of hospitalized infants with moderate bronchiolitis was undertaken to determine whether the use of albuterol by nebulization enhances physiologic or clinical recovery.

Methods.—Fifty-two patients younger than 24 months of age had moderately severe, acute viral bronchiolitis. The minimum clinical appearance of the children included mild irritability when touched, with occasional crying but ability to be consoled; moderate retractions, including obvious intercostal, supraclavicular, or subcostal retractions with moderate distress; and moderate wheezing or diffuse expiratory wheezes with scattered early inspiratory wheezes (Table 1). The patients received either nebulized albuterol or normal saline placebo for 72 hours. Survival analysis and improvement in oxygen saturation during hospitalization were the primary outcome measures. Measurements of improvement in oxygen saturation, accessory muscle use, and wheezing were taken to assess the time required to reach pre-established discharge criteria. Actual length of hospital stay was also recorded. A comparison of adverse outcomes between the 2 groups was conducted.

Results.—Mean improvement in oxygen saturation at baseline, at 24 hours, or during hospitalization did not differ between the albuterol and placebo groups. Significant improvement in oxygen saturation over time was demonstrated in both groups, but there was no significant difference in improvement between the 2 groups. As defined by improvement in oxygen saturation, accessory muscle use, or wheezing, there was no difference in time to reach discharge criteria between the 2 groups. Length of hospital stay and the frequency of adverse outcomes also did not differ between the 2 groups.

TABLE 1.—Clinical Score*

General appearance	0	Asleep
	1	Calm, content, happy, and/or interactive
	2	Mildly irritable when touched, occasional crying, but able to be consoled
	3	Moderately irritable, difficult to console, less interactive
	4	Extremely irritable, cannot be comforted, crying throughout examination, or not interactive
Accessory muscle use	0	No retraction
	1	Mild retractions (mild intercostal supra, and/or subcostal retractions, but minimal distress)
	2	Moderate retractions (obvious intercostal, supraclavicular, and/or subcostal retractions with moderate distress)
	3	Severe retractions (severe intercostal supraclavicular and subcostal retractions with marked distress)
Wheezing	0	No wheezing or crackles
	1	Wheezing (scattered, end-expiratory wheezes or crackles only)
	2	Moderate wheezing (diffuse expiratory wheezes ± scattered early inspiratory wheezes)
	3	Severe wheezing (diffuse inspiratory and expiratory wheezing

*Adapted from Schuh et al.
(Courtesy of Dobson JV, Stephen-Grogg SM, McMahon SR, et al: The use of albuterol in hospitalized infants with bronchiolitis. *Pediatrics* 101:361-368. Copyright 1998, by the American Academy of Pediatrics. Reproduced by permission of *Pediatrics*.)

Conclusion.—In infants with acute, moderate bronchiolitis, nebulized albuterol therapy does not appear to enhance recovery or attenuate severity of illness, as evidenced by improvement in oxygen saturation, length of hospital stay, or time to meet standardized discharge criteria.

▶ Do you currently routinely use nebulized albuterol in treating your patients hospitalized with moderately severe (clinical score greater than 2, see Table 1) bronchiolitis? If so, this study should challenge you to think about how you manage your patients with bronchiolitis, if not to change your practice. This study is well constructed, with unequivocal results, and it merits your attention.

W.W. Dexter, M.D.

Neutrophil CD11b Expression as a Diagnostic Marker for Early-onset Neonatal Infection

Weirich E, Rabin RL, Maldonado Y, et al (Natl Inst of Allergy and Infectious Disease, Bethesda, Md; Stanford Univ, Calif)
J Pediatr 132:445–451, 1998   14–11

Introduction.—At a cost of more than $800 million, 300,000 newborns are treated for infections every year. There are 17 infants treated for nonspecific signs for each infant who has a confirmed infection. A series of risk factors are being sought to dictate clinical decisions aimed at prevention or anticipatory treatment of neonatal infection. Within 5 minutes of exposure to bacterial products such as endotoxin in vitro, there is an increase of CD11b, a member of the β-integrin family of adhesion proteins. It may be an early postsurgical predictor of sepsis in adults. Neonatal neutrophils stimulated with lipopolysaccharide increase surface expression of CD11b proportionately to that of adults, to an unregulated level in infected neonates. This can be detected by flow cytometry. Whether neutrophil surface expression of CD11b predicts early-onset infection or suspected infection in at-risk infants was assessed.

TABLE 2.—Data Summary

Outcome Group	Total in Each Group	No. Cultured	No. Positive by Culture	Neutrophil CD11b >60	Peak Serum CRP >1
Infection confirmed°	7			7	5
Bacterial	5	106	5	5	5
Viral	2	11	2	2	0
Infection suspected	17			16	15
No infection	82			0	2
Total	106			25	22

(Courtesy of Weirich E, Rabin RL, Maldonado Y, et al: Neutrophil CD11b expression as a diagnostic marker for early-onset neonatal infection. *J Pediatr* 132:445–451, 1998.)

Methods.—Flow cytometry of whole blood samples was used to determine CD11b expression on peripheral blood neutrophils. There were 106 at-risk infants admitted to the neonatal intensive care unit, and blood was obtained and stained with antibodies detecting CD11b and CD15. Simultaneous recordings of blood for culture, blood counts, and C-reactive protein (CRP) determination were also made.

Results.—There were 7 infants with positive bacterial or viral cultures, known as a confirmed infection (Table 2). Seventeen infants had clinical signs of infection, but negative cultures, known as suspected infection. No clinical signs and negative cultures were found in 82 infants, known as no infection. In infants with confirmed infection, neutrophil CD11b was elevated. In those with suspected infection, it was elevated in 94% of infants, and in those with no infection, there was no elevation. For diagnosis of neonatal infection at initial evaluation, the negative predictive value was 100%, the positive predictive value was 99%, the sensitivity was 96% and the specificity was 100%. Peak CRP levels correlated with CD11b levels. At the time of admission, CD11b was elevated in all 5 infants with proven bacterial infection, whereas CRP was normal in 3 of these 5 until the second day in the neonatal intensive care unit. Elevated CD11b was found in both infants with positive viral cultures, but the CRP levels remained within normal limits. There was a 99% negative predictive value of neutrophil CD11b for identifying suspected or confirmed infection.

Conclusion.—For exclusion of early-onset neonatal infection, this assay for neutrophil CD11b is a promising test. In the population of neonates at risk for early-onset infection, this assay may reduce hospital and antibiotic use, if validated prospectively.

▶ Severe neonatal infection, although uncommon, can be devastating and difficult to clinically ascertain. For years in my institution, we have relied on the CRP and CBC as markers of early-onset neonatal infection. However, as the authors note, these can be misleading, both in identifying and excluding infection. Relying on these tests, then, can lead to both undertreatment or overtreatment—far more commonly the latter. Although the neutrophil CD11b assay remains somewhat unproven, it seems quite promising. Share this information with your neonatology colleagues and stay tuned. We may soon have a better tool to detect early-onset neonatal infection.

W.W. Dexter, M.D.

A Multicentre Study on Behalf of the European Society of Paediatric Gastroenterology and Nutrition Working Group on Acute Diarrhoea: Early Feeding in Childhood Gastroenteritis

Sandhu BK, Isolauri E, Walker-Smith JA, et al (Royal Hosp for Sick Children, Bristol, England; Univ of Tampere, Finland; Royal Free Hosp, London; et al)
J Pediatr Gastroenterol Nutr 24:522–527, 1997   14–12

Background.—In children with gastroenteritis, dehydration needs to be corrected and hydration maintained using an optimal oral rehydration solution (ORS). Nutritional repair is also a goal in the management of such children. Several studies published in the past 15 years have shown that "regrading" need not be done slowly, and that after initial oral rehydration therapy (ORT), full age-appropriate feeding is well tolerated in children older than 6 months, with no adverse effects. However, 2 risk factors—age and diarrheal severity—merit caution. The effects of ORS and early or late feeding on the duration and severity of diarrhea, weight gain, and complications in weaned infants were investigated in a multicenter European study.

Methods.—Two hundred thirty children with gastroenteritis were enrolled in the study. By random assignment, 134 patients received early feeding (group A) and 96, late feeding (group B). The most common pathogen in both groups was rotavirus.

Findings.—The average amount of ORS taken in the first 4 hours was comparable in the 2 groups. Number of watery stools and the occurrence of vomiting did not differ between groups in this rehydration phase. Four to 24 hours after rehydration, group A had a significantly higher mean weight gain than group B (Fig 1). Group B consumed more ORS than

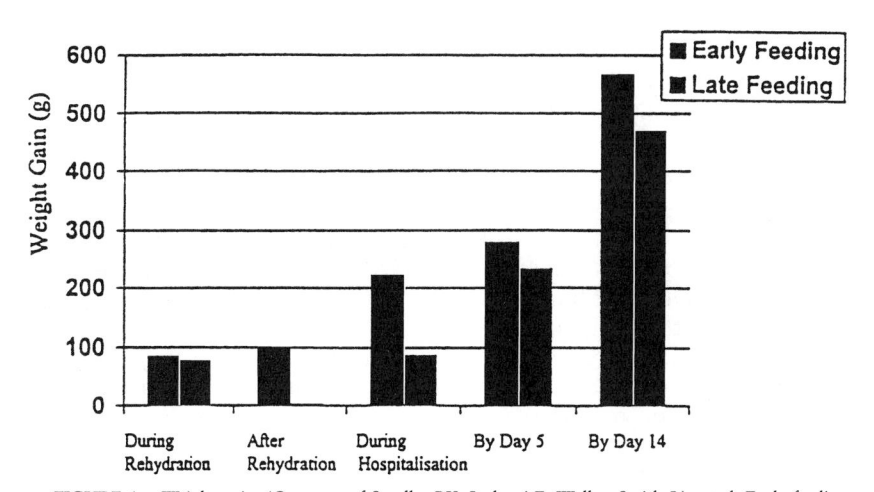

FIGURE 1.—Weight gain. (Courtesy of Sandhu BK, Isolauri E, Walker-Smith JA, et al: Early feeding in childhood gastroenteritis: A multicentre study on behalf of the European Society of Paediatric Gastroenterology and Nutrition Working Group on Acute Diarrhoea. *J Pediatr Gastroenterol Nutr* 24:522–527, 1997.)

group A, but the total amount of fluid intake was comparable. The 2 groups did not differ significantly in plasma sodium, potassium, or bicarbonate levels. Net weight gain during hospitalization was significantly greater in group A. By days 5 and 14, weight gain was similar in the 2 groups. Four children in each group needed IV fluids by day 4, none of whom had significant lactose intolerance.

Conclusions.—Continuation of feeding during gastroenteritis is beneficial. For mildly to moderately dehydrated children, optimal management consists of oral rehydration with ORS in the first 4 hours, followed by resumption of normal feeding. Breast-feeding should be resumed. Supplementing the usual feeds with ORS, 10 mL/kg per liquid stool, as necessary, will prevent further dehydration.

▶ This multicenter trial really confirms a direction in which we have all been, I hope, moving. The description of withholding feedings of youngsters with gastroenteritis as "enforced starvation" captures the negative impact of this practice. The evidence that oral rehydration is effective treatment for the dehydration that follows the vomiting and diarrhea associated with gastroenteritis is unequivocal.[1] The evidence for early resumption of normal feedings is accumulating. The results of this randomized trial lends support to this practice. Rehydrate them and then let them eat, and stop "enforced starvation" for gastroenteritis.

W.W. Dexter, M.D.

Reference

1. 1996 Year Book of Family Practice, p 212.

Perinatal Transmission of Human Papillomavirus in Infants: Relationship Between Infection Rate and Mode of Delivery
Tseng C-J, Liang C-C, Soong Y-K, et al (Chang Gung Med College, Taipei, Taiwan)
Obstet Gynecol 91:92–96, 1998   14–13

Introduction.—While it is well established that human papillomavirus (HPV) is transmitted sexually, it can also be transmitted perinatally. The presumed source of neonatal infection and anogenital disease is through the infected birth canal, but the relationship between the mode of delivery and perinated HPV transmission is still unknown. The transmission rate of HPV in newborn infants born to HPV-positive mothers was determined, as well as the relationship between perinatal HPV transmission and mode of delivery (cesarean vs. vaginal).

Methods.—There were 160 pregnant women selected who had vaginal delivery and 141 who had cesarean delivery. The presence of HPV types 16 and 18 DNA sequences, using the polymerase chain reaction, was assessed in the buccal and genital swabs of neonates born to HPV-positive mothers.

Results.—Among the pregnant women, the overall frequency of HPV 16/18 infection was 22.6%. There was a 39.7% overall frequency of HPV transmission from HPV 16/18–positive mothers to newborns at birth. When infants were delivered vaginally, there was a significantly higher rate of HPV 16/18 infection than when infants were delivered by cesarean (51.4% vaginal vs. 27.3% cesarean). No significant difference in the incidence of perinatal HPV infection between HPV types 16 and 18 was present in either the vaginal delivery group or the cesarean delivery group. Between the buccal and genital sites, there were no significant differences. There were no differences between male and female infants overall.

Conclusions.—After vaginal delivery, neonates are at higher risk for exposure to HPV than after cesarean delivery. An important determinant for perinatal HPV transmission may be viral load, but it does not appear to influence the persistence of infection. A longitudinal investigation of newborn infants with HPV infection should be conducted to determine the persistence of the transmission and any clinical importance it may have.

▶ We have lived through the changing recommendations regarding maternal herpes simplex and the decision to perform a prophylactic cesarean section to prevent neonatal infection. As HPV becomes better recognized—especially types 16 and 18 that are associated with cervical cancer—the issue of perinatal transmission is bound to develop. This study from Taiwan, with reasonable sample sizes, documents perinatal transmission of HPV types 16 and 18 in substantial numbers. Although cesarean delivery was protective, the rate of perinatal transmission was 27% even with surgery. The clinical importance of perinatal transmission of HPV is unknown. No recognized neonatal infection exists except for the development of warts. Early infection with HPV may confer protective immunity, or it may simply heighten risk by giving a longer period of chronic infection. Look for this issue to evolve as we gain a better understanding of this and other chronic viral infections.

J.E. Scherger, M.D., M.P.H.

Sudden Infant Death Syndrome

Abandoning Prone Sleeping: Effect on the Risk of Sudden Infant Death Syndrome
Skadberg BT, Morild I, Markestad T (Univ Hosp of Bergen, Norway)
J Pediatr 132:340–343, 1998

Objective.—Whereas it is known that the prone sleeping position is a risk factor for sudden infant death syndrome (SIDS), the effect on the SIDS rate of totally abandoning the prone sleeping position is unknown. The long-term effects of an intervention campaign to avoid prone sleeping on the SIDS mortality rate and on parents' choice of sleeping position for young infants were evaluated in a Norwegian population-based case-reference study.

Methods.—After implementation in 1990 of an intervention program to avoid prone sleeping, the number of SIDS deaths (sudden and unexpected death between 1 week and 1 year after birth) during 1993 through 1995 was recorded. Five hundred families with infants aged 2–6 months were randomly selected as the reference group.

Results.—During the study period, there were 6 unexplained, sudden deaths for a SIDS rate of 0.3 per 1,000 live births. One infant usually slept in the prone position, 3 were placed in the prone position in their last sleep, and 1 was found dead in the prone position. One infant died when the carriage tilted and it was stuck between the bottom and the wall. Five infants had shown signs of fever or upper respiratory distress. Five of 6 mothers of SIDS infants smoked during pregnancy and after delivery vs. 29% of mothers in the reference group. Mothers of SIDS infants had significantly less education than mothers in the reference group. Excluding the 2 apparently accidental deaths, the SIDS rate was 0.2 per 1,000 live births. In the reference group, only 7 (1.4%) infants usually slept prone, 49.1% slept supine, 24.7% slept on the side and supine, and 0.6% slept supine and prone. Significantly more rural than urban infants slept prone. Significantly more infants put to sleep on their side changed position during sleep. At least once during the last week before the questionnaire was filled out, 59.4% of infants had been found with their heads covered.

Conclusions.—The intervention program to avoid the prone sleeping position decreases the rate of SIDS. The side-sleeping position is the least stable. About half the infants slip under the covers when sleeping.

▶ This large population-based study from Norway provides dramatic evidence that prone sleeping position is a major factor in SIDS. A decline from 3.5 SIDS deaths per 1,000 live births to 0.3 per 1,000 is most impressive, largely because of a campaign directed at abandoning prone sleeping for infants. These numbers are comparable to the decline in Reye's syndrome that has occurred worldwide as a result of the abandonment of giving aspirin to children. Other factors such as maternal smoking remain important in the causation of SIDS, but this evidence is so compelling that every health care provider to infants should discuss sleeping positions with the parents.

J.E. Scherger, M.D., M.P.H.

SIDS: Counseling Parents to Reduce the Risk
Carroll JL, Siska ES (Johns Hopkins Children's Ctr, Baltimore, Md; SIDS Network—Pennsylvania Connection, York)
Am Fam Physician 57:1566–1572, 1998   14–15

Background.—The incidence of sudden infant death syndrome (SIDS) has been declining in the United States, a change brought about by public education on risk factors for the syndrome. When no physiologic abnormalities were able to be identified in infants whose deaths were attributed to SIDS, researchers examined external factors, such as sleeping position

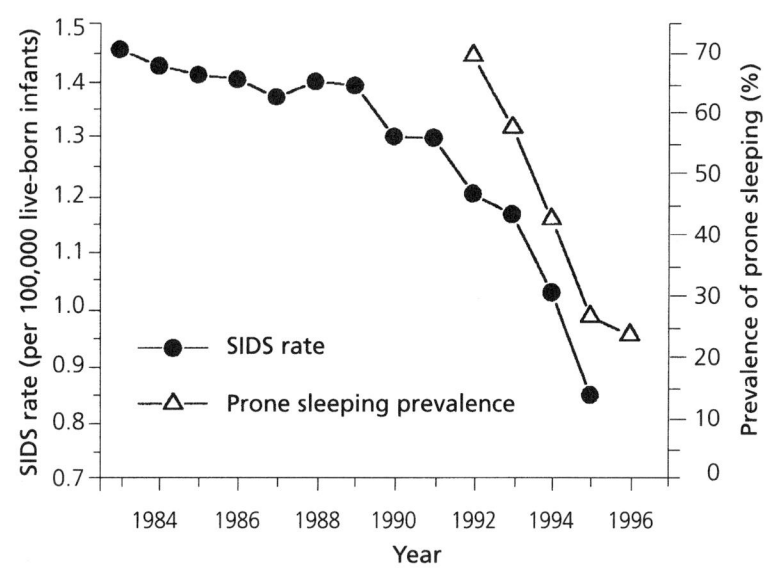

FIGURE 1.—Sudden infant death syndrome rate vs. prone sleeping rate in the United States, 1983 to 1995 (1995 data are preliminary). *Abbreviation: SIDS,* sudden infant death syndrome. (Courtesy of Carroll JL, Siska ES: SIDS: Counseling parents to reduce the risk. *Am Fam Physician* 57:1566–1572, 1998. Published by the American Academy of Family Physicians.)

and exposure to cigarette smoke. Public education about risk factors led to a striking decline in SIDS rates.

Risk-Reduction Measures.—Available scientific research supports having healthy babies sleep in the supine position, not exposing babies to cigarette smoking during pregnancy and after birth, and avoiding potentially hazardous bedding materials. Breast feeding rather than bottle feeding may also offer protection. Reports from many countries suggest that changing babies from the stomach to the back for sleeping results in a substantial decline in the SIDS rate (Fig 1).

Smoking cessation counseling is an important part of prenatal care, both for the expectant mother and the father. Soft bedding material and soft crib toys should be avoided because they may increase the risk of carbon dioxide rebreathing. Infants should not be swaddled in bed or tucked in tightly. Home monitoring devices are recommended for infants considered to be at high risk for sudden death because of medical conditions and for the siblings of SIDS victims. The physician should pay special attention to parents who have already lost a child to SIDS.

Discussion.—Family physicians can further reduce the incidence of SIDS, the major cause of death in infants under the age of 1 year, by educating parents about the risk factors for the syndrome: prone sleeping position, exposure to cigarette smoke, and a potentially hazardous sleeping environment.

▶ The worldwide decline in SIDS is a great success story and testimony to the power of public education. Although there is still more research to be done regarding underlying causes and prevention programs, family physicians may counsel their new parents with some confidence regarding the avoidance of SIDS. Avoiding a prone sleeping position is the most important part of health education, followed by the avoidance of cigarette smoke exposure and sleeping environments consisting of soft bedding material. Despite these measures, some SIDS deaths will occur, and family physicians play a critical role in providing counseling and support to these families.

J.E. Scherger, M.D., M.P.H.

Heavy Caffeine Intake in Pregnancy and Sudden Infant Death Syndrome
Ford RPK, and the New Zealand Cot Death Study Group (Community Child and Family Service, Christchurch, New Zealand; Univ of Auckland, New Zealand; Univ of Otago, New Zealand)
Arch Dis Child 78:9–13, 1998   14–16

Objective.—Because caffeine crosses the placental barrier leading to low birth weight and spontaneous abortion in some studies, it is theorized that maternal caffeine consumption may increase the risk of SIDS. In a nationwide case-control study, parents of SIDS infants were surveyed to evaluate the effect of maternal caffeine use on the incidence of SIDS.

Methods.—The New Zealand Cot Death Study, conducted between 1987 and 1990, surveyed parents of 393 SIDS infants and 1,592 controls regarding maternal caffeine consumption in the first and third trimesters. Heavy caffeine consumption was defined as 400 mg/day or greater (4 cups/day or greater).

Results.—More mothers of SIDS infants than control infants, in both the first and third trimester, were heavy caffeine drinkers (30% vs. 18%, and 31% vs. 18%, respectively). Compared with non–heavy caffeine users, heavy caffeine users had a significantly higher risk of having a SIDS infant (odds ratio, 1.65).

Conclusions.—Heavy caffeine use (400 mg/day or greater) during the first and third trimesters significantly increases the risk of SIDS. Caffeine use is a modifiable behavior, and reducing caffeine intake during pregnancy can reduce the incidence of SIDS.

▶ Moderate caffeine consumption (equivalent of 3 or fewer cups of coffee per day) has been found to be of no risk in pregnancy. This study from New Zealand, where the SIDS incidence has been higher than most countries, suggests that heavier caffeine consumption is associated with an increased risk of SIDS (odds ratio 1.65). While this risk is very small compared with maternal smoking, it lends some evidence to the recommendation that most things should be used in moderation, especially during pregnancy.

J.E. Scherger, M.D., M.P.H.

Weather Temperatures and Sudden Infant Death Syndrome: A Regional Study Over 22 Years in New Zealand
Schluter PJ, Ford RPK, Brown J, et al (Healthlink South, Christchurch, New Zealand; New Zealand Meteorological Service)
J Epidemiol Community Health 52:27–33, 1998   14–17

Objective.—Because SIDS occurs more frequently in the winter, there is speculation that local climate and weather patterns may affect the incidence of SIDS. The possible relationship between weather and SIDS was examined retrospectively in an epidemiologic study in Canterbury, New Zealand.

Methods.—The 786 SIDS deaths occurring between 1968 and 1989 were investigated for season effects, temperature changes during the day, rate of change of temperature during the day the preceding 8 days, the rate of change of temperatures between successive days preceding and including the designated day, and the susceptibility of infants aged 12–52 weeks vs. younger infants. The Kolmogorov-Smirnov test was used to make specific pair-wise comparisons between temperature distributions.

Results.—There were 545 of 8,036 days when 1 or more SIDS deaths occurred. There were more SIDS deaths in months with colder minimum temperatures and on winter days with relatively stable temperatures. Variation between day effects had little or no effect on the SIDS incidence. Infants 12 weeks or older were more likely than younger infants to die of SIDS on days with small hourly temperature changes.

Conclusion.—There is a strong seasonal and temperature effect on the SIDS rate. After a cold period, the risk of SIDS was increased when temperatures warmed, and there was little hourly variation in temperature.

▶ Watch out for those warmer days that happen right after a cold spell. New Zealand has had the highest incidence of SIDS in the world, possibly associated with prone sleeping on soft surfaces such as comforters or sheepskins. This study covers 22 years, where most of these risk factors have been abandoned and the incidence of SIDS has declined. However, the information here on weather is interesting, but its clinical significance is uncertain.

J.E. Scherger, M.D., M.P.H.

Injury

Predictors of Injury Mortality in Early Childhood
Scholer SJ, Mitchel EF Jr, Ray WA (Vanderbilt Univ, Nashville, Tenn)
Pediatrics 100:342–347, 1997   14–18

Objective.—Injuries are the leading cause of death in children aged 1 to 4 years. Although certain maternal sociodemographic characteristics have been linked to fatal childhood injuries, whether these factors are independent or associated is not known. The association between maternal/infant

*Risk score:
Maternal education	Points
≥ 16 years	0
13-15 years	1
12 years	2
< 12 years	3
Maternal age	
> 30 years	0
26-30 years	1
20-25 years	2
< 20 years	3
# of other children	
None	0
One	1
Two	2
≥ Three	3

Injury Mortality Rate (per 100 000 child years)

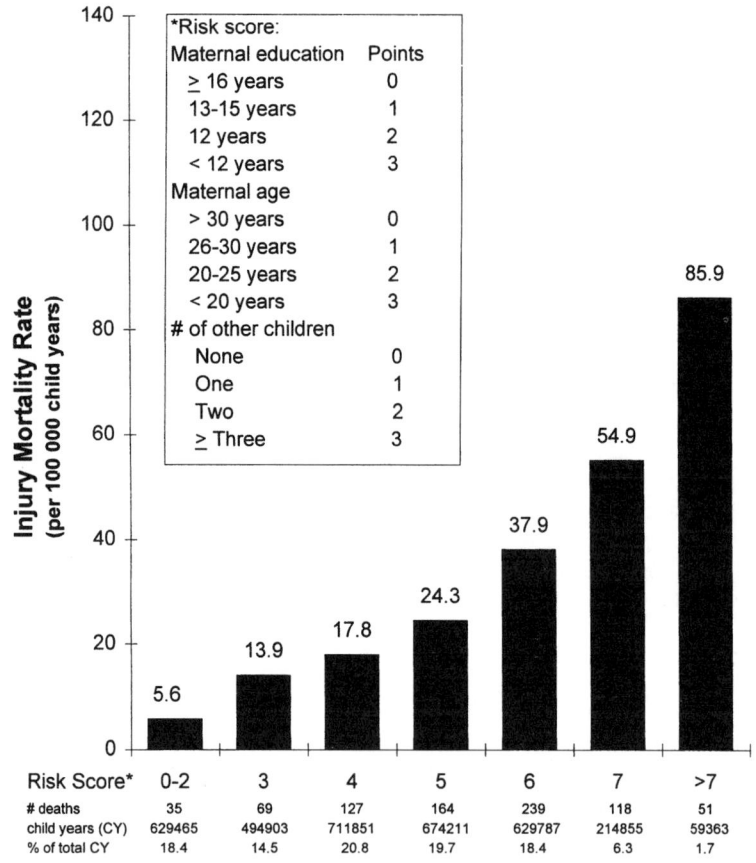

Risk Score*	0-2	3	4	5	6	7	>7
rate	5.6	13.9	17.8	24.3	37.9	54.9	85.9
# deaths	35	69	127	164	239	118	51
child years (CY)	629465	494903	711851	674211	629787	214855	59363
% of total CY	18.4	14.5	20.8	19.7	18.4	6.3	1.7

FIGURE 1.—Children's Injury Risk Score, ages 0 through 4 years. The effect of maternal factors (education, age, and number of other children) on injury mortality rate for children 0 through 4 years of age. *Risk score calculation based on maternal education (16 years or more, 0 points; 13–15 years, 1 point; 12 years, 2 points; less than 12 years, 3 points), age (more than 30 years, 0 points,; 26–30 years, 1 point; 20–25 years, 2 points; less than 20 years, 3 points), and number of other children (none, 0 points; one, 1 point; two, 2 points; three or more, 3 points). Numbers above bars represent the injury mortality rate (per 100,000 child years) for children with the corresponding risk score. (Courtesy of Scholer SJ, Mitchel EF Jr, Ray WA: Predictors of injury mortality in early childhood. *Pediatrics* 100:342–347, 1997. Reproduced with permission from *Pediatrics*.)

characteristics and mortality from injury for a large population of children 0 through 4 years of age was investigated to identify maternal/infant characteristics that are independent risk factors for mortality, to study risk factors for these children, and to determine whether maternal/infant characteristics can predict high-risk populations.

Methods.—Birth certificates were obtained for all children aged 0 to 4 years between Jan. 1, 1985, and Dec. 31, 1994, in the state of Tennessee. Maternal age, race, education, neighborhood income, parity, use of prenatal care, residence, infant's sex, and gestational age were recorded. Death certificates were obtained for all children who died during the study period.

Results.—Of 1,035,504 children, 803 died of injuries. This rate of 23.5 per 100,000 child years compares well with the estimated U.S. rate of 25 per 100,000. According to multivariate analysis, maternal education, number of other children, and maternal age were associated with a 50% or more increased risk of death (Fig 1). Race and income were not significantly associated with increased risk of death from injury. Children of unmarried mothers or children who were born prematurely had relative risks of death from injury of 1.78 and 1.50, respectively. The 3 characteristics identified as increasing the risk of death from injury were used to stratify children into 7 risk categories. Children in the high-risk category had an injury mortality rate more than 15 times higher than children in the low-risk category. The number of potentially preventable deaths, assuming that the mortality rate for all children could be reduced to the lowest rate, was calculated to be 614 (76.3%).

Conclusion.—Maternal education, age, and parity were associated with increased risk of death from injury in children aged 0 to 4 years. Most of these deaths can be prevented.

▶ Before reviewing this study, if I had been presented with a K-type question about the relationship of injury mortality in young children to age, parity, and education, I am not sure I would have answered "all of the above." There clearly are holes in this study. The authors did not look at many other variables that almost certainly have some effect on this. Nevertheless, with any other process that leads a "cause of death" list, we devote significant time and energy to attempting to modify risk factors (for example, heart disease and seat belt laws). These issues are, or should be, included in our health screening examinations. The association between age, parity, and maternal education and mortality is quite strong. This is compelling evidence to include these items in your risk assessment and anticipatory guidance teaching. It is compelling enough that I hope this evidence is also included in our policy debates about the allocation of health, education, and welfare dollars.

W.W. Dexter, M.D.

Injuries to Children in the United States Related to Trampolines, 1990–1995: A National Epidemic
Smith GA (Ohio State Univ, Columbus)
Pediatrics 101:406–412, 1998

Introduction.—Trampoline-related injuries have been reported since the 1950s, but relatively few studies have focused on these injuries among children. The epidemiology of trampoline-related injuries among children 18 years and younger was described using data collected from the United States Consumer Product Safety Commission (CPSC).

Methods.—Population projections from the Bureau of the Census for January 1993, the midpoint of the 6-year study period, were used to calculate trampoline-related injury rates per 100,000 U.S. children 18 years and younger. Type of injury was grouped according to categories of the National Electronic Injury Surveillance System of the CPSC.

Results.—During the 6-year study period, an estimated 249,400 trampoline-related injuries were treated in children 18 years and younger at hospital emergency departments in the United States. The number of injuries in this age group increased by 98% from 1990 (29,600) to 1995 (58,400). Boys and girls were equally represented, and the median age of injured children was 10 years (Fig 2). Increases from 1990 to 1995 were greatest (127%) among those aged 13–18 years. Injuries to the extremities predominated in all age groups and accounted for more than 70% of all injuries. Lower extremity injuries predominated in the older (13–18 years) age group, whereas upper extremity injuries were more common in chil-

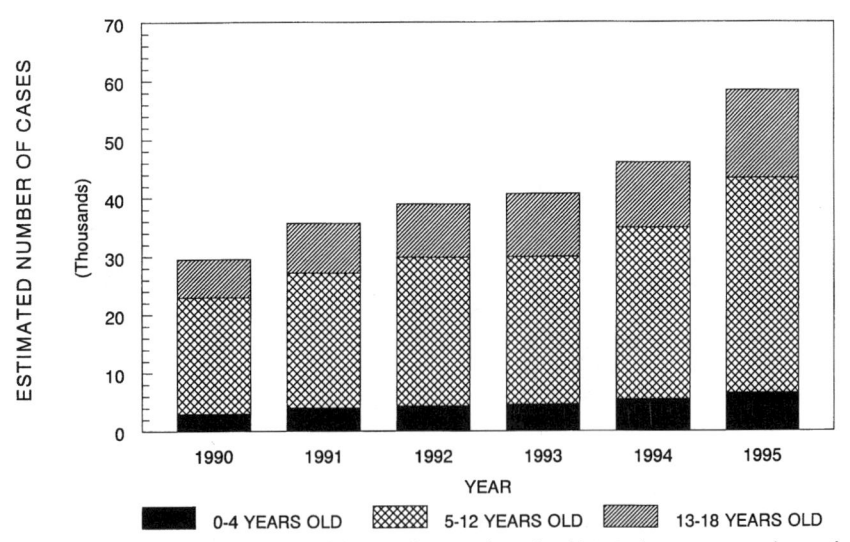

FIGURE 2.—Estimated number of children with trampoline-related injuries by age group and year of injury. (Courtesy of Smith GA: Injuries to children in the United States related to trampolines, 1990–1995: A national epidemic. *Pediatrics* 101:406–412. Copyright 1998 by the American Academy of Pediatrics. Reproduced with permission from *Pediatrics*.)

FRACTURE OR DISLOCATION 83.4%

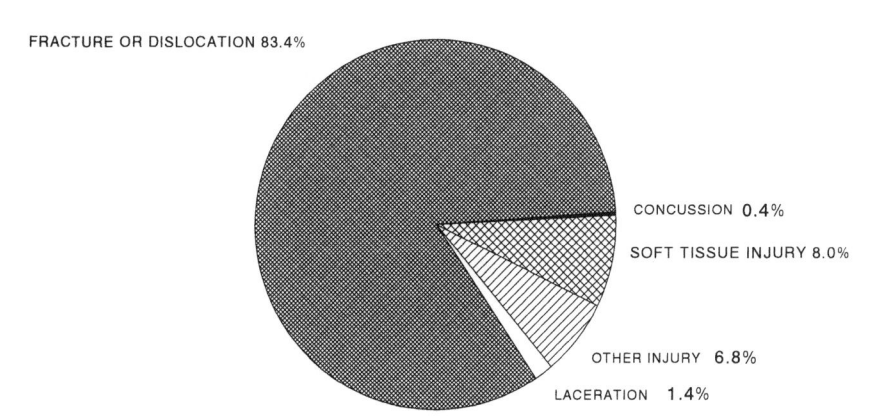

CONCUSSION 0.4%

SOFT TISSUE INJURY 8.0%

OTHER INJURY 6.8%

LACERATION 1.4%

FIGURE 5.—Percent of children with trampoline-related injuries admitted to the hospital or transferred to another hospital by type of injury. (Courtesy of Smith GA: Injuries to children in the United States related to trampolines, 1990–1995: A national epidemic. *Pediatrics* 101:406–412. Copyright 1998 by the American Academy of Pediatrics. Reproduced with permission from *Pediatrics*.)

dren younger than 5 years. There was a significant association between upper extremity injury and fractures or dislocations, so that younger children had a high rate of fractures and dislocations. The most common injuries among children admitted to hospital or transferred to another hospital were fractures or dislocations (Fig 5).

Conclusions.—The popularity of trampolines has been growing, despite a 1977 recommendation by the American Academy of Pediatrics (AAP) that trampolines be banned as part of physical education programs in schools. In a 1981 statement, the AAP cautioned that trampolines should never be used in the home setting. Some injuries have caused paralysis or were fatal.

▶ During the past few years, trampolines have reappeared—and have done so in nearly half of my own neighborhood backyards! The data presented in this study, pulled from the National Electronic Injury Surveillance System, (NEISS) are alarming. The prohibitive number of injuries in trampolining is why this school sport was discontinued many years ago. The NEISS data, while relatively sensitive, does miss injuries that are not seen in the emergency department. Thus it may, in fact, underreport injuries sustained in trampolining. Keep in mind, though, that there is a real problem with data such as NEISS in describing injury patterns. True injury risk cannot be ascertained because there is no denominator. Clearly, there has been a huge increase in the number of trampoline-related injuries in the past few years. However, the number of participants or exposures may, in fact, be so great (compared with the number of injuries) that the risk of injury may be comparatively small—especially when compared with various contact collision sports such as high school football. That said, I don't buy it. This is a dangerous activity (83% of injuries are fractures and dislocations!). Even a fraction of this number of injuries has caused towns and cities to pull out playground equipment, and schools to discontinue organized and supervised sports. Should we ban the recreational sales of trampolines? Possibly. A few liability suits will, I suspect, get that ball rolling. In the meantime, prevent, prevent, prevent: urge your friends, neighbors, and patients to exercise extreme caution. At the least, any use should be very well supervised.

W.W. Dexter, M.D.

Preparticipation Examinations

Profile of Preparticipation Cardiovascular Screening for High School Athletes

Glover DW, Maron BJ (St. Luke's Hosp, Kansas City, Mo; Minneapolis Heart Inst Found, Minn)
JAMA 279:1817–1819, 1998
14–20

Objective.—Interest in preparticipation screening for competitive high school athletes is increasing because of reports of sudden death in young athletes as a result of unsuspected cardiovascular disease. Preparticipation screening procedures available to high school athletes were assessed for adequacy.

Methods.—Guidelines, requirements, and screening measures of high school athletic associations from 50 states and the District of Columbia were reviewed and compared with the 1996 American Heart Association (AHA) consensus panel guidelines on screening.

Results.—Whereas all jurisdictions except Rhode Island require an examination prior to athletic participation, 8 states do not have recommended history and physical questionnaire guidelines. Important cardiovascular items were included in 0% to 56% of state forms, and only 26 states required parental verification and approval of histories. Specific heart problems were addressed on only 5% to 37% of physical examination forms. Of 39 states with history and physical examination questionnaires, 16 had not revised their forms in more than 5 years and 6 had not revised their forms in more than 10 years. Seventeen of 43 state forms contained at least 9 of 13-AHA recommended items. Five of 50 states requiring preparticipation screening had no specific recommendations or requirements regarding examiners. Eleven states allow for practitioners with little or no cardiovascular training, and 25 allow examination by nonphysicians. Only 33 states recommend annual preparticipation screening.

Conclusion.—Preparticipation as it is currently being practiced in United States high schools is unlikely to screen out potentially lethal cardiovascular problems effectively. Critically important guidelines are often missing. It is recommended that national standards be developed for preparticipation screening of high school athletes.

▶ In 1996, the AHA used a consensus panel for the development of guidelines for screening athletes before participation in high school athletics. This survey studied the 50 states to determine the level of compliance with these guidelines.

I found the study to be disturbing. A number of common problems known to be associated with increased cardiovascular risk are not included in the preparticipation screening of athletes. Because most high schools accept the state-recommended screening protocols, the authors recommend that we be proactive in assuring that the protocol used in our state meets AHA guidelines. In addition, if you have responsibility for a high school athletic program or simply do preparticipation physicals in your office, you need to include the items listed in the table in this article as part of the screening.

R.C. Davidson, M.D., M.P.H.

The Preparticipation Physical Examination: Mayo Clinic Experience With 2,739 Examinations
Smith J, Laskowski ER (Mayo Clinic Rochester, Minn)
Mayo Clin Proc 73:419–429, 1998

Objective.—The risk of competition injuries and adverse cardiac events in young athletes has spurred interest in providing preparticipation physical examinations (PPEs) as part of a community sports medicine program. The 3-year results of PPEs performed on 2,739 high school athletes at the Mayo Clinic Sports Medicine Center are presented to identify medical and orthopedic problems of sufficient severity to place an athlete at risk, to educate physicians and residents, to improve community access to sports medicine care, and to establish the Sports Medicine Center as a base for Sports medicine education and treatment.

Methods.—Between May 1992 and August 1995, 2,739 athletes were examined by physicians and residents from the Departments of Physical Medicine and Rehabilitation, Orthopedics, Family Medicine, and Internal Medicine using the station system. On completion of the examination, athletes were classified as cleared for participation in sports, not cleared (NC), or cleared with follow-up recommended (CFU).

Results.—There were 327 (11.9%) athletes classified as CFU and 53 (1.9%) as NC. Athletes classified as CFU had vision problems (53.5%), musculoskeletal abnormalities (27.8%), cardiac abnormalities or hypertension (5.2%), or other abnormalities (13.5%). Athletes classified as NC had musculoskeletal abnormalities (43.4%), cardiac problems or syncope (18.9%), vision problems (13.2%), seizures (7.5%), testicular problems or hernia (7.5%), or other problems (9.5%). The time-efficient station examination system has been used in other sports preparticipation studies.

Conclusion.—The Mayo Sports Medicine Clinic PPE using the station system is an efficient and effective way of identifying abnormalities in young athletes. The abnormalities found most in athletes classified as either NC or CFU were vision or musculoskeletal.

▶ I have included this article as it is a succinct presentation of the performance and yield of the sports preparticipation evaluation. The findings here are generally accepted averages in sports medicine and echo the experience we have had in our group (n ≈1,500) over the years. Here are a few take-home points and tips. It is extremely difficult to screen for cardiac abnormalities. A thorough history is the cornerstone for this screening. The preparticipation monograph cited by the authors[1] was crafted by a number of national primary care and sports medicine organizations. It is an excellent guide and should serve as the foundation for all screening programs. The questionnaire is thorough and easy to use. In our program, we limit the stations to vital signs and vision screening. The review of the history and the rest of the examination is performed by a single provider who can use the added time to ask some of the more sensitive questions, which can be extremely difficult in the usual station-type setting. We also insist on including the athlete's family doctor in the loop for follow-up of any conditions or problems identified and by sending a copy of our form to their office.

W.W. Dexter, M.D.

Reference

1. American Academy of Family Physicians, American Academy of Pediatrics, American Medical Society for Sports Medicine, American Orthopaedic Society for Sports Medicine, American Osteopathic Academy of Sports Medicine: *Preparticipation Physical Evaluation*, 2nd ed. Minneapolis: The Physican and Sportsmedicine, 1997.

Screening for Hypertrophic Cardiomyopathy in Young Athletes
Corrado D, Basso C, Schiavon M, et al (Univ of Padua, Italy; Natl Health Service, Padua, Italy)
N Engl J Med 339:364–369, 1998   14–22

Introduction.—Cardiovascular disease is the most common cause of sudden death in athletes. For athletes older than age 35 years, atherosclerotic coronary artery disease is the most common cause of sudden death; hypertrophic cardiomyopathy has been implicated as the cause of death in about one third of younger competitive athletes. Early identification of abnormalities by screening before athletes participate in competitive sports may prevent sudden death. Since 1971, Italian law has required that every athlete undergo annual clinical evaluation before participating in competitive sports. The effectiveness of this strategy on the prevention of hypertrophic cardiomyopathy was assessed in athletes in the Veneto region of Italy.

Methods.—Sudden deaths among athletes and nonathletes 35 years or younger were prospectively studied in the Veneto region of Italy from 1979 to 1996. The causes of death between athletes and nonathletes were reviewed and pathologic findings were compared to clinical histories and electrocardiograms. Cardiovascular reasons for disqualification from sports competition were analyzed. A consecutive series of 33,735 young athletes from Padua, Italy, who underwent preparticipation screening during the same time period were observed.

Results.—Of 269 young people with sudden death, 49 (18.2%) were competitive athletes, mean age, 23 years, (44 males, 5 females). The most common causes of sudden death in these athletes were 22.4%, arrhythmogenic right ventricular cardiomyopathy; 18.4%, coronary atherosclerosis; and 12.2%, anomalous origin of a coronary artery. One death (2%) in young competitive athletes was caused by hypertrophic cardiomyopathy; in young nonathletes, the rate was 7.3% (16 deaths). Hypertrophic cardiomyopathy was found during preparticipation examination in 22 athletes (0.07%) and accounted for 3.5% of cardiovascular reasons for disqualification. None of the athletes who were disqualified because of hypertrophic cardiomyopathy died during a mean follow-up of 8.2 years.

Conclusion.—Hypertrophic cardiomyopathy was a rare cause of death in young competitive athletes in Italy who underwent preparticipation screening. It is possible that sudden death was prevented in athletes who were screened and disqualified before participating in competitive sports.

▶ Last year Dr. Scherger reviewed an article describing sudden death in athletes.[1] Screening for the entities that cause this, particularly for hypertrophic cardiomyopathy (HCM) in young athletes, has become a hot topic over the past few years. Fortunately, as this study from Italy demonstrates, HCM is very uncommon. It can be, however, a fatal condition in vigorously exercising children, and the consensus is we should screen for this disorder. But what is the best method for screening? Performing routine EKGs and/or echocardiograms has not proved to be either useful or cost effective. A reasonable list of recommendations based on the AHA Guidelines is described in a recent *JAMA* article by Glover and Maron.[2] They looked at screening requirements state by state and found most to be less than adequate. A careful history and physical examination remain the gold standard. For a good review of the overall preparticipation examination, see "The Preparticipation Physical Examination: Mayo Clinic Experience with 2,739 Examinations."[3] I firmly recommend purchasing the monograph cited in the commentary and basing your preparticipation evaluation on that document.

W.W. Dexter, M.D.

References

1. Maron BJ, Shirani J, Poliac LC, et al: Sudden death in young competitive athletes: Clinical demographic and pathological profiles. *JAMA* 276:199–204, 1996.
2. Glover D, Maron B: Profile of preparticipation cardiovascular screening for high school athletes. *JAMA* 279:1817–1819, 1998.
3. Smith J, Laskowski ER: The preparticipation physical examination: Mayo Clinic experience with 2,739 examinations. *Mayo Clin Proc* 73:419–429, 1998.

Miscellaneous

Preschool Speech and Language Screening: Further Validation of the Sentence Repetition Screening Test

Sturner RA, Funk SG, Green JA (Johns Hopkins Univ, Baltimore, Md; Univ of North Carolina, Chapel Hill; Univ of Connecticut, Storrs)
J Dev Behav Pediatr 17:405–413, 1996   14–23

Background.—Federal law mandates identification and remediation of communication problems that would interfere with schooling. One speech and language screening test, the Sentence Repetition Screening Test (SRST), is both brief and validated in kindergarten-aged children. To extend the validity of this test, investigators evaluated the SRST in a group of prekindergarten children.

Methods.—Participants were solicited at kindergarten registration in a rural North Carolina County. During registration, parents completed a questionnaire and made appointments for the screening of their children. Within 2 weeks, 343 children, aged 54–66 months, were tested using the SRST. The SRST consists of 15 sentences repeated by the child after tester demonstration (Fig 2). Morphemes and phonemes are scored. The average test time is 3 minutes. A stratified sample of 76 children were recalled for further testing by the Bankson and Illinois Test of Psycholinguistic Abilities and the Arizona Articulation Proficiency Scale (AAPS) within 2 months. Five months later, kindergarten teacher assessments were obtained.

RUN WITH ME
WHO WERE THOSE MEN?
PUSH THE BROWN BUTTON
THANK YOU FOR MY PRESENT
LOOK AT THE LAZY CLOWN
ISN'T THAT A FUNNY SKY?
THIS IS A SUNNY DAY
WHAT IS SHE LOOKING FOR?
SOME BLUE BIRDS ARE EATING THE SEED
THERE IS A BIG BALL IN THE BOX
IT IS NOT TIME TO GO TO SCHOOL
THEY WALKED INTO THE STORE TO BUY HIS BOOKS
I DON'T KNOW WHY HE'S CRYING
NOW I'LL PLAY WITH CARS AND TRUCKS
WE SAW FLYING FISH AT THE ZOO

FIGURE 2.—Sentence repetition screening items. The underlined letters correspond to the phonemes that are scored for articulation. The actual score sheet includes boxes below these phonemes for scoring and boxes above all morphemes for separately scoring any omissions. (Courtesy of Sturner RA, Funk SG, Green JA: Preschool speech and language screening: Further validation of the sentence repetition screening test. *J Dev Behav Pediatr* 17(6):405–413, 1996.)

Results.—With a prevalence of 11%, SRST language outcome prediction had a sensitivity of 0.62, a specificity of 0.91, a predictive validity of 0.44, an overreferral rate of 8.4%, and an underreferral rate of 4%. With a prevalence of 11%, SRST articulation outcome prediction had a sensitivity of 0.57, a specificity of 0.95, a predictive validity of 0.75, an overreferral rate of 3.7%, and an underreferral rate of 8.3%. Global parent and teacher ratings resulted in high overreferral rates compared with the SRST.

Conclusions.—The brief SRST, which had been validated as an assessment of communication skills in kindergartners, was validated for a group of preschool-aged children. As this test can be administered in 3 minutes, it would be useful for routine screening by pediatricians.

▶ This is a validation study of a simple office-based screening procedure for potential language problems in preschool children. Similar to previous studies, this study showed that the SRST is a valid screening tool for identifying speech problems. The simple sentences included in Figure 2 were shown to be fairly sensitive in identifying speech problems and had a very high specificity (greater than 90%) for identifying children who had trouble with articulation.

R.C. Davidson, M.D., M.P.H.

Variation of Bone Age Progression in Healthy Children
Benso L, Vannelli S, Pastorin L, et al (Universitá di Torino, Italy; Instituto di Statistica Medicae Biometria Università di Milano, Italy)
Acta Paediatr Suppl 423:109–112, 1997   14–24

Background.—Whether the observed general trend in bone age progression can be applied to individuals is important. Factors affecting the rate of skeletal maturation and the utility of skeletal maturation measures to assess individuals were studied.

Methods.—Four hundred seven Italian boys, aged 7 to 12 years, underwent bone age assessment. These measures were correlated with auxological variables.

Findings.—Using the radius-ulna-short bones (RUS) technique, bone age velocity was found to be greater in the Italian boys than for the UK reference standards. Considerable interindividual dispersion around the mean was noted. Bone age velocity was poorly correlated with height velocity. The correlation between skeletal and pubertal maturation was minimal. Slight positive correlations were observed between bone age velocity and height standard deviation score and between bone age velocity and body mass index. Bone age estimations using RUS were greater than those with the carpus (Fig 2).

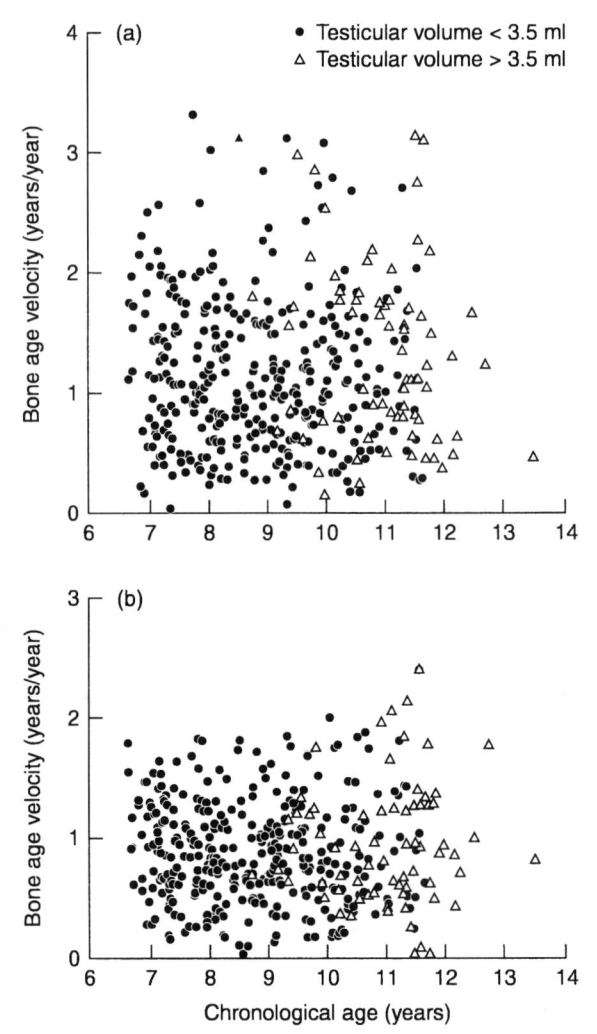

FIGURE 2.—Bone-age velocity vs. chronological age, by testicular volume, using (a) Tanner-Whitehouse 2 (TW2) radius-ulna-short bones and (b) TW2 carpal bones in 407 normal healthy boys. (Courtesy of Benso L, Vannelli S, Pastorin L, et al: Variation of bone age progression in healthy children. *Acta Paediatr Suppl* 423:109–112, 1997.)

Conclusions.—The interindividual deviation in measured bone ages was marked in this study. This variability makes it difficult to relate data on an individual basis to other measures of growth and maturation.

▶ I know that bone age, or bone age velocity, measurements are not everyday tests in family practice. This article suggests to me that perhaps even fewer such tests should be ordered. I had the misimpression that we could identify normal from abnormal, but the tremendous variability these investigators found among normal boys calls into question our use of these tests to consider an individual patient's growth.

M.A. Bowman, M.D., M.P.A.

Renal Function After Short-term Ibuprofen Use in Infants and Children
Lesko SM, Mitchell AA (Boston Univ)
Pediatrics 100:954–957, 1997

Objective.—Although ibuprofen is not associated with renal failure in children, the possibility of less severe renal impairment has not been studied. The possibility of impaired renal function in febrile children after short-term use of ibuprofen was evaluated in a randomized, double-blind, controlled trial.

Methods.—Between February 1991 and June 1993, 97 children received a suspension of acetaminophen (12 mg/kg), 103 received a suspension of ibuprofen (5 mg/kg), and 88 children received a suspension of ibuprofen (10 mg/kg). Blood urea nitrogen (BUN) and creatinine levels were measured at baseline and after nonsteroidal anti-inflammatory drug (NSAID) administration. Children were followed up for 4 weeks.

Results.—Admission BUN and creatinine levels were 4.1 μmol/L and 43 μmol/L, respectively, for children receiving 5 mg/kg ibuprofen, 3.8 and 41 for those receiving 10 mg/kg ibuprofen, and 3.9 and 43 for those receiving acetaminophen. The prevalence of BUN values greater than 6.4 mmol/L and creatinine levels greater than 62 μmol/L did not vary with NSAID or dosage. Mean creatinine level and prevalence of elevated BUN in children with dehydration were 44 μmol/L and 14%, respectively, and did not vary with NSAID or dosage.

Conclusion.—BUN and creatinine levels in children given short-term ibuprofen are not significantly higher than in children taking acetaminophen.

▶ I have a healthy respect for the potential adverse effects of ibuprofen and other NSAIDs. Having had several adult patients over the years go into (fortunately, completely reversible) renal failure after taking ibuprofen, I am cautious about recommending its use and I monitor patients who take it on a long-term basis. In children, I find that ibuprofen works well in reducing fever and pain, and I prescribe its use fairly often. Parents often ask about ibuprofen's safety profile in children, and I admit to having some doubts, particularly in dehydrated kids. This study goes a long way in reassuring me about the safety profile, from a renal standpoint, of short-term use of ibuprofen in children, even those who are dehydrated.

W.W. Dexter, M.D.

Therapeutic Misadventures With Acetaminophen: Hepatotoxicity After Multiple Doses in Children

Heubi JE, Barbacci MB, Zimmerman HJ (Children's Hosp Med Ctr, Cincinnati, Ohio; George Washington Univ, Washington, DC; Armed Forces Inst of Pathology, Washington, DC)
J Pediatr 132:22–27, 1998

Background.—With the recognition that aspirin plays a pathogenetic role in Reye's syndrome, acetaminophen has become widely used for relief of pain and fever in children. However, acetaminophen is hepatotoxic in single doses of greater than 140 mg/kg. Few reports have described liver toxicity occurring with multiple overdoses of this common drug. Children with hepatotoxicity resulting from multiple doses of acetaminophen were described.

Patients.—Forty-seven such cases were identified from a review of the literature, reports to the Food and Drug Administration, and the experience of a children's hospital. The patients ranged in age from 5 weeks to 10 years; 22 were 2 years old or younger. Acetaminophen dosage, estimated in 39 patients, ranged from 60 to 420 mg/kg/day. The duration of administration, estimated from 33 subjects, was 1 day to 6 weeks. Acetaminophen preparations intended for adults were given to 52% of patients. The patients had a mean peak serum aspartate aminotransferase level of 10,225 IU/L and a mean serum alanine aminotransferase level of 7,355 IU/L. These were significantly higher than the values reported for a sample of 12 children with hepatic failure unrelated to acetaminophen. Thirty patients had information permitting estimation of the time since the last dose of acetaminophen; in 22 of these cases, the serum acetaminophen level exceeded the toxic range for acute ingestion. Among 43 reported cases, the mortality rate was 55%. Another 4 patients survived after orthotopic liver transplantation.

Conclusion.—Repeated overdose of acetaminophen can lead to hepatotoxicity in children. The repeated overdoses alter the metabolic pathway, affecting the development of hepatic injury. These children have very high liver enzyme levels with fulminant hepatic failure and serum acetaminophen levels beyond the toxic range. The true frequency of this acetaminophen hepatotoxicity caused by multiple overdoses is unknown. Physicians must advise parents on the safe use of acetaminophen, including judicious use of antipyretic medications.

▶ Acetaminophen has long been regarded as a safe medication which may be used by parents for their children for the nonspecific treatment of fever and pain. Many parents have a strong need to do something for their ill children, and repeated doses of Tylenol are often given for spurious reasons. This article and many other recent ones report the potentially serious and sometimes fatal liver toxicity that can result from high doses of acetaminophen. Parents need to be given clear instructions regarding individual dosing and maximum daily dosing; they should also be discouraged from frequent acetaminophen use.

J.E. Scherger, M.D., M.P.H.

Assessment of Adenoidal Obstruction in Children: Clinical Signs Versus Roentgenographic Findings
Paradise JL, Bernard BS, Colborn DK, et al (Univ of Pittsburgh, Pa; Children's Hosp of Pittsburgh, Pa)
Pediatrics 101:979–986, 1998   14–27

Introduction.—A common condition of childhood is chronic nasal obstruction attributable to large adenoids. However, few children with nasal obstruction complain of difficulty in nasal breathing. Mouth breathing and hyponasal speech have been the classic physical signs considered indicative of adenoidal nasal obstruction. A study was conducted to determine whether the presence and degree of adenoidal nasal obstruction in children can be assessed satisfactorily by simple clinical means and whether it correlates with roentgenographic assessments.

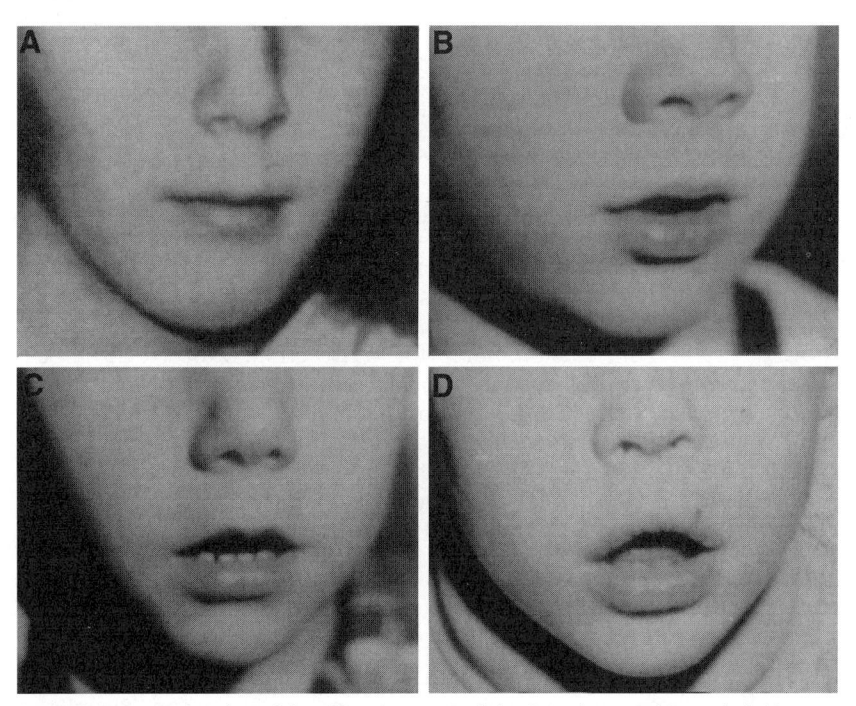

FIGURE 1.—Grades of mouth breathing: **A**, none; **B**, slight; **C**, moderate; and **D**, marked. (Courtesy of Paradise JL, Bernard BS, Colborn K, et al: Assessment of adenoidal obstruction in children: Clinical signs versus roentgenographic findings. *Pediatrics* 101:979–986, 1998. Reproduced with permission from *Pediatrics*.)

Roentgenographic Ratings in 1033 Subjects

□ No obstruction
▨ Borderline obstruction
■ Obstruction

Nasal Obstruction Index

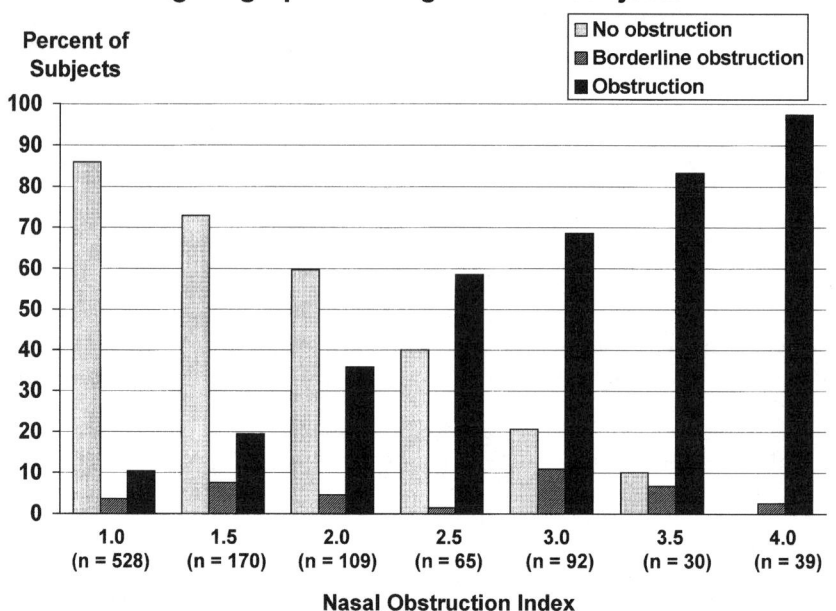

| | 1.0 (n = 528) | 1.5 (n = 170) | 2.0 (n = 109) | 2.5 (n = 65) | 3.0 (n = 92) | 3.5 (n = 30) | 4.0 (n = 39) |

FIGURE 3.—Relationships between clinical assessments of nasal obstruction and roentgenographic assessments of nasopharyngeal airway patency. (Courtesy of Paradise JL, Bernard BS, Colborn K, et al: Assessment of adenoidal obstruction in children: Clinical signs versus roentgenographic findings. *Pediatrics* 101:979–986, 1998. Reproduced with permission from *Pediatrics*.)

Methods.—A 4-point scale, ranging from "none" to "marked," was used to rate the degree of children's mouth breathing (Fig 1) and speech hyponasality and was called the Nasal Obstruction Index. Classifications of lateral soft-tissue roentgenograms of the nasopharynx were based on assessment of adenoid size and of nasopharyngeal airway patency that showed either no obstruction, borderline obstruction, or obstruction. Levels of interobserver and intraobserver agreement concerning the classifications were also determined. Correlations in individual children between clinical rating and roentgenographic ratings of nasal/nasopharyngeal obstruction were determined. The roentgenographic ratings were used as the gold standard in the calculation of predictive values of clinical ratings.

Results.—In the study 235 children were measured for mouth breathing and 648 children were measured for speech hyponasality; weighted κ values for interobserver agreement ranged from 0.84 to 0.91. Two hundred seven children were assessed roentgenographically, and the value for interobserver agreement in assessing nasopharyngeal airway status was 0.92 whereas the intraobserver agreement for 191 children was 0.88. For concordance between Nasal Obstruction Index values and roentgenographic ratings in 1,033 children, the Kendall's τ *b* value was 0.51. At the lower and upper extremes of 1.0 and 3.5 or more, the Nasal Obstruction

Index values were highly predictive of concordant roentgenographic ratings (Fig 3).

Conclusion.—Reliable and reasonably valid assessment of the presence and degree of adenoidal obstruction of the nasopharyngeal airway can be provided by standardized clinical ratings of the degree of children's mouth breathing and speech hyponasality. At the extremes of either marked obstruction or no obstruction, these clinical assessments are particularly valid. To establish the presence of adenoidal obstruction, clinical assessment alone may be insufficient; however, when findings are unequivocally negative, clinical assessment can suffice to rule out adenoidal obstruction with a high degree of confidence.

▶ Here is a clinically useful study. We all see kids who breathe through their mouths and have the (usually parental) complaint of "always sounding stuffed up." This is a quick and reliable technique for assessing obstruction, especially for ruling out significant obstruction. I certainly agree that further work-up is necessary if operative measures are under consideration. This technique is also simple; use the degree of mouth breathing (pictured in Fig 1) with a few standard phrases (see abstract) with nose open and nose pinched.

W.W. Dexter, M.D.

Evaluation of Boys With Marked Breast Development at Puberty
Sher ES, Migeon CJ, Berkovitz GD (Johns Hopkins Univ, Baltimore, Md)
Clin Pediatr (Phila) 37:367–372, 1998   14-28

Introduction.—About 60% of all boys have gynecomastia, a part of normal male puberty. Over a period of 6 months to 1 year, the gynecomastia usually regresses and the extent of breast tissue is limited. An imbalance between androgen and estrogen concentrations appears to be the cause of pubertal gynecomastia, but in some boys breast development is marked and persistent, and a complete evaluation is indicated for these boys. The endocrine function in 60 boys who had marked breast development at puberty was evaluated. The clinical characteristics that distinguished boys with no etiologic factors from boys of similar age with the problem were determined.

Methods.—During a 10-year period there were 60 boys older than 9 years who had breast development greater than 4 cm in diameter around the time of puberty. Height, weight, sexual development, and extent of gynecomastia were recorded. A determination was made from blood of luteinizing hormone, follicle-stimulating hormone, testosterone, and estradiol. Testosterone and estradiol were assayed with radioimmunoassay.

TABLE 1.—Clinical Characteristics of Subjects With Gynecomastia of Known Etiology

Etiology	Onset of Gynecomastia (Year)	Sexual Hair at Evaluation (Tanner Stage)	Age at Evaluation (Year)	Karyotype	LH (mIU/mL)	FHS (mIU/mL)	T (nmol/L)	E_2 (pmol/L)
Klinefelter's syndrome	10.0	V	17.9	47,XXY	47.8	60.5	4.92	140
Increased aromatase	10.0	III	11.9	46,XY	7.7	5.0	1.12	228
Partial androgen insensitivity	10.3	V	13.4	46,XY	22.5	12.9	33.7	143
XX Male	11.4	IV	14.4	46,XX	33.6	33.9	9.81	158
Primary testicular failure	11.6	V	17.5	46,XY	23.0	20.0	26.6	220
Fibrolamellar hepatocarcinoma	12.3	II	13.8	—	<2.0	4.0	2.01	389
Klinefelter's syndrome	16.8	V	19.3	47,XXY	67.6	62.0	7.94	—
Normal values for prepubertal child	—	—	—	—	<5.0	<5.0	<0.69	<46
Normal values for adult male	—	—	—	—	3.9–18	1.5–16	9.55–30.4	36.8–220

Abbreviations: LH, luteinizing hormone; T, testosterone; E2, estradiol.
(Courtesy of Sher ES, Migeon CJ, Berkovitz GD: Evaluation of Boys With Marked Breast Development at Puberty. *Clin Pediatr* 37:367–372, 1998.)

Results.—In 7 boys, an endocrine abnormality was identified, which included Klinefelter's syndrome; 46, XX maleness; primary testicular failure; partial androgen insensitivity; fibrolamellar hepatocarcinoma; and increased aromatase activity (Table 1). Underlying medical problems were found in 8 boys, 5 of whom had neurologic disorders. Significant idiopathic gynecomastia, otherwise known as macromastia, was found to be the cause in the remaining 45 boys. These boys were taller and heavier than average.

Conclusion.—It is unusual to find pathologic causes of marked pubertal gynecomastia. An endocrine evaluation of all affected boys is called for because of the potential for significant health problems among boys with marked breast development. Greater body mass than other boys of similar age was found in boys with marked idiopathic breast development, which may contribute in part to their breast development.

▶ Although this study is from a referral clinic and reaffirms that many boys with breast development at puberty are endocrinologically normal, it also shows that there is a significant rate of abnormalities in teenage boys with males who had large breast development (greater than 4 cm in diameter), sometimes called "macromastia." Fifteen of 60 boys had either hormonal causes (n = 7) or underlying medical problems (n = 8), including diabetes, cystic fibrosis, or neurologic disorders (seizures, hydrocephalus, and venous malformations). Most of those with gynecomastia of unknown origin were tall and obese. Evaluation of macromastia includes a good history and physical examination (particularly looking for signs of Klinefelter's syndrome or testicular atrophy) and measurement of serum luteinizing hormone, follicle-stimulating hormone, testosterone, and estradiol.

M.A. Bowman, M.D., M.P.A.

Students' Acquisition and Use of School Condoms in a High School Condom Availability Program
Schuster MA, Bell RM, Berry SH, et al (Univ of California, Los Angeles)
Pediatrics 100:689–694, 1997   14–29

Objective.—Whether the various condom-availability programs offered by high schools are being used is not known. A high school program making condoms available without parental consent or gatekeepers was studied to determine whether students knew about it, how they reacted to it, and which students used it.

Methods.—Students in grades 9 through 12 filled out an anonymous survey form about sexual activity and condom use 1 year after the program was established in 1 racially and socioeconomically diverse Los Angeles community high school.

Results.—Surveys were completed by 1,112 students (51% male), representing 59% of eligible students and evenly distributed among the 4 grades. Awareness of the school condom program was high, with 88% of students knowing about it and 74% understanding that parental consent was not required. Almost half (48%) of the responders had taken condoms from the school and another 5% had obtained them for someone else. Boys were more likely than girls (60% vs. 45%) to have obtained condoms. Blacks were most likely and Asian and Pacific Islanders were least likely to have obtained condoms. Nonvirgins were more likely than virgins to have obtained condoms (70% vs. 38%), and students who had had sexual relations were more likely to obtain condoms than those who had not had sexual relations (71% vs. 37%). A significant number of students used condoms for other than sexual activity, such as putting them on or putting them on a partner, on fingers, or on a banana. Of those having vaginal intercourse, 41% of the boys and 26% of the girls had obtained condoms from school. Support for the condom program was high, with 88% agreeing that the school should give out condoms, 75% saying they liked the way the school ran the program, 65% desiring more distribution locations in the school, and 68% wanting vending machines in restrooms. Most students strongly opposed requiring parental permission, with 79% of students reporting that they would use condoms less often if parental permission were required. Thirteen percent of the students believed that having condoms available at school made it harder to refuse sex, whereas 71% disagreed.

Conclusion.—Student reaction to this high school condom-availability program was positive at 1 year.

▶ The provision of condoms to high school students is debated vigorously in many communities. By providing them, do we, in effect, sanction sexual activity? Although I counsel my patients about abstinence, my teaching and experience would suggest otherwise. Ultimately, whether condoms are provided or not, young people have always, and will always, engage in sexual activities. There is no argument that condoms aren't a cost-effective tool in preventing pregnancy and disease. This study points out that if high school–aged young men and women have access to condoms, they will use them. This is preventive medicine at its most basic, on a community-based level, and it deserves our support.

W.W. Dexter, M.D.

Educational and Occupational Outcome of Hyperactive Boys Grown Up
Mannuzza S, Klein RG, Bessler A, et al (Long Island Jewish Med Ctr, New Hyde Park, NY; New York State Psychiatric Inst, Columbia Univ, NY)
J Am Acad Child Adolesc Psychiatry 36:1222–1227, 1997   14–30

Background.—Attention deficit–hyperactivity disorder (ADHD), a very prevalent diagnosis in childhood, adversely affects academic performance and other areas of child functioning. Little is known regarding the adult outcome of this disorder. The long-term educational achievement and occupational rank of men who had a diagnosis of ADHD in childhood were reported.

Methods.—White boys of average intelligence and with ADHD diagnosed clinically according to systematic criteria at a mean of 7 years of age were followed up prospectively, for a period ranging from 15 to 21 years. At a mean age of 24 years, 85 probands (82% of the original cohort) and 73 control subjects (94% of the original group) were interviewed by trained clinicians.

Findings.—The ADHD group had completed significantly less formal schooling (about 2 years) than the control subjects. The ADHD individuals also had lower-ranking occupations than control subjects. Adult mental status did not explain these differences.

Conclusions.—Childhood ADHD appears to predispose boys to certain disadvantages in adulthood. The presence of this diagnosis continues to affect important functional domains unassociated with the current psychiatric diagnosis.

▶ I was sensitized to this problem while working with a furniture builder some years ago whose son was in treatment for ADHD. It was perfectly obvious to me that the father had the same problem, but it was unrecognized. In addition, despite his obviously superior intelligence, he had experienced lower educational achievement and lower occupational status than he had set out to achieve (although he built wonderful furniture!). This study fuels the ongoing debate about recognizing and treating adult ADHD. Would effective treatment extending from childhood into adulthood make a difference? Unfortunately, there is as yet no answer.

A.O. Berg, M.D., M.P.H.

15 Women's Health

Overview

Randomized controlled trials: Abstracts 15–12, 15–19, 15–20, 15–21, 15–24, 15–26, 15–27, 15–28, and 15–35

Breast Cancer

- Diet, nutrition, and exercise and breast cancer risk
- Weight and breast cancer risk
- *BRCA1* mutations in the general population
- Uterine side effects of tamoxifen
- Vitamin E and hot flashes in breast cancer survivors
- Hospital volume and breast cancer survival
- Effect of Nancy Reagan's mastectomy on choice of treatment for breast cancer
- Breast cancer survival in HMO and fee-for-service settings
- Sonographic features of cysts

Cervical Cancer

- Cervical cancer screening in women with and without hysterectomies
- Cost-effectiveness of diagnosis and management of SIL
- Use of the endocervical brush after endocervical curettage
- Follow-up of patients with abnormal Pap smears
- False-positive cervicovaginal cytology
- Order of sampling and Pap smear quality
- PAPNET screening

Polycystic Ovary Syndrome

- Late endocrine effects of ovarian electrocautery
- Metformin therapy

Premenstrual Syndrome

- Sertraline and dysphoric disorder
- Calcium carbonate treatment
- Effect of gonadal steroids on behavior

Emergency Contraception and Abortion

- Self-administered emergency contraception
- Expectant management vs. curettage for spontaneous abortion
- Effect of NSAIDs on effectiveness of misoprostol

Menopause

- Bone changes and carotid atherosclerosis in postmenopausal women
- Dietary soy and hot flashes

Hormone Replacement Therapy

- Androgen effects on estrogen use
- Lack of estrogen effect of a Chinese herbal treatment
- Patient-specific decisions about hormone replacement therapy
- Bleeding as a predictor of endometrial hyperplasia
- Effects of cyclic vs. combined hormone replacement therapy on bleeding

Miscellaneous

- Routine digital rectal examination as part of the pelvic examination
- Protocol for pessary management
- Epidemiology of repeat ectopic pregnancy
- Depot leuprolide and endometriosis

Breast Cancer

Population Attributable Risk for Breast Cancer: Diet, Nutrition, and Physical Exercise

Mezzetti M, La Vecchia C, Decarli A, et al (Istituto Europeo di Oncologia, Milan, Italy; Università degli Studi di Milano, Milan, Italy; Centro di Riferimento Oncologico, Aviano, Itlay)
J Natl Cancer Inst 90:389–394, 1998   15–1

Background.—Currently, the most recognizable risk factors for breast disease have to do with reproduction and menstruation. However, these risks are not modifiable. The proportion of breast cancer cases in Italy attributable to modifiable risk factors—diet, alcohol intake, physical activity, and body mass index—was estimated to help focus prevention strategies.

Methods.—Data were obtained from an Italian case-control study that involved 2,569 case subjects with breast cancer and 2,588 control subjects. The original study was conducted from June 1991 to April 1994. β-carotene, vitamin E, and alcohol intakes were analyzed, as well as physical activity and body mass index (for postmenopausal subjects), using unconditional multiple logistic regression models. From this, risks of breast cancer for certain populations were determined as were multivariate odds ratios.

Results.—The attributable risk for high alcohol intake (greater than 20 g/day) was 10.7% (95% confidence interval [CI], 4.4% to 17.0%). The risk for low β-carotene intake was 15.0% (95% CI, 7.4% to 22.9%), and for low vitamin E intake (less than 8.5 mg/day) was 8.6% (95% CI, −0.4% to 17.5%). For low physical activity levels, the attributable risk was 11.6% (95% CI, −0.1% to 23.3%). The risk factors that were most significant for premenopausal women were alcohol and β-carotene intake. The greatest risk for postmenopausal women was being overweight (10.2%; 95% CI, 0.2% to 20.2%). Twenty-eight percent of cases were accounted for by β-carotene and alcohol intake. Thirty-two percent of cases were accounted for by β-carotene intake and physical activity (95% CI, 14.3% to 49.8%). Thus, 33% of cases were explained by these 3 factors.

Conclusions.—The potentially modifiable risk factors associated with breast cancer account for approximately one third of breast cancer cases in the population studied. This suggests many theoretical routes for prevention of the disease.

▶ Is breast cancer a preventable disease? We commit a lot of resources to the secondary prevention of breast cancer with mammographic screening and with clinical and self-breast examination—all are controversial. Primary prevention, when possible, is always the best approach. This case-control study adds to the accumulating evidence that points to modifiable and nonmodifiable risk factors for this disease. This type of model works well for heart disease and is showing promise for breast cancer. The keys to primary prevention of so many disease entities are coming into focus: diet and exercise. In our reductionist approach to so many of the problems that confront us in medicine, the search continues to precisely define these risk factors—modifiable and nonmodifiable. I am beginning to wonder, however, if this approach is, to some degree, obscuring the real solution to primary prevention of breast cancer and other disease processes, which is, at once, both simple and vexedly complicated: diet and exercise.

W.W. Dexter, M.D.

Dual Effects of Weight and Weight Gain on Breast Cancer Risk
Huang Z, Hankinson SE, Colditz GA, et al (Harvard School of Public Health, Boston; Harvard Medical School, Boston; Brigham and Women's Hosp, Boston)
JAMA 278:1407–1411, 1997
15-2

Background.—There appears to be a relationship between body weight and breast cancer risk and survival, but no clear and consistent positive association between body weight and breast cancer has been confirmed. Although most studies have examined the effect of body weight at diagnosis, adult weight gain may be a better variable for assessing adiposity and its metabolic consequences. Data from a cohort study of nurses who were followed up for 16 years were used to examine body mass index (BMI) at age 18 years and at midlife, as well as adult weight change in relation to breast cancer incidence and mortality.

Methods.—The Nurses' Health Study cohort included 121,700 female nurses aged 30–55 years who responded to mailed health questionnaires in 1976. Follow-up surveys were sent every 2 years to identify newly diagnosed breast cancer cases and update information on risk factors. Excluded from this study were women with any cancer other than nonmelanoma skin cancer and those with incomplete baseline data on risk factors. The 95,256 women in the present analysis were categorized according to current BMI and BMI at age 18 years.

Results.—By 1992, 1,000 premenopausal and 1,517 postmenopausal invasive breast cancers were identified in the cohort. A higher current BMI was associated with a lower incidence of breast cancer among premenopausal women. Among postmenopausal women, a higher BMI was minimally associated with increased breast cancer incidence. A stronger positive relationship was present among postmenopausal women who had never used hormone replacement therapy (relative risk [RR], 1.59 for BMI greater than 31 kg/m^2 vs. 20 kg/m^2 or less; 95% confidence interval [CI], 1.09–2.32). A higher BMI at age 18 years was associated with lower breast cancer incidence both before and after menopause. Although weight gain after age 18 years was not related to the incidence of breast cancer before menopause, weight gain after age 18 years was positively associated with breast cancer incidence after menopause. This relationship was strongest among women who never used hormones (RR, 1.99; 95% CI, 1.43–2.76 for weight gain greater than 20 kg vs. no weight gain). Among postmenopausal women, both current BMI and weight gain after age 18 years were strongly associated with death from breast cancer.

Conclusions.—The expected adverse effect of excess body fat on breast cancer risk in postmenopausal women may be partially offset by a protective effect of being overweight in early adulthood. Adult weight gain, however, increases the risk of both breast cancer incidence and mortality after menopause. Women who avoid weight gain as an adult, especially those who do not use hormone replacement therapy, may reduce their risk of postmenopausal breast cancer.

▶ The Nurses' Health Study is a long-term, large, ongoing surveillance study that is providing some very intriguing data. This study seems to provide another compelling reason to encourage our adult patients to stay fit and avoid adult weight gain. The authors consider this a modifiable risk factor for breast cancer. Theoretically, given their data, I would agree. Practically, it is a tough one to modify. I was surprised at the negative relationship between a higher BMI (age younger than 18 years) and breast cancer risk. Upon closer inspection of this study, I am left with more questions than answers. Although they looked at hormone use, the authors did not look for other associations with BMI that might provide a subset of patients at higher risk.

The salient point: adult weight gain appears to increase breast cancer risk; it is a point worth including in your health care maintenance visit.

W.W. Dexter, M.D.

***BRCA1* Mutations and Breast Cancer in the General Population: Analyses in Women Before Age 35 Years and in Women Before Age 45 Years With First-Degree Family History**
Malone KE, Daling JR, Thompson JD, et al (Fred Hutchinson Cancer Research Ctr, Seattle)
JAMA 279:922–929, 1998

Background.—Although studies of high-risk families with multiple early-onset breast cancers have been valuable for determining the type and spectrum of germline mutations on the *BRCA1* gene, such research does not provide guidance to women with modest family history profiles. General population studies are needed to assess the *BRCA1* mutation frequency in women perceived to be at high risk and to develop profiles of women most likely to be carriers.

Methods.—Two categories of women hypothesized to be at increased risk of carrying mutations were studied: those with breast cancer diagnosed before the age of 35 years, and those diagnosed before 45 years and with a first-degree family history of breast cancer. Subjects were drawn from 2 population-based, case-control studies.

Findings.—Of 193 women with breast cancer diagnosed before age 35 years (none selected on the basis of family history status), 6.2% had germline *BRCA1* mutations. Of 208 women diagnosed before age 45 years with a first-degree family history, 7.2% had germline *BRCA1* mutations. Both groups included variations in mutation frequency noted by age and family history. Mutation frequency declined as age at diagnosis increased. Greater proportions of mutations were seen in patients with at least 1 relative diagnosed as having breast cancer before 45 years of age, in patients with greater numbers of affected relatives, and in patients with a family history of ovarian cancer. The frequency of mutations did not vary by bilateral breast cancer family history. Seventy-one control women with a first-degree family history had no frameshift or nonsense mutations, though missense changes of unknown significance were observed in both case and control subjects.

Conclusions.—In this study, women with *BRCA1* germline mutations did not have a common family history profile. A large percentage of the women with a first-degree breast cancer family history and of the women with a breast cancer diagnosis before age 35 did not have germline *BRCA1* mutations. Thus, although early-onset disease and a strong family history of breast cancer may be useful guidelines for checking *BRCA1* status, it may be difficult to develop *BRCA1* mutation screening criteria for women with modest family history profiles.

▶ This is 1 of 2 articles published in the same issue of *JAMA* that provided the first data on *BRCA1* mutations in typical populations, as opposed to data from populations of patients already known to be at extremely high risk. This article is a case-control study of women at moderate risk, finding that those few with *BRCA1* mutations lack a common family history profile. The second study, also using a case-control design, found only 3 (1.4%) of 211 women with breast cancer had *BRCA1* mutations.[1] I currently chair an expert panel working on the issue of *BRCA1* screening in primary care, and we used these two articles to conclude that screening is definitely not ready for widespread application, despite its increasing availability. Our panel also found that the data supporting the interventions proposed for those with mutations (e.g., prophylactic mastectomy, increased screening) are of very poor quality. This is clearly an area to watch closely, but it would be misguided to recommend screening and case finding based on the data we have so far.

A.O. Berg, M.D., M.P.H.

Reference

1. Newman B, Mu H, Butler LM, et al: Frequency of breast cancer attributable to BRCA1 in a population-based series of American women. *N Engl J Med* 1998; 279:915–921.

Uterine Side Effects of Tamoxifen: A Need for Systematic Pretreatment Screening
Berlière M, Charles A, Galant C, et al (Catholic Univ of Louvain, Brussels, Belgium)
Obstet Gynecol 91:40–44, 1998   15–4

Introduction.—The risk for endometrial cancer appears to be increased with tamoxifen, perhaps 2 to 3 times greater than in women with breast cancer not treated with tamoxifen. In women at high risk for breast cancer, tamoxifen is being studied as a preventive agent, but its side effects should be evaluated carefully before its extensive use as a preventive treatment. The effect of tamoxifen on the endometrium was studied in postmenopausal women with breast cancer. Women at higher risk for endometrial cancer on the basis of gynecologic pretreatment were identified.

Methods.—There were 264 postmenopausal women with breast cancer who underwent pelvic ultrasound in a 3-year period. If ultrasound abnormalities were detected, outpatient hysteroscopy and endometrial biopsy were performed. Before treatment with tamoxifen was started at 20 mg/day and annually thereafter, initial endometrial evaluation was done. Endometrial lesions and endometrial hyperplasia were focused on. There were 2 categories of endometrial hyperplasia: hyperplasia without cytologic atypia and hyperplasia with cytologic atypia. Adenocarcinoma in situ was defined as well-differentiated endometrial carcinoma confined to the endometrial mucosa without myometrial invasion.

Results.—Asymptomatic endometrial lesions were diagnosed in 46 women (17.4%) before starting tamoxifen, and 2 were atypical lesions. Women with initial lesions and those without initial lesions were followed up separately. In women with lesions initially, compared with those without, the incidence of atypical lesions was significantly higher at 3 years of follow-up. Among 9 women with lesions initially, there were 3 lesions, vs. 1 lesion among 51 women who did not have lesions initially.

Conclusion.—On the basis of endometrial evaluation before tamoxifen therapy, a group of subjects at high risk can be defined. Because of the high incidence of severe atypical lesions, these women should be followed up carefully.

▶ The authors found that patients with uterine abnormalities detected through vaginal ultrasound screening prior to starting tamoxifen were more likely to develop further significant abnormalities in the next 3 years in spite of treatment of the initial abnormality. This is logical, although it is based on small numbers (only 4 [3.9%] patients developed atypical lesions in the next 3 years). The authors conclude that all patients should be prescreened. This is not necessarily logical, and I do not believe this paper presents enough data to determine if prescreening makes sense. However, it is clear that it would take very large numbers of patients to truly study this, since the rate of development of uterine cancer during tamoxifen therapy, while higher than without tamoxifen, is still quite low. The authors noted that 2 asymptomatic patients had cancers prior to tamoxifen treatment, which later might have been falsely attributed to the treatment itself.

M.A. Bowman, M.D., M.P.A.

Prospective Evaluation of Vitamin E for Hot Flashes in Breast Cancer Survivors
Barton DL, Loprinzi CL, Quella SK, et al (Mayo Clinic and Found, Rochester, Minn; Carle Cancer Ctr, Urbana, Ill; Illinois Oncology Research Assoc Community Clinical Oncology Program, Peoria, Ill; et al)
J Clin Oncol 16:495–500, 1998

Background.—Many breast cancer survivors have hot flashes. Although these can generally be treated with estrogen and progesterone, some physicians and patients are concerned with using these hormones. Vitamin E, which has been said to alleviate these symptoms, was examined as a treatment for hot flashes.

Methods.—Women older than 18 years with a history of breast cancer were studied. These patients also reported hot flashes at least 14 times per week for a 1-month period. Baseline hot flashes were determined using 1 week of data. Patients were then randomly assigned to receive either 800

IU of vitamin E daily or placebo for 4 weeks. During a second 4-week period, former placebo patients were given vitamin E and vice versa. Study participants filled out daily questionnaires regarding the frequency of hot flashes and potential vitamin E side effects. There were 125 total participants, 105 of whom completed the trial.

Results.—No patients showed vitamin E toxicity. Crossover analysis demonstrated that vitamin E treatment yielded an average of 1 less hot flash per day. However, patients did not notice this difference, as they did not prefer vitamin E to the placebo (32% vs. 29%, respectively).

Conclusion.—Although vitamin E administration was associated with a significant though small reduction in hot flash frequency in breast cancer patients, this reduction was not clinically significant.

▶ This is a great example of a study that makes medical sense and even shows statistically significant "benefits," but where the patients failed to appreciate the improvement. The most important clinical outcomes for interventions are those that patients would notice and care about, regardless of the improvements measured by objective/statistical methods. Yet there are other more compelling reasons for patients to consider taking vitamin E, so, based on these findings, it's still worth discussing with your patients who have had breast cancer. They just should not expect much symptomatic improvement.

A.O. Berg, M.D., M.P.H.

Hospital Volume Differences and Five-Year Survival From Breast Cancer
Roohan PJ, Bickell NA, Baptiste MS, et al (New York State Dept of Health, Albany)
Am J Public Health 88:454–457, 1998   15–6

Introduction.—Both patient and hospital characteristics have an effect on the treatment and outcome of patients with breast cancer. The use of breast-conserving surgery, radiation therapy, and other services varies among hospitals of different sizes, location, and teaching status. The effect of hospital volume on long-term survival was examined in a study of breast cancer surgery performed in New York hospitals.

Methods.—The study cohort consisted of 47,890 women hospitalized for breast cancer between 1984 and 1989. Excluded from the cohort were patients whose records showed race other than white or black, race unknown, invalid geographic information, and/or unknown stage of cancer. Data from the New York State Cancer Registry and Social Security Administration death files identified 6,952 deaths resulting from breast cancers. The 266 hospitals in the state that perform breast cancer surgery were classified according to volume: very low (10/yr), low (11–50/yr), moderate (51–150/yr), and high (more than 150/yr). Age was categorized as younger than 50 years, 50 through 64 years, 65 through 74 years, and older than 75 years. Socioeconomic status was classified as low, middle, or high.

Results.—Five-year survival was significantly higher for patients receiving care at high-volume hospitals, and this was the case for each cancer stage: in situ, localized, regional, and metastatic. Although teaching status was closely and positively related to high volume, teaching status did not yield additional survival advantage. Patients receiving care at very low-volume hospitals had a 60% higher risk of death than patients receiving care at high-volume hospitals. Risks of dying were also increased at low- and moderate-volume hospitals vs. high-volume hospitals and in women aged 75 years or older. After adjustment for cancer stage and other variables, women in the oldest age group had a 60% higher risk of death when treated with breast-conserving surgery rather than with a mastectomy. Other factors associated with increased risk of death were advanced cancer stage, comorbid conditions, black race, and low socioeconomic status.

Conclusions.—The effect of high hospital surgical volume on 5-year breast cancer survival was large and clinically significant. This effect was consistent across all cancer stages and after adjustment for many relevant risk factors. The risk ratios of the 4 hospital volume categories had narrow confidence intervals with almost no overlap, supporting a distinct dose-response effect of volume on survival.

▶ These are scary findings because the number of cases in "low volume" hospitals is similar to that in countless small hospitals across the country. This study joins a growing number (and we should expect many more) linking hospital characteristics to the outcomes of care. We are already seeing studies examining the next level down of outcomes attributable to individual physicians and surgeons. The impact of measuring and reporting outcomes on the eventual configuration of our health care system cannot be overstated. Studies like this one make it very, very clear that lives are at stake and that hospitals (and physicians) will be accountable.

A.O. Berg, M.D., M.P.H.

Effect of Nancy Reagan's Mastectomy on Choice of Surgery for Breast Cancer by US Women
Nattinger AB, Hoffmann RG, Howell-Pelz A, et al (Med College of Wisconsin, Milwaukee; Univ of Texas, Galveston)
JAMA 279:762–766, 1998

15–7

Introduction.—The influence of public figures on popular behavior is well known. It is believed that celebrities can influence health care behavior, thus we see celebrity endorsements for promoting safe sex and avoiding illegal drugs. There is little documentation regarding the effect of celebrity role models on medical care or health behaviors. There was a sharp drop in breast-conserving surgery (BCS) in late 1987 that was not related to any publications in the medical literature or lay press that questioned the effectiveness of BCS. It was associated with the choice of a modified radical mastectomy after open biopsy for Nancy Reagan on October 17, 1987. Reported is the first known investigation of the influence of a celebrity (Reagan) on national medical practice (treatment of breast cancer).

Methods.—Data on 82,230 women, aged 30 years and older, with diagnoses of local or regional breast cancer was taken from the Surveillance, Epidemiology, and End Results tumor registry from 1983 to 1990. The other data source was Medicare Part A, from which information was gathered regarding 80,057 women, aged 65–79 years, who received inpatient surgery for local or regional breast cancer in 1987 or 1988. The percentage of BCS use vs. mastectomy over time was assessed.

Results.—Compared with the situation in the quarter before Reagan's mastectomy, women were 25% less likely to undergo BCS in the 2 quarters after her operation. The BCS rate returned to baseline in subsequent quarters. The reduction in BCS was significant in white women and was most prominent in women aged 50–79 years living in the central and southern regions of the United States. It was most sustained in women living in areas with lower levels of income and education.

Conclusion.—This example of the influence of Nancy Reagan's mastectomy on choice of surgery for breast cancer in women in the United States suggests that medical care can be influenced substantially by celebrity role models. This is particularly true among persons who demographically resemble the celebrity and those of lower income and educational status.

▶ This article confirms the fact that our patients are paying attention to the health problems of celebrities. We can all recall events that seem to have increased (if only temporarily) attention to problems ranging from prostate cancer screening to HIV infection to depression and suicide to alcohol and drug abuse. It is quite rare to have data documenting the size of the effect. Note, however, that the percent reduction is based on a relatively small baseline percentage, making the results ("a 25% reduction") sound more impressive than they are. The absolute reduction was on the order of 5%. I take from this that physicians need to be paying attention to the health problems of celebrities because their patients are doing so.

A.O. Berg, M.D., M.P.H.

Breast Cancer Survival and Treatment in Health Maintenance Organization and Fee-for-service Settings
Potosky AL, Merrill RM, Riley GF, et al (Natl Cancer Inst, Bethesda, Md; Health Care Financing Administration, Baltimore, Md; Group Health Cooperative of Puget Sound, Seattle; et al)
J Natl Cancer Inst 89:1683–1691, 1997   15–8

Background.—As more patients receive their health care via HMOs, data are becoming available for comparison with the traditional fee-for-service (FFS) system. Ten-year survival rates and types of treatment for women with breast cancer who were enrolled in an HMO or an FFS system were compared.

Methods.—The 13,358 women enrolled (all 65 years of age) had been treated for primary breast cancer between 1985 and 1992. For HMO enrollees, tumor registries were reviewed to identify 1,424 subjects from the San Francisco-Oakland area and 580 subjects from the Seattle-Puget Sound area. Medicare records from these 2 areas were reviewed to identify 5,752 and 5,602 subjects respectively in the FFS system. The data were adjusted for tumor stage, comorbid conditions, and sociodemographic factors to allow comparisons of differences in survival and in treatment between the 2 health care systems.

Findings.—Subjects in HMOs tended to be younger at diagnosis and the breast cancer was significantly more likely to be diagnosed at an earlier tumor stage than for patients in the FFS setting. Diagnosis with stage 1 disease occurred in 47% of HMO subjects in both geographic areas, and in 43% of FFS subjects in San Francisco-Oakland and 37% of FFS subjects in Seattle-Puget Sound. Subjects in the FFS system were significantly more likely to have comorbid conditions (12% to 13%) than those in the HMO (slightly more than 8%). Breast-conserving surgery occurred significantly more often in subjects in HMOs than in patients in FFS systems (odds ratios, 1.55 for San Francisco-Oakland and 3.39 in Seattle-Puget Sound). Furthermore, subjects undergoing breast-conserving surgery were significantly more likely to receive radiotherapy if they were enrolled in an HMO (odds ratios 2.49 in San Francisco-Oakland and 4.62 in Seattle-Puget Sound). The HMO:FFS ratio of cancer-related mortality risk was 0.71 in the San Francisco-Oakland area and 1.01 in Seattle-Puget Sound area.

Conclusions.—Treatment differences favored the HMO system over the FFS system. Women in HMOs typically were treated at an earlier age and disease stage, more often underwent breast-conserving therapy, and more often received adjuvant radiotherapy. Furthermore, long-term survival for subjects in the HMO system was at least as good as that for subjects in the FFS system. These data provide reassurance about patient care outcomes in managed care settings.

▶ Managed care organizations (MCOs) have been hammered over the last couple of years around many issues, especially those related to "customer" satisfaction. Legislators at state and federal levels are falling all over themselves passing laws that would change the way MCOs work and interact with the public. In all the controversy, we need to be sure that we not lose sight of the fact that MCOs do some things very well and at lower cost. This study persuasively shows that outcomes for breast cancer are, if anything, better in MCOs than in the private sector. One can be sure that there is an opportunity cost if MCOs maintain outcomes at lower cost; something has to "give." One of the big debates in the next few years is how much patients are willing to "pay" in foregone services and amenities to save money on their health care insurance, provided that outcomes can be maintained.

A.O. Berg, M.D., M.P.H.

Sonographic Features of Mammary Oil Cysts

Harvey JA, Moran RE, Maurer EJ, et al (Univ of Virginia, Charlottesville)
J Ultrasound Med 16:719–724, 1997   15–9

Objective.—Mammary oil cysts form when fat cells are disrupted, usually by injury, resulting in formation of a macroscopic pool of oil. Inflammation and later fibrosis develop. On mammography oil cysts appear as a radiolucent mass. Their appearance on sonography has been less well studied. Results of a retrospective review of the sonographic appearance of mammary oil cysts and of the role of ultrasonography in evaluation are discussed.

Methods.—Between 1988 and 1995, sonograms were performed on 15 patients with oil cysts in 26 breasts. Lesion echogenicity, wall appearance, and presence of posterior acoustic enhancement or shadowing were reviewed and compared by 3 radiologists.

Results.—Three patients had a sonogram to evaluate radiodense mammographic nodules, and 12 had a palpable mass, 8 with a history of surgery or trauma. Ultrasonography was performed in 7 patients to evaluate a lump when mammography was not definitive. Five patients had ultrasonography performed before mammography for a palpable mass. Oil cysts had a variable appearance. Two looked like simple apocrine cysts having posterior acoustic enhancement, and 3 had anechoic portions mimicking an intracystic mass. Most oil cysts were hypoechoic (65%), had smooth walls (88%), and no posterior characteristics (50%).

Conclusion.—The sonographic appearance of mammographic oil cysts is variable and may resemble that of an intracystic mass. A circumscribed hypoechoic mass without acoustic enhancement is characteristic of an oil cyst, particularly when the patient has a history of breast injury or trauma.

▶ I included this article because I did not know about mammary oil cysts. The authors saw 26 in 7 years at the University of Virginia, which would make the condition uncommon, but not rare. Three of the patients had no recalled trauma, but the condition is generally seen after trauma and is benign. If the patient did know of trauma, it would be important to let the reading/performing physician be aware of that.

M.A. Bowman, M.D., M.P.A.

Cervical Cancer

Cervical Cancer Screening Among Women With and Without Hysterectomies

Eaker ED, Vierkant RA, Konitzer KA, et al (Univ of Wisconsin, Madison)
Obstet Gynecol 91:551–555, 1998   15–10

Objective.—Whether women who have had a hysterectomy benefit from Pap testing is controversial. The rates of Pap testing in women with a total hysterectomy for various reasons were compared with rates for women who had not had a hysterectomy.

Methods.—In a retrospective study of a cohort of age-matched women with and without hysterectomy in the Marshfield Epidemiologic Study Area, the annual Papanicolaou test rate for women with total hysterectomy for benign reasons (n = 197), total hysterectomy for malignancy (n = 75), supracervical hysterectomy (n = 43), and no hysterectomy (n = 315) were compared.

Results.—Women having hysterectomy because of malignancy were significantly older than women having hysterectomy for benign conditions. The mean follow-up was 5.4 years for women with hysterectomies for benign conditions, 5.2 years for malignant conditions, and 29.3 years for supracervical hysterectomies. Women aged 45 years or less with hysterectomies for malignant reasons had a significantly higher Pap test rate (0.79 tests per year) than women having hysterectomies for benign reasons (0.29 tests per year) and a nonsignificantly higher test rate than women with supracervical hysterectomies. For older women, the rates were significantly different (0.45 [malignancy], 0.19 [benign] and 1.39 [supracervical] tests per year. Women with hysterectomies for benign conditions had significantly fewer tests (mean difference, −0.34 tests per year) compared with women having a hysterectomy for malignancy (mean difference, 0.87 tests per year) and unexposed women (mean difference, −0.03 tests/year).

Conclusion.—Although women with hysterectomies for benign conditions had significantly fewer Pap tests than women with hysterectomies for malignant conditions, they are probably receiving 2 or 3 times as many Pap tests as are needed.

▶ More than 50% of women who have had hysterectomies for benign reasons were receiving unnecessary Pap smears. This does not surprise me, because it is what I have seen in practice. I know I sometimes do these unnecessary tests myself, usually because patients so strongly believe they should get them (ingrained over many years of seeing physicians annually for Pap smears). Another reason is the woman's uncertainty of the reason for the hysterectomy. I also perform Pap smears on women who have a history of abnormal Pap smears without actual cervical cancer; I am not sure if this is appropriate or not.

M.A. Bowman, M.D., M.P.A.

Cost-Effectiveness Analysis of Diagnosis and Management of Cervical Squamous Intraepithelial Lesions
Cantor SB, Mitchell MF, Tortolero-Luna G, et al (Univ of Texas, Houston; Univ of Texas, Austin)
Obstet Gynecol 91:270–277, 1998
15–11

Objective.—Although colposcopy is the treatment of choice, because of its sensitivity, for women with abnormal Papanicolaou smear tests, it shows poor specificity. Fluorescence spectroscopy is being tested as a tool for diagnosing cervical precancer. Five strategies for diagnosis and treatment of cervical squamous intraepithelial lesions (SILs) were compared for cost-effectiveness using a decision-analytic model.

Methods.—The strategies were (1) the cost-effectiveness of colposcopy followed by loop electrosurgical excision procedure (LEEP) if high-grade SILs were found on second-visit biopsy; (2) see-and-treat colposcopy (using LEEP on first visit, if necessary); (3) spectroscopically directed biopsy if high-grade SILs were found on second-visit biopsy; (4) see-and-treat spectroscopy (using LEEP on first visit; similar to see-and-treat colposcopy); and (5) see-and-treat spectroscopy and colposcopy together and treatment with LEEP in 1 visit. The number of appropriately treated, inappropriately treated, or missed patients were determined in a hypothetical cohort of 100 patients with an abnormal Papanicolaou test.

Results.—See-and-treat spectroscopy was the least expensive, and the least effective strategy costing $160,479 to detect accurately 31.55 per 100 patients with precervical cancer. Colposcopy-directed biopsy was the most expensive strategy costing $311,808 to detect 45.78 per 100 patients. Adding the see-and-treat option to both techniques increased the effectiveness to 46.05 per 100 patients at a cost of $285,133. Compared with see-and-treat spectroscopy, the combination of see-and-treat colposcopy and spectroscopy showed weak dominance, whereas colposcopy showed strong dominance (i.e., an unusually high cost-effectiveness ratio). The incremental cost-effectiveness ratio for see-and-treat spectroscopy and colposcopy was $8,596 per patient with cervical precancer. Sensitivity analysis using fluorescence spectroscopy demonstrated a significant cost-savings.

Conclusion.—The specificity of colposcopy and savings per patient diagnosed with precervical cancer are improved when followed by fluorescence spectroscopy. Fluorescence spectroscopy increases the diagnostic efficacy of precervical cancer at a significant cost saving.

▶ The treatment of cervical lesions has become very expensive and time consuming with the new technologies of colposcopy, LEEP, and other modalities. Women with low-grade cervical pathology are frequently visiting physicians every few months for expensive procedures resulting in yearly health care costs exceeding the national average for all patients. This study addresses the cost-effectiveness of management of cervical SIL lesions and recommends spectroscopy as a less expensive alternative. The diagnosis and management of cervical lesions is an area that is evolving and requires further study in a primary care setting to achieve the right balance of patient observation and intervention.

J.E. Scherger, M.D., M.P.H.

A Randomized Controlled Trial to Evaluate the Use of the Endocervical Brush After Endocervical Curettage

Tate KM, Strickland JL (Univ of Missouri Kansas City School of Medicine)
Obstet Gynecol 90:715–717, 1997
15–12

Introduction.—To evaluate the presence of disease in the endocervical canal, endocervical curettage, usually with the Kevorkian endocervical curette, is performed. Up to 28% of the time, however, this curette is inadequate for such evaluation. Insufficient sampling results in increased cost and inconvenience for the patient. An effective tool for increasing adequacy of a Papanicolaou smear is the endocervical brush. With the endocervical brush, the rate of inadequate sampling is 8.5% or less. A study was conducted to determine whether use of the endocervical brush increases the yield of endocervical tissue on an endocervical curettage specimen.

Methods.—There were 124 women with abnormal Papanicolaou smears who underwent colposcopy and biopsy. The Kevorkian endocervical curette was used to perform endocervical curettages. Endocervical curettage tissue was then collected with either a curette (62 women) or an endocervical brush (62 women). Pathologists reviewed the specimens.

Results.—In the women who had sampling with a curette (the control group), 6 of the 58 endocervical curettage specimens contained insufficient endocervical tissue for pathologic diagnosis. None of the samples from the endocervical brush group were insufficient. There was a statistically significant difference between the 2 groups.

Conclusion.—The number of insufficient samples was decreased by adding use of the endocervical brush to endocervical tissue sampling at colposcopy. A valuable addition to this diagnostic tool is the endocervical brush method of collection of an endocervical curettage specimen from the canal after use of the Kevorkian curette. The use of this brush for obtaining an endocervical curettage specimen, is recommended. The number of insufficient samples was decreased from 10% to 0% when use of the endocervical brush was added to endocervical tissue sampling.

▶ Although I have not seen another study to verify the findings of the authors, their method seems simple, straightforward, and quite effective. After using the curette to collect an endocervical sample during colposcopy, the authors simply used a standard endocervical brush to collect the specimen from the canal, rather than relying on the curette alone. With this method, none of the patients had an inadequate sample from the endocervical curettage. Although only a small percentage of the patients agreed to enter the study (for reasons unclear to me), I cannot think of how this would have affected the study outcome, as those who agreed to participate were randomized in a standard fashion. Thus, I think it is reasonable to incorporate this method into practice now.

M.A. Bowman, M.D., M.P.A.

Efforts to Improve the Follow-up of Patients With Abnormal Papanicolaou Test Results

Block B, Branham RA (Shadyside Hosp, Pittsburgh, Pa)
J Am Board Fam Pract 11:1–11, 1998

Background.—Following up women with abnormal Papanicolaou test results can be difficult. Return rates for repeat testing and colposcopy are poor. The efficacy of a protocol consisting of educational input, logistic

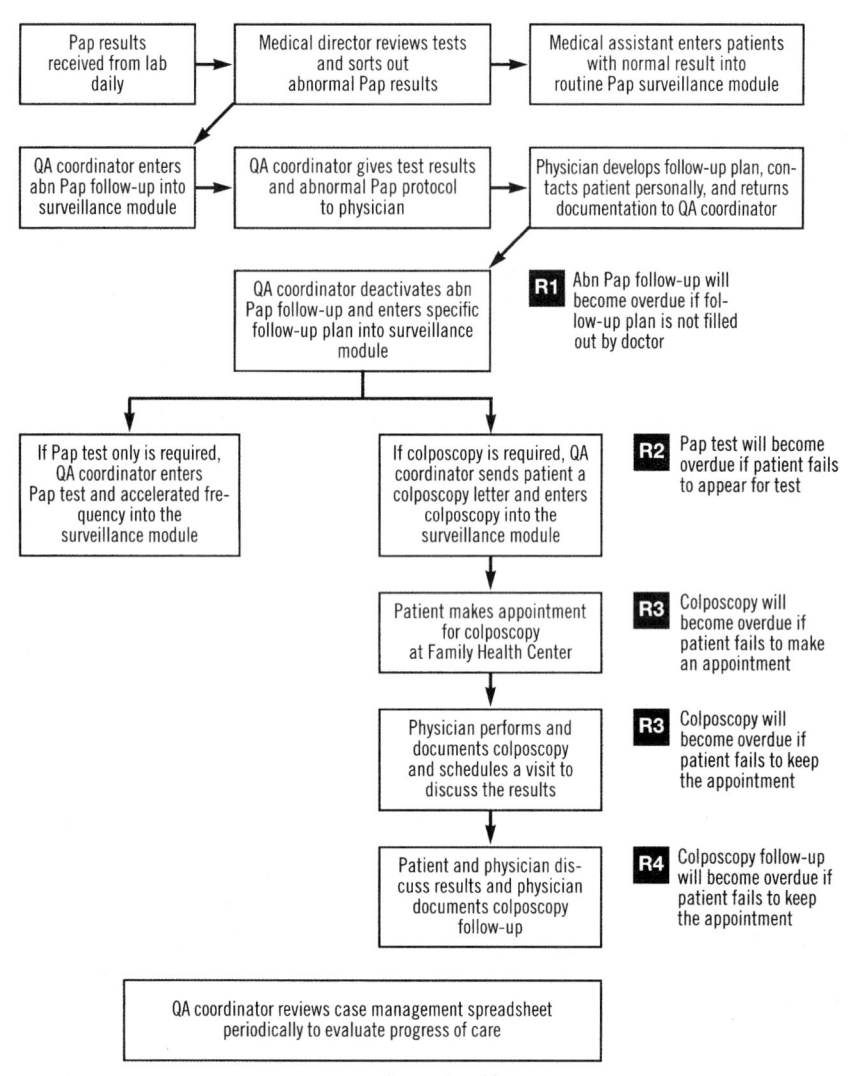

FIGURE 2.—Case management system used in study. *Abbreviations: Pap*, Papanicolaou, *QA*, quality assessment, *abn*, abnormal. (Courtesy of Block B, Branham RA: Efforts to improve the follow-up of patients with abnormal Papanicolaou test results. *J Am Board Fam Pract* 11:1–11, 1998.)

aids, transportation assistance, and automated prompting in improving follow-up care of women with abnormal Papanicolaou test results was reported.

Methods.—Of 1,796 women undergoing Papanicolaou testing between 1994 and 1996, 147 (8%) had abnormal findings. Eighty-three percent had dysplasia; 16%, atypia; and 1%, carcinoma in situ. All patients were followed up according to protocol.

Findings.—The overall success and colposcopy rates markedly increased. In 1990, before the protocol was implemented, 36% of patients with abnormal results were overdue for follow-up, compared with only 13% in 1996. Twenty percent of patients assigned to repeat Papanicolaou testing failed to return, compared with 10% assigned to colposcopy. At the colposcopy clinic, missed appointments dropped from 56% in 1993 to 12% in 1996. Colposcopic biopsy was found to be much more effective than Papanicolaou testing for detecting precursors of cervical cancer at follow-up (Fig 2).

Conclusion.—The new protocol dramatically improved the outcome of this cervical cancer screening program. Educational programs, formalized approaches to care, transportation assistance, and reminder systems were an integral part of this successful protocol.

▶ I spend a good deal of time giving talks about the science of prevention, tirelessly pointing out that the science is only the first step. The real challenge is turning the science into effective practice. This article documents the success of an aggressive program to improve Papanicolaou smear follow-up, using an automated system that most group practices should be able to emulate. The full flow diagram is reproduced in Figure 2, which is taken from the article. Much of the arguing about prevention has to do with which services should be offered, ignoring the fact that there are no physician practices achieving 100% success in preventive interventions that everyone already agrees on, like Papanicolaou smears. This study shows that a well-managed approach can lead to dramatic improvements.

A.O. Berg, M.D., M.P.H.

False Positive Cervicovaginal Cytology: A Follow-up Study
Anderson MB, Jones BA (St John Hosp, Detroit)
Acta Cytol 41:1697–1700, 1997
15–14

Background.—Although colposcopic biopsy is the standard by which cervicovaginal cytologic findings are judged, errors can occur. Follow-up data were obtained for patients initially classified as having false positive results when subsequent cervical biopsy did not detect abnormality, to determine whether later studies did reveal abnormalities.

Study Design.—All patients who had cervical biopsy between January 1990 and December 1992 within 3 months of cytology were reviewed.

TABLE 1.—Cervicovaginal Cytology and Histology Results After Noncorrelating Smear and Biopsy of 53 Patients With Follow-up

Diagnosis	Cytology n	(%)	Histology n	(%)
WNL or benign cellular changes	24*	(45)	2†	(4)
ASCUS	9	(17)	0	
SIL of indeterminate degree	5	(9)	4	(7)
LSIL	9	(17)	6	(11)
HSIL	5	(9)	7	(13)

Note: Twelve patients had both positive cytologic and histologic results.
*Four patients with negative cytologic findings had positive biopsy results.
†Both patients had positive follow-up cytologic findings.
Abbreviations: WNL, within normal limits; ASCUS, atypical squamous cells of undetermined significance; SIL, squamous intraepithelial lesion; LSIL, low-grade SIL; HSIL, high-grade SIL.
(Courtesy of Anderson MB, Jones BA: False positive cervicovaginal cytology: A follow-up study Acta Cytol 41:1697–1700, 1997.)

Cases with positive cytology and negative biopsy findings were identified. Follow-up diagnostic studies were obtained from medical records.

Findings.—From January 1990 to December 1992, 31,233 cervicovaginal cytology specimens were processed. A colposcopic biopsy was performed within 3 months in 1,242 cases. Of these, 68 were considered to be cytologic false positive results. Follow-up cytologic or histologic studies were available for 53 of these patients. Of those 53 patients, 33 had subsequent positive findings. This group included 24 patients with squamous intraepithelial lesion, which indicated a sampling error at initial biopsy, and 9 with atypical squamous cells of unknown significance (Table 1).

Conclusions.—In this study group, 45% of those patients who were initially categorized as having false positive cytologic and biopsy findings had subsequent evidence of squamous intraepithelial lesion. Follow-up remains important for patients with a discrepancy between cervical cytologic findings and initial biopsy findings, because many of these patients have abnormalities that are revealed on subsequent studies.

▶ I feel the authors modestly overstate their results. From my perspective, follow-up cervical smears with squamous intraepithelial lesions remain insufficient to say that the original biopsy was wrong—biopsy evidence should still be the gold standard, although not necessarily realistic in practice as it might require conization or hysterectomy. Their methodology did not use a gold standard, but the intermediary of colposcopic biopsy or cervical smear. However, I do agree with the authors' conclusions that patients with positive cervical smears and negative biopsy results may well have positive biopsy results in the relatively short-term future and need "diligent follow-up." The quick appearance of positive results of biopsy may result from original biopsy sampling errors, from interpretive errors, or because these high-risk patients subsequently have new areas of abnormalities. Patients with "false positive" smears should have careful follow-up, often requiring additional biopsies.

M.A. Bowman, M.D., M.P.A.

Order of Endocervical and Ectocervical Cytologic Sampling and the Quality of the Papanicolaou Smear

Eisenberger D, Hernandez E, Tener T, et al (Allegheny Univ, Philadelphia)
Obstet Gynecol 90:755–758, 1997
15–15

Objective.—Whether the order in which endocervical and ectocervical samples are collected affects the quality of the smear has not been studied well. Whether the order of cell collection influences the proportion of smears with air-drying artifact, the number of smears obscured by blood, or the endocervical cell detection rate was investigated.

Methods.—Five hundred brush-first smears and 500 spatula-first smears were collected and reviewed by in-house cytotechnologists. Abnormal slides were reevaluated.

Results.—Smears were considered limited for interpretation if they did not contain endocervical cells or mucus, if they were obscured by blood, if they were too thick, if there was inflammation, or if there was an air-drying artifact. There were 405 (81%) adequate brush-first smears and 410 (82%) spatula-first smears. The brush-first groups had significantly more smears satisfactory but obscured by blood (n = 22) than did the spatula-first group (n = 3). In the spatula-first group, there were significantly more low-grade or high-grade squamous intraepithelial lesions (n = 55, 11%) than in the brush-first group (n = 35, 7%).

Conclusion.—Better quality (fewer smears obscured by blood) Papanicolaou smears are obtained first with the use of the Ayre spatula, and then with the use of the endocervical brush.

▶ I have experimented with the order of the cytologic sampling myself, and decided that it usually worked better to do the cytobrush last. What I noticed is that there was frequently bleeding from the cytobrush, making it difficult to ensure adequate sampling. However, these authors found no difference in the rate of adequate smears, only in the rate of squamous intraepithelial lesions. Whether the higher rate of squamous intraepithelial lesions noted with the spatula-first group resulted from obscuring blood in the cytobrush-first group, the methodology of varying the sampling by season of the year, or some other reason, is unclear to me. I hope additional work will be done to verify that the spatula-first increases the rate of detection of important lesions.

M.A. Bowman, M.D., M.P.A.

PAPNET-assisted Rescreening of Cervical Smears: Cost and Accuracy Compared With a 100% Manual Rescreening Strategy

O'Leary TJ, Tellado M, Buckner S-B, et al (Armed Forces Inst of Pathology, Washington, DC)
JAMA 279:235–237, 1998

Objective.—Because a significant number of cervical abnormalities are missed in conventional cytologic examinations, new cost-effective, more specific, and more sensitive cervical cancer screening techniques are needed. Results are presented of a study assessing the effectiveness and cost-effectiveness of a computer-assisted rescreening system (PAPNET, Neuromedical Systems Inc., Suffern, NY)) in identifying cellular abnormalities in Pap smears previously diagnosed as "within normal limits" or "benign cellular changes" after both primary screening and a second manual rescreening, and comparing this cost with that of completely manual rescreening.

Methods.—PAPNET was used to rescreen 5,478 Pap smears of female Air Force service members and dependents, aged 12 to 88, taken between 1994 and 1995. Rescreened Pap smears reclassified as abnormal were evaluated by a consensus panel of 3 pathologists and 3 cytotechnologists. The proportion of PAPNET smears designated and confirmed as abnormal and the costs of rescreening were determined.

Results.—Of the 1,614 (29%) slides requiring rescreening, 448 (8%) were designated as possibly abnormal. Eleven of these smears were reviewed again by the consensus panel, and 5 were reclassified as atypical squamous cells of undetermined significance (ASCUS) and 1 as atypical glandular cells of undetermined significance (AGCUS). In the latter case, 2 subsequent Pap smears showed low-grade squamous intraepithelial neoplasia. Two women whose smears were designated ASCUS subsequently had normal Pap smears. The remaining 3 could not be located. Manual screening took 3 times as long as PAPNET screening. It cost $5,825 to $33,781 for each additional ASCUS or AGCUS finding and $17,475 to $101,343 for each additional case of low-grade squamous intraepithelial neoplasia diagnosed.

Conclusion.—PAPNET identified a few more cases of cervical cancer than did manual screening but at a significant cost.

▶ We need a cervical cancer screening technique that has improved specificity and lower cost, not just increased sensitivity with higher cost and little change in outcome. Thus, I have not yet been impressed with the various new screening techniques that have recently arisen, and this article reinforces that PAPNET is not worth the cost and effort for the bulk of cervical cancer screening. I found it interesting that PAPNET did not always find endocervical cells when they were present. I agree with the authors that what we most need to improve cervical cancer screening is to do Pap smears on women who have not had them.

M.A. Bowman, M.D., M.P.A.

Polycystic Ovary Syndrome

Late Endocrine Effects of Ovarian Electrocautery in Women With Polycystic Ovary Syndrome

Gjønnæss H (Aker Univ Hosp, Oslo, Norway)
Fertil Steril 69:697–701, 1998   15–17

Introduction.—Since the original description of ovarian electrocautery, pregnancy rates near 80% were found in women with polycystic ovary syndrome, and successful ovulation was up to 96%, with resultant decreases in serum concentrations of androgens and luteinizing hormones. The duration of the endocrine changes produced by ovarian electrocautery in women with polycystic ovary syndrome was examined. It was also determined whether late endocrine changes were dependent on body weight.

Methods.—Through the laparoscope, ovarian electrocautery was performed on 165 infertile women with polycystic ovary syndrome. Before the operation and at defined intervals thereafter, blood was sampled. Sampling was performed 1 week before the menstrual period after the establishment of regular cycles. Determinations were made of serum concentrations of hypophyseal and ovarian hormones, including sex hormone-binding globulin.

Results.—A significant decrease in androgens and gonadotropins was seen after ovarian electrocautery for polycystic ovary syndrome, and there was a clear shift from anovulation to ovulatory cycles. There was an increase in sex hormone-binding globulin. The effects were seen to continue for many years. Two thirds of the women were still ovulating after 18–20 years. In normal-weight women, the ovulation rate did not differ significantly from that in overweight women, and the rates were practically identical after 10–20 years (Table 1).

Conclusion.—Ovarian function, including androgen production, is normalized with ovarian electrocautery for polycystic ovary syndrome. The

TABLE 1.—Body Weight and Persistence of Ovulation After Ovarian Electrocautery

Observation Period	Normal Weight	Overweight	All	P Value
3 mo	78 (21/27)	65 (13/20)	72 (34/47)	NS
1 y	89 (24/27)	65 (11/17)	80 (35/44)	NS
3 y	79 (19/24)	50 (10/20)	66 (29/44)	<0.05
10 y	68 (17/25)	71 (12/17)	69 (29/42)	NS
>10 y	80 (12/15)	69 (11/16)	74 (23/31)	NS

Percent ovulation rate*

*Numbers in parentheses represent total number of ovulators/total number of women in the observation periods.
Abbreviation: NS, not significant.
(Courtesy of Gjønnæss H: Late endocrine effects of ovarian electrocautery in women with polycystic ovary syndrome. *Fertil Steril* 69:697–701. Copyright 1998, with kind permission from Elsevier Science Ltd, The Boulevard, Langford Lane, Kidlington OX5 1GB.)

results seem to be stable for 18–20 years. Ovarian electrocautery did not appear to increase the risk of early menopause.

▶ It is not clear when we should use electrocautery of the ovary for polycystic ovary syndrome. I was impressed that so many patients had normalized ovarian function, including long-term decreases in androgens, and a fairly high fertility rate, for 18–20 years. Electrocautery is supposed to create fewer adhesions than the former wedge resections have. Unfortunately, the authors did not report on the rate of obesity, diabetes, or cholesterol abnormalities. If these rates also normalized, should we use the procedure early, and not only as a late therapy for those patients wishing fertility?

M.A. Bowman, M.D., M.P.A.

Metformin Therapy Improves the Menstrual Pattern With Minimal Endocrine and Metabolic Effects in Women With Polycystic Ovary Syndrome
Morin-Papunen LC, Koivunen RM, Ruokonen A, et al (Univ Central Hosp of Oulu, Finland)
Fertil Steril 69:691–696, 1998 15–18

Introduction.—Characterized by chronic anovulation, elevated androgen levels, signs of hyperandrogenism, enlarged cystic ovaries, and obesity, polycystic ovary syndrome may also cause metabolic disturbances. Decreased insulin sensitivity was found among lean and obese women with polycystic ovary syndrome. A previous study of only 8 weeks' duration showed an improvement in insulin sensitivity, associated with decreases in serum luteinizing hormone and androgens, in women with polycystic ovary syndrome. In obese women with polycystic ovary syndrome, the clinical, hormonal, and biochemical effects of 4–6 months of metformin therapy were determined.

Methods.—Twenty obese women with polycystic ovary syndrome were treated with 0.5 g of metformin 3 times daily for 4–6 months. During the treatment, assessments of clinical symptoms, menstrual pattern, and hirsutism, as well as serum concentrations of sex steroids, sex hormone-binding globulin, gonadotropins, and lipids, were made.

Results.—During therapy, more regular cycles were experienced by 11 women (68.8% of the women with menstrual disturbances). There were no changes in body mass index, blood pressure, or hirsutism. After 2 months of treatment, the mean testosterone level decreased significantly, but by 4–6 months it had returned to the starting level. Free testosterone levels decreased significantly during the treatment. In the levels of other sex steroids or lipids measured at 4–6 months of treatment, there were no significant changes.

Conclusion.—The majority of women tolerate metformin therapy well. Especially in obese women with polycystic ovary syndrome, and in those who have menstrual disturbances, metformin therapy may be clinically useful. With regard to testosterone levels, the effect may be transitory, and women with hirsutism did not seem to benefit from metformin therapy.

▶ Metformin seems to be a potentially attractive therapy for the insulin-resistance often seen in polycystic ovary syndrome. Based on some earlier reports, I had selectively used metformin for patients and found, as these authors did, that the patients had more normalized periods. This therapy seems preferable to using recurrent progesterone or birth control pills to help prevent the endometrial cancer that can go with prolonged absence of menses in polycystic ovary syndrome with hyperstimulation of the uterus. I was hoping that metformin might also help with obesity or lipid abnormalities, but this study of 20 patients did not confirm these potentials. Nor was hirsutism improved. It would seem that metformin may prevent or delay the onset of diabetes in these patients, but this is not yet known. Of course, a return of menstruation may mean a return of fertility, and metformin would not be recommended early in pregnancy; thus, fertility issues must be considered carefully.

M.A. Bowman, M.D., M.P.A.

Premenstrual Syndrome

Symptomatic Improvement of Premenstrual Dysphoric Disorder With Sertraline Treatment: A Randomized Controlled Trial
Yonkers KA, for the Sertraline Premenstrual Dysphoric Collaborative Study Group (Univ of Texas, Dallas; Univ of Buffalo, NY; Univ of Pennsylvania, Philadelphia; et al)
JAMA 278:983–988, 1997
15–19

Objective.—Premenstrual dysphoric disorder (PMDD) includes psychological symptoms of depression, anxiety, and mood swings that can be severe enough to lead to functional impairment in 3% to 5% of menstruating women. Selective serotonin reuptake inhibitors (SSRIs) have been shown to be effective in combating depressive symptoms. The efficacy of sertraline, an SSRI, in the treatment of mood, behavioral, and physical symptoms of PMDD and in changing functional impairment was investigated in a large multisite, randomized, double-blind, placebo-controlled trial.

Methods.—Women aged 24–45 years at 12 university-affiliated outpatient psychiatric and gynecology clinics underwent 2 screening cycles (n = 447) and 1 cycle of single-blind placebo (n = 277). Those with a diagnosis of PMDD of 2 years or more were randomly allocated to receive either placebo (n = 122) or sertraline hydrochloride (50–150 mg/day) (n = 121), beginning on day 1 of menses and continuing throughout the cycle. Outcome was measured using The Daily Record of Severity of Problems, Hamilton Rating Scale for Depression, Clinical Global Impression Scale, and Social Adjustment Scale.

Results.—Two hundred women completed the study. On patients' self-reports, the sertraline group showed significantly more improvement than did the placebo group with daily symptom scores decreasing by 32% and 11%, depressive symptoms improving by 32% and 13%, and physical symptoms improving by 32% and 8%. The sertraline group showed significantly more improvement than the placebo group in functional impairment (38% vs. 13%), interference with hobbies and social activities (38% vs. 17%), and problems in relationships (42% vs. 15%). Treatment-related adverse events were reported by 75% of the sertraline group and 58% of the placebo group and resulted in the withdrawal of 8% and 2%, respectively. The sertraline group had significantly more nausea, diarrhea, and decreased libido than did the placebo group.

Conclusion.—Women treated for PMDD with sertraline had significant improvement in depressive and physical symptoms and in feelings of anger and irritability.

▶ Chalk up another potential indication for use of the SSRI antidepressants. Note that the study sample was taken from volunteers recruited through advertising and from referrals, and that more than half indicating interest did not meet study criteria. Although sertraline was certainly more effective than placebo (32% vs. 8% amelioration of symptoms), it is also true that more than two thirds of the patients did not benefit. This and the need to take the medication constantly to prevent symptoms that are intermittent are important disincentives for using it as a first-line treatment.

A.O. Berg, M.D., M.P.H.

Calcium Carbonate and the Premenstrual Syndrome: Effects on Premenstrual and Menstrual Symptoms
Thys-Jacobs S, and the Premenstrual Syndrome Study Group (St. Luke's-Roosevelt Hosp Ctr, NY)
Am J Obstet Gynecol 179:444–452, 1998   15–20

Background.—Recently, it has been suggested that calcium deficiency may underlie premenstrual syndrome (PMS) and that calcium supplementation may be therapeutic for PMS symptoms. A trial was undertaken to evaluate the efficacy of calcium carbonate as a treatment for the symptoms of PMS.

Methods.—Healthy, premenopausal women, aged 18 to 45 years, were recruited from 12 health centers to participate in a randomized, double-blind, placebo-controlled study of the effect of calcium supplementation on the symptoms of PMS. Participants were screened for willingness to comply and PMS severity. Each of 720 women were then prospectively screened during 2 menstrual cycles for good general health; normal laboratory findings; regular menstrual cycles; discontinuance of use of analgesics; and the occurence of PMS, using the PMS diary. The 497 women who were admitted to the treatment phase of the trial were randomized to receive 1,200 mg elemental calcium per day (TUMS E-X) or placebo for 3 menstrual cycles. Participants recorded daily symptoms, symptom severity, medication compliance, side effects, and menstrual bleeding. They were contacted biweekly by telephone and through monthly follow-up visits. All 466 participants with a valid screening and treatment cycle were included in the efficacy analysis. The primary outcome measure was the symptom complex score. The primary efficacy measure was the difference between the symptom complex score with treatment vs. placebo. There were no demographic or symptomatic differences between the 2 groups.

Results.—During the luteal phase of the treatment cycle, there was a significantly lower average symptom complex score in the calcium-treated group for the second and third treatment cycles—especially the third—compared with the placebo group. By the third treatment cycle, calcium treatment resulted in an overall 48% reduction from baseline in the total and individual symptom scores. There was also a 30% reduction in PMS symptoms in the placebo group in the third menstrual cycle.

Conclusion.—This large trial showed that calcium carbonate was effective for treatment of the symptoms of PMS. Calcium supplementation should be considered a therapeutic alternative in the management of PMS. Further research is required into optimal dose and duration of this therapy. Calcium supplementation has the additional benefit of reducing osteoporosis risk in women who may be calcium deficient.

▶ I suspect you have read about this in the papers: Calcium improves premenstrual syndrome. A definitive, highly effective cure for PMS remains elusive, although antidepressants clearly help the subgroup of sufferers with a strong affective component. Most of our treatments provide a modest amount of relief, and the same can be said of the calcium treatment in this article: There was an overall 48% reduction in total symptom scores, compared with a 30% reduction with placebo, by the third treatment cycle. No effects were seen in the first treatment cycle. The effects were seen across all types of symptom groups, although fatigue and insomnia did not seem to improve. The medication was reportedly well tolerated. I like this potential treatment compared with the alternatives because it is inexpensive, over-the-counter, and serves a dual purpose as women need more calcium for the prevention of osteoporosis than they traditionally get in the United States.

The study is generally well designed and carried out. The compliance rate was impressive and unlikely to be obtained in practice. The women were taking large quantities of calcium—2 TUMS E-X twice a day for 1,200 mg of elemental calcium. There was no attempt to identify the original calcium intakes of the women, and I wonder how that would effect the results. Women would need to be told that they would have to take the calcium for at least 3 months to see the results. No long-term follow-up was undertaken in this study.

M.A. Bowman, M.D., M.P.A.

Differential Behavioral Effects of Gonadal Steroids in Women With and in Those Without Premenstrual Syndrome

Schmidt PJ, Nieman LK, Danaceau MA, et al (Natl Inst of Mental Health, Bethesda, Md; Natl Inst of Child Health and Human Development, Bethesda, Md)

N Engl J Med 338:209–216, 1998

Introduction.—It is believed that the premenstrual syndrome (PMS) is triggered by hormone-related events that occur before the midluteal phase of the menstrual cycle. The role of estrogen and progesterone in PMS was assessed.

Methods.—Twenty women with PMS and 15 controls without PMS with a mean age of 37 years (range 27–45 years) underwent hormone

TABLE 2.—Symptom Ratings During the Administration of Leuprolide and Leuprolide Plus Hormone Replacement in 10 Women With Premenstrual Syndrome and 15 Normal Women*

Symptom and Group	Leuprolide Alone Week 2	Week 3	Leuprolide + Hormone Replacement Week 2	Week 3	P Value†
		Mean ±SD			
Sadness					
Women with premenstrual syndrome	1.2±0.3	1.2±0.2	2.0±0.8	2.2±0.9‡§	0.003
Normal women	1.2±0.3	1.2±0.3	1.2±0.2	1.2±0.3	
Anxiety					
Women with premenstrual syndrome	1.3±0.3	1.2±0.2	2.0±0.6	2.1±0.9‡§	0.01
Normal women	1.2±0.2	1.2±0.3	1.1±0.2	1.1±0.1	
Bloating					
Women with premenstrual syndrome	1.2±0.2	1.2±0.2	2.2±1.1	2.3±1.1‡§	0.10
Normal women	1.1±0.2	1.2±0.2	1.3±0.5	1.2±0.3	
Food cravings					
Women with premenstrual syndrome	1.5±0.8	1.5±0.7	1.3±0.5	1.6±1.0	0.30
Normal women	1.1±0.1	1.1±0.1	1.3±0.2	1.2±0.3	
Impaired function					
Women with premenstrual syndrome	1.2±0.2	1.3±0.3	1.7±0.7	1.8±0.8‡§	0.10
Normal women	1.2±0.4	1.2±0.3	1.1±0.3	1.2±0.4	
Irritability					
Women with premenstrual syndrome	1.3±0.2	1.4±0.5	2.1±0.7	2.2±0.8‡§	0.02
Normal women	1.3±0.4	1.3±0.3	1.3±0.2	1.3±0.3	

*Scores range from 1 (symptoms not present) to 6 (symptoms present in the extreme). The Bonferroni *t*-test was used for all post hoc comparisons. All *P* values are two-tailed. When consistent with hypothesized interactions between study groups and study phase, selected trend differences were assessed with post hoc comparisons. For this analysis, symptoms during estradiol and progesterone therapy were averaged, given the absence of main or interactive effects of the month of treatment.
†The *P* value is for the interaction between treatment (leuprolide alone or leuprolide plus hormone replacement), study group (women with premenstrual syndrome or normal women), and week by repeated-measures analysis of variance.
‡*P* < 0.05 for the comparison with leuprolide alone at week 3 in women with premenstrual syndrome.
§*P* < 0.05 for the comparison with leuprolide plus hormone replacement at week 3 in normal women.
(Reprinted by permission of *The New England Journal of Medicine*, from Schmidt PJ, Nieman LK, Danaceau MA: Differential behavioral effects of gonadal steroids in women with and in those without premenstrual syndrome. *N Engl J Med* 338:209–216. Copyright 1998, Massachusetts Medical Society. All rights reserved.)

assays of plasma progesterone and estradiol. Women with PMS were randomly assigned to receive 3 monthly injections of either the gonadotropin-releasing hormone agonist leuprolide acetate (3.75 mg) or an equal volume of saline placebo in double-blind fashion. In a follow-up trial, women with PMS whose symptoms responded to ovarian suppression in the first 3 months continued to receive leuprolide for another 3 months to evaluate the effect on mood of separately adding back physiologic doses of estradiol and progesterone for 4 weeks. Controls participated in a similar protocol. Patients were followed up using daily self-reports and biweekly rater-administered symptom-rating scales.

Results.—The 10 women with PMS who received leuprolide had a significant reduction in symptoms, compared with baseline values and values for 10 females receiving placebo. Women with PMS who received leuprolide plus estradiol or progesterone had a significant recurrence of symptoms. The 15 controls and 5 females given placebo hormone during continued leuprolide administration had no changes in mood (Table 2).

Conclusions.—Women with PMS had fewer symptoms during ovarian suppression, and recurrence of symptoms during ovarian steroid hormone replacement. Normal females did not have mood changes with either manipulation. These findings suggest that normal plasma concentrations of gonadal steroids in susceptible women can trigger an abnormal deterioration in mood.

▶ These investigators used an ingenuous study design to show that women with classic PMS who respond to leuprolide have short-term hypersensitive responses to normal levels of hormones. The response was primarily increased sadness and irritability. Of particular interest was that this response occurred with either estradiol or progesterone, for all of those thinking that one hormone or the other was the cause of the problem. Leuprolide, the gonadotropin-releasing hormone used in this study to reduce premenstrual symptoms, cannot be used long-term as a solo medication because of the development of artificial menopause and osteoporosis. This study may not apply to women who do not respond to gonadotropin-releasing hormones (perhaps one third to one half of patients with PMS), and reconfirms that there may actually be more than one cause of premenstrual syndrome. The study results also cannot be used to indicate the response to the long-term use of hormones.

M.A. Bowman, M.D., M.P.A.

Emergency Contraception and Abortion

The Effects of Self-administering Emergency Contraception
Glasier A, Baird D (Edinburgh Healthcare Natl Health Service Trust Family Planning and Well Woman Services, Scotland; Univ of Edinburgh, Scotland)
N Engl J Med 339:1–4, 1998
15–22

Introduction.—Up to 1.7 million unintended pregnancies and 0.8 million abortions could be prevented by the use of emergency postcoital contraception, which has been licensed in the United Kingdom since 1984. Because the method must be prescribed by a physician and taken within 72 hours after intercourse, many women who know that it is available underuse it. With short notice, it may be hard to arrange a medical consultation. A study was undertaken to investigate how women might behave if emergency contraception were more readily available and what the effect would be on the number of unintended pregnancies.

Methods.—The treatment group consisted of 553 women who were given a replaceable supply of hormonal emergency contraceptive pills to take home. They were compared with a control group of 530 women who were to visit a physician for emergency contraception. Detailed information at follow-up was given by 379 women in the treatment group (69%) and by 326 women in the control group (62%).

Results.—Emergency contraception was used by 180 women in the treatment group (47%). Of those who returned the questionnaire, 98% used the emergency contraception correctly. No serious adverse effects were found. In the control group, 87 women (27%) used emergency contraception at least once. Emergency contraception was not more likely to be used repeatedly by the women in the treatment group. Both groups used other methods of contraception in a similar fashion. There were 18 unintended pregnancies in the treatment group and 25 unintended pregnancies in the control group.

Conclusion.—No harm resulted when emergency contraception was made more easily obtainable. The rate of unwanted pregnancies may be reduced by this practice. Women who were given the opportunity to keep the tablets at home found that emergency contraception was a useful addition to their contraceptive options.

▶ This article suggests that giving selected women greater control of emergency contraception could lead to fewer unwanted pregnancies (although, admittedly, this result was not statistically significant). Use of the emergency contraception by the participants seems high, particularly since most were also using another form of contraception (primarily condoms). This may result from the unrepresentative group of patients, primarily those who had recently had an abortion or had recently used emergency contraception. The authors say that the pills were available without prescription, but that is not correct—the pills were just provided in advance of their potential need. In fact, giving patients a prescription but not the actual pills, as might be done in practice, could also result in lower rates of use than found in this study. All of the women received follow-up examinations, and it is unclear whether this plan would work as well as a means of contraception in real-world practice.

M.A. Bowman, M.D., M.P.A.

Expectant Management Versus Elective Curettage for the Treatment of Spontaneous Abortion

Hurd WW, Whitfield RR, Randolph JF Jr, et al (Univ of Michigan, Ann Arbor)
Fertil Steril 68:601–606, 1997   15–23

Objective.—With the advent of new technology, a threatened abortion can now be detected as early as 6 to 7 weeks after the last menstrual period. No studies have evaluated the optimal management methods for an impending abortion in the presence of a closed cervix. Whether the amount of uterine tissue present was prognostic for the risk of complications associated with curettage or expectant observation was assessed by evaluating the treatment and outcome of every impending abortion diagnosed during a 5-year period.

Methods.—Between January 1, 1990 and December 1, 1994, records of 197 pregnancies determined to be nonviable were examined for mode of presentation, gestational age at first symptom, diagnosis, treatment, and incidence of complications. Patients with a closed cervix were treated expectantly or with elective curettage. Retrospectively pregnancies were divided into those having significant uterine tissue (intrauterine gestational sac larger than 10 mm in mean diameter) and those having minimal intrauterine tissue. Complications were compared between the 2 groups.

Results.—There were 13 spontaneous abortions and 26 ectopic pregnancies that were excluded from the analysis. The remaining 158 patients were diagnosed as having impending abortions before the abortion occurred. There was minimal intrauterine tissue in 89 patients and significant intrauterine tissue in 69. In this latter group, 39 underwent curettage, and 30 were managed expectantly. Six in this group later requested curettage and were excluded from the analysis. There were no complications in the group with minimal intrauterine tissue, regardless of whether they were managed expectantly or underwent curettage. Nine (37%) of 24 patients with significant intrauterine tissue treated expectantly had complications, including a missed abortion, a septic abortion, an incomplete abortion requiring emergency curettage, and a transfusion. One woman who underwent curettage had a uterine perforation.

Conclusion.—Expectant treatment is appropriate for women with impending abortions and minimal intrauterine tissue. In patients with significant intrauterine tissue, the risk of complications is significantly lower with elective curettage than with expectant management.

▶ Using the retrospective cutoff of a 10 mm gestational sac, these authors conclude that women with a nonviable first-trimester nonectopic pregnancy, associated with more than minimal intrauterine tissue but a closed cervix, should receive an elective uterine curettage rather than expectant observation, due to the higher rate of complications. However, the "complication" of expectant management was that 7 of 9 patients needed curettage and 2 had slow resolution of a missed abortion. I would only consider that 1 of the expectant group had a major complication, i.e., the 1 who had a septic abortion. Thus, my conclusion would be that expectant management is still okay, as long as one understands that curettage may be needed. Major issues with the methodology were that the patients were not randomized, but curettage was based on patient and physician preference; all patients were being treated for infertility; and the cutoff of 10 mm was chosen after the fact. Certain patients (certain conception dates, human chorionic gonadotropin decreasing to less than 1,000; gestation less than 6 weeks) were presumed to have minimal intrauterine tissue without vaginal ultrasound. I feel new diagnostic technologies have made it easier to follow women with spontaneous abortions expectantly.

M.A. Bowman, M.D., M.P.A.

Effect of Nonsteroidal Anti-inflammatory Drugs on the Action of Misoprostol in a Regimen for Early Abortion
Creinin MD, Shulman T (Univ of Pittsburgh, Pa)
Contraception 56:165–168, 1997   15–24

Objective.—Analgesia for pain during medical abortion has not been well discussed. Whereas nonsteroidal anti-inflammatory drug (NSAID) use does not block prostaglandin action, some investigators are concerned that NSAIDs may inhibit uterine cramping. Use of NSAIDs in 3 medical abortion trials involving methotrexate and misoprostol was reviewed.

Methods.—The 3 trials included 416 women with a gestational age of 56 days or less having an elective abortion who received misoprostol alone or 50 mg/m^2 of methotrexate IM on day 1 followed in 7 days by 800 µg of misoprostol vaginally. Misoprostol was repeated if abortion did not occur. Patients were instructed to take ibuprofen or acetaminophen for cramping as needed and were also given a prescription for acetaminophen with codeine phosphate (300 mg/30 mg) or a comparable narcotic. Pain control and time to abortion were recorded.

Results.—Within 24 hours, 215 women aborted, whereas 59 required a second dose of misoprostol (Table 1). Only 32 of 145 women who did not take an NSAID aborted ($P = 0.002$).

TABLE 1.—Nonsteroidal Anti-inflammatory Drug Use After Misoprostol Administration for Abortion

| | Abortion After First Dose of Misoprostol |||| Abortion After Second Dose of Misoprostol ||||
| | Yes || No || Yes || No ||
	n	%	n	%	n	%	n	%
NSAID	132	53.7	114	46.3	27	48.2	29	51.8
NSAID not used	83	48.8	87	41.2	32	22.1	113	57.9

Abbreviation: NSAID, nonsteroidal anti-inflammatory drug.
(Reprinted by permission of the publisher from Creinin MD, Shulman T: Effect of nonsteroidal anti-inflammatory drugs on the action of misoprostol in a regimen for early abortion. *Contraception* 56:165–168, Copyright 1997 by Elsevier Science Inc.)

Conclusion.—Nonsteroidal anti-inflammatory drug use after misoprostol does not interfere with pregnancy expulsion in women having elective abortions.

▶ There is reluctance to use NSAIDs for pain control during medical abortions using misoprostol, although theoretically they should not inhibit the action of the prostaglandin already administered. This article looks at women who used NSAIDs (including aspirin) for pain control and the outcome. The data support no negative influence on the success rate of the medical abortion. Thus, physicians involved with these patients can suggest NSAIDs for pain control as desired, although the authors suggest waiting until the misoprostol has been administered.

M.A. Bowman, M.D., M.P.A.

Menopause

Bone Changes and Carotid Atherosclerosis in Postmenopausal Women
Uyama O, Yoshimoto Y, Yamamoto Y, et al (College of Nursing Art and Science Hyogo, Akashi, Japan)
Stroke 28:1730–1732, 1997   15–25

Background.—Because life expectancy has increased, most postmenopausal women will experience osteoporosis and atherosclerotic disease. These diseases are currently considered unrelated. The relationship between bone mineral density (BMD) and carotid wall US findings was investigated.

Methods and Findings.—Thirty women, aged 67–85, were studied. High-resolution B-mode US was performed. Severity of carotid atherosclerosis was assessed by plaque score. Dual-energy radiograph absorptiometry was done to determine BMD. In a multiple linear regression analysis, plaque score was found to be significantly associated with total cholesterol level and with low total BMD.

Conclusions.—These data indicate that osteoporosis and carotid atherosclerosis, a major cause of ischemic cerebrovascular disease, are related. Sunlight deprivation from immobilization (caused by cerebral arteriosclerosis) combined with a decreased dietary intake of vitamin D may be responsible for osteoporosis in women with severe carotid atherosclerosis.

▶ In this group of postmenopausal Japanese women who were basically nonsmokers and nondrinkers, bone mass was inversely related to carotid plaque formation, and plaque formation was related to total cholesterol (as expected). The authors conjecture about potential links through vitamin D, but I suspect that estrogens are more important, because estrogens increase bone mass, improve lipid profiles, and may decrease atherosclerosis. Exercise could also be important. Regardless of the etiology, the finding of either osteoporosis or atherosclerosis in our postmenopausal women should make us think about the other condition, so we can appropriately provide therapy and prevention.

M.A. Bowman, M.D., M.P.A.

The Effect of Dietary Soy Supplementation on Hot Flushes
Albertazzi P, Pansini F, Bonaccorsi G, et al (Univ of Ferrara; Ferrara Research Consortium; Univ of Bologna, Italy)
Obstet Gynecol 91:6–11, 1998   15–26

Objective.—Because of the risk of breast cancer and venous thromboembolism, hormone replacement therapy (HRT) is contraindicated in some women. There is little relief from menopausal symptoms for these women. In Japan, where soy is a dietary staple, less than 25% of women complain of hot flushes, compared with 85% of North American women. Results of a short-term, randomized, double-blind, placebo-controlled pilot study of the effect of a soy-enriched diet on severe hot flushes are reported.

Methods.—Women, aged 45 to 62, experiencing hot flushes received either 60 g of isolated soy protein daily ($n = 51$) or 60 g of placebo daily ($n = 53$) for 12 weeks. Women were assessed at baseline and at 4, 8, and 12 weeks. Patients kept diaries and recorded number of daily hot flushes and night sweats prestudy and throughout the study period and rated other menopausal symptoms, including paresthesia, insomnia, nervousness, melancholia, vertigo, weakness, arthralgia, headaches, palpitation, and formication. Weight and blood pressure were measured. Changes in symptoms were analyzed statistically.

Results.—Forty patients taking soy and 39 patients taking placebo completed the study. Women taking soy had a significant 26% reduction in average number of hot flushes by week 3, a 33% reduction by week 4, and a 45% reduction by the end of week 12. The placebo group experienced a 30% reduction in the average number of hot flushes by the end of week 12. The difference between groups was significant at week 12 (Fig 1). There were 11 women in the soy group and 14 in the placebo group who did not complete the study. Most discontinued because of gastrointestinal side effects and food intolerance (7 in each group).

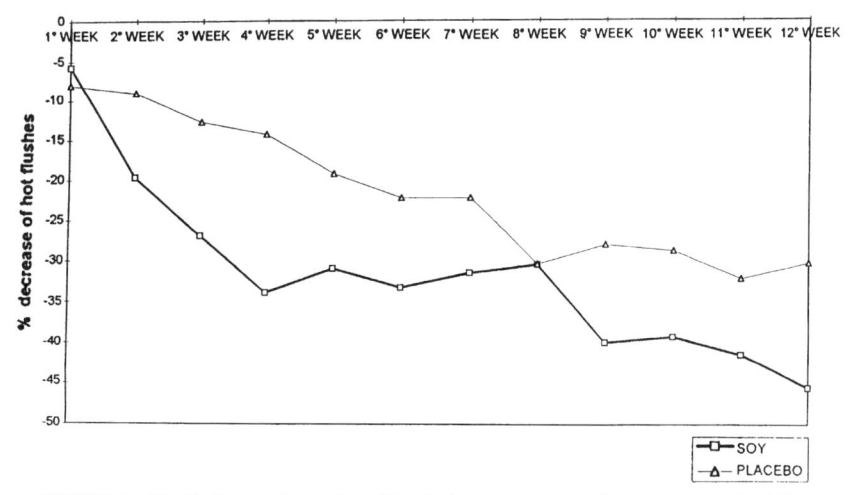

FIGURE 1.—Weekly decrease in number of hot flushes; score expressed as percentage. The difference between soy and placebo was always significant after week 2, with the exception of week 8. (Courtesy of Albertazzi P, Pansini F, Bonaccorsi G, et al: The effect of dietary soy supplementation on hot flushes. *Obstet Gynecol* 91:6–11, 1998. Reprinted with permission from The American College of Obstetricians and Gynecologists.)

Conclusion.—Menopausal women on a soy diet had a significant reduction in the number of daily hot flushes.

▶ Another topical alternative-medicine study, one which shows positive results. This is a well-designed study of Italian women with a large number of hot flushes. There was a 30% reduction in hot flushes with placebo, a common level of response; the response level to soy was a 45% reduction in hot flushes at 3 months. The effect of soy can be helpful, but may not be dramatic, nor as great as that of estrogens. Perhaps higher doses of soy would be more successful, as the dose used was about one third the typical daily consumption in Japan. There was no comparison to estrogens, and there is little clinical data on soy's ability to mimic other estrogenic effects, such as on cardiovascular disease. Kupperman index of other menopausal symptoms showed no improvement.

M.A. Bowman, M.D., M.P.A.

Hormone Replacement Therapy

Vasodilator Effects of Estrogen Are Not Diminished by Androgen in Postmenopausal Women
Sarrel PM, Wiita B (Yale Univ, New Haven, Conn; Solvay Pharmaceuticals Inc, Marietta, Ga)
Fertil Steril 68:1125–1127, 1997   15–27

Background.—Previous studies suggest that androgen, when used in combination with estrogen therapy, relieves symptoms such as dyspareunia, loss of libido, and hot flushes in postmenopausal women. A group of postmenopausal women who wanted relief from these symptoms were given estrogen-androgen therapy or estrogen therapy to determine the vasoactive effect of these treatments.

Method.—Twenty women underwent esterified estrogen or esterified estrogen and methyltestosterone treatment for 8 weeks. All test subjects had used Estrace, Premarin, or Estraderm treatment for at least 12 months before the study. At baseline, 4, and 8 weeks, laser Doppler velocimetry was performed on the fingertips and vagina to determine blood flow responses. The blood flow velocities of the vagina and area under the curve (AUC) of the fingertips were recorded.

Results.—The area under the curve of the fingertips and the vaginal blood flow velocities were greater in the androgen group. However, the difference between groups was not statistically significant.

Conclusion.—The addition of androgen to estrogen treatment seems to increase postocclusion fingertip blood flow and does not diminish enhanced vascular reactivity resulting from estrogen treatment.

▶ This is a hopeful finding, but it is an intermediary effect, not the real effect we want. As testosterone levels are known to fall in menopause, testosterone is increasingly used in postmenopausal women to help with primarily libido issues and could help with other postmenopausal problems. However, effects on heart disease are unknown and concerning. I am not prescribing testosterone for women yet, but think there may be hope of doing so if the correct doses are ascertained and available, and if additional studies can identify safety (two big 'ifs'). This small study suggests that vaginal and fingertip vasodilation may not fall when testosterone is used in conjunction with estrogen. However, there were only 20 women, and the vasodilation fell in the estrogen-only group at 4 weeks for some unknown reason.

M.A. Bowman, M.D., M.P.A.

Does Dong Quai Have Estrogenic Effects in Postmenopausal Women? A Double-blind, Placebo-controlled Trial
Hirata JD, Sweirsz LM, Zell B, et al (Kaiser Permanente Med Ctr, Oakland and Richmond, Calif)
Fertil Steril 68:981–986, 1997   15–28

Background.—Alternative therapy is very popular in the United States and yet many of these treatments have not been examined scientifically for effectiveness. The effect of dong quai, a Chinese herbal remedy used to treat symptoms associated with menopause was examined to determine whether this herbal therapy has an effect on the internal production of estradiol or estrone as determined by examination of vaginal and endometrial linings.

Method.—Seventy-one postmenopausal women who were screened for various medical conditions and who exhibited frequent night sweats or vasomotor flushes were given randomized dong quai or placebo treatment. Dong quai recipients took the equivalent of 4.5 g of the root per day. Test subjects were examined at 6, 12, and 24 weeks. All visits included endometrial US. At the initial visit and the twelfth-week visit, blood pressure, serum estrogen levels, and vaginal cells were evaluated. At week 24, blood pressure and weight were also measured. If a greater than 5 mm endometrial thickness was determined through endometrial US at the final visit, endometrial biopsy was performed. Participants kept journals recording the vasomotor episodes they experienced and were also evaluated using the Kupperman index, which ranks menopausal symptom complaints as nonexistent, mild, or severe. Significance of difference between the placebo and dong quai groups was determined using t-test and χ^2 test.

Results.—Six test subjects receiving placebos dropped out of the study before test completion as did 4 receiving dong quai. Test subjects could not accurately tell whether they were taking the placebo or the actual drug. All test subjects reported mild side effects including burping, headaches, and gas. Statistically significant differences were not recorded in the vaginal maturation index, frequency of vasomotor flushes, the endometrial thickness, or in the Kupperman index.

Conclusion.—This test suggests that dong quai administered in isolation does not relieve menopausal symptoms any more readily than a placebo. Endometrial proliferation did not occur as a result of administering dong quai. Hence, the herbal therapy does not seem to increase the production of estradiol or estrone.

▶ With alternative medicine popular among the lay public and the media, it is also attracting the attention of physicians. Dong quai is widely used for menopause and is reported to calm the symptoms. This study included sufficient women and lasted for long enough (6 months) to provide good data. In addition, the authors considered several types of outcomes, both symptoms and the important signs of vaginal maturation and endometrial thickness. Although dong quai is often used with other herbs in China, it has often been used in the United States as a solo medication. This study should be replicated by others, but does not suggest dong quai will be effective for menopausal symptoms.

M.A. Bowman, M.D., M.P.A.

Patient-specific Decisions About Hormone Replacement Therapy in Postmenopausal Women
Col NF, Eckman MH, Karas RH, et al (Tufts Univ, Boston; Univ of Massachusetts, Worcester; Fallon Health Care System, Worcester, Mass)
JAMA 277:1140–1147, 1997

Objective.—Whereas heart disease kills 233,000 women annually, hip fracture 65,000, and breast cancer 43,000, women often fear breast cancer more. A study was designed to assist patients and physicians in deciding whether or not to administer hormone replacement therapy (HRT) by estimating the patient's risk factors for various diseases.

Methods.—The computer program DECISION MAKER using a Markov model was used to examine the benefits and risks of taking HRT in 2 hypothetical identical cohorts of women, 1 cohort taking HRT and the other not taking HRT. Risk factors and disease incidence were coupled using published regression models to estimate the lifetime risk of development of coronary heart disease (CHD), breast cancer, hip fracture, and endometrial cancer. Estimates of the impact of HRT on disease incidence were examined as a function of duration of exposure. Mortality rates were calculated from survival tables.

Results.—Use of HRT should increase life expectancy for most women by as long as 41 months depending on the individual risk primarily for CHD and breast cancer. Women with at least 1 risk factor for CHD, including a smoking history, high blood pressure, high cholesterol, early menarche, and first-degree relative with breast cancer would be expected to gain at least 1 year from HRT. The only women who would not live longer are those at lowest risk for CHD and hip fracture and highest risk for breast cancer, such as 2 first-degree relatives with breast cancer. The results for black women paralleled those for white women but were 10% to 25% lower.

Conclusion.—The benefit of HRT on reducing the incidence of CHD outweighs the risk of breast cancer in all women except those with 2 first-degree relatives with breast cancer.

▶ This mathematical model suggests that almost all menopausal women would gain 3 years of life expectancy by taking HRT. Because CHD is a more common cause of death, just 1 risk factor for heart disease outweighed having first-degree relatives with breast cancer. Only women with 2 first-degree relatives with breast cancer and risk factors for neither hip fracture nor heart disease would not benefit from HRT, which is fewer than 1% of women. The benefit for black women is lower, and not as supported by specific data. Recent developments, however, may mean that eventually we will be using new forms of HRT that do not even raise the risk of breast cancer but maintain benefits for heart disease and bone mass.

M.A. Bowman, M.D., M.P.A.

Is Bleeding a Predictor of Endometrial Hyperplasia in Postmenopausal Women Receiving Hormone Replacement Therapy?
Pickar JH, for the Menopause Study Group (Wyeth-Ayerst Research, Philadelphia; Eastern Virginia Med School, Norfolk)
Am J Obstet Gynecol 177:1178–1183, 1997   15–30

Objective.—Unopposed estrogen therapy can result in endometrial hyperplasia in postmenopausal women. Because endometrial hyperplasia can progress to endometrial cancer, a progestin is now commonly added to

TABLE 5.—Predictability of Irregular Bleeding With or Without Spotting as an Indicator of Endometrial Hyperplasia in Treatment Groups A, B, and E

Regimen/Test	Last 30 Days	Bleeding/Spotting Last 60 Days	Last 90 Days
Continuous combined HRT			
Positive predictor	1/101 = <1%	1/137 = <1%	1/164 = <1%
Negative predictor	443/444 = 99.8%	411/412 = 99.8%	386/387 = 99.7%
Unopposed estrogen (CE)			
Positive predictor	46/100 = 46.0%	49/116 = 42.2%	49/126 = 38.9%
Negative predictor	167/177 = 94.4%	157/164 = 95.7%	148/155 = 95.5%

NOTE: Values are number of women.
Abbreviations: HRT, hormone replacement therapy; CE, conjugated estrogens.
(Courtesy of Pickar JH, for the Menopause Study Group: Is bleeding a predictor of endometrial hyperplasia in postmenopausal women receiving hormone replacement therapy? *Am J Obstet Gynecol* 177:1178–1183, 1997.)

hormone replacement therapy in postmenopausal women with a uterus. The predictive value of bleeding patterns and endometrial histologic data from the Menopause Study Group and of biopsy results for endometrial hyperplasia was evaluated.

Methods.—The Menopause Study Group trial was a double-blind, prospective, parallel, controlled study of 1,724 nonhysterectomized postmenopausal women randomly assigned to treatment with continuous combined conjugated estrogens (0.625 mg) and medroxyprogesterone acetate (2.5 or 5.0 mg), treatment with cyclic combined conjugated estrogens and medroxyprogesterone acetate (5.0 or 10.0 mg), or conjugated estrogens alone for 13 cycles. Vaginal bleeding and spotting episodes were recorded in a daily diary. Incidences of irregular bleeding episodes were compared with histologic endometrial changes.

Results.—Of the 62 patients with diagnosed endometrial hyperplasia, 57 (92%) were in the unopposed conjugated estrogens group. Women with endometrial hyperplasia in the unopposed conjugated estrogens group had significantly more bleeding days than did women without hyperplasia. The predictive value of amenorrhea to predict a nonhyperplasia diagnosis was 99.7% to 99.8% (Table 5). With women taking continuous or cyclic medroxyprogesterone acetate, irregular bleeding was not associated with hyperplasia.

Conclusions.—Whereas irregular bleeding is associated with endometrial hyperplasia in women taking unopposed estrogens, it is not associated with endometrial hyperplasia in women receiving either cyclic or continuous progestin as part of hormone replacement therapy.

▶ This article reaffirms that postmenopausal unopposed estrogen is associated with a substantial rate of development of hyperplasia (about 20% within 1 year), but also provides helpful information about the implications of bleeding in women on various regimens including estrogens and progesterones. The number of days of bleeding was associated with hyperplasia in the estrogen-only group, but not in the combined regimens. Thus, bleeding in women taking concurrent estrogen and progesterone is not a marker for hyperplasia. However, the rate of development of hyperplasia in the 4 different types of estrogen and progesterone regimens was quite low. Admittedly, this makes it difficult to know when or whether to check for hyperplasia in women on the combination regimens. One other reminder from the study was that some women on estrogen-only developed hyperplasia but had amenorrhea.

M.A. Bowman, M.D., M.P.A.

Unexpected Vaginal Bleeding and Associated Gynecologic Care in Postmenopausal Women Using Hormone Replacement Therapy: Comparison of Cyclic Versus Continuous Combined Schedules

Ettinger B, Li D-K, Klein R (Kaiser Permanente Med Care Program, Oakland, Calif)
Fertil Steril 69:865–869, 1998   15–31

Objective.—Women using cyclic hormone replacement therapy (HRT) experience 3 times the rate of unexpected vaginal bleeding than non-HRT users and require additional gynecologic resources. Medical records were retrospectively reviewed to compare gynecologic care received by postmenopausal women receiving cyclic HRT with care received by those using continuous HRT.

Methods.—Episodes of unexpected vaginal bleeding were compared in 284 women (154 new users) using continuous combined HRT and 306 women (154 new users) using cyclic HRT. Patients were followed up for an average of 2 years.

Results.—The unexpected vaginal bleeding rate for new users was a significant 67% higher than among previous users (35 vs. 21 visits). Among all women, there was no difference in unexpected vaginal bleeding episodes between those using cyclic HRT and those using continuous combined HRT. There was no difference between groups after adjusting for age, previous use of HRT, and time since menopause. Among new users of cyclic HRT, 38.3% had more than 1 visit for unexpected vaginal bleeding and 12.3% had more than 1 endometrial biopsy compared with 41.6% and 20.1%, respectively, for women using continuous combined HRT. The risk of 1 visit or more for unexpected vaginal bleeding for cyclic HRT users compared with continuous combined HRT users was 1.7 in the first 6 months, 1.4 in the next 6 months, 1.2 in the second year, and 0.9 in the third year. The relative risk of endometrial biopsy during the same respective periods was 2.6, 2.6, 1.8, and 1.2.

Conclusion.—Although unexpected vaginal bleeding for women using cyclic and continuous combined HRT consumes a considerable amount of gynecologic resources for the first 2 years, the care required for women using continuous combined HRT diminishes thereafter. The decline in the requirement for gynecologic resources for women using cyclic HRT is considerably slower.

▶ Gosh, this was even worse than I thought. Even after 2 years of treatment almost half of women on cyclic regimens had visits for unexpected bleeding and 15% had endometrial biopsies per year. The continuous regimens were better but still had a substantial rate of visits and biopsies. Given the rate of endometrial cancers in women on any regimen including regular progestins, the rate of endometrial biopsies seems very high and very low yield. I wonder if better education of the women about the substantial rate of bleeding would decrease the numbers of visits, and better education of the physicians could decrease the rate of biopsies.

M.A. Bowman, M.D., M.P.A.

Miscellaneous

Diagnostic Utility of the Digital Rectal Examination as Part of the Routine Pelvic Examination
Campbell KA, Shaughnessy AF (Harrisburg Family Practice Residency Program, Pa)
J Fam Pract 46:165–167, 1998   15–32

Introduction.—The digital rectal examination (DRE) has become a standard aspect of the routine pelvic examination in women of all ages, despite a lack of evidence of the diagnostic utility of this examination. Some studies report that women may postpone or defer pelvic examinations because of discomfort associated with the DRE. The diagnostic yield of routine DRE in healthy younger women was retrospectively assessed.

Methods.—The study setting was a family practice center affiliated with a residency program and serving a largely white, middle-class, suburban population. Approximately 2,000 pelvic examinations are performed at the center each year. Charts reviewed were those of women younger than 40 years who had a routine DRE during a routine pelvic examination; excluded were patients examined by residents. Chart abstractors categorized DRE results as positive, negative, or not performed. Positive findings were characterized as diagnostic, confirmatory, or incidental. Accuracy of findings was determined by a chart review for further workup.

Results.—The review identified 357 eligible charts; 327 were available for analysis, and 272 of these had DREs documented. There were 8 (3%) findings: 7 were incidental (hemorrhoids, stool in rectum, and a vaginal scar), and 1 was confirmatory (colitis). The DREs yielded no diagnostic findings.

Discussion.—The diagnostic yield of these 272 routine DREs performed in women younger than 40 years during a routine pelvic examination had a diagnostic yield of zero. Although the DRE is an inexpensive test, its low diagnostic yield and discomfort argue for discontinuing the DRE as part of a routine pelvic examination.

▶ Should this study change your practice? Perhaps, perhaps not. Why not? The methodology is weak, as is the premise that women are avoiding pelvic exams because of the discomfort of the DRE. Nevertheless, I applaud the authors for looking critically at the utility of a component of the physical examination that certainly is uncomfortable and may not be providing us with useful information. Personally, I have long since ceased including this maneuver as a routine part of the physical examination of healthy, asymptomatic young women. I would like to see a more controlled investigation of this. In the meantime, these results should, at least, cause one to reassess the utility of the routine DRE in this population.

W.W. Dexter, M.D.

A Simplified Protocol for Pessary Management
Wu V, Farrell SA, Baskett TF, et al (Dalhousie Univ, Halifax, Nova Scotia, Canada)
Obstet Gynecol 90:990–994, 1997   15–33

Background.—Physicians and patients may perceive pessaries as inconvenient and, thus, be reluctant to use them in the management of pelvic prolapse. A simplified protocol for pessary use was described.

Methods.—One hundred ten women with symptomatic pelvic organ prolapse who chose pessary management were enrolled in the prospective study. The mean age was 65 years. The patients had an initial pessary fitting and were checked again at 2 weeks. Thereafter, the patients were seen only every 3 to 6 months for follow-up.

Findings..—Seventy-four percent of the women were fitted successfully. Sixty-six percent using a pessary for more than 1 month still used the pessary after 12 months. Fifty-three percent of these patients were still using the pessary after 36 months. Prolapse severity did not predict the likelihood of pessary failure, except for women with complete vaginal eversion. Women with stress incontinence were less likely to have a successful fitting and more likely to choose surgical treatment. Neither current hormone use nor substantial perineal support predicted a greater likelihood of successful pessary fitting. No serious complications occurred.

Conclusion.—Pessaries are a safe long-term option for the management of pelvic prolapse, with no need for frequent pelvic examinations. This simplified protocol may enhance the appeal of this treatment modality.

▶ I have successfully prescribed pessaries for my patients, and I think this article is a reminder that pessaries can be a safe, effective, and well-liked long-term alternative to surgery for a significant number of women with symptomatic pelvic prolapse. The authors had success even with a complete vaginal eversion! The authors reported that the patients preferred to have the physicians remove and clean the pessaries every few months, but my patients have all performed their own home self-care after instruction in the office (similar to instruction for diaphragm use).

The authors did not report on the rate of improvement in urinary symptoms after pessary fitting, which would have been interesting. The cube pessary had a high rate of vaginal erosions (5 of 6), whereas the ring pessary had a low rate (3 of 101). Remember to think of the pessary.

M.A. Bowman, M.D., M.P.A.

Epidemiology of Repeat Ectopic Pregnancy: A Population-based Prospective Cohort Study
Skjeldestad FE, Hadgu A, Eriksson N (Norwegian Univ, Trondheim, Norway; Natl Ctrs for Disease Control and Prevention, Atlanta, Ga; Orkdal Hosp, Orkanger, Norway)
Obstet Gynecol 91:129–135, 1998   15–34

Background.—Studies of the effect of ectopic pregnancy on subsequent fertility have been problematic. Pregnancy outcomes after the first (index) ectopic pregnancy were further investigated, with a focus on risks during the index pregnancy which might be associated with a repeat event.

Methods.—Six hundred ninety-seven women aged 37 years or younger at the time of their first ectopic pregnancy were studied. None had had tubal surgery before the index pregnancy. The women were followed up for 1 to 17 years. Three hundred fifty-three women had a total of 555 pregnancies.

Findings.—Pregnancy order was the strongest correlate of the subsequent occurrence of ectopic pregnancy. The frequency of repeat ectopic

TABLE 4.—Odds of Repeat Ectopic Pregnancy in Subsequent Pregnancies

	Adjusted OR	95% CI
Pregnancy order		
1st subsequent	11.8	2.0, 68.0
2nd subsequent	3.0	0.5, 21.1
3rd or more subsequent	1.0	Reference
Repeat ectopic pregnancy		
1 repeat (2nd) ectopic pregnancy	9.5	2.5, 36.6
No repeat (1st) ectopic pregnancy	1.0	Reference
Status at index ectopic pregnancy		
Age (y)		
≤24	3.1	1.1, 8.9
≥25	1.0	Reference
Infectious pathology*		
Yes	2.7	1.5, 5.0
No	1.0	Reference
Have started infertility work-up		
Yes	2.3	1.0, 5.1
No	1.0	Reference
Conceived with intrauterine device		
In situ at index pregnancy		
Yes	0.4	0.1, 0.9
No	1.0	Reference

*Defined as either adhesions or macroscopic damage to the contralateral tube or both.
Abbreviations: OR, odds ratio; CI, confidence interval.
(Courtesy of Skjeldestad FE, Hadgu A, Eriksson N: Epidemiology of repeat pregnancy: A population-based prospective cohort study. *Obstet Gynecol* 91:129–135, 1998. Reprinted with permission from The American College of Obstetricians and Gynecologists.)

pregnancy declined by one third for each pregnancy from the first to the third. Women diagnosed as having infectious pathology had a risk of another ectopic pregnancy almost 3 times greater than that among women without infectious pathology. Other variables associated with repeat ectopic pregnancy were age of 24 years or less at the index pregnancy, history of repeat ectopic pregnancy, initiation of infertility work-up, and conception with an intrauterine device at the index pregnancy. Surgical procedure was not related to repeat ectopic pregnancy (Table 4).

Conclusions.—Assisted reproduction should be considered for women who have had 2 ectopic pregnancies. After 2 ectopic pregnancies, the chance of a completed intrauterine pregnancy was only about 4%.

▶ This study took over 15 years, included a large number of ectopic pregnancies in women under age 37 (n = 697), and had a follow-up rate of 93%, for which I admire the authors. These are terrific data, and can be helpful in decision-making for patients with ectopic pregnancies. While treatment of ectopic pregnancy is increasingly medical for small, unruptured ectopics, it was reassuring that surgical method was not associated with variation in outcome. Overall, about half of the patients who had an ectopic pregnancy became pregnant again. The highest-risk pregnancy for repeat ectopic pregnancy was the first one; the overall rate of future ectopic pregnancies (for those who became pregnant) was 12%. Age below 24, infectious pathology (defined as adhesions or macroscopic damage of the contralateral tube), and infertility were associated with a higher rate of a future ectopic pregnancy. An ectopic developing during the use of an intrauterine device was associated with fewer future ectopic pregnancies, suggesting the causative factors related to the intrauterine device are temporary. For women with 2 ectopic pregnancies, the chance of another pregnancy proceeding to term was only about 4% (although the number in this group was small), suggesting such women should consider other alternatives.

M.A. Bowman, M.D., M.P.A.

Leuprolide Acetate Depot and Hormonal Add-back in Endometriosis: A 12-Month Study
Hornstein MD, for the Lupron Add-Back Study Group (Harvard Med School, Boston; Univ of California, Los Angeles; Univ of Illinois, Chicago)
Obstet Gynecol 91:16–24, 1998   15–35

Background.—Gonadotropin-releasing hormone (GnRH) agonists are effective for the treatment of endometriosis-associated pelvic pain, but their use is limited by hypoestrogenic side effects, such as bone mineral density loss and vasomotor symptoms. To minimize bone loss, bone-sparing agents can be added-back to the regimen. The efficacy and safety of the GnRH agonist leuprolide acetate in depot suspension, alone and in combination with 3 add-back regimens, was examined in women with endometriosis-associated pelvic pain.

Study Design.—This multicenter, randomized, double-blind, 1-year trial included 201 healthy women. Participants were aged 18–43 years, had regular menstrual cycles, and a history of symptomatic endometriosis. All participants received an IM injection of 3.75 mg of Lupron Depot every 4 weeks for 52 weeks. The 51 patients in group A received placebo instead of progestin and estrogen. The 55 patients in group B received daily oral norethindrone acetate and placebo instead of estrogen. The 47 patients in group C received norethindone and daily 0.625 mg of oral conjugated equine estrogens. The 48 patients in group D received daily oral norethindrone and daily 1.25 mg of conjugated equine estrogens. All patients took calcium supplements. All 4 groups were matched demographically. Patients were seen before therapy and then every 4 weeks for 52 weeks. At each visit, dysmenorrhea and pelvic pain were assessed, and serum was obtained for estradiol assessment. Before therapy and at 24 and 52 weeks, a complete physical examination was performed, lipid profiles were obtained, and bone mineral density of the lumbar spine was assessed.

Findings.—By the eighth week of therapy, all 4 groups had significant improvement in pelvic pain. More group D patients terminated the study early because of inadequate symptomatic improvement. Group A had significant bone density loss, whereas bone density was preserved in all 3 of the groups with the add-back regimens.

Conclusions.—This large, 1-year, multicenter, randomized, double-blind clinical trial demonstrated that the GnRH agonist, leuprolide acetate depot, can be safely and effectively used to treat the pain of endometriosis for at least 1 year, when used with an add-back regimen containing norethindrone acetate alone or in combination with 0.625 mg of conjugated equine estrogens daily. These regimens reduce pelvic pain, while alleviating hypoestrogenic symptoms and preserving bone density.

▶ In this study of the use of leuprolide acetate for endometriosis, there were 201 patients in 4 separate study groups completed at 26 sites. Important variables were considered, including bone mass, lipids, and symptoms. All groups had improvement in overall symptoms, although all groups also had a substantial rate of the development of hot flashes, with the leuprolide only group having a much higher rate of hot flashes. The leuprolide only group lost bone mass and the group taking the higher dose of estrogen had a borderline significant increase in bone mass. All groups had adverse changes in lipid profiles, with a decrease in high-density lipoprotein cholesterol and increase in low-density lipoprotein cholesterol. The group taking 1.25 mg of conjugated estrogens with progesterone as compared to lower dose estrogen or progesterone only had a higher dropout rate because of lack of improvement, although all groups had a substantial dropout rate. All the authors had some relationship to the drug company making leuprolide acetate. Leuprolide acetate with hormonal add-back seems like a reasonable option for endometriosis, but patients will need to be well informed of the risks and benefits.

In a separate study by different investigators using nafarelin (also funded by the manufacturers), intermittent treatment, i.e., using 3 months of treatment after about a 1-year lapse from previous treatment, helped with symptoms while maintaining bone mass.[1] This was an open-label study, and all women had normal bone mass at the beginning of the study. The effects on lipids were not studied.

M.A. Bowman, M.D., M.P.A.

Reference

1. Adamson GD, Heinrichs WL, Henzl MR, et al: Therapeutic efficacy and bone mineral density response during and following a three-month re-treatment of endometriosis with nafarelin (Synarel). *Am J Obstet Gynecol* 177:1413–1418, 1997.

16 Pregnancy

Overview

Randomized controlled trials: Abstracts 16–1, 16–3, 16–13, and 16–17

Prenatal Issues

- Low-dose iron supplementation
- Risk of neural tube defect
- Low-dose aspirin in the prevention of preeclampsia
- *Helicobacter pylori* and hyperemesis gravidarum
- What is normal blood pressure in pregnant women?
- Treatment of miscarriage
- Variations in evaluation and treatment of preterm labor

Gestational Diabetes

- Selective screening
- Use of a high carbohydrate diet before the oral glucose tolerance test
- Two articles on unrecognized prepregnancy diabetes and diabetes after delivery
- Health status of women 3 to 5 years after gestational diabetes

Labor and Delivery

- Use of terbutaline for external cephalic version
- Vacuum extraction and neonatal cephalohematoma
- A scoring system to decide about vaginal birth after cesarean section
- Rising cesarean section rates

Pregnancy Outcomes

- Pelvic muscle exercise and transient incontinence
- Outcomes in morbidly obese women
- Outcomes in anxious women
- Outcomes of women with gestational diabetes

Obstetric Health Services

- Why family physicians deliver babies
- Midwifery and birth outcomes

Prenatal Issues

Iron Supplementation in Pregnancy: Is Less Enough? A Randomized, Placebo Controlled Trial of Low Dose Iron Supplementation With and Without Heme Iron
Eskeland B, Malterud K, Ulvik RJ, et al (Univ of Bergen, Norway; Haukeland Univ, Bergen, Norway)
Acta Obstet Gynecol Scand 76:822–828, 1997   16–1

Introduction.—Iron supplementation in pregnancy is controversial. There is concern that iron supplementation could aggravate a pathologic hemoconcentration in pregnancy. In addition, the possible negative interaction of iron with the absorption of other nutrients (zinc, magnesium) and dose-dependent side effects of iron supplementation are reasons for prescribing iron at the lowest effective dose. The efficacy of low-dose iron supplementation with and without a heme component prescribed during the second half of pregnancy was assessed in a randomized, double-blind, placebo-controlled trial.

Methods.—Ninety women were randomly assigned to receive daily doses of either heme iron (27 mg of elemental iron with a heme iron component), non-heme iron, or placebo. Participants underwent testing throughout pregnancy and 8 and 24 weeks postpartum for red cell indices and iron status markers (s-ferritin, s-iron, total iron binding capacity, and erythrocyte protoporphyrin).

Results.—The hematologic effects were similar in the 2 iron treatment groups. Hemoglobin fell below 110 g/L in 25% of supplemented women, compared with 52% of women who received placebo. It fell below 100 g/L in no women in the supplemental iron group and 14% of women in the placebo group. At the end of pregnancy, iron status was significantly superior for all measured parameters in the heme iron group, compared with placebo. Differences between the iron groups were nonsignificant, probably because of small sample size. From the start of pregnancy to postpartum, the percentage of women with empty iron stores decreased from 14% to 8% in the heme iron group, increased from 3% to 27% in the non–heme iron group, and increased from 21% to 52% in the placebo group.

Conclusions.—A daily dose of 27 mg of elemental iron, containing a heme component, administered in the second half of pregnancy helps prevent depletion of iron stores after delivery in most women. Equivalent doses of pure inorganic iron were somewhat less effective, but the sample size was too small to demonstrate significance.

▶ Unnecessarily high doses of iron have their drawbacks. Iron overload is not a healthy condition, even for pregnant women. This article from Norway shows that many women will have adequate iron stores by simply taking a single low-dose pill beginning at 20 weeks' gestation. While not addressed in this article, iron supplementation postpartum, particularly with substantial blood loss, would also be important. If pregnant women do not enter pregnancy with iron deficiency anemia, and do not have a history suggestive of low iron stores, I do not give iron supplementation beyond what is in a prenatal vitamin.

J.E. Scherger, M.D., M.P.H.

Risk for Neural Tube Defect–Affected Pregnancies Among Women of Mexican Descent and White Women in California
Shaw GM, Velie EM, Wasserman CR (March of Dimes Birth Defects Found, Emeryville, Calif)
Am J Public Health 87:1467–1471, 1997   16–2

Background.—Neural tube defects are common congenital anomalies with substantial ethnic and geographic differences in prevalence. A previous study reported a 50% or more increased risk for neural tube defect-affected pregnancies among Latina women compared with white women. This risk was further investigated.

Methods.—Data were obtained from a population-based case-control study of fetuses and live-born infants with neural tube defects in a cohort born between 1989 and 1991 in California. The mothers of 538 infants and fetuses with neural tube defects and the mothers of 539 normal infants were interviewed.

Findings.—Women of Mexican descent had a risk for neural tube defect-affected pregnancy about twice as high as that among white women, with an odds ratio of 1.9. Mexico-born Latina women had a 2.4 odds ratio compared with that of white women. The risk for U.S.-born Mexican women was not markedly greater than that for whites. The greater risk among Mexico-born Latina women could not be attributed to differences in the many parental characteristics and exposures studied.

Conclusions.—The risk for neural tube defect-affected pregnancy is substantially higher in Mexico-born Latina women than in white women. The increased risk is relevant to the population burden of neural tube defects, as nearly 20% of all California births are to Mexican women born in Mexico.

▶ We know that diet, and specifically folic acid, is very important in the prevention of neural tube defects. This study shows that Mexican-American women born in the United States do not have a higher risk compared to other U.S.-born women; however, women born in Mexico have a 2 times higher risk for babies with neural tube defects. Folic acid is contained in green leafy vegetables, along with seafood and meats of higher quality (less fat). The traditional diet in Mexico (tortillas, refried beans, and higher fat meats) is likely to be less adequate in folic acid. More research needs to be done to help certain ethnic groups provide adequate folic acid in their diets along with promoting the recommendation for vitamin supplementation in women of childbearing age.

J.E. Scherger, M.D., M.P.H.

Low-dose Aspirin to Prevent Preeclampsia in Women at High Risk

Caritis S, and the National Institute of Child Health and Human Development Network of Maternal-Fetal Medicine Units (Univ of Pittsburgh, Pa; Univ of Tennessee, Memphis; Univ of Alabama, Birmingham; et al)
N Engl J Med 338:701–705, 1998

Objective.—Large trials studying low-dose aspirin to prevent preeclampsia showed that preeclampsia developed in only 2.5% to 7.6% of women taking placebo. The failure to detect a beneficial effect may have been the result of including women at low risk for preeclampsia who do not benefit from low-dose aspirin. Results of a double-blind, randomized, placebo-controlled trial to determine whether aspirin therapy reduces the incidence of preeclampsia in high-risk women was reported.

Methods.—Thirteen centers identified 2,539 women at high risk for preeclampsia because of pregestational insulin-treated diabetes mellitus (n = 471), chronic hypertension (n = 774), multifetal gestations (n = 688), and previous preeclampsia (n = 606). Between weeks 13 and 36 of pregnancy, women were given either 60 mg of aspirin (n = 1,273) or placebo (n = 1,266) once daily until delivery.

Results.—Nineteen women in the aspirin group and 17 women in the placebo group did not complete the study. The incidence of preeclampsia was similar in both the aspirin (18%) and placebo (22%) groups and between individual risk groups. Risk was lowest for mothers with multifetal gestations and highest for mothers with hypertension. Whereas aspirin significantly reduces the incidence of preterm birth from 18.6% to 17.5%, the difference is not clinically significant.

Conclusions.—Aspirin did not significantly lower the preeclampsia rate in high-risk women and did not reduce a preterm birth rate in a clinically significant manner.

▶ Just when we thought we had a breakthrough in preventing dreaded preeclampsia, further scientific work reveals that low-dose aspirin is probably a false hope. The authors and *The New England Journal of Medicine* are to be commended for persisting with further research to dispel what was felt to be a scientific breakthrough. Negative results that cause us to abandon a treatment are just as important in medical science as a new therapy apparently demonstrated through credible research.

J.E. Scherger, M.D., M.P.H.

Hyperemesis Gravidarum Associated With *Helicobacter pylori* Seropositivity
Frigo P, Lang C, Reisenberger K, et al (Univ Hosp of Vienna)
Obstet Gynecol 91:615–617, 1998   16–4

Background.—Hyperemesis gravidarum, a severe form of morning sickness, is characterized by weight loss, ketonemia, and electrolyte imbalance. Increased serum steroid hormone and human chorionic gonadotropin levels are thought to have a role in this condition. An increased accumulation of fluid caused by increased steroid hormones in pregnant women may lead to a shift in pH, which may result in subclinical *Helicobacter pylori* infection. The possible relationship between *H. pylori* infection and hyperemesis gravidarum was explored.

Methods.—One hundred five patients with hyperemesis gravidarum were studied prospectively. Concentrations of *Helicobacter* serum IgG in this group were compared with those in asymptomatic gravidas matched by gestational week.

Findings.—Serum IgG concentrations were positive in 90.5% of the patients with hyperemesis and in 46.5% of the control subjects. This difference was significant. Mean index percentages of the IgG titers were 74.2% and 24.3% in the hyperemesis and control groups, respectively.

Conclusion.—Infection with *H. pylori* appears to be associated with hyperemesis gravidarum. However, treatment to eradicate *H. pylori* at the time of organogenesis is problematic.

▶ Severe and prolonged vomiting remains an important problem in obstetric care, resulting in temporary disability and frequent hospital admissions. Why some women get this condition and others don't has been a mystery. This study suggests that *H. pylori* may be playing a role. *Helicobacter pylori* has recently emerged as the major cause of peptic ulcer disease. This ubiquitous organism is difficult to eradicate, and triple therapy may not be feasible during pregnancy. We must clarify the role of this organism in gastric disease and develop preventive strategies to help susceptible patients, and in this instance before pregnancy.

J.E. Scherger, M.D, M.P.H.

Ambulatory Blood Pressure Monitoring in Pregnancy: What Is Normal?
Brown MA, Robinson A, Bowyer L, et al (Univ of New South Wales, Kogarah, Australia)
Am J Obstet Gynecol 178:836–842, 1998   16–5

Background.—Although pregnant women have their blood pressure checked at each office visit, the "white coat" effect may affect such readings. This effect results in readings that are higher than would be found with the woman at home and out of the clinic. To determine the normal range of out-of-the-clinic blood pressure values, these authors used ambulatory blood pressure monitoring in women at different stages of pregnancy.

Methods.—Twenty-four hour ambulatory blood pressure monitoring was used in 259 women at any or all of 4 stages of gestation: 9 to 17 weeks, 18 to 22 weeks, 26 to 30 weeks, and more than 30 weeks. Thus, data were measured cross-sectionally, for a total of 276 successful monitoring sessions. None of the subjects had chronic or known "white coat" hypertension. Differences between 4 office determinations and 3 ambulatory determinations were averaged to provide an estimate of the "white coat" effect. Upper limits of normal were defined as 2 SDs above the mean.

Findings.—At all stages of pregnancy, ambulatory blood pressure measurements were significantly higher (by 11 to 12 mm Hg systolic and by 5 to 11 mm Hg diastolic) than values measured in the clinic. Also, throughout pregnancy, measurements while the patient was asleep were significantly lower (by 12% to 14% for systolic and by 18% to 19% for diastolic) than when the patient was awake. Blood pressure varied slightly throughout pregnancy, from 9 to 13 mm Hg while the subject was awake and by 8 to 13 mm Hg while the subject was sleeping. Upper limits of normal awake blood pressure for the 4 gestational stages (9 to 17 weeks, 18 to 22 weeks, 26 to 30 weeks, and more than 30 weeks) were 130/77, 132/79, 133/81, and 135/86 mm Hg, respectively.

Conclusions.—Blood pressure normally rises slightly as pregnancy progresses. Furthermore, the diurnal variations in blood pressure (significantly lower at night) are similar to fluctuations seen in nonpregnant patients. Ambulatory blood pressure readings were actually significantly higher than those measured in the clinic, probably because of increased daytime activity and perhaps some measure of device error (early in the study, the ambulatory monitoring device tended to overestimate blood pressure values). In any case, these data provide reference values for normal blood pressure during pregnancy.

▶ The authors point out that blood pressure measurement is the most frequently performed test on pregnant women, yet very little is known about the normal blood pressure changes of pregnancy. This large study from Australia documents that blood pressure changes substantially during pregnancy. The most practical finding is that diastolic blood pressure generally increases up to 11 mm Hg between the beginning and end of pregnancy. I had generally thought that blood pressure would decrease during pregnancy because of expanded intravascular volume, and that even mild increases could be a warning sign for preeclampsia. I will no longer consider modest increases in diastolic blood pressure during pregnancy as unusual.

J.E. Scherger, M.D., M.P.H.

Treatment of Miscarriage: Current Practice and Rationale
Hemminki E (Natl Research and Development Centre for Welfare and Health, Helsinki)
Obstet Gynecol 91:247–253, 1998
16–6

Objective.—Health service use during miscarriage and medical treatment of miscarriage in Finland and the rationales behind them are reviewed in a descriptive study of treatment practices.

Methods.—In 1994 a survey was mailed to a representative sample of 3,000 Finnish women, aged 18 to 44 years to determine if they had sought medical care for miscarriage between 1990 and 1994. Treatment practices were compared with recommended practices in textbooks. Data for years 1969 through 1989 were compared with data from years 1990 through 1994.

Results.—Of 2,189 responders, 326 (15%) reported 1 or more miscarriages: 166 (51%) during years 1969 through 1989, and 96 (29%) during the years 1990 through 1994. Sixty-four (20%) were included but had missing data on the year. In 1988 and 1995, 84% and 88%, respectively had an evacuation operation. Most textbooks recommended hospitalization, physician care, and routine evacuation. There were no studies that addressed how to deal with completed miscarriages, service provisions, routine evacuations, or immediate evacuation or expectant management of missed abortions. Trials tested different evacuation methods but had ill-defined study groups or were poorly controlled.

Conclusion.—There are no controlled studies of treatment of miscarriage. Clinical trials are needed to provide pregnant women with bleeding problems with the best available information about when to contact health care professionals.

▶ This study shows that our treatment of miscarriage is not evidence based. The almost routine use of hospital visits and uterine evacuation procedures is both expensive and sometimes traumatic for the woman. For years, I have favored an approach of expectant management of these patients with good results. I was delighted to see this article reviewing the literature and being critical of the lack of evidence for the common practice of intervention. The treatment of miscarriage would be a ripe area of study for family physicians active in maternity care.

J.E. Scherger, M.D., M.P.H.

Variations Between Family Physicians and Obstetricians in the Evaluation and Treatment of Preterm Labor

Hueston WJ (Univ of Wisconsin, Madison; Eau Claire Family Practice Residency, Wis)
J Fam Pract 45:336–340, 1997

Background.—Though there are significant differences in maternity care provided by family physicians and obstetricians, outcomes are equally good. The approaches of family physicians and obstetricians when assessing and managing women with preterm contractions or labor were compared.

Methods.—A questionnaire was sent to a random sample of obstetricians and family practitioners in 10 states. Fifty-four percent in active practice completed and returned the questionnaire.

Findings.—When asked about their 3 most common treatment strategies for women with preterm labor, family physicians listed beta agonists and hydration more often than did obstetricians. Obstetricians were more likely to use magnesium sulfate and nifedipine. For the treatment of women with preterm contractions and no cervical changes, obstetricians were more likely to give either of the 2 short-term tocolytic therapies, whereas family physicians were more likely to use less aggressive approaches. After adjustment for facility type and years of experience, family physicians were about half as likely as obstetricians to use tocolytics in women with contractions but no cervical changes.

Conclusions.—Obstetricians appear to be more likely to use more aggressive therapy to treat women with premature contractions but no cervical changes. It is unlikely that patient preferences would affect the choice of treatment for preterm labor.

▶ Clinical guidelines and standards of care are an effort to provide greater consistency in patient care for common conditions. Ideally, one would hope that family physicians active in obstetrics would practice the same standards of care as obstetricians in the treatment of conditions such as preterm labor. The study by Hueston shows that obstetricians tend to be more aggressive with preterm labor, particularly with the use of magnesium sulfate, and with patients without changes in the cervix. If one defines labor as contractions resulting in cervical change, this would suggest that obstetricians may be overdiagnosing preterm labor and overtreating such patients. This study is a reminder that family physicians should focus on evidence-based medicine and a careful consideration of practice guidelines rather than mimicking the behavior of obstetricians.

J.E. Scherger, M.D., M.P.H.

Gestational Diabetes

Selective Screening for Gestational Diabetes Mellitus
Naylor CD, for the Toronto Trihospital Gestational Diabetes Project Investigators (Sunnybrook Health Science Centre, North York, Ont, Canada; Univ of Toronto; Toronto Hosp; et al)
N Engl J Med 337:1591–1596, 1997   16–8

Objective.—Screening all pregnant women for gestational diabetes mellitus is expensive, time-consuming, and uncomfortable for patients. Furthermore, the merits of detecting and treating this condition are difficult to demonstrate. Results of a prospective study evaluating if the efficiency of screening could be enhanced, by considering the patients' risk of gestational diabetes based on their clinical characteristics, are presented.

Methods.—The 3,131 pregnant women in the study were randomly allocated to the derivation or validation group. Risk factors of the derivation group—age, race, body mass index, parity, family history of diabetes, and adverse obstetrical history—were used to establish new screening strategies based on clinical scores that divided women into 3 risk groups: low, intermediate, and high. Low-risk women would not be screened and intermediate-risk women would receive the usual care. Women with plasma glucose levels of 130 mg/dl or high-risk women with plasma glucose levels of 128 mg/dl would receive universal screening. The strategies were evaluated by using the validation group.

Results.—According to multivariate analysis, age, race, and body mass index were independent predictors of gestational diabetes mellitus. The new strategy allowed 34.7% of women to avoid screening. The new strategy detected between 81.2% and 82.6% of women with gestational diabetes, with false-positive rates of 15.4% and 16.0%. Usual care detected 78.3% of women with gestational diabetes, with a false-positive rate of 17.9%.

Conclusion.—The new strategies taking women's clinical characteristics into account allow efficient and accurate screening for gestational diabetes mellitus in pregnant women.

▶ During the 1980s, the dominant thinking was that all pregnant women needed to be screened for gestational diabetes, since risk scoring and selective screening would miss too many cases. Women with very little likelihood for gestational diabetes were having to go through the sometimes unpleasant process of an oral glucose challenge. This article reflects a trend back toward selective screening, a welcome trend to physicians delivering pregnancy care. But physicians must remain vigilant in making the diagnosis of gestational diabetes, and consider screening in all patients.

J.E. Scherger, M.D., M.P.H.

Does a High Carbohydrate Preparatory Diet Affect the 3-Hour Oral Glucose Tolerance Test in Pregnancy?

Entrekin K, Work B, Owen J (Univ of Alabama, Birmingham; Med College of Georgia, Augusta)
J Matern Fetal Med 7:68–71, 1998

16–9

Objective.—The clinical benefits of a high carbohydrate diet consumed for 3 days before a glucose tolerance test (GTT) for gestational diabetes have not been established. This recommendation was prospectively tested at a university hospital outpatient obstetric clinic.

Methods.—A total of 354 pregnant women with elevated blood sugar screening tests were studied. The women were divided into 3 groups: the Carbo group ($n = 108$) ate 150 g or more of carbohydrate per day for 3 days; the Candy group ($n = 105$) consumed 6 Snickers candy bars per day for 3 days; and the Ad Lib group ($n = 141$) ate their usual diets for 3 days before taking a GTT. Whole-blood glucose values were determined at 1, 2, and 3 hours. The outcome measure was the incidence of gestational diabetes mellitus among the 3 groups.

Results.—According to the GTT, 29% of the Carbo group, 28% of the Ad Lib group, and 28% of the Candy group had gestational diabetes. Glucose values at 1, 2, and 3 hours were similar among groups (Table 3).

Conclusions.—The type of preparatory diet does not affect the results of the GTT in pregnancy.

▶ Old conventions are hard to replace. Certain protocols, however inconvenient, have a way of persisting. The oral GTT has largely been removed from medical practice except in pregnancy, where it remains the gold standard for diagnosing gestational diabetes. Preparing a patient for a GTT, with the recommendation of 3 days of a high carbohydrate diet, has always been filled with uncertainty as to its importance and compliance. This study suggests that the 3-day carbohydrate loading is not necessary before a GTT in pregnancy because it has no impact on the laboratory values. Simplifying the oral GTT in pregnancy will help with its use, and lessen the temptation to diagnose gestational diabetes only on the basis of screening tests.

J.E. Scherger, M.D., M.P.H.

TABLE 3.—Mean (SD) Blood Sugar Values of Women Assigned to 1 of 3 Preparatory Diets for the Glucose Tolerance Test

	Carbo	Ad Lib	Candy	P
Fasting	82 (13)	79 (12)	80 (13)	.36
1-hour	151 (36)	153 (37)	149 (38)	.72
2-hour	130 (34)	131 (35)	130 (35)	.91
3-hour	104 (28)	103 (33)	103 (36)	.99

Abbreviation: SD, one standard deviation.
(Courtesy of Entrekin K, Work B, Owen J: Does a high carbohydrate preparatory diet affect the 3-hour oral glucose tolerance test in pregnancy? *J Matern Fetal Med* 7:68–71, 1998.)

Studies of Postnatal Diabetes Mellitus in Women Who Had Gestational Diabetes: Part 1. Estimation of the Prevalence of Unrecognized Prepregnancy Diabetes Mellitus
Beischer NA, Wein P, Sheedy MT, et al (Univ of Melbourne, Australia; Mercy Hosp for Women, Melbourne, Australia)
Aust N Z J Obstet Gynaecol 37:412–419, 1997   16–10

Objective.—The number of women with gestational diabetes (GD) who were glucose intolerant before pregnancy is unknown. The proportion of GD caused by undiagnosed prepregnancy diabetes and an estimate of the prevalence of undiagnosed prepregnancy diabetes mellitus in women in the state of Victoria, Australia were determined.

Methods.—A glucose tolerance test (GTT) was performed in 57,563 women due to deliver at Mercy Hospital for Women during the past 25 years. Gestational diabetes was defined as a 1-hour plasma glucose value of 9.0 mmol/L or greater and a 2-hour value of 7.0 mmol/L or greater. Women were followed after delivery, 4 to 6 weeks later, and at 1 year if the GTT was abnormal or at 2 years if it was not.

Results.—Gestational diabetes was diagnosed in 4,243 deliveries in 3,730 women. A GTT was performed after 2,957 deliveries. Diabetes was diagnosed in 59 women within 6 months of delivery and in 55 by postnatal GTT. Ketosis developed in 3 women during pregnancy and in 1 woman at 11 weeks after delivery. Considering pregnancy and postpregnancy GTT, it would appear that 53% of the women (31 of 59) had unrecognized prepregnancy diabetes mellitus.

Conclusion.—The prevalence of unrecognized diabetes is estimated at 1 in 1,031 women of child-bearing age.

Studies of Postnatal Diabetes Mellitus in Women Who Had Gestational Diabetes: Part 2. Prevalence and Predictors of Diabetes Mellitus After Delivery
Wein P, Beischer NA, Sheedy MT (Univ of Melbourne, Australia; Mercy Hosp for Women, Melbourne, Australia)
Aust N Z J Obstet Gynaecol 37:420–423, 1997   16–11

Objective.—Mercy Hospital for Women in Melbourne, Australia performs a glucose tolerance test (GTT) on all pregnant women and repeats the test 6 weeks after delivery in all women with gestational diabetes (GD). Whether GD is a risk factor for postnatal diabetes mellitus is not known. The prevalence and predictors of postnatal diabetes mellitus was determined in 3,730 women with GD diagnosed in 57,563 consecutive pregnancies.

Methods.—The definition of GD as determined in 2.5% of the population was a 1-hour plasma glucose level of 9.0 mmol/L or greater and a 2-hour value of 7.0 mmol/L or greater. The associations between severity of GD based on the antenatal GTT, fetal macrosomia, insulin requirement during pregnancy, maternal age, country of birth, and booking status in women with GD who had diabetes mellitus vs. those who did not were analyzed. The GD was classified by severity as grade 1 (1-hour plasma glucose level of 9.0 mmol/L or greater and a 2-hour value of 7.0 mmol/L or greater); grade 2 (1-hour plasma glucose level of 10.0 mmol/L or greater and a 2-hour value of 7.8 mmol/L or greater); grade 3 (2-hour value of 8.9–12.1 mmol/L or greater); and grade 4 (fasting 7.8 mmol/L or greater or 2-hour 12.2 mmol/L or greater).

Results.—Gestational diabetes was diagnosed in 3,730 women during 4,243 pregnancies (5% of deliveries). Diabetes mellitus was diagnosed in 59 women (2%) within 6 months after delivery. Two had grade 1 GD postnatally, 8 had grade 2, 18 had grade 3, and 30 had grade 4. Only 10.6% of women with GD who needed insulin had postnatal diabetes mellitus. The severity of GD, Asian origin, and 1-hour plasma glucose value during the antenatal GTT were risk factors for postnatal diabetes mellitus. For every 1 mmol/l increase in antenatal GTT, the risk of postnatal diabetes mellitus increased 47%.

Conclusion.—Severity of GD, Asian origin, and 1-hour plasma glucose value during the antenatal GTT were significant and independent predictors of postnatal diabetes mellitus.

▶ This large study (Abstracts 16–10 and 16–11) from Australia shows that some women with a diagnosis of GD actually have unrecognized prepregnancy diabetes mellitus. Even though this population may represent only 2% of pregnancies regarded as complicated by GD, this percentage may contribute to findings of complications not generally attributed to GD. Prepregnancy diabetes mellitus has many risk factors for pregnancy, whereas GD is associated with only macrosomia and consequent birth complications. This large study also underscores the importance of a follow-up GTT in patients with GD.

J.E. Scherger, M.D, M.P.H.

Self-Perceived Health Status of Women Three to Five Years After the Diagnosis of Gestational Diabetes: A Survey of Cases and Matched Controls

Feig DS, Chen E, Naylor CD, et al (Sunnybrook Health Science Centre, Toronto; Univ of Toronto)
Am J Obstet Gynecol 178:386–393, 1998   16–12

Objective.—A survey was mailed to women with and without gestational diabetes, identified by the Toronto Tri-Hospital Gestational Diabetes Project, to measure their self-rated health status on the SF-36 and their anxieties about their own health and that of the children born from the index pregnancy.

Methods.—Surveys were mailed to 139 women diagnosed with gestational diabetes between September 1989 and March 1992 and to 406 age-, delivery date-, race-, and family history-matched control subjects in a randomized, prospective, analytic cohort study.

Results.—Sixty-five usable case and 197 usable control subject surveys were returned. Fourteen women with gestational diabetes did not recall having it, and 11 control subjects said they had had gestational diabetes at some time. SF-36 health scores were significantly lower for women with gestational diabetes than for control subjects (68.9 vs. 73.8). When women with gestational diabetes who denied having it and control subjects who said they had had gestational diabetes were excluded, the differences were no longer significant (70.9 vs. 74.4). Compared with control subjects, women with gestational diabetes were significantly more worried about their own health (99 vs. 109), rated their child as significantly less healthy than children of control subjects (103.8 vs. 111.6), and worried that they were significantly more likely to have diabetes (70.09 vs. 73.38). Women's worry about their health was negatively correlated with diabetes prevention behavior. Compared with control women, women with diabetes were significantly more likely to believe they were at increased risk for the development of diabetes.

Conclusion.—Compared with control women, women diagnosed with gestational diabetes viewed their health and the health of their children as poorer.

▶ Disease labels have a profound effect on a patient's self-perceived sense of health and well being. Because of the low specificity of common screening tests for gestational diabetes, many pregnant women are given this diagnosis without actually having the disease. This study suggests that a diagnosis of gestational diabetes does produce long-term consequences in how women view their own health status. We must be mindful that a short-term focus on care during pregnancy does have long-term effects. Disease labels should only be given out when they truly exist.

J.E. Scherger, M.D., M.P.H.

Labor and Delivery

A Randomized Placebo-controlled Evaluation of Terbutaline for External Cephalic Version
Fernandez CO, Bloom SL, Smulian JC, et al (Univ of Texas, Dallas; UMDNJ, New Brunswick, NJ)
Obstet Gynecol 90:775–779, 1997

Introduction.—External cephalic version has resurfaced with ongoing pressures to decrease cesarean delivery rates. Only 2 randomized, placebo-controlled trials have assessed the effects of tocolysis. The effects of subcutaneous terbutaline on the success rate of term external cephalic version were evaluated in women with singleton noncephalic gestations.

Methods.—One hundred three women were randomly assigned to receive either subcutaneous terbutaline, 0.25 mg, or placebo. External cephalic version was attempted at 15–30 minutes after injection. External cephalic version was discontinued after 3 attempts, for patient discomfort, if there was fetal heart rate deceleration, or when successful. Patients were discharged home and followed up weekly thereafter. Outcome measures included initial success of external version, presentation in labor, route of delivery, and indications for operative delivery.

Results.—External cephalic version was achieved in 27 of 52 women (52%) receiving terbutaline and 14 of 51 (27%) receiving placebo (a significant difference). Four (15%) and 3 (21%) of the successful versions in the terbutaline and placebo groups, respectively, spontaneously reverted to breech presentation. During labor, there were 24 (46%) and 13 (25%) cephalic presentations in the terbutaline and placebo groups, respectively. For women with successful versions, the cesarean delivery rates were 11 of 41 (27%). For failed versions, the rate was 58 of 62 (94%).

Conclusions.—The initial success rate of versions and the rate of cephalic presentations in labor were significantly increased and the rate of cesarean deliveries was significantly reduced with subcutaneous administration of terbutaline before attempted version in women at term with noncephalic presentation.

▶ External version is a technique that may be performed by family physicians using ultrasound, reducing the frequency of breech presentation at term, and reducing the rate of cesarean section. This nice study shows that a subcutaneous dose of terbutaline may be helpful in relaxing the uterus and increasing the rate of successful versions.

J.E. Scherger, M.D., M.P.H.

Neonatal Cephalohematoma From Vacuum Extraction
Bofill JA, Rust OA, Devidas M, et al (Univ of Mississippi, Jackson)
J Reprod Med 42:565–569, 1997
16–14

Background.—The rupture of a diploic or emissary vessel in the potential space between the periosteum and the outer edge of the fetal skull can result in a neonatal cephalohematoma. Cephalohematomas are more common after vacuum-assisted vaginal delivery than after forceps or spontaneous births. The factors predisposing to the development of cephalohematoma after vacuum extraction are not known.

Methods and Findings.—At 34 or more weeks' gestation, 322 women were assigned randomly to delivery by vacuum delivery using the intermittent or continuous technique. Cephalohematomas occurred in roughly equal numbers in the 2 groups. Cephalohematoma was significantly associated with station at point of application, increasing asynclitism, and increasing application to delivery time. In a stepwise multiple logistic regression analysis, only the last 2 factors were significant. Nonsignificant factors included gestational age, birth weight, instrumental rotation, and previous vaginal delivery.

Conclusions.—Increasing asynclitism appears to be the only predelivery factor predisposing to neonatal cephalohematoma after vacuum-assisted delivery. Cephalohematoma formation was more likely to develop as the duration of vacuum application increased during delivery. However, only 28% of the neonates in this series had cephalohematoma when the time to vacuum application to delivery exceeded 5 minutes.

▶ This study looked at 2 techniques of vacuum extraction, continuous and intermittent. The continuous pressure technique is new and not generally described in protocols for vacuum extraction. Cephalohematoma and other scalp trauma are the greatest risks with vacuum extraction, and providers such as family physicians may be timid in its use. This study shows that the total amount of time that the vacuum cup is in contact with the fetal head is the most important variable in causing damage, and continuous extraction does not increase the risk over intermittent technique. Also, continuous pressure may have the advantage of facilitating rotation of the fetal head. Family physicians may be encouraged to consider continuous application of a vacuum extractor in patients, particularly those needing head rotation, but they should also be aware that prolonged application increases risk. The Advanced Life Support in Obstetrics course, sponsored by the American Academy of Family Physicians, recommends that the vacuum not be applied greater than 30 minutes.[1]

J.E. Scherger, M.D., M.P.H.

Reference

1. American Academy of Family Physicians. Advanced Life Support in Obstetrics Course Syllabus, "Forceps and Vacuum Extraction," Third Edition, 1996, pp 137–147.

Vaginal Birth After Cesarean Delivery: An Admission Scoring System
Flamm BL, Geiger AM (Kaiser Permanente Med Ctrs, Southern California Region, Riverside)
Obstet Gynecol 90:907–910, 1997   16–15

Background.—Though vaginal birth after cesarean (VBAC) has been shown to be safe, complications are apparently more likely to occur in women who have an unsuccessful trial of labor. In the current study, a scoring system was developed to predict the likelihood of vaginal birth in patients undergoing a trial of labor after previous cesarean delivery using factors known at admission.

Methods.—A trial of labor was attempted in 5,022 women assigned randomly to score derivation and score testing groups. Multivariate logistic regression modeling was applied to score derivation group data to develop a predictive scoring system for vaginal birth. This system was then tested using data from the testing group.

TABLE 2.—Admission Characteristics and Assigned Score Points Predicting Successful Vaginal Birth After Cesarean (Score Development Group)

Characteristic	β Coefficient	Odds Ratio	95% CI	Score Points*
Age under 40	0.95	2.58	1.55, 4.3	2
Vaginal birth history				
Before and after first cesarean	2.21	9.11	2.18, 38.04	4
After first cesarean	1.22	3.39	2.25, 5.11	2
Before first cesarean	0.43	1.53	1.12, 2.10	1
None	referent			0
Reason other than FTP for first cesarean	0.66	1.93	1.58, 2.35	1
Cervical effacement at admission				
>75%	1.00	2.72	2.00, 3.71	2
25%–75%	0.58	1.79	1.31, 2.44	1
<25%	referent			0
Cervical dilation 4 cm or more at admission	0.77	2.16	1.66, 2.82	1

CI = confidence interval; FTP = failure to progress.
*Select one value, which may be zero, from each of the 5 categories.
(Courtesy of Flamm BL, Geiger AM: Vaginal birth after cesarean delivery: An admission scoring system. *Obstet Gynecol* 90:907–910, 1997. Reprinted with permission from The American College of Obstetricians and Gynecologists.)

Findings.—Five variables significantly affected mode of birth and were included in the weighted scoring system (Table 2). Rates of successful VBAC ranged from 49% in women with scores of 0 to 2 to 95% in those with scores of 8 to 10. Increasing score and an increasing probability of VBAC were correlated linearly (Table 3).

Conclusions.—This scoring system may be useful for counseling patients about the option of VBAC. Such information may be especially helpful for patients opting for trial of labor but beginning to doubt this choice after labor has begun.

TABLE 3.—Performance of Admission Score

	Score Development Group			Score Testing Group		
Score	Number With Score	% VBAC	% Cesarean	Number With Score	% VBAC	% Cesarean
0 to 2	120	41.7	58.3	114	49.1	50.9
3	346	59.2	40.8	329	59.9	40.1
4	605	64.3	35.7	595	66.7	33.3
5	664	79.1	20.9	660	77.0	23.0
6	354	87.6	12.4	360	88.6	11.4
7	183	93.4	6.6	189	92.6	7.4
8 to 10	142	99.3	0.7	158	94.9	5.1
Total	2414	74.2	25.8	2405	74.9	25.1

VBAC = Vaginal birth after cesarean.
(Courtesy of Flamm BL, Geiger AM: Vaginal birth after cesarean delivery: An admission scoring system. *Obstet Gynecol* 90:907–910, 1997. Reprinted with permission from The American College of Obstetricians and Gynecologists.)

▶ I generally do not pay attention to scoring systems in pregnancy because they have a miserable record of being more useful than clinical judgment. However, the lead author of this article, Bruce Flamm, has great experience with vaginal birth after cesarean delivery. While virtually all patients deserve a trial of labor after previous cesarean section, the data provided by Flamm and Geiger in this large study would provide useful predictive value for both physicians and patients.

J.E. Scherger, M.D., M.P.H.

A Cut Above: The Rising Caesarean Section Rate in New Zealand
Bulger T, Howden-Chapman P, Stone P, et al (Wellington School of Medicine, New Zealand)
N Z Med J 111:30–33, 1998   16–16

Objective.—The cesarian section rate (CSR) is rising worldwide. Because of the increased risks to mother and infant and the increased cost of cesarian deliveries, the trends in frequency of cesarian section (CS) were examined in New Zealand.

Methods.—The demographics for women having a CS for the period 1988/89 to 1994/95 were compared with published information for 1983/84.

Results.—The CSR increased from 9.6% in 1983/84 to 11.6% in 1988/89 to 15.3% in 1994/95. Failure to progress accounted for 28% of CSs, and previous CS for 19%. These combined with fetal distress and breech presentation accounted for 67% of CSs. The number of CSs increased with age of the mother across all ethnic groups, with Maori women having the lowest CSR. The reasons for the increases are not clear. The increase in repeat CSR is partially the result of concern over uterine rupture which, studies have demonstrated, occurs in less than 1% of cases. Almost all women having CSs were satisfied, and almost half would do it again. Hospital programs for lowering the CSR have been more successful than national programs.

Conclusions.—The CSR is increasing for reasons that are not entirely clear. Hospital-based programs to lower the rate are more successful than national initiatives.

▶ I included this article because of its marked contrast from the U.S. data. In the United States, the CSR peaked at near 25% in the early 1990s and has now declined to about 21%. Most authorities are recommending a target CSR of about 15%. It is interesting that in New Zealand, a rise from 9.6% to 15.3% over 10 years (1984–1994) has been met with alarm. Because CS is safer for the mother and baby than most complicated vaginal deliveries, and increased infant monitoring during labor raises the CSR, a target in developed countries of around 15% is a reasonable goal. The United States and New Zealand appear to be approaching this mean from opposite directions.

J.E. Scherger, M.D., M.P.H.

Pregnancy Outcomes

Effect of Pelvic Muscle Exercise on Transient Incontinence During Pregnancy and After Birth

Sampselle CM, Miller JM, Mims BL, et al (Univ of Michigan, Ann Arbor; Kent State Univ, Ohio)
Obstet Gynecol 91:406–412, 1998

Background.—Vaginal birth has a major effect on the development of urinary incontinence, although pregnancy with cesarean birth may also be a risk factor. In nonpregnant, incontinent women, pelvic muscle exercise has been shown to increase muscle strength and decrease urine loss. There is little information about the effect of pelvic muscle exercise on urinary incontinence in women in their childbearing years.

Methods.—In a prospective, randomized trial, 72 pregnant women were assigned to a treatment group where they received instruction in pelvic muscle exercise or to a control group which received routine care with no instruction in pelvic muscle exercise. The women completed a questionnaire concerning symptoms of urinary incontinence, and pelvic muscle strength was measured with an instrumented gynecologic speculum. Data were obtained at 20 weeks and 35 weeks of gestation, and at 6 weeks, 6 months, and 12 months after birth.

Results.—Data were reported for 46 women who had either vaginal or cesarean birth and for a subsample of 37 women who had vaginal birth. Longitudinal data were reported for women who provided complete data throughout the study. Women in the treatment group have decreased symptoms of urinary incontinence; significant effects from treatment were seen at 35 weeks of gestation and at 6 weeks and 6 months post partum. A significant interaction between time and treatment for urinary incontinence was shown by a repeated measures analysis of variance. Initial pelvic muscle strength had a significant effect on pelvic muscle strength during pregnancy and after birth; pelvic muscle strength at 20 weeks of gestation was a significant predictor of strength at 12 months post partum. Women in the treatment group had greater pelvic muscle strength at 6 weeks and 6 months post partum than did women in the control group, but this difference was not statistically significant.

Discussion.—Based on these findings, the authors recommend that women receive instruction in pelvic muscle exercise before and after birth. Because of the importance of baseline pelvic muscle strength, it is also recommended that pelvic muscle strength be evaluated in women who are planning a first pregnancy and that those with muscle weakness be encouraged to perform pelvic muscle exercise.

▶ It is nice to know that the exercises we request women to do during and after pregnancy actually work. Even though this study relied on self-reported data, the decrease in incontinence is impressive.

J.E. Scherger, M.D., M.P.H.

Pregnancy Outcome and Weight Gain Recommendations for the Morbidly Obese Woman

Bianco AT, Smilen SW, Davis Y, et al (Mount Sinai Med Ctr, New York; New York Univ)
Obstet Gynecol 91:97–102, 1998

16–18

Objective.—Although the prevalence of morbid obesity is increasing in women of child-bearing age and obesity is a risk factor for poor infant and maternal outcomes, there is little information about the effect of the amount of gestational weight gain on pregnancy outcome in obese women. Results were reported of a retrospective cohort study comparing perinatal morbidity and neonatal outcome in morbidly obese and nonobese women and investigating the effect of gestational weight gain on pregnancy in morbidly obese women.

Methods.—The effect of gestational weight on pregnancy was compared in 613 morbidly obese women and 11,313 nonobese controls, aged 20 to 34 years, who delivered between 1988 and 1995. Multiple regression analysis was used to evaluate associations between obesity and race, parity, clinic service, substance abuse, and pre-existing medical conditions.

Results.—Morbidly obese women were more likely to be black or Hispanic, parous, attending a clinic, substance abusers, and having preexisting medical conditions than nonobese women. Morbidly obese women gained an average of 20 pounds, whereas nonobese women gained an average of 31.4 pounds. Morbidly obese women were at higher risk for gestational diabetes (odds ratio [OR], 3.2), pregnancy-induced hypertension (OR, 3.6), placental abruption (OR, 1.4), fetal distress (OR, 1.3), meconium (OR, 1.3), failure to progress (OR, 2.6), and cesarean section (OR, 2.3). These risk factors for morbidly obese patients were not affected by gestational weight gain, although these patients were significantly more likely than controls to have infants who were large for gestational age and required neonatal ICU admission.

Conclusion.—Gestational weight gain in morbidly obese women adversely affects neonatal, but not perinatal, outcome. Morbidly obese women should not gain more than 25 pounds during pregnancy to avoid delivering a large-for-gestational-age infant.

▶ The increased risk of morbidly obese pregnant women is well known. What is not well understood is the degree to which gestational weight gain may increase or decrease these risks. This retrospective study of over 600 morbidly obese women, compared with a much larger control group, documented the risks and showed that these were not affected by gestational weight gain. However, I recommend that obese women gain less than the recommended 22–28 lbs during pregnancy to not let weight gain during pregnancy worsen the maternal obesity. This study shows that lower than generally recommended weight gains are safe in obese women, i.e., they do not increase the risk of a low–birth weight neonate. I have achieved great patient satisfaction in helping obese pregnant women gain just 10–15 lbs during their pregnancy.

J.E. Scherger, M.D., M.P.H.

Obstetric Outcome in 100 Women With Severe Anxiety Over Childbirth
Sjögren B, Thomassen P (Karolinska Hosp, Stockholm; Södersjukhuset, Stockholm)
Acta Obstet Gynecol Scand 76:948–952, 1997   16–19

Background.—About 20% of pregnant women have fear of delivery, and many of these women request cesarean section. In Sweden, the rate of cesarean section performed for psychosocial indications increased from 0.57% to 1.45% of all births from 1983 to 1989. The rate of cesarean section in absolute numbers increased from about 680 to 1,700 per year during the same period. A recent study has reported that fear of delivery primarily results from lack of trust and self-confidence and a fear of death, pain, and loss of control. A treatment model based on individual psychological and obstetric support was evaluated.

Methods.—The obstetric outcomes of 100 women referred because of severe anxiety over childbirth and 100 control subjects were evaluated. A detailed obstetric and psychological history was obtained, and interested women were referred to a psychotherapist. Most women maintained contact with a psychosomatic gynecologist to discuss the psychological and obstetric aspects of childbirth.

Results.—Women in the study group had a higher rate of psychic problems than those in the control group. Of the 100 women in the study group, 68 initially requested cesarean section. After psychological intervention, 38 of these women agreed to vaginal delivery and 30 had an elective cesarean section. Another 13 women had a cesarean section for obstetric or mixed reasons. There was a low complication rate, which was similar in both groups. Women in the study group who had vaginal delivery had a higher rate of induction of labor, a higher rate of epidural and pudendal anesthesia, and shorter labor time. The savings from the fewer cesarean sections performed more than made up for the cost of psychological therapy.

Discussion.—A 50% reduction in the number of cesarean sections performed for psychosocial indications was seen after an individualized treatment program of psychological and obstetric support for women with severe fear of childbirth, making them similar to a control group. The cost of the psychological treatment was less than the savings from the fewer cesarean sections performed. The advantages of an emotionally satisfying delivery, with positive effects on the mother-child relationship, cannot be expressed in economic terms.

▶ One of the pleasures of being an editor for the YEAR BOOK OF FAMILY PRACTICE is reviewing the interesting and practical studies done in Sweden.

This article describes 100 women who worry those of us providing childbirth services. Does extreme fear of childbirth complicate pregnancy? This study shows that these women generally have a good outcome and that psychosocial support may help most of them have a successful vaginal delivery.

J.E. Scherger, M.D., M.P.H.

Pregnancy Outcomes in Women With Gestational Diabetes Compared With the General Obstetric Population
Casey BM, Lucas MJ, McIntire DD, et al (Univ of Texas, Dallas)
Obstet Gynecol 90:869–873, 1997   16–20

Background.—Gestational diabetes complicates 1% to 3% of all pregnancies. Authorities disagree about the significance of gestational diabetes in women without concomitant fasting hyperglycemia. Pregnancy outcomes in a homogeneous group of women with glucose intolerance were compared with those of women without this disorder.

Methods.—Data on all women with singleton cephalic-presenting neonates giving birth at 1 center between 1991 and 1995 were retrospectively analyzed. Of 61,209 nondiabetic women, 874 were given a diagnosis of class A_1 gestational diabetes.

Findings.—Women with class A_1 gestational diabetes were significantly older, heavier, of greater parity, and more often Hispanic than those without. Hypertension was present in 17% and 12%, respectively. Thirty percent of the women with gestational diabetes and 17% of those without had cesarean deliveries. Also significant was the between-group difference in the incidence of shoulder dystocia: 3% and 1%, respectively. Infants born to women with gestational diabetes were significantly larger, which explained the increase in dystocia. There was a 12% attributable risk for large-for-gestational-age infants in women with class A_1 gestational diabetes.

Conclusion.—Excessive fetal size is the main effect of class A_1 gestational diabetes. Large size can increase the risk of difficult labor and delivery. About 1 in 8 women with class A_1 gestational diabetes mellitus will give birth to a large-for-gestational-age infant because of glucose intolerance.

▶ This article reinforces the fact that gestational diabetes does not carry all of the many complications that overt diabetes brings to a pregnancy. The singular outcome that gestational diabetes brings is macrosomia, with its attendant intrapartum complications such as shoulder dystocia. Patients with gestational diabetes should be monitored carefully in late pregnancy for hypertension and other problems that all pregnant women are monitored for.

J.E. Scherger, M.D., M.P.H.

Miscellaneous

Why Family Physicians Deliver Babies
Roberts RG, Bobula JA, Wolkomir MS, et al (Univ of Wisconsin, Madison; Med College of Wisconsin, Milwaukee)
J Fam Pract 46:34–40, 1998
16–21

Background.—Family physicians attend about 500,000 of the 4 million births in the United States annually, are better distributed geographically than obstetricians, and have a smaller percentage of patients with preterm labor who have epidural anesthesia, episiotomy, instrument delivery, or cesarean section. The percentage of family physicians who deliver infants has decreased from 37% in 1980 to 26% in 1993. This decrease may have negative effects on the health of pregnant women and their newborns. The role of family physicians in prenatal care is important for the 25% of Americans who live in rural areas, where family physicians make up two thirds of maternity caregivers. The reasons why family physicians choose to deliver infants were explored.

Methods.—A questionnaire was mailed to 1,300 family physicians who attended continuing education courses in pregnancy. Respondents were identified as (1) those who had always delivered infants; (2) those who had previously not delivered infants, but had recently started to or planned to; and (3) those who had never delivered infants, or who had stopped doing so. The responses of the first 2 groups were contrasted with the responses of the third group.

Results.—Of the 1,300 mailed questionnaires, 575 were returned and considered for analysis. There were 421 physicians in group 1, 92 physicians in group 2, and 62 physicians in group 3. The responses did not vary among geographic regions. The most common reasons for choosing to deliver infants were personal enjoyment, adequate obstetric training in residency, desire to care for younger families, and experience with supportive obstetricians during residency. The most common reasons for choosing not to deliver infants were unacceptable lifestyle, community saturation of maternity caregivers, fear of lawsuits, and lack of need to build a practice.

Discussion.—These findings show that family physicians who choose to deliver infants often do so for personal enjoyment and that those who do not deliver infants have concerns about the lifestyle of a maternity caregiver. External factors also affected these decisions. Family physicians who had had experiences with supportive obstetricians during residency were more likely to choose to deliver infants. Family physicians who wish to practice obstetrics may be more attracted to practices that treat younger patients or patients from communities that accept family physicians in the role of a maternity caregiver.

▶ This article was a breath of fresh air in a year that has shown some decline in the number of family physicians providing obstetric care. Despite ever-increasing technology, liability concerns, and pressure from obstetricians and hospital staff, family physicians who deliver infants continue to show a high degree of personal enjoyment.

J.E. Scherger, M.D., M.P.H.

Midwifery Care, Social and Medical Risk Factors, and Birth Outcomes in the USA

MacDorman MF, Singh GK (Ctrs for Disease Control and Prevention, Hyattsville, Md; Univ of Kansas, Topeka)
J Epidemiol Community Health 52:310–317, 1998   16–22

Objective.—The infant mortality rate in the United States is twice as high as that of number-one ranked Japan, primarily because of barriers to prenatal and perinatal care for many pregnant women. Many have advocated the increasing use of midwives to provide needed care at lower costs so long as the use of midwives does not compromise the care of mothers and infants. Birth outcomes and infant mortality rates for births in the United States delivered by physicians and certified nurse midwives were compared.

Methods.—Multivariate logistic regression was used to compare the risks of infant mortality and low birth weight for singleton vaginal births at 35–43 weeks' gestation delivered by physicians or nurse midwives during 1991. Women with similar sociodemographic and medical risks were studied.

Results.—Physicians delivered 94.7% of births and certified nurse midwives, 4.1% of births. The infant mortality rate was 53.4% lower for certified nurse midwives than for physicians for all births, and 13.9% lower for singleton vaginal deliveries. The percentage of low birth weight and preterm births was significantly higher for physicians than for certified nurse midwives. Certified nurse midwives delivered a greater percentage of at-risk mothers. Certified nurse midwives had a 19% lower adjusted risk of infant mortality, a 33% lower risk of neonatal mortality, and a 31% lower risk of delivering a low–birth weight infant than did physicians. The average birth weight for midwife-assisted births was 37 g higher than for physician-assisted births. Postneonatal mortality rates were similar.

Conclusions.—Use of certified nurse midwives is a safe and less expensive alternative to maternity care, particularly for disadvantaged mothers.

▶ This large national study documents the excellent outcomes for certified nurse midwives in obstetric care. Although questions always remain regarding patient mix and referral of higher-risk patients, the bottom line is that the birth outcomes from midwifery care are excellent. Family physicians active in obstetric care should consider working with midwives to provide high-quality care. It is always good to be associated with professionals who have such excellent results.

J.E. Scherger, M.D., M.P.H.

17 Other Clinical Issues

Overview

Randomized controlled trials: Abstracts 17–14, 17–15, and 17–20

Cancer

- A 20-year report card of cancer in the United States
- Aspirin in the prevention of colorectal cancer
- Patient treatment preferences and prognosis
- Cancer risk among offspring of childhood cancer survivors
- Cough as an indicator of lung cancer

Ethics and End-of-Life Issues

- Physician and patient attitudes toward drug company gifts
- The ethics of controversial screening tests
- Bedside rationing and the patient's best interests
- Patient and physician roles in end-of-life decisions
- Physician-assisted suicide and euthanasia in the United States

Patient Compliance

- Financial incentives to achieve compliance
- Dosage frequency and compliance

Alternative and Complementary Medicine

- Why patients use alternative medicine
- Therapeutic touch

Miscellaneous

- Pain in seriously ill hospitalized adults
- Adverse drug reactions in hospitalized patients
- Antinuclear antibody testing as a screen for rheumatic diseases
- Publication bias for reporting positive results
- Effects of students on ambulatory encounters
- Gowning and patient satisfaction

Cancer

Cancer Incidence and Mortality, 1973–1995: A Report Card for the U.S.
Wingo PA, Ries LAG, Rosenberg HM, et al (American Cancer Society, Atlanta, Ga; Natl Cancer Inst, Bethesda, Md; Ctrs for Disease Control and Prevention, Hyattsville, Md; et al)
Cancer 82:1197–1207, 1998   17–1

Objective.—Cancer incidence and mortality declined between 1990 and 1995 for the first time since record keeping began in the 1930s.

Methods.—Cancer incidence, mortality rates, and short-term trends were reported for whites, blacks, Asians and Pacific Islanders, and Hispanics.

Results.—Whereas incidence rates increased by 1.2% per year between 1973 and 1990, rates declined nonsignificantly by 0.7% per year during 1990–1995, with decreases in incidence of cancers of the lung, prostate, colon/rectum, urinary bladder, and leukemia. Incidences of lung, colon/rectum, and urinary bladder cancers decreased significantly. Female breast cancer incidence was no longer increasing significantly during this period. After significant annual increases in death rates for all sites of 0.4% per year between 1973 and 1990, rates declined significantly by 0.5% per year during 1990–1995. Death rates from the 4 leading cancers—lung, female breast, prostate, and colon/rectum—declined significantly between 1990 and 1995, with the decline in combined rates in males being greater than the decline in females.

Conclusions.—These results and trends indicate that efforts to control and new methods of treating cancer are working.

▶ This "report card" documents a decline in cancer incidence and mortality for the first time. In last year's YEAR BOOK OF FAMILY PRACTICE, I commented on an article by Bailar[1] who was skeptical about "gains" in cancer control, arguing for more research into primary and secondary prevention. This article, documenting modest improvements in cancer incidence and mortality in the early 1990s, does not change the validity of Bailar's analysis. Cancer incidence and mortality are still higher today than in 1973. This article does suggest that we turned a corner around 1990, and it will be of critical interest to see whether the trend continues. Whether the improvements can be attributed to prevention or treatment is still very much at issue.

A.O. Berg, M.D., M.P.H.

Reference

1. 1998 YEAR BOOK OF FAMILY PRACTICE, p 357.

Aspirin Use and Colorectal Cancer: Post-Trial Follow-up Data From the Physicians' Health Study
Stürmer T, Glynn RJ, Lee I-M, et al (Harvard Med School, Boston)
Ann Intern Med 128:713-720, 1998

Introduction.—Observational studies have reported that the use of aspirin and other nonsteroidal anti-inflammatory drugs (NSAIDs) reduces colorectal cancer incidence or mortality. The Physicians' Health Study, however, found no association between aspirin and colorectal cancer after 5 years of low-dose aspirin. In the current analysis, the follow-up period of the Physicians' Health Study was extended to a mean of 12 years.

Methods.—Two hypotheses were tested in the Physicians' Health Study: that the risk of cardiovascular disease is reduced by taking 325 mg aspirin on alternate days and that the incidence of cancer is decreased by taking 50 mg of β-carotene taken on alternate days. The aspirin arm of the trial was stopped early (January 1988) and the β-carotene arm continued until December 1995, its scheduled completion. Participants were male physicians aged 40 to 84. This analysis used all confirmed incident cases of colorectal cancer and all cases of colorectal cancer reported until October 25, 1995.

Results.—Colorectal cancer was diagnosed in 341 study participants, 173 in the aspirin group and 168 in the placebo group. Over 12 years of follow-up, assignment to low-dose aspirin was associated with a relative risk for colorectal cancer of 1.03. When the aspirin arm of the trial was discontinued because of the beneficial effects on cardiovascular disease, physicians could choose aspirin or placebo to take with the β-carotene. For those who used aspirin frequently after 1988, the relative risk for colorectal cancer was 1.07.

Conclusion.—Both randomized and observational analyses of data from the Physicians' Health Study fail to show an association between the use of aspirin and the incidence of colorectal cancer. Clinicians should be cautioned about using aspirin or other NSAIDs for the primary prevention of colorectal cancer.

▶ The aspirin debate has gone on for quite awhile, but this study—now up to a 12-year follow-up—adds to a growing consensus that aspirin has no protective effect for colorectal cancer. There are some limitations to the methods because the randomized trial lasted for only 5 of the 12 years, but using conservative assumptions the analysis virtually rules out a clinically important protective effect. For all of aspirin's other potential benefits in primary and secondary prevention, I think we can cross colorectal cancer off the list for now.

A.O. Berg, M.D., M.P.H.

Relationship Between Cancer Patients' Predictions of Prognosis and Their Treatment Preferences
Weeks JC, Cook EF, O'Day SJ, et al (Dana-Farber Cancer Inst, Boston; Brigham and Women's Hosp, Boston; Univ of California, Los Angeles; et al)
JAMA 279:1709–1714, 1998   17–3

Introduction.—Because most metastatic solid tumors are incurable and life expectancy is short, patients often need to choose between cancer-directed therapy and supportive care. Therapy aimed at life extension may have toxic side effects and reduce quality of life during the patient's final weeks or months. Researchers hypothesized that patients with terminal cancer would prefer comfort care if they had an accurate understanding of their prognosis.

Methods.—Study participants were 917 adults hospitalized at 5 teaching institutions in the United States with stage III or IV non–small-cell lung cancer or colon cancer metastatic to liver. All were enrolled in phases 1 and 2 of the Study to Understand Prognoses and Preferences for Outcomes and Risks of Treatments (SUPPORT). The process of decision making and patient outcomes was described in phase 1, a prospective observational study. Phase 2 tested the effect of an intervention in which physicians were provided with information about both prognosis and patient preferences and in which a nurse attempted to facilitate communication to enhance decision making.

Results.—The patient group was 84% white and 62% male; average patient age was 62. Sixty-one percent had lung cancer and 39% had metastatic colon cancer. Five hundred patients (55%) had died at 6 months of follow-up. Patients who thought they would live for at least 6 months were more likely (odds ratio [OR] 2.6) to favor life-extending therapy than those who thought there was at least a 10% chance that they would not survive 6 months. This OR was 8.5 among patients who estimated their 6-month survival probability at greater than 90% but whose physicians' prognosis was quite poor (less than 10% 6-month survival probability). Physicians estimated prognosis quite accurately, whereas patients overestimated survival duration. Six-month survival was no better for patients who chose aggressive treatment than for those who chose comfort care.

Discussion.—Results of the phase 2 SUPPORT intervention trial show that providing prognostic information to physicians did not change patterns of care in these terminally ill patients. To minimize futile therapy, physicians need to inform patients better about prognosis and make sure that their patients hear and understand this information.

▶ This study conveys a sad message that we would do well to heed. Patients with terminal cancer tend to overestimate their chances for survival, with a direct effect on their decision making. Although offering hope has long been one of the physician's most venerated tools in caring for patients with cancer, studies like this one make it equally clear that leading patients to overestimate chances for survival can induce them to accept therapies that are not truly in their best interests. Hope needs to be conveyed in the context of the facts.

A.O. Berg, M.D., M.P.H.

Risk of Cancer Among Offspring of Childhood-Cancer Survivors
Sankila R, for the Association of the Nordic Cancer Registries and the Nordic Society of Paediatric Haematology and Oncology (Finnish Cancer Registry, Helsinki; Danish Cancer Society, Copenhagen; Univ Hosp, Lund, Sweden; et al)
N Engl J Med 338:1339–1344, 1998   17–4

Background.—An increasing number of survivors of childhood cancer are reaching reproductive age and having their own children. The risk of cancer (other than retinoblastoma) in the children of these survivors has not been established.

Methods.—Data on 5,847 children of 14,652 survivors of childhood cancer in Denmark, Finland, Iceland, Norway, and Sweden were analyzed. The offspring were followed up for 86,780 person-years.

Findings.—Forty-four malignant neoplasms were diagnosed in the offspring. The standardized incidence ratio was 2.6. Seventeen neoplasms were retinoblastomas, for a standardized incidence ratio of 37. The second most common primary site was the brain and CNS, with a standardized incidence ratio of 2.0. Excluding 4 cases of cancer likely to be hereditary and 2 subsequent cancers in children with hereditary retinoblastoma, there were 22 sporadic cancers, for a standardized incidence ratio of 1.3.

Conclusions.—The risk of cancer among the children of survivors of childhood cancer appears to be small and limited to the offspring of survivors whose cancer was diagnosed before the age of 10 years. Thus, survivors of childhood cancer should not be discouraged from having children for fear that their children may be at increased risk of cancer.

▶ The quality of this study is sufficiently high that we should treat their simple finding as a "fact." If the statistics hold, most family practices have several survivors of childhood cancer among their patients. This study reassures us that as these patients reach reproductive age, no additional nonhereditary cancer risk for their offspring has been detected.

A.O. Berg, M.D., M.P.H.

Prolonged Cough and Lung Cancer: The Need for More General Practice Research to Inform Clinical Decision-making

Liedekerken BMJ, Hoogendam A, Buntinx F, et al (Univ of Maastricht, The Netherlands; Univ of Leuven, Belgium)
Br J Gen Pract 47:505, 1997

Introduction.—Certain signs and symptoms ("key symptoms"), such as macroscopic hematuria and anal blood loss, are considered to indicate a high likelihood of a disease. Prolonged cough is generally believed to be a key symptom indicative of lung cancer. Focusing on general practice, a meta-analysis was performed to determine the diagnostic value of prolonged (more than 6 weeks) cough for the subsequent diagnosis of lung cancer.

Methods.—Data were collected via a MEDLINE search (1966–1995) and a careful screening of the references of all papers retrieved. Included in the analysis were all articles that reported on the relationship between prolonged coughing and the diagnosis of lung cancer in a cohort of patients.

Results.—A single study, published in 1977, reported the data of all cells of the 2-by-2 table required for calculating all basic indicators of diagnostic value: sensitivity, specificity, and positive and negative predictive value. The study, which included 6,027 patients from a specialized setting, showed a high negative predictive value (0.99) for prolonged cough as an indicator of lung cancer, a low positive predictive value (0.03), a sensitivity of 0.48, and a specificity of 0.71. One additional study calculated sensitivity only (0.33).

Conclusion.—No general practice-based study that reported basic data for estimating the diagnostic value of prolonged cough was found in the literature. The teaching of general practice should be based on research performed within general practice rather than in teaching hospitals.

▶ This meticulous literature review failed to find any evidence whatsoever regarding the predictive value of cough as an indicator of lung cancer in primary care. It should make all of us pause as we consider the immense amount of research that could be conducted, correlating all of the hundreds of historical facts and physical examination findings with specific conditions. Medical practice has been built for hundreds of years in reverse, answering the question: What historical facts and physical findings accompany already-recognized disease? I believe that one of the potential benefits of the new interest in "evidence-based" medicine will be to force us to think more often in the right direction: If a patient can be linked to a particular historical or physical finding, what is the likelihood that that patient has a specific condition?

A.O. Berg, M.D., M.P.H.

Ethics and End-of-Life Issues

A Comparison of Physicians' and Patients' Attitudes Toward Pharmaceutical Industry Gifts
Gibbons RV, Landry FJ, Blouch DL, et al (Washington Hosp Ctr, DC; Univ of Health Sciences, Bethesda, Md)
J Gen Intern Med 13:151–154, 1998   17–6

Introduction.—Gifts are commonly made to physicians by the pharmaceutical industry, a practice which is considered controversial. Pharmaceutical companies are thought to be spending more than $8,000 per physician per year. A guideline of the American College of Physicians states: "Gifts, hospitality, or subsidies offered to physicians by the pharmaceutical industry ought not to be accepted if acceptance might influence or appear to influence the objectivity of clinical judgment." Previous studies have not compared whether patients and their physicians agree on the appropriateness and influence of pharmaceutical industry gifts. Physicians' and patients' attitudes toward pharmaceutical gifts were compared.

Methods.—There were 268 surveyed physicians, 100 randomly selected patients, and 96 patients in a convenience sample who completed a survey in which they were asked to rate 10 pharmaceutical gifts on whether the gifts were appropriate for physicians to accept and whether the gifts were likely to influence prescribing.

Results.—Gifts were believed to be less appropriate and more influential by patients than by physicians. About half of the patients knew that such gifts were given to physicians; of those who did not know, 24% indicated that their perception of the medical profession had been altered with this knowledge. When asked if their own physician accepted gifts from pharmaceutical companies, 53% said they didn't know, 27% said yes, and 20% said no. A belief that gifts might influence prescribing was a predictor for patients feeling that gifts were inappropriate. Knowledge of guidelines was the best predictor for physicians feeling that gifts were inappropriate.

Conclusion.—Pharmaceutical gifts were felt to be more influential and less appropriate by patients than by physicians. When deciding whether to accept particular gifts, physicians may want to consider this. Physician behavior may be changed by broader dissemination of guidelines. The potentially different viewpoints of patients and physicians should be considered in future guidelines.

▶ This article shows persuasively that patients and physicians have different views of pharmaceutical industry gifts. Does it surprise you that nearly a third of patients in this study thought that the gift of a pen or coffee mug would influence prescribing behavior (compared with 8% of physicians)? It did me. On the face of it, the test of "would you be willing to have these arrangements generally known?" appears to be inadequate. The authors comment that this test probably overestimates the appropriateness of gifts as viewed by patients. Our residency practice no longer accepts "detailing" visits from pharmaceutical representatives, but pens, paper pads, and "knick-knacks" (I don't know what else to call them) are somehow still ubiquitous in the office. Are these items as noninfluential as we think? What do our patients think when they see us use them?

A.O. Berg, M.D., M.P.H.

Ethical Considerations in the Provision of Controversial Screening Tests
Doukas DJ, Fetters M, Ruffin MT IV, et al (Univ of Michigan, Ann Arbor; Baylor Medical College, Houston)
Arch Fam Med 6:486–490, 1997   17-7

Objective.—Patients who request screening tests with dubious benefits may be creating an ethical dilemma for their physicians. Screening recommendations of insurance companies, the media, public advocacy groups, and patients are often at variance. Ethical approaches for managing the difficult circumstance of a patient-initiated request for a screening test with controversial benefits were reviewed.

An Evidence-based Approach to Early Detection.—Most tests do not meet minimal criteria for screening accuracy and effectiveness. Physicians are not obligated to provide treatment that has not been shown to be beneficial.

Potential Biases and Screening.—Screening guidelines sometimes reflect the biases of the groups that develop them. Public advocacy groups and the media frequently report anecdotal evidence or results of uncorroborated studies.

Moral Arguments in the Provision of a Screening Test.—Physicians can use preventive ethics to dissuade patients from making uninformed decisions. Physicians should determine whether patients are seeking controversial screening tests because of fear, misinformation about effectiveness, or peace of mind. Physicians should also counsel patients about the risk of unnecessary injury or further invasive testing resulting from a false positive test. Physicians should also make it clear to patients that no test can assure zero risk of disease. Physicians are under no obligation to provide treatment that has a dubious benefit.

Conclusion.—Patients who insist on a screening test with controversial benefits create an ethical dilemma for physicians. Physicians can take a preventive ethics approach to patient education to maintain trust and provide realistic expectations.

▶ One of the most common questions I am asked when presenting recommendations from the U.S. Preventive Services Task Force is how to say no to a patient who requests a screening test that is not supported by scientific evidence. The question is even harder to answer if the test is also being performed routinely by other physicians, or worse, has been advertised in the lay press. The family physician ethicists writing this article clarify the ethical issues, emphasizing that for screening tests, as for any other medical care, physicians cannot be compelled to offer services that run counter to their best scientific judgment. In my view, physicians collectively would pay a high price in lost integrity if it became the common expectation that physicians were willing to perform any professional service that the patient wanted, regardless of its scientific merits.

A.O. Berg, M.D., M.P.H.

Does Bedside Rationing Violate Patients' Best Interests? An Exploration of "Moral Hazard"
Ubel PA, Goold S (Univ of Pennsylvania, Philadelphia; Univ of Michigan, Ann Arbor)
Am J Med 104:64–68, 1998

Background.—Bedside rationing has been defined as the withholding, by a physician, of a medically beneficial service on the basis of that service's cost to someone other than the patient. Both opponents and proponents of bedside rationing agree that the patient's best interests are violated when beneficial services are withheld. The implications for physicians of such a moral hazard were reviewed.

Moral Hazard.—A $100 blood test may detect a painful disease in a group of individuals, each of whom has a 1/10,000 risk for the disease. One patient, who would have to pay only $5 as a copayment to receive the test, asks his physician to order it. The physician knows that the overall cost of this test is $1 million per disease detected. It is clearly in the patient's best interest to spend $5 on the test, but the actual cost of $100 will be picked up by others.

Potential Means of Dealing With the Moral Hazard Dilemma.—By eliminating health care insurance for all above some minimum income, patients would be more likely to examine the cost of care carefully and make their own judgment of the value of a particular test or service. The economic inefficiencies of health insurance, however, protect patients from the catastrophic expenses of treating unpredictable serious illness. The physician's dilemma might also be removed were patients required to pay for discretionary services. Difficulties in this scenario would be the need to agree upon necessary vs. discretionary services and the patient's ability to make informed, optimal choices. A patient might also choose health care insurance that would pay, or not pay, for the most costly services. Among other problems with this approach, patients may find themselves having opted out of potentially life-saving treatments.

The Morality of Bedside Rationing.—Because health insurance raises health expenditures beyond what is desirable, acceptable ways need to be found to ration health care. The focus needs to be on marginally beneficial services that people would not be willing to pay for were it not for insurance-caused moral hazard. Rationing is morally preferable to diverting funds away from valued to marginally valued health services, and the physician may be in the best position to make bedside rationing decisions.

Our society needs to do more to decide what health care is necessary for everyone and what is discretionary.

▶ The inadvisability of rationing at the bedside has been such an ethical article of faith for the last dozen years that this novel argument suggesting the opposite is a real show-stopper. The authors make a provocative case, although their remedies (eliminate health insurance, eliminate health insurance for discretionary services, or decide on coverage at the time of enrollment) are blue-sky thinking for the present. I view this article, though, as one more argument in favor of payment systems and structures that remove this "moral hazard" from medical practice. We have already practiced (uncomfortably) with it too long.

A.O. Berg, M.D., M.P.H.

Patient and Physician Roles in End-of-Life Decision Making
Johnston SC, and the End-of-Life Study Group (Univ of Kansas, Wichita)
J Gen Intern Med 13:43–45, 1998   17–9

Objective.—Results demonstrate serious shortcomings in end-of-life decisions and the medical care provided. The quality of discussions and decisions involving patients and their doctors must improve. A multicenter, cross-sectional survey involving randomly selected primary care patients and physicians in 8 United States communities was conducted between January and May 1992 to determine the roles of patient, physician, and family in end-of-life decisions.

Methods.—Participants included 329 adult outpatients (74 black, 140 male), aged 19 to 94 years, who completed an 83-item questionnaire and

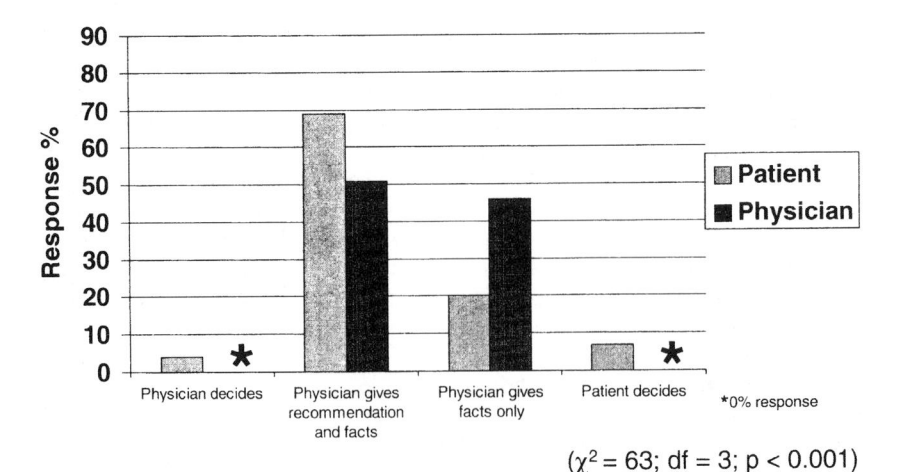

$(\chi^2 = 63; df = 3; p < 0.001)$

FIGURE 2.—How should the patient and the physician share the decision-making process? (Courtesy of Johnston SC, and the End-of-Life Study Group: Patient and physician roles in end-of-life decision-making. *J Gen Intern Med* 13:43–45, 1998. Reprinted by permission of Blackwell Scienec, Inc.)

272 primary care physicians (236 white, 60 female), aged 27 to 90 years, who completed a 58-item questionnaire. Responses of patients and physicians were compared statistically.

Results.—The average Karnofsky score was 90. Patients rated their health as excellent (8%), very good (22%), good (33%), fair (28%), or poor (7.6%). Physicians were practicing internal medicine (49%), family medicine (45%), or general medicine (5%). Although most patients and physicians believed that the patient was responsible for making end-of-life decisions, significantly more physicians believed that the patient was responsible. Patients were significantly more likely to prefer shared end-of-life decisions (Fig 2).

Conclusion.—Patients prefer to share end-of-life decisions with physicians. Physicians need to be made aware of this preference.

▶ This provocative article adds a fresh dimension to the debates regarding end-of-life decisions by focusing on the difference between patients and physicians on the issue of shared decision making. Figure 2, taken from the article, illustrates the problem well. It shows that most patients want advice in addition to the facts, something that causes discomfort for some physicians. The easy answer to this dilemma, it seems to me, is first, to raise the question of end-of-life planning more routinely with patients, but, second, to ask patients early on whether they are seeking facts, advice, or both.

A.O. Berg, M.D., M.P.H.

A National Survey of Physician-assisted Suicide and Euthanasia in the United States

Meier DE, Emmons C-A, Wallenstein S, et al (Mount Sinai School of Medicine, NY; Univ of Chicago; Univ of Rochester, NY)
N Engl J Med 338:1193–1201, 1998   17–10

Introduction.—In the United States, strong arguments are heard for and against easing the legal constraints on physician-assisted suicide. A majority of people favor legalization, according to public-opinion polls. Little relation to the range of clinical circumstances in which physicians care for patients who are near the end of life is borne by the proposed regulatory guidelines. A representative sample of physicians with a high likelihood of caring for dying patients were surveyed to assess the prevalence of requests for assistance with euthanasia or suicide and the physicians' compliance with these requests.

Methods.—Questionnaires were mailed to 3,102 physicians in the 10 specialties in which doctors are most likely to receive requests from patients for assistance with suicide or euthanasia, and 1,902 physicians completed the questionnaire, a response rate of 61%.

Results.—Eleven percent of the physicians said there were circumstances in which they would be willing to speed a patient's death by prescribing medication under current legal constraints. A lethal injection would be provided by 7%. Thirty-six percent of physicians said they would hasten a patient's death by prescribing medication if it were legal, and 24% said they would provide legal injection if it were legal. A request for assistance with suicide was reported by 18.3% of physicians. A request for lethal injection was received by 11.1% of physicians. At least 1 prescription to be used to hasten death was written by 16% of the physicians receiving such requests, or 3.3% of the entire sample. One lethal injection was administered by 4.7% of physicians.

Conclusion.—Requests for physician-assisted suicide and euthanasia were reported by a substantial proportion of physicians in the United States in the specialities surveyed, and such requests have been complied with by about 6% of physicians.

▶ This article provides the best national data on physician-assisted suicide and euthanasia that I have seen. Survey studies are always limited by response rate and the hazards of self-report, especially on sensitive topics like these; but the sampling strategy here was meticulous and the analysis conservative, so I believe the results. Your response to the findings will depend on which side of the fence you prefer. Those who are opposed to physician participation in suicide or euthanasia under any circumstances will be appalled by the surprisingly large number of physicians who have participated or say they would. Those who support physician involvement in these end-of-life decisions will be encouraged both by the number of physicians who seem willing to think about it, and by the number of physicians who have been asked about it by patients. This debate, like so many others, boils down to 2 opposing philosophies: making life decisions based on utilitarian principles of what the majority wants vs. a deontological approach appealing to some external standard. In this respect, the public opinion polls favor the utilitarian view of easing legal constraints; physician groups are still overwhelmingly on the side of maintaining a principle based on an external, professional standard. I have no personal doubt that the pressures to ease restraints will continue from both outside and inside the profession. It is a windy debate that family physicians cannot escape. Articles like this one provide a periodic check on the windspeed.

A.O. Berg, M.D., M.P.H.

Patient Compliance

Should We Pay the Patient? Review of Financial Incentives to Enhance Patient Compliance
Giuffrida A, Torgerson DJ (Univ of York, England)
BMJ 315:703–707, 1997   17–11

Objective.—Noncompliance with appointments or medication is a problem that affects the quality of medical care and wastes resources. The most common interventions applied to increase patient compliance include mail or telephone reminders. The effectiveness of financial incentives to enhance patients' compliance with medication and medical appointments was investigated in a literature review.

Methods.—Medline, Embase, PsychLit, EconLit, and the Cochrane Database of Clinical Trials were searched, as were the reference lists of articles retrieved, for quantitative data regarding the effect of financial incentives in the form of cash, coupons, lottery tickets, toys, meal or bus tokens, vouchers, or gifts on compliance. The proportions of compliant patients in the intervention and control groups were estimated as were the odds of compliance. Degree of compliance was compared with incentive offered. The number of patients that needed to be treated to improve compliance by 1 patient was calculated.

Results.—Eleven randomized studies were found and reviewed. Ten of the studies showed that financial incentives improved compliance more than other types of incentives. Only 1 study set in a pediatric clinic showed improved compliance with a nonfinancial incentive.

Conclusion.—Financial incentives are significantly more effective in improving compliance than are other types of incentives. Financial incentives may be more cost-effective than other interventions to improve compliance.

▶ I have previously heard of using financial incentives to increase compliance, although I have not personally tried paying patients directly. I have suggested that patients use their own financial incentives—put $2 in a jar each day they do not smoke, for example, until they reach a preset amount for a desired item. Although these authors report that results of 10 of 11 studies were positive, only 5 studies had any confidence intervals that did not include 1; in other words, the results were often not statistically significant. However, I suspect, regardless of the study quality, financial incentives can work if the dollar amount is high enough. If insurance companies or HMOs pay, this is essentially transferring dollars from one insured individual to another, but even this may be reasonable if it lowers overall costs to everyone. Family physicians could also consider financial incentives to patients under risk contracts; unfortunately, there are few data to indicate the specifics of how to do so, such as the amount and for what conditions.

M.A. Bowman, M.D., M.P.A.

Impact of Dosage Frequency on Patient Compliance
Paes AHP, Bakker A, Soe-Agnie CJ (Universiteit Utrecht, The Netherlands)
Diabetes Care 20:1512–1517, 1997   17–12

Background.—Patient compliance in taking prescriptions is a crucial element in the effectiveness of drug therapy. The effect of dosage frequency on patient compliance was investigated.

Method.—Ninety-one patients with diabetes being treated with oral antidiabetic agents participated in this 6-month study. which utilized Medication Event Monitoring System containers to record the number of

TABLE 1.—Compliance and Dosage

Dosage	Compliance (%)	Range (%)	95% CI
Once daily	98.7 ± 18.6	19–123	92.8–104.7
Twice daily	83.1 ± 24.9	9–109	74.7–91.5
Three times daily	65.8 ± 30.1	7–102	49.1–82.5

Note: Data are means ±SD, unless otherwise indicated.
Abbreviation: CI, confidence interval.
(Courtesy of Paes AHP, Bakker A, Soe-Agnie CJ et al: Impact of dosage frequency on patient compliance. *Diabetes Care* 20:1512–1517, 1997.)

tablets taken at any time. The information gained from this device was used in combination with data from a patient questionnaire to determine compliance. The following criteria were used to determine compliance: (1) percentage of prescribed medication used during the study period; (2) percentage of days in which the prescribed dosage was taken properly (1, 2, or 3 times per day); and (3) percentage of medication taken within 25% of the time of prescription intervals.

Results.—The percentage of prescribed medication taken by test subjects ranged from 7% to 123%, with a mean of 74.8 ± 26.0%. The regimen compliance ranged from 0% to 97% with a mean of 67.2 ± 30.0%. For patients taking 1 dose per day, the average compliance was 79%. For those taking 3 doses per day, compliance dropped to 38%. Thus, compliance was inversely proportional to the number of daily doses prescribed. With more doses, there was less compliance (Table 1). The most common type of noncompliance was dose omission. However, 34.7% of test subjects used more medicine than was prescribed and nearly 40% of all patients with 1 prescribed dose per day took more than their prescribed amount of medication.

Conclusion.—Because compliance has been shown to increase with fewer numbers of prescribed dosages, it seems reasonable to prescribe only 1 dosage of medications per day. However, it has also been shown that lowering the dosages of medicine taken per day increases the likelihood of taking extra doses of medication. Thus, the prescribed number of drug dosages should be based not on compliance issues but on the therapeutic range of the drug.

▶ New electronic devices provide new insights to compliance. As we generally suspected, compliance was better for once-a-day medication, modestly worse for twice-a-day medication, and probably uncomfortably low for 3 times a day. However, for each frequency, there was at least 1 patient who took more than was prescribed, and this happened most frequently for the once-a-day medications—40% of the patients had taken more tablets than prescribed. Almost no patients took 3 times a day medication close to an every 8-hour schedule; instead, they took the medication with meals. A big disadvantage of the once-daily schedule was that more of these patients had days with no medication. Thus, depending on the type of medication, a twice-daily dose may be an overall better alternative, or compliance aids should be used to determine whether the daily dose was already consumed. And so, the hackneyed phrase, "more study needed" applies...

M.A. Bowman, M.D., M.P.A.

Alternative and Complementary Medicine

Why Patients Use Alternative Medicine: Results of a National Study
Astin JA (Stanford Univ, Palo Alto, Calif)
JAMA 279:1548–1553, 1998   17–13

Introduction.—It was reported in 1993 that 34% of adults in the United States used at least 1 unconventional form of health care within the previous year. Subsequent reports in the United States and abroad support the prevalent use of alternative health care practices. Possible predictors of alternative health care use were investigated.

Methods.—The following 3 theories regarding why individuals use alternative medicine were evaluated: (1) dissatisfaction with conventional treatment; (2) need for personal autonomy and control over health care decisions; and (3) philosophical congruence with the patient's values, worldview, spiritual/religious philosophy, or beliefs about the nature and meaning of health and illness. A random sample of 1,500 individuals was selected to complete an extensive mail survey regarding use of alternative health care, perceived benefits and risks of the therapies, health beliefs and attitudes, views toward and experiences with conventional medicine, political beliefs, and worldview.

Results.—There was a 69% (1,035 of 1,500 individuals) response rate. Predictors of alternative health care use were higher education, poorer health status, a holistic orientation to health, having had a transformational experience that changed the individual's worldview, classification in a cultural group identifiable by their commitment to environmentalism, commitment to feminism, interest in spirituality and personal growth psychology, and any of the following health problems: anxiety, back problems, chronic pain, or urinary tract problems. Only 4.4% reported that they relied primarily on alternative therapies.

Conclusion.—Individuals used alternative health care practices primarily because they were more congruent with their own values, beliefs, and philosophical orientations toward health and life. Dissatisfaction with conventional medicine and need for personal control were not major determinants for use of alternative medicine. The finding of only 4.4% of individuals relying primarily on alternative therapies suggests that alternative therapies are used in conjunction with, rather than instead of more conventional treatment.

▶ The late 1990s has been a time of resurgence for unconventional therapies. For many complex social and cultural reasons, many patients are not satisfied with modern medicine despite its great success and powerful therapies. This important study shows that individuals are using unconventional therapies not primarily out of a rejection of modern medicine, but to expand their health-seeking behaviors into therapies congruent with their health beliefs and culture. It is important for family physicians to both understand and respect such health-seeking behavior.

J.E. Scherger, M.D., M.P.H.

A Close Look at Therapeutic Touch
Rosa L, Rosa E, Sarner L, et al (Questionable Nurse Practices Task Force, Loveland, Colo; Natl Therapeutic Touch Study Group, Loveland, Colo; Quackwatch Inc, Allentown, Pa)
JAMA 279:1005–1010, 1998

Introduction.—Therapeutic touch is a widely used nursing practice rooted in mysticism but alleged to have a scientific basis. Many medical problems are claimed to be healed or improved by manual manipulation of a "human energy field" that is perceptible above the patient's skin. This practice's theory and technique require a "human energy field" to impart any therapeutic benefit to a patient. A clinical trial would test whether practitioners can perceive "human energy fields" as tingling, pulling, throbbing, hot, cold, spongy, or tactile as taffy. It was determined whether therapeutic touch practitioners could actually perceive a "human energy field."

Methods.—Twenty-one practitioners with therapeutic touch experience for 1–27 years were tested. They were asked to state whether the investigator's unseen hand hovered above their left hand or their right hand. Placement of the investigator's hand was determined by flipping a coin. Seven practitioners were tested 20 times each and 14 practitioners were tested 10 times each.

Results.—In only 123 (44%) of 280 trials, practitioners of therapeutic touch identified the correct hand, which is close to what would be expected with random chance. The practitioner's score and length of experience had no significant correlation. If therapeutic touch practitioners could reliably detect a human energy field, the study would have demonstrated this, according to the statistical power of this experience. The practitioners would have been able to locate the investigator's hand 100% of the time, if therapeutic touch were valid. Chance alone would result in a score of 50%.

Conclusion.—The investigator's "energy field" could not be detected by 21 experienced therapeutic touch practitioners. The claims of therapeutic touch are groundless and further professional use is unjustified, based on the failure of these practitioners to substantiate their most fundamental claim.

▶ This article began as a science project of a girl aged 9 years. I first heard about it on public radio and believe that it fully deserves all the attention it has received. It is a great reminder that high-quality research can be done without a $1 million National Institutes of Health grant; and it gives hope for all parents of 9-year-olds that science projects can be fun and useful. This article also shows that the scientific study of alternative and complementary therapies requires only creativity and modest investment. The devastating findings have already generated a bitter debate, but I think the burden of proof has now shifted to the proponents of therapeutic touch.

A.O. Berg, M.D., M.P.H.

Miscellaneous

Patient Empowerment and Feedback Did Not Decrease Pain in Seriously Ill Hospitalized Adults
Desbiens NA, Wu AW, Yasui Y, et al (Univ of Tennessee Memphis, Chattanooga; Johns Hopkins Univ, Baltimore, Md; Fred Hutchinson Cancer Research Ctr, Seattle; et al)
Pain 75:237–246, 1998   17–15

Objective.—There is a high prevalence of pain in terminally ill patients. Because the belief is that this pain is treatable, a pain intervention program based on effective cognitive and psychological approaches for reducing pain was delivered by nurse clinicians trained in pain assessment, education, and control. Feedback of patients' pain experience to physicians and nurses was instituted as part of a randomized trial.

Methods.—Between January 1992 and January 1994, a pain intervention program was delivered at 5 U.S. tertiary care academic centers to 2,652 terminally ill patients. The usual care was administered to a control group of 2,152 terminally ill patients. Specially trained nurse clinicians assessed patients' pain, educated them about pain control, told them they could have their pain controlled, and encouraged them to speak with their doctors about their pain. Family members of patients unable to communicate were trained via the intervention program. The pain level and level of satisfaction with pain control were assessed during hospitalization, at 2 months, 6 months, and at after-death interviews with surrogates.

Results.—Almost 51% of patients reported some pain. Although 79.8% of intervention patients reported contact with a nurse clinician, few received a specific type of pain intervention, and pain was reported by 43.4% of patients at discharge. Only 20% of these patients received a specific type of pain intervention. With the remainder, it was reported that maximum efforts were already being made (37%), or the patient was satisfied with the efforts (19%), or both (34%). The intervention group had slightly more pain than the control group. After adjusting for baseline pain risk, there was a small but clinically significant increase in the risk of pain in the intervention group (odds ratio [OR], 1.15; 95% confidence interval [CI], 1.00–1.33). Pain satisfaction was not increased in the intervention compared with the control group (OR, 1.12; 95% CI, 0.91–1.39). There were no significant differences in the level of pain or satisfaction with pain control at any time point. Surrogates of patients who died reported that two fifths of patients had extreme or moderately severe pain in the last 3 days of life.

Conclusions.—The pain intervention program was unsuccessful in treating pain in terminally ill patients. Pain control in terminally ill patients remains a problem that needs to be more effectively dealt with. Intensive pain strategies need to be developed to address this ongoing problem.

▶ These findings are very disappointing. The intervention here was state-of-the-art and about as intensive as we are likely to see in a hospital setting. Some would have us believe that all pain is controllable if physicians and nurses would just do their job properly. Two other provocative articles showing the dimensions of the problem in primary care and in nursing homes are also worth reading.[1,2] Collectively these results inject realism into what, in recent years, has been an overly optimistic view of what is possible in pain control. We still have much to learn about how to provide adequate pain relief.

A.O. Berg, M.D., M.P.H.

References

1. Gureje O, Von Korff M, Simon GE, et al: Persistent pain and well being. A World Health Organization study in primary care. *JAMA* 280:147–151, 1998.
2. Bernabei R, Gambessi G, Lapane K, et al: Management of pain in elderly patients with cancer. *JAMA* 279:1877–1881, 1998.

Incidence of Adverse Drug Reactions in Hospitalized Patients: A Meta-analysis of Prospective Studies
Lazarou J, Pomeranz BH, Corey PN (Univ of Toronto)
JAMA 279:1200–1205, 1998

Introduction.—Now that a recent bill passed by the U.S. Senate requires pharmaceutical companies to provide adverse drug reaction (ADR) information to consumers, public attention is focused on ADRs. A meta-analysis of prospective studies from which ADR incidences were obtained was conducted. Serious and fatal ADRs, which represent the great impact of drug therapy, were evaluated.

Methods.—Thirty-nine prospective studies of ADRs over a period of 32 years were part of the meta-analysis. The incidence of ADRs occurring in the hospital and the incidence of ADRs causing admission to hospital were combined to obtain the overall incidence of ADRs in hospitalized patients. Errors in drug administration, overdose, noncompliance, therapeutic failures, drug abuse, and possible adverse reactions were excluded. Those reactions that required hospitalization, were permanently disabling, or resulted in death were considered serious.

Results.—There was a 6.7% overall incidence of serious ADRs, with a 0.32% incidence of fatal ADRs in hospitalized patients. Serious ADRs were estimated at 2,216,000 in 1994, with fatal ADRs estimated at 106,000; making ADRs between the 4th and 6th leading cause of death after heart disease, cancer, stroke, pulmonary disease, and accidents, and ahead of pneumonia and diabetes.

Conclusion.—There was an extremely high incidence of serious and fatal ADRs in U.S. hospitals. These data suggest that ADRs represent an important clinical issue, although these results must be viewed with circumspection, because of heterogeneity among studies and small biases in the samples.

▶ This article reports a messy meta-analysis of messy underlying studies, yet the authors make a convincing case that their findings, if anything, underestimate the incidence of ADRs (as defined by the authors). Still, the claim that ADRs are the 4th to 6th leading cause of death should be carefully scrutinized. These are not "new" deaths; they are currently accounted for in other categories such as heart disease, cancer, and stroke. Should a cancer patient's death that appears to be caused by a chemotherapeutic agent be attributed to the cancer or to the drug? For this analysis, the authors went with the drug. I agree with the authors that ADRs are probably too common. We physicians are programmed in training to overestimate the benefits of treatments and to underestimate adverse effects. If this article causes us to consider the possibility of adverse effects of treatment more carefully, and gives our patients the courage to ask about them more frequently, the authors have done their job.

A.O. Berg, M.D., M.P.H.

Usefulness of Antinuclear Antibody Testing to Screen for Rheumatic Diseases
Malleson PN, Sailer M, Mackinnon MJ (Univ of British Columbia, Vancouver, Canada; British Columbia's Children's Hosp, Vancouver, Canada)
Arch Dis Child 77:299–304, 1997   17–17

Background.—As antinuclear antibodies are often found in the sera of children with rheumatic disease, the indirect immunofluorescence antinuclear antibody (FANA) test is frequently used as a screening tool for pediatric rheumatic disease. The usefulness of the FANA test, using human laryngeal epithelial carcinoma cells as a nuclear substrate, as a screening tool for pediatric rheumatic disease was investigated.

Study Design.—A retrospective review was performed of all FANA tests performed on sera from 1,369 children at British Columbia's Children's Hospital from March 1991 to July 1995. The serum sample was tested to its end point with doubling dilutions. A diagnosis of any chronic inflammatory arthropathy, connective tissue disease, or vasculitis was considered to be a diagnosis of rheumatic disease.

Findings.—In those children who were diagnosed with a rheumatic disease, FANA tests were positive in 67%, compared with 64% of those with a diagnosis of nonrheumatic disease. More girls than boys had a high titer FANA positivity, independent of their rheumatic disease status. At a

TABLE 3.—Characteristics of the Indirect Immunofluorescence Antinuclear Antibody Test for Screening for Rheumatic Diseases

FANA Endpoint Titre	Sensitivity	Specificity	Positive Predictive Value	Negative Predictive Value
≥1:1280	0.18	0.98	0.80	0.74
1:640	0.24	0.96	0.69	0.75
1:320	0.32	0.88	0.53	0.76
1:160	0.42	0.75	0.41	0.76
1:80	0.53	0.60	0.36	0.76
1:40	0.63	0.47	0.33	0.75
1:20	0.67	0.36	0.30	0.73

Note: Figures are for girls and boys combined.
(Courtesy of Malleson PN, Sailer M, Mackinnon MJ: Usefulness of antinuclear antibody testing to screen for rheumatic diseases. *Arch Dis Child* 77:299–304, 1997.)

serum dilution of 1:40, a positive FANA test had a sensitivity of 0.63 and a positive predictive value of 0.33 for rheumatic disease (Table 3). For systemic lupus erythematosus, mixed connective tissue disease, or overlap syndrome, the FANA test had a sensitivity of 0.98, but a positive predictive value of 0.10.

Conclusion.—A negative FANA test means that a diagnosis of pediatric systemic lupus erythematosus or mixed connective tissue disease is unlikely, but a positive test is a poor predictor of these diagnoses. If the FANA test is to be used as a screening test for pediatric rheumatic disease, a higher initial titer, such as 1:160, should be used to eliminate the many false positives and reduce costs. Whether the FANA test should be replaced with an anti-DNA antibody test for screening pediatric patients for rheumatic disease should be examined in clinical studies.

▶ I included this article to remind us (myself most of all) to be careful and selective in ordering a FANA test. Too often, this test is used as a screening tool in patients with symptoms that might be related to a connective tissue process. Particularly in children, this test is difficult to interpret and, thus, can be unreliable. Although negative test results are reassuring, the incidence of false positives is quite high. The results of this study drive home the point that the FANA test should really be used for confirming a clinical suspicion, not as a screening device.

W.W. Dexter, M.D.

Effect of the Statistical Significance of Results on the Time to Completion and Publication of Randomized Efficacy Trials
Ioannidis JPA (NIH, Bethesda, Md)
JAMA 279:281–286, 1998

17–18

Background.—Concern has been raised that clinical studies with negative findings may never be published and that this may result in a distorted view of the optimal practice of medicine. The current study investigated whether time to completion and publication of randomized phase 2 and 3 trials are affected by the statistical significance of results.

Methods.—The analysis included 109 randomized efficacy trials done by 2 multicenter groups studying HIV infection between 1986 and 1996. Total enrollment was 43,708 patients. The time from the start of enrollment to completion of follow-up and time from completion of follow-up to peer-reviewed publication were analyzed.

Findings.—Median time from the start of enrollment to publication was 5.5 years. This period was significantly longer for trials with nonsignificant findings (6.5 years) than for those with results favoring the experimental arm (4.3 years). This difference was primarily due to difference in the time from completion to publication. On average, trials with significant results favoring any arm completed follow-up significantly earlier than those with nonsignificant results. Long-protracted trials often had low event rates, failing to achieve statistical significance, whereas trials terminated early had significant findings. Studies with positive findings were submitted for publication significantly faster than those with negative findings. The former were also published more rapidly than the latter.

Conclusions.—Even within highly efficient multicenter trial groups, efficacy trials with statistically significant findings are published faster than those with nonsignificant results. Most of this time lag occurs after the study has been completed.

▶ This is one of the best articles I've seen documenting the oft-feared but little-documented problem of publication bias, where a "positive" result showing that an intervention works better than another is likely to be published sooner than a "negative" result where the interventions are more nearly equivalent. Other research shows that "later" for many negative studies becomes "never." I see this as a serious and fundamental problem in the way that the research enterprise is conducted. Over time it means that medical practice becomes more and more intervention-oriented because that's what most published studies will support. Evidence-based medicine depends on the publication of evidence. If the negative half of evidence is under-represented in published reports, we are working with only half of the picture.

A.O. Berg, M.D., M.P.H.

Direct Observation of Community-based Ambulatory Encounters Involving Medical Students
Frank SH, Stange KC, Langa D, et al (Case Western Reserve Univ, Cleveland, Ohio; Henry Ford Health System, Detroit)
JAMA 278:712–716, 1997   17–19

Objective.—As medical student education has shifted from inpatients tertiary settings to community-based ambulatory primary care practices, physician productivity has decreased. The impact of the medical student on the process of patient care was studied.

Methods.—Research nurses observed physician behavior and services rendered during patient visits and administered a patient exit questionnaire and a physician questionnaire in a cross-sectional, multimethod study in 16 community-based family practice offices accepting medical students. Use of clinical time was assessed using the Davis Observation Code. Patient satisfaction was measured during 452 outpatients visits with and without medical students using the Medical Outcomes Study 9-item visit rating scale.

Results.—Medical students were involved in 83 visits. Students were significantly more likely to see Medicaid patients and minority patients than white patients or patients with private insurance. When medical students were involved, physicians spent more time setting visit expectations, and less time taking histories, providing feedback, and answering patients' questions. There was no significant difference in time spent in other physician behavior categories. The amount of time the physician spent with the patient was similar with (10.3 minutes) or without (9.9 minutes) a medical student present. Medical student involvement did not change patient satisfaction. Physicians spent significantly more time discussing problems of other family members when medical students were involved.

Conclusion.—The presence of a medical student changed the content but not the total time the physician spent with the patient nor did it alter the patient's level of satisfaction. Students were significantly more likely to see Medicaid patients and minority patients.

▶ Many family physicians have students with them at least part-time, contributing greatly to medical student education. This article is reassuring and consistent with my experience. I did not believe that medical students made me more inefficient, but it does depend on how the experience is arranged. This article also does not note that physicians spend additional educational time with the student, often after seeing patients, thus contributing to the overall cost of the experience. Like the authors, I am not clear on how to assess the higher portion of poor and minority patients seen by the students, although it is of concern.

M.A. Bowman, M.D., M.P.A.

Gowning: Effects on Patient Satisfaction

Meit SS, Williams D, Mencken FC, et al (West Virginia Univ, Morgantown)
J Fam Pract 45:397–401, 1997

Background.—Gowning status may affect patients' trust in their physician and the overall duration of the clinic visit. The effects of gowning on patient satisfaction were investigated.

Methods.—Fifteen hundred patients were assigned randomly to gown or nongown status when they arrived for their clinic visit. After inclusion criteria were applied, 895 patients participated in the study. Four hundred fifty-five (51%) completed the Trust in Physician Scale. Data on total time from check-in to check-out were recorded.

Findings.—Gowning status had no significant effect on patients' trust in their physician or clinic visit duration. No significant interactions occurred with gowning status, patient sex, physician sex, patient age, or patient education. Younger patients and patients seeing a physician for the first time were significantly less trustful of their physician.

Conclusions.—Gowning status appears to be unrelated to patients' trust in their physician and satisfaction with care. Duration of clinic visit was also unassociated with gowning status.

▶ This is one of those issues that would have been hard to credit before customer satisfaction entered medical care. Paying attention to the physical and psychological comfort of patients, while always an issue, was never as prominent as it has become in recent years. Satisfying the customer has become an acknowledged goal of the medical encounter. Thus, it makes sense that we should seek to understand whether the little rituals that are part of clinical practice have an effect on patient satisfaction. Those that have an adverse impact on satisfaction will be examined more closely. Here's one that requires no intervention: Gowning early or late has no effect on satisfaction.

A.O. Berg, M.D., M.P.H.

18 Health Policy and Economics

Overview

Randomized controlled trial: Abstract 18–13

Issues in Primary Care
- Community dimensions of primary care practice
- A hidden system of primary care?
- Case management in primary care
- Practice style and patient outcome
- Expenditures and mortality related to primary care vs. specialty physicians as personal physicians
- Equity in allocating resources to primary care
- Methods of compensating primary care physicians in medical groups

Health System Issues
- Gatekeeping
- Physicians' views of health plans
- Physician satisfaction with HMO and fee-for-service practice
- Insurance and continuity as predictors of outcome
- Follow-up of 1989 graduates

Quality, Outcomes, and Peer Review
- Education for physicians and patient outcome
- Quality comparison of physician office and commercial laboratories
- Effects of consumer reports on patient care
- Reliability and validity of peer review

Issues in Primary Care

The Four Community Dimensions of Primary Care Practice
Pathman DE, Steiner BD, Williams E, et al (Univ of North Carolina, Chapel Hill; Univ of Missouri-Columbia)
J Fam Pract 46:293–303, 1998

18–1

Background.—Although there is support for the community playing a larger role in the work of physicians, it is unclear how physicians should be involved in the community. This study proposed and tested an organizing framework that identified 4 categories of community health-related activities appropriate for physician involvement.

Methods.—A random sample of 500 young primary care physicians in the United States was mailed a questionnaire. Respondents reported on their confidence in performing each of 15 specific community health-related activities. Factor analysis was used to test the hypothesis that physician involvement in the community can be grouped into the 4 proposed categories. Predictors of involvement were identified using ordinary least-squares regression models.

Results.—The response rate was 66.6%. Factor analysis showed that the specific community activities fit neatly into the 4 proposed categories. This provided a means of validating the distinctiveness of each of the categories. Respondents reported a range of community involvement. A surprising finding was that physicians who worked with minority and poor patient populations reported less community involvement. Physicians treating more patients covered by an HMO or capitated health plans also reported less community involvement. The four types of community activities for physician involvement were (1) identifying and intervening in the health problems of the community, (2) responding to the specific health issues of local cultural groups, (3) coordinating community health resources, and (4) assimilating into the community and local organizations.

Discussion.—It was disturbing to find that demographic indicators of greater socioeconomic need of patients and community did not predict greater physician involvement in any of the 4 categories. These findings support the hypothesis that physicians have a 4-part role in the health care issues of the community. This and similar studies may help physicians recognize how they can meet the expectation that they approach their work with a community perspective.

▶ Primary care, including family practice, offers the potential for the convergence of public health and community medicine within clinical practice. This article nicely describes four practical dimensions of a community oriented primary care physician. Medical students and residents should be trained to develop this perspective and carry it into their practice. What is disturbing from this article is that primary care physicians in managed care settings and those serving underserved populations were the least likely to report such community involvement. Somehow, population based financing for care needs to translate into community oriented practice.

J.E. Scherger, M.D., M.P.H.

The Generalist Role of Specialty Physicians: Is There a Hidden System of Primary Care?
Rosenblatt RA, Hart LG, Baldwin L-M, et al (Univ of Washington, Seattle; Health Care Financing Administration, Region X, Seattle)
JAMA 279:1364–1370, 1997

18–2

Introduction.—Although many specialist physicians argue that they can provide the same comprehensive care as primary care physicians, there is debate about the extent to which specialists incorporate elements of primary care into their ambulatory patient practice. A cross-sectional study was conducted to examine the question, using data on ambulatory care recorded in Part B of the Washington State Medicare Claims Database in 1994 and 1995.

Methods.—Patients included in the study were 373,505 Medicare beneficiaries 65 or older who made office visits to the study physicians. Core attributes of primary care examined were continuity (the majority-of-care relationship, with a single physician providing more than 50% of all ambulatory visits to 1 patient during the study period), comprehensiveness (the ability of the physician to address a broad range of patient problems), and preventive care (influenza immunization was recorded).

Results.—The patients had an average of 7.48 outpatient visits per year, and most saw both generalists and specialists; 9.6% had seen only generalists and 14.7% only specialists. Medical specialists had a majority-of-care relationship with only 7.8% of their patients and surgical specialists only 5.2%. In contrast, approximately half (49.8%) of all ambulatory visits to general internists and family physicians were made by majority-of-care patients. The rate of influenza immunization was higher in patients who received the majority of their care from generalists (55.4%) than for those who received their majority of care from medical (47.7%) or surgical (39.6%) specialists.

Conclusion.—A substantial proportion of elderly patients see only specialists for their care, but most specialist physicians do not assume the principal care responsibility for such patients. Immunization rates are lower for patients who receive the majority of their care from specialists; exceptions are pulmonologists and rheumatologists.

▶ This important article by a leading family medicine research team at the University of Washington describes the fundamental differences between the care given by primary care physicians and specialists. As many people receive all of their health care through specialists, there are often gaps in the basic services they should receive. This study documents that, in general, people who use specialists as their personal physicians receive less optimal care than those who use generalist physicians and are less likely to receive important preventive services.

J.E. Scherger, M.D., M.P.H.

Case Management Programs in Primary Care
Ferguson JA, Weinberger M (Indiana Univ, Indianapolis)
J Gen Intern Med 13:123–126, 1998

18-3

Background.—Managed care agencies are supposed to provide incentives for disease prevention and cost reduction. One potential mechanism for providing cost-effective care is "case management," specialized programs to treat high-risk and high-use patients. To determine whether these programs are cost-effective and achieve their clinical goals, a literature review was performed.

Methods.—The English language literature from 1985–1997 was searched on MEDLINE and HealthSTAR using the Medical Subject headings *case management, patient care planning, patient-centered care, disease management, care management, and managed care programs.* Only articles reporting results from randomized controlled interventions targeting adult patients with nonfatal, nonpsychiatric illness were included. A descriptive summary is presented.

Findings.—A total of 9 studies met the conditions for inclusion. Of these 9 studies, 4 targeted patients with a specified condition and 5 targeted a heterogeneous group of patients. Three interventions were supervised by a medical subspecialist and 6 by generalists. Two studies were performed at multiple sites and the rest at single sites. Of the 7 studies which examined impact on health resource use, only 2 found a positive effect. Both of these successful programs targeted patients with 1 specified disease. All 6 studies which examined patient-centered outcomes reported positive results. However, of the 3 studies that examined cost, none reported significant savings.

Conclusions.—A review of the existing literature on the case management approach to health care does not provide a clear endorsement of these programs and their impact on health resource use. Although patient-centered variables were reportedly improved, the cost was not specified. Multisite, longitudinal trials with long-term follow-up are required to determine the role of the case management approach in our health care system.

▶ If your local health maintenance organizations are like mine, case management nurses are common. This article verifies that case management is yet another medical intervention that has been widely incorporated with essentially no supporting data. The authors could find only 7 randomized controlled trials and little consistency in outcomes. Basically, patients liked the programs, but at what cost? I suspect case management programs will evolve into yet another attempt at reducing medical care costs.

M.A. Bowman, M.D., M.P.A.

Physician Practice Styles and Patient Outcomes: Differences Between Family Practice and General Internal Medicine
Bertakis KD, Callahan EJ, Helms LJ, et al (Univ of California, Davis)
Med Care 36:879–891, 1998

Objective.—Comparisons of family practices and internal medicine practices have suffered from patient selection bias and physician responses that reflected ideal rather than actual practice. Results of a prospectively randomized clinical trial to determine the differences in patient outcomes between family practice and internal medicine, to measure quantitatively how the style of the physician-patient relationship differs between the specialties, and to determine how differences in practice style may systematically lead to differences in patient outcome are discussed.

Methods.—A total of 509 nonpregnant new patients (193 male), mean age 41.3 years, at the University of California, Davis Medical Center, were randomly allocated to the family practice or general medicine clinic. The ethnic distribution was 62.7% white, 22.2% black, 8.3% Hispanic, 3.5% Asian, and 3.3% Native American. Patients were followed for 1 year and then asked to fill out an exit questionnaire including a self-reported health status (Medical Outcomes Study, Short Form-36) and patient satisfaction. Practice styles were assessed using the Davis Observation Code.

Results.—Questionnaires were completed by 417 patients. There were no significant differences between the 2 groups in change in health status. Patient satisfaction increased significantly and similarly for both groups. At the initial visit, internal medicine physicians spent significantly more time with patients than family practice physicians. Family practice physicians devoted significantly more time to health behavior and counseling (15.2% and 1.2% vs. 12.6% and 0.5%). Internal medicine physicians focused more on the technical aspects of medical care whereas family practice physicians spent more time on health behaviors. Patient activation efforts were significantly more likely to occur with healthier patients, patients who were less satisfied with health care in general, women patients, and with more educated patients. Counseling was significantly correlated with a positive change in health status. Emphasis on patient activation was significantly correlated with a positive change in patient satisfaction, whereas a technical practice style was negatively and significantly correlated with patient satisfaction.

Conclusion.—Physician behavior rather than practice style significantly influence patient satisfaction. A practice emphasizing counseling was predictive of a positive change in health status and a practice style emphasizing patient activation predicted improved patient satisfaction.

▶ Greater involvement of the patient (called patient activitation) and greater counseling were the major determinants of improved patient satisfaction and health status, respectively. These activation and counseling processes were performed more frequently by the residents who were in family practice than internal medicine residencies. We all know that patients must assist in taking responsibility for their health to maximize outcomes; compliance is important. With all these statements, the differences in actions by the residents and in the patient outcomes were still small although statistically significant. I would hope our beliefs and actions were more obviously different with greater improvements in outcome.

M.A. Bowman, M.D., M.P.A.

Primary Care Physicians and Specialists as Personal Physicians: Health Care Expenditures and Mortality Experience
Franks P, Fiscella K (Univ of Rochester, NY)
J Fam Pract 47:105–109, 1998   18–5

Background.—Managed care has brought the role of the primary care physician to the fore, while restricting patient access to specialists. Some research has suggested that specialty care may be superior to that provided by primary care physicians. To examine this issue, health care expenditures and 5-year mortality rates were compared between patients who reported a primary care physician and those who reported a specialist as their personal physician.

Study Design.—Data were obtained from the Household Survey component of the National Medical Expenditure Survey. This component consisted of a 1-year panel survey of about 35,000 people in 14,000 civilian households. Information was collected in 1987 on medical care, health expenditures, health insurance, health status, and health care access. This analysis included respondents who were at least 25 years of age and reported at least 1 physician as a usual source of care. Five-year mortality data were obtained from the National Death Index. Study data included age, sex, race, education, income, and geographical region. Participants identified their personal physician as either a primary care physician or specialist. Total annual health care expenditures and 5-year mortality rates were compared for these 2 groups.

Findings.—Of the 13,837 eligible respondents, 12,213 reported a primary care physician as their personal physician. Those who reported a primary care physician as their personal physician were more likely to be female, white, and rural and to report fewer medical diagnoses and have higher health perceptions, as well as lower annual health care expenditures and lower 5-year mortality rates. After adjustments for demographics, health insurance, reported diagnoses, health perceptions, and smoking status, those who reported a primary care physician as their personal physician had 33% lower annual adjusted health care expenditures and lower adjusted 5-year mortality rates than those who had a specialist as their primary care physician.

Conclusions.—This large study based on the National Medical Expenditure Survey indicated that having a primary care physician as ones personal physician is associated with lower health care expenditures and reduced mortality rates. The role of the primary care physician appears to be cost effective. More research on the optimal integration of primary and specialty care is needed for the appropriate allocation of health care resources.

▶ This is the article to read when you are feeling beat up over declining revenues, increased paperwork, and the other hassles of our medical care system. Yes, family doctors make a difference. Patients who reported a primary care physician, rather than a specialist, as their personal care physician had a substantially lower mortality rate, even after adjusting for many other factors. The average annual cost of care was also lower. The study had a large number of patients, and the information on mortality rates was from a 5-year benchmark. The study was based on self-report, and the severity of illness may not have been fully accounted for in the multiple regression analysis. Providing care across conditions and over time improve outcomes.

M.A. Bowman, M.D., M.P.A.

Taking Equity Seriously: A Dilemma for Government From Allocating Resources to Primary Care Groups
Bevan G (London School of Economics and Political Science)
BMJ 316:39–43, 1998
18–6

Background.—In Great Britain, the Labor government has announced its intention to eliminate 2 types of health care inequities: clinical and financial. Because of endemic variations in medical practice, it is not possible to eliminate both types of inequities simultaneously. The government will have to choose which type of inequity it should eliminate.

Implications of Eliminating Clinical Inequity.—Giving priority to clinical equity implies physician referral autonomy. Constraints would only apply to general practitioners using the same provider. Rationing would occur through waiting times defined by clinicians, which would override the ability to pay. Financial equity would be discarded. Variation in medical practice would be the rule.

Implications of Eliminating Financial Inequity.—Giving priority to financial equity requires creating budgets for primary care groups. Clinical inequity could then be reduced by the use of evidence-based medicine and surveillance of medical care variation.

Conclusions.—Because of endemic variations in medical practice, it is not currently possible to eliminate both clinical and financial inequity simultaneously in health care in Great Britain. Eliminating financial inequity first permits variation in medical practice to be examined, which may lead to clinical equity. Epidemiologists, general practitioners, and hospitals must work together to understand variation in medical practice and to determine the appropriate allocation of medical resources.

▶ For those who think that being a general practitioner in Britain is a homogeneous situation, this article is most instructive. There is no doubt that financial incentives guide physician behavior, no matter how well-meaning physicians are in the care of their patients. Britain is experimenting with financial incentives in an effort to reduce costs or provide more appropriate services. Continuous high quality physician education, along with a minimization of financial incentives and an environment of quality improvement and accountability, are the principles to move toward more uniform quality care.

J.E. Scherger, M.D., M.P.H.

Primary Care Physician Compensation Method in Medical Groups: Does It Influence the Use and Cost of Health Services for Enrollees in Managed Care Organizations?
Conrad DA, Maynard C, Cheadle A, et al (Univ of Washington, Seattle)
JAMA 279:853–858, 1998

Objective.—There have been few studies that have evaluated the impact of financial incentives for physicians on the general use and cost of health services. The relationship between the method of compensating the primary care physician (PCP) and the use and estimated cost of health services for adult enrollees of managed care organizations (MCOs) is investigated.

Methods.—Surveys of clinical practices were mailed to PCPs in 76 medical groups (3 or more physicians) in the state of Washington to determine whether use and cost of health care services were affected by the method of compensation provided to the physician. Five different compensation methods were used to assess measures of cost and use, and the effect of each was analyzed using least squares regression.

Results.—Surveys were completed by 62 (82%) medical groups with a total of 200,931 patients, aged 1 or more years, and 865 PCPs. The main outcome measures were total visits, hospital stay, and estimated yearly cost per member. There was no significant association between compensation, cost, and use according to multiple regression analysis. Enrollee age, sex, plan benefit level, and physician age were significantly associated with compensation method, cost, and use. Women incurred 77% more costs and had 4.7% more visits than men. Patient benefit levels and physician age had smaller but still significant effects on use and costs.

Conclusion.—Many factors can potentially influence PCP behavior. The PCP compensation method by itself does not have a signficant effect on cost and use of health care services for managed care enrollees whose PCP practices within a medical group. Future studies should examine the robustness of this finding in other settings and as managed care evolves over time.

▶ This is a welcome study suggesting that primary care physicians practice medicine similarly regardless of compensation method. Many have exaggerated the degree to which physician behavior is driven by financial incentives. As more physicians work in large medical groups with financial arrangements close to a base salary, the public may be reassured that the frequency of visits and expenditures for care resemble national norms in such settings.

J.E. Scherger, M.D., M.P.H.

Health System Issues

Is Gatekeeping Better Than Traditional Care? A Survey of Physicians' Attitudes

Halm EA, Causino N, Blumenthal D (Harvard Med School, Boston)
JAMA 278:1677–1681, 1997   18–8

Introduction.—In the restructuring of the health care system, primary care physicians as gatekeepers have become a central element in orchestrating and controlling the health care of its enrollees, which includes referrals to specialists, hospitalizations, and other expensive services. The expectations of gatekeepers is that they can (1) increase the quality of care by increasing coordination and (2) reduce costs. Previous studies have not separated the effects of gatekeeping as an administrative arrangement from the confounding effects of different payment mechanisms such as capitation.

Methods.—There were 330 physicians who served as primary care gatekeepers and traditional providers and who were surveyed to assess their attitudes about the effects of gatekeeping compared with traditional care in terms of the quality of patient care, administrative work, appropriateness of resource use, and cost.

Results.—Control of costs, frequency, and appropriateness of preventive services and knowledge of a patient's overall care were considered to be the positive effects of gatekeeping compared with traditional care by physicians. The negative effects of gatekeeping, according to the physicians, were the increased paperwork and telephone calls, the inaccessibility to specialists, the inability to order expensive tests and procedures, a decrease in overall quality of care, less freedom to make clinical decisions, the poorer quality of physician-patient relationships, less time spent with patients, and less appropriate use of hospitalizations and laboratory tests. The survey revealed that 7% of physicians were of mixed opinion, 21% said gatekeeping was worse, 40% said gatekeeping was the same as traditional care, and 32% rated gatekeeping as better than traditional care. Fewer years in clinical practice, generalist training, and experience with gatekeeping and HMO plans were all factors related to the rating of gatekeeping as positive.

Conclusion.—Positive and negative effects of gatekeeping were identified by physicians. Gatekeeping was considered to be better than or comparable with traditional care arrangements by 72% of physicians overall.

▶ This article might surprise some physicians who have assumed that mandatory gatekeeping models are considered to be negative by patients and physicians alike. Physicians in general, but especially primary care physicians, realize the benefit of having health care coordinated by a single primary care physician who knows the patient well over time. Patient choice has been discovered to be a critically important American value during the transitions of managed care. Gatekeeping is not a positive term, but receiving health care by and through a primary care physician is a time-honored and important model for delivering health care.

J.E. Scherger, M.D., M.P.H.

Are All Health Plans Created Equal? The Physician's View

Borowsky SJ, Davis MK, Goertz C, et al (Minneapolis Veterans Affairs Med Ctr; Univ of Minnesota, Minneapolis; Hennepin County Med Ctr, Minneapolis)
JAMA 278:917–921, 1997

Introduction.—Consumer surveys and data from the Health Plan Employer and Data Information Set effort provide information about the cost and quality of care in health plans. Physicians may be a valuable source of such information, but their input is infrequently sought. Physicians who were providers from 3 health plans (100 physicians per plan) in Minnesota were surveyed regarding their views on health plan practices.

Methods.—Likert-type items were used to assess health plan practices that promote or impede delivery of high-quality care. Physicians were asked to rate the 3 plans.

Results.—Of surveys sent to 300 physicians, 249 (84%) were returned. Less than 20% of physicians gave plans the highest rating for health care practices that promote delivery of high-quality of care. Barriers to delivery of high-quality care were associated with adequate time to spend with patients, covered benefits and copayment structure, and utilization management practices. Generalists tended to assign higher ratings than specialists for quality of primary care.

Conclusions.—Physician surveys can be used to reveal strengths and weaknesses of health plans. Consumers and purchasers of health care can benefit from physician ratings of health plan practices that promote or impede delivery of high-quality care.

▶ Health plans seem preoccupied with patient satisfaction surveys and focusing on the opinions of patients in making decisions. This article graphically shows that asking the doctors may also be very important. Physicians have very different views on the quality of health plans, and such views may be frequently expressed to patients, individually and in groups. It would be wise for health plans to take care of their physicians with the same concern that they address the preferences of patients.

J.E. Scherger, M.D., M.P.H.

Changing Nature of Physician Satisfaction With Health Maintenance Organization and Fee-for-Service Practices
Schulz R, Scheckler WE, Moberg DP, et al (Univ of Wisconsin—Madison)
J Fam Pract 45:321-330, 1997   18-10

Introduction.—Health maintenance organizations are the predominant form of managed care. Earlier research in Dane County, Wisconsin, indicated that physicians did not undergo a sudden drop in autonomy as a result of experience with HMOs. Physician satisfaction with HMOs was evaluated and compared with that of fee-for-service (FFS) practices to determine factors that contribute to satisfaction in an HMO-dominated environment.

Methods.—Cross-sectional surveys were used in 1986 and 1993 to query all Dane County physicians in active practice. Physician overall support for HMO development, satisfaction with the work situation, and clinical freedom within HMO and FFS practices were compared for the 2 periods.

Results.—There were significantly more physicians supportive of the development of HMOs in 1993 than in 1986. Primary care physicians were significantly more satisfied with HMO practice, perceived clinical freedom in HMO practice, and satisfaction with autonomy and resources. Perceived satisfaction and freedom with FFS practice was significantly lower in 1993 than 1986 for hospital-based and referral specialists, but not primary care physicians. Mean levels of satisfaction with FFS practices were higher in 1986 and 1993, compared with that of HMOs for the 2 time points. Satisfaction with Medicare practice was assessed in 1993 only and was significantly lower than satisfaction observed with HMO or FFS practice.

Conclusions.—Primary care physicians were more satisfied than subspecialists with HMOs because of HMO-generated income and the expanded clinical freedom. The decline in satisfaction with FFS practice among primary care physicians and subspecialists might be related to diminishing clinical freedom from indemnity carriers.

▶ The change to organize delivery systems from the cottage industry of independent practice is progressing inexorably in the United States. Physicians who have been in practice for the past 10-20 years might be called a transition generation. This article shows that physicians are becoming comfortable with new delivery systems and are beginning to realize that organized health plans with prepayment of health care to populations have definite advantages.

J.E. Scherger, M.D., M.P.H.

Insurance or a Regular Physician: Which Is the Most Powerful Predictor of Health Care?
Sox CM, Swartz K, Burstin HR, et al (Harvard School of Public Health, Cambridge, Mass; Brigham and Women's Hosp, Boston)
Am J Public Health 88:364–370, 1998

Introduction.—Some individuals with health care insurance do not have a regular, ongoing relationship with a physician, whereas others who are uninsured do have such a relationship. The lack of a regular physician is a predictor of both poor access to care and poor outcome. This study hypothesized that the lack of a regular physician is a more powerful barrier to health services access than is insurance status.

Methods.—Study sites were the adult emergency departments of 5 urban teaching hospitals in the Boston area. Those eligible for the study were aged 18 to 64, were not retired, and did not have Medicare or "other" insurance. Complaints selected for enrollment eligibility were abdominal pain, asthma or chronic obstructive pulmonary disease, chest pain, hand laceration, head trauma, and vaginal bleeding. Medical records were reviewed and patients were interviewed to determine their socioeconomic and demographic background, insurance status, and the presence of co-morbid conditions.

Results.—During a 1-month period, 1,952 of 4,325 patients seen in the emergency departments with 1 of the 6 complaints met other eligibility criteria. In multivariate analysis, the lack of a regular physician was a more consistent and stronger predictor of poor access to care than was insurance status. Patients without a regular physician were at greater risk for delay in seeking care, for no physician visits in the last year, and for no emergency department visits in the last year. Black patients, uninsured patients, and those who had changed insurance were more likely to delay seeking care. Among patients with a regular physician, both uninsured and privately insured patients had equally good access to health care. But even for privately insured patients, the lack of a regular physician was a predictor of poor access.

Conclusion.—Each of 3 measures of poor access to care—delay in seeking emergency care, no physician visits in the previous year, and no emergency department visits in the previous year—was more strongly predicted by the lack of a regular physician than by insurance status. Access to health services can be improved by directing patients to choose a regular physician.

▶ Having a regular physician removes a major barrier to receiving routine health care. This study from the Harvard School of Public Health provides information regarding the importance of having a regular physician. Insurance status has been described as an important predictor with respect to access to care. This study shows that having a regular physician has a greater influence on health care behavior than does insurance status.

J.E. Scherger, M.D., M.P.H.

The Class of 1989 and Physician Supply in Canada
Ryten E, Thurber AD, Buske L (Association of Canadian Med Colleges, Ottawa; Canadian Post-MD Education Registry, Ottawa, Ont, Canada; Canadian Medical Assoc, Ottawa, Ont, Canada)
Can Med Assoc J 158:723–728, 1998   18–12

Objective.—To determine whether the physician supply in Canada was outstripping the demand, a 7-year longitudinal study was conducted to assess migration and specialty choices and patterns of post-MD training of 1,722 MDs from the class of 1989.

Methods.—Graduates of Canada's 16 medical schools were tracked every year from their graduation in 1989 to the spring of 1996. Data were analyzed statistically.

Results.—As of 1996, 1,300 (75.5%) of the 1,722 graduates were practicing in Canada, 216 (12.5%) were residency or fellowship training in Canada, 193 (11.2%) were in another country and 15 were no longer in medicine. Of those practicing in Canada, 878 (57.9%) were in general or family medicine, and 638 (42.1%) were specialists or in specialty training. Approximately 2/3 of graduates still lived in the same province in 1995 to 1996 that they lived in before entering medical school. All Canadian provinces except Ontario, Quebec, British Columbia, and the territories, experienced migration losses. Few graduates migrated to Newfoundland or Saskatchewan.

Interpretation.—Approximately three fourths of graduates were in practice in Canada in 1995–96. Most were practicing general or family medicine. Internal migration was significant, resulting in migration losses from most provinces. Given these migration losses, the number of physicians required for self-sufficiency will be considerably below what will be needed in the foreseeable future.

▶ Physician workforce data from our large neighbor to the north is of interest to the United States. The United States is facing a physician surplus in many areas and migration of physicians from Canada to the United States is common. This study documents that almost 12% of newly trained Canadian physicians migrate from their country, most commonly to the United States. In addition, Canada has the same difficulty as the United States with a maldistribution problem. The positive news from Canada is that almost 60% of graduates from this class were in family practice. If Canada does indeed have a physician shortage, changes in the United States may result in the development of a reverse migration.

J.E. Scherger, M.D., M.P.H.

Quality, Outcomes, and Peer Review

Impact of Education for Physicians on Patient Outcomes
Clark NM, Gong M, Schork MA, et al (Univ of Michigan, Ann Arbor; Columbia Univ, New York; NIH, Bethesda, Md)
Pediatrics 101:831–836, 1998   18–13

Introduction.—It is not known whether education for practicing physicians would change their clinical behavior. When it comes to chronic conditions such as asthma, in which a long-term partnership between patient and clinician is established, data about the link between clinician education and patient outcomes may be valuable. The effects of an interactive seminar based on theoretic principles of self-regulation on general practice pediatricians and their patients with asthma were examined to determine whether there was improvement in the physicians' clinical treatment of asthma and in their patient-teaching and communication behavior. The parents of the children with asthma also judged the performance of the physicians.

Methods.—Seventy-four general practice pediatricians were assigned to a program group or a control group. Five months after the program, 93% provided follow-up information. At baseline 637 of the patients participated, and in a 22-month window after the intervention 74% provided follow-up data.

Results.—Addressing patients' fears about medicines, reviews of written instructions, provision of a sequence of education messages, writing down how to adjust medications at home when symptoms change, and reports of spending less time with patients were found more often in physicians who were in the program group (Table 1). Parents reported more often that physicians in the program group were likely to be reassuring, described as a goal that the child be fully active, and gave information to relieve specific worries. These parents reported more often that they knew how to make management decisions at home after a visit with the physician. Patients from the program group were more likely to have received a prescription for inhaled anti-inflammatory medicine and to have been asked by the physician to demonstrate how to use a metered-dose inhaler. Significantly fewer nonemergency office visits were made by children seen by program physicians. Fewer visits for follow-up of an episode of symptoms were also made by this group. There were no differences between the 2 groups in emergency department visits and hospitalizations. Children treated by program physicians and placed on a regimen of inhaled corticosteroids had fewer symptoms and fewer follow-up visits, nonemergency physician office visits, emergency department visits, and hospitalizations.

Conclusion.—There were shorter patient-physician encounters, more favorable patient responses to physicians' actions, less health care use, and

TABLE 1.—Postprogram Differences in Pediatricians' Behavior*

Variable	Adjusted Mean of Treatment Group†	Adjusted Mean of Control Group†	P Value (ANCOVA)
Treat newly diagnosed patients with inhaled antiinflammatory therapy	67.77%	56.27%	.044
Address specific fears about the new medication	5.14	4.68	.026
Give written instructions for later reference about using the medication	4.52	3.91	.058
Go over the instruction for the new medication	5.04	4.43	.01
Write down for the family how to adjust the medicine when symptoms change	4.30	3.46	.001
Provide guidelines for patients to use to adjust therapy when clinical conditions change	80.39%	65.34%	.003
Time spent on a visit for a newly diagnosed child with asthma (in minutes)	22.8	27.1	.007

*Analysis of covariance with baseline data as a covariate. No significant differences between treatment and control groups at baselines were identified for these variables.
†Likert type response format, where 1 = never and 6 = always.
(Courtesy of Clark NM, Gong M, Schork A, et al: Impact of Education for Physicians on Patient Outcomes. *Pediatrics* 101:831–836, 1998. Reproduced with permission.)

a significant impact on the prescribing and communications behavior of physicians as a result of the interactive seminar based on theories of self-regulation.

▶ I did not select this article because it shows that continuing medical education can effect physician behavior—which it does—but because it reinforces that a theory the authors call "self-regulation" has positive benefits for patients. A whole book has been written on this theory.[1] Here is a summary: Giving patients a sense of control and responsibility for their own health and the education to implement this control improves their ability to manage their health. In this case, physicians, through active learning, could in turn help their patients to effectively self-manage, without spending more time with the patients.

M.A. Bowman, M.D., M.P.A.

Reference

1. Bandura A: *Social Foundations of Thought and Action.* Englewood Cliffs, NJ, Prentice-Hall, 1986.

Are Physicians' Office Laboratory Results of Comparable Quality to Those Produced in Other Laboratory Settings?

Hurst J, Nickel K, Hilborne LH (Univ of California, Los Angeles; RAND, Santa Monica, Calif)
JAMA 279:468–471, 1998

Objective.—In 1995, California mandated that all laboratories conform with the Clinical Laboratory Improvement Amendments standards (CLIA) passed by Congress in 1988. The quality of laboratory testing, measured by proficiency testing (PT) scores, was compared for licensed California clinical laboratories (non-POLs), physicians' office laboratories (POLs) that employ licensed medical technologists, and physicians' office laboratories that do not employ licensed medical technologists.

Methods.—PT performance data for 1996, for all 1,110 California clinical laboratories taking part in the American Association of Bioanalysts proficiency testing program, were compared for total cholesterol, triglycerides, serum glucose, potassium, TSH digoxin, erythrocyte counts, leukocyte counts, prothrombin time, infectious mononucleosis, and urine cultures. Performance was evaluated in each of the 3 laboratory groups as (1) overall rates of "unsatisfactory" (single testing event failure), (2) "unsuccessful" (repeated testing event failure); and (3) rates of "unsatisfactory" performance by testing event for each group of hematology and chemistry analytes combined.

Results.—The overall rates of unsatisfactory and unsuccessful performance were 21.5% and 4.4%, respectively, for POLS, 14.0% and 1.8%, respectively, for POLs employing medical technologists, and 8.1% and 0.9%, respectively, for non-POLs. The unsuccessful rate for POLs was 4 times that of non-POLs and 2 times that of POLs employing medical technologists,

Conclusion.—The unsuccessful rate for POLs was significantly higher than the unsuccessful rates for non-POLs and for POLs using licensed medical technologists. Less education, training, and supervision may account for these differences. Laboratory directors must understand the importance of the regulations and conscientiously supervise analytical personnel to ensure the integrity of the total testing process.

▶ The CLIA regulations have greatly reduced the amount of laboratory work done in physician offices. Most physicians have assumed that they were providing quality laboratory testing in their offices despite the lack of rigorous standards usually given to licensed laboratories. This study suggests that physician office laboratory results were unsatisfactory with respect to quality more than other laboratory settings. Physicians wanting to provide laboratory testing in their office will need to ensure that they are meeting the highest standards of care.

J.E. Scherger, M.D., M.P.H.

Consumer Reports in Health Care: Do They Make a Difference in Patient Care?

Longo DR, Land G, Schramm W, et al (Univ of Missouri, Columbia; Missouri Dept of Health, Jefferson City)
JAMA 278:1579–1584, 1997   18–15

Background.—Consumer reports are a standardized way in which patients can compare the quality and range of services of health care providers. Such reports can provide both individuals and groups with important comparative information for improving patient care and for marketing their services. This article reports the influence of an obstetrics consumer report on the willingness of Missouri hospitals to begin new obstetric and child care programs.

Methods.—Data from 90 hospitals offering obstetric services were gathered, including information on the length of stay, number of births, cesarean section rate, vaginal birth after cesarean rate, neonatal mortality rates, and patient satisfaction. The data were collated, and the consumer report was published; then 1 year later, the hospitals were surveyed to see whether the consumer report prompted any implemented or planned changes in services. Of the 88 hospitals that still offered obstetric services, 82 responded to the survey (93%).

Findings.—Of those hospital administrators surveyed (typically the obstetric nurse supervisor), 24% found the guide unhelpful, 29% were neutral, and 46% rated the guide useful in examining their own services. Hospitals that had low or average patient satisfaction ratings were more likely to have changed or were more likely to be considering a change in policies than were hospitals with higher patient satisfaction ratings. The biggest areas for change were as follows: when the guide was published, 34 programs did not offer follow-up services, 42 did not offer car seats, 33 did not have a formal transfer agreement, 33 did not have a lactation consultant, and 15 did not offer tubal ligations. After the report's publication, 17 of 34 programs (50%) began offering follow-up services, 18 of 42 (43%) began a car seat program, 13 of 33 (39%) created a formal transfer agreement, 6 of 18 (33%) began a breast-feeding education program, and 2 of 15 (13%) began offering tubal ligations. In most situations, the hospital decided to institute a new program because a competitor in the same market already offered a similar program. In fact, hospitals in the most competitive markets were twice as likely to change policies or add new procedures as hospitals in noncompetitive situations. Policy changes, such as a reduction in the cesarean delivery rate and an increase in the vaginal birth after cesarean rate, were in the direction of improving outcomes. Furthermore, hospitals with lower patient satisfaction rates were more likely to plan to change or have changed their policies.

Conclusions.—Publication of the consumer guide had a substantial impact on the types of obstetric services provided. Changes were most evident in competitive markets and in hospitals that scored low on a given measure in comparison with the other hospitals. The improvements in clinical factors such as cesarean delivery rates indicate that hospitals actually changed their medical practices in response to the guide's publication. In summation, consumer guides can improve the quality of care and the marketability of health care services.

▶ This study pulled together quite an astonishing group of "outcome" measures related to a not-very-complicated consumer intervention. The authors correctly point out that all the changes cannot be ascribed solely to the consumer intervention because several other factors that could have had an effect were happening at the same time (e.g., other national and state reports). Still, the availability of the other materials to the average consumer and hospital was small. The authors make a compelling case that the intervention made the difference. This is health policy reform conducted on a large scale and a small budget. I am certain that these results will stimulate countless similar efforts in other states and settings.

A.O. Berg, M.D., M.P.H.

Peer Review of the Quality of Care: Reliability and Sources of Variability for Outcome and Process Assessments
Smith MA, Atherly AJ, Kane RL, et al (Univ of Minnesota, Minneapolis)
JAMA 278:1573–1578, 1997
18–16

Introduction.—Many quality assurance strategies use peer review of quality of care, but poor interrater reliability is a major limitation. The interrater reliability of outcome and process measures was compared in a population of frail older adults, and systematic sources of variability contributing to poor reliability were identified.

Methods.—Patients were randomly selected from the Program for All-Inclusive Care of the Elderly, which capitates and co-ordinates acute and long-term care services for frail older adults at a number of sites. Participants were 313 elderly individuals. Their medical records for a 1-year period were retrospectively reviewed by 8 certified geriatricians and 6 certified geriatric nurse practitioners. Outcomes were examined using structured implicit judgments and explicit questions on specific aspects of patient outcome and a summary judgment on overall outcome.

Results.—Two reviews of 180 of the charts yielded a total of 493 completed reviews. Eight tracer conditions examined were present in the following percentages of charts: arthritis (61%) bathing problems (80%), dementia (60%), hypertension (58%), urinary incontinence (55%), constipation (49%), depression (40%), and malnutrition (38%). Outcome measures exhibited higher interrater reliability than process measures. Five of the outcome measures, but none of the process measures, achieved fair to good (greater than 0.40) reliability. Factors contributing to poor reliabilities for process measures were the reviewers' inability to differentiate among cases with respect to quality of management, systematic bias from individual reviewers, and systematic bias related to the reviewer's professional training.

Conclusion.—Quality of care is difficult to evaluate for elderly patients with multiple chronic illnesses. In a managed care setting, such patients may be particularly vulnerable to undertreatment as a means of cost containment. Factors influencing reliability of outcome and process assessments need to be recognized so that quality of care measures are more accurate.

▶ Quality is the buzzword, and quality measurement tools are everywhere. Physicians tend to assume that a "tool" accurately measures what it says it does. This article, critically evaluating the reliability of outcome and process assessments, suggests otherwise. In my view, quality assessment tools should be critically evaluated and validated before being applied. As with all kinds of other rules and recommendations, it is usually left to the "end" user (that is, the physician) to discover, often too late, that the thing doesn't work as intended. Family physicians already need to be critical evaluators of individual research studies and clinical practice guidelines. We also need to become savvy consumers of quality assessment tools. We should not accept tools that have not been adequately tested for reliability and validity. Further, we should aim for measures of clinical outcomes that patients would notice and care about, not tools that simply measure the process of care.

A.O. Berg, M.D., M.P.H.

Subject Index

A

Abdominal
  symptoms and *Helicobacter pylori*, in children, 275
Abortion, 336
  early, misoprostol in, effect of nonsteroidal anti-inflammatory drugs on action of, 338
  spontaneous, expectant management *vs.* elective curettage for, 337
Abuse
  child, further, after Munchausen syndrome by proxy, nonaccidental poisoning, and nonaccidental suffocation, 220
  concept of, validating, 205
  domestic, management guidelines when male and female partners are patients of same physician, 206
  emotional, effects on health indicators, in women, 205
Acarbose
  vs. metformin in dietary-treated type 2 diabetics, 73
Acebutolol
  long-term effects on sexual function, in men and women, 6
Acetaminophen
  combined with aspirin and caffeine for migraine, 257
  hepatotoxicity from multiple doses, in children, 300
  after misoprostol for early abortion, 338
  use and excessive warfarin anticoagulation, 43
Acquired immunodeficiency syndrome (*see* AIDS)
Actinic
  damage, sunscreens in prevention of, 149
Activity
  physical (*see* Physical, activity)
Acyclovir
  oral, switching from prescription to over-the-counter status, 113
Adenoidal
  obstruction, in children, 301
Adenotonsillar
  hypertrophy, chronic, amoxicillin/clavulanate for, in children, 273
Admission
  scoring system to predict vaginal delivery after cesarean delivery, 367

Adolescent
  allergy in, penicillin, amoxicillin, and cephalosporin, diagnosis of, 129
  athletes
    high school, preparticipation cardiovascular screening for, 292
    screening for hypertrophic cardiomyopathy in, 294
  back pain in, 177
  fibromyalgia syndrome in, 180
  gynecomastia in, in boys, 303
  high school, condom availability program for, students' acquisition and use of condoms in, 305
  knee injuries in, correlation of arthroscopic and clinical findings with MRI findings in, 188
  obese, morbidly, effects of high-protein, low-fat ketogenic diet on, 59
  urban, effect of HIV counseling and testing on sexually transmitted diseases and condom use in, 104
  urinalysis in, screening dipstick, 110
Adverse drug reactions
  incidence in hospitalized patients, 394
Aerobic
  demands of lawn mowing in coronary artery disease patients, 228
  exercise
    blood pressure and, 2
    training, effect on aerobic fitness, immune indices, and quality of life in HIV-positive patients, 103
  fitness of HIV-positive patients, effect of exercise training on, 103
Affluent older population
  depressive symptoms among, 212
African Americans (*see* Blacks)
Age
  bone, progression, variation in healthy children, 297
  headache and, tension-type, 254
Aging
  skin, premature, ultraviolet light-induced, pathophysiology of, 151
AIDS, 102
  (*See also* HIV)
  in HIV-infected injection drug users, prognostic indicators for, 109
Air
  travel-associated barotrauma, oral pseudoephedrine *vs.* topical oxymetazoline in prevention of, 262

Airflow
  sports nasal strips and, 263
Airway(s)
  disease, reactive, 121
  response to allergen, skin sensitivity to allergen does not accurately predict, 125
  upper, abnormal resistance during sleep, and hypertension, 4
Albumin
  excretion rate in type 2 diabetics, long-term effects of simvastatin on, 75
Albuterol
  in hospitalized infants with bronchiolitis, 277
Alcohol
  dependence, naltrexone in management of, 204
  intake
    folate and vitamin B_6 intake and, and risk of coronary heart disease in women, 14
    high, and risk of breast cancer, 311
  problem, screening for, 198
  use, 198
    mortality among middle-aged and, in U.S. and Russia, 202
    mortality among middle-aged and elderly and, in U.S., 200
Alfuzosin
  /antibiotics for chronic prostatitis, 166
Algorithm
  for administering subcutaneous heparin for deep venous thrombosis, 40
Allergen
  airway response to, skin sensitivity to allergen does not accurately predict, 125
Allergic
  asthma, skin sensitivity to allergen does not accurately predict airway response to allergen in, 125
Allergy, 121
  food, multiple, in breastfed infants, 127
  penicillin, amoxicillin, and cephalosporin, diagnosis of, 129
Alpha-blockers
  /antibiotics for chronic prostatitis, 166
Alternative
  medicine, 391
  why patients use, 391
Alzheimer's disease, 194
  special care units, residence in, effects on functional outcomes, 195
  tacrine in, 196
Ambra
  grisea D6 in homeopathic preparation for vertigo, 261

Ambulatory
  encounters, community-based, involving medical students, 397
Amitriptyline
  in fibromyalgia syndrome in children and adolescents, 182
Amlodipine
  long-term effects on sexual function, in men and women, 6
  vs. fosinopril in hypertensive type 2 diabetics, 70
Amoxicillin
  allergy, diagnosis of, 129
  /clavulanate for chronic adenotonsillar hypertrophy, in children, 273
Anamirta
  cocculus D4 in homeopathic preparation for vertigo, 261
Androgen(s)
  decrease after ovarian electrocautery for polycystic ovary syndrome, 329
  insensitivity, partial, and marked breast development in boys at puberty, 305
  lack of effect on vasodilator effects of estrogen in postmenopausal women, 341
Anesthesia
  topical, vs. ring block and dorsal penile nerve block for neonatal circumcision, 171
Angiotensin
  -converting enzyme inhibitors
    cancer risk with, 26
    for prevention of renal failure in insulin-dependent diabetics, 61
Antibiotics
  /alpha-blockers for chronic prostatitis, 166
  effect on reconsultation for acute lower respiratory tract illness, 117
  prophylactic, for tick bites and Lyme disease, 93
Antibody
  testing, antinuclear, to screen for rheumatic diseases, in children, 395
Anticoagulant
  service, nurse specialist, cost and effectiveness of, 41
Anticoagulation, 40
  warfarin, excessive, acetaminophen and other risk factors for, 43
Antidepressant
  use in nursing homes, effects of restraint intervention and OBRA '87 regulations on, 217

Antifungal
  preparations, anti-inflammatory activity of, 152
  products, prescribing by nondermatologists vs. dermatologists, 158
Antigen
  prostate-specific antigen screening in elderly men, and preferences and informed consent, 167
Antihypertensive
  drugs
    effects on sexual function, long-term, in men and women, 6
    intracerebral hemorrhage and, 249
Anti-inflammatory
  activity of antifungal preparations, 152
  drugs, nonsteroidal
    misoprostol action in early abortion and, 338
    topical, quantitative systematic review of, 186
    ulcers related to, omeprazole vs. misoprostol for, 132
    ulcers related to, omeprazole vs. ranitidine for, 134
Antinuclear
  antibody testing to screen for rheumatic diseases, in children, 395
Antioxidant(s), 239
  vitamins
    effect on transient impairment of endothelium-dependent brachial artery vasoactivity after single high-fat meal, 241
    in prevention of cardiovascular disease, 239
Antiretroviral
  therapy initiation in HIV infection, improved survival after, 108
Anxiety
  disorder, social, paroxetine for, 219
  severe, over childbirth, and obstetric outcome, 372
Aorta
  elasticity, effect of chronic garlic intake on, in elderly, 244
Apnea
  sleep, obstructive
    blood pressure and, effect of avoidance of supine position during sleep on, 3
    hypertension and, 4
Apolipoprotein
  B levels as risk factor for ischemic heart disease, 51

Appendix
  CT of, effect on treatment and use of hospital resources, 148
Aromatase
  activity, increased, and marked breast development in boys at puberty, 305
Artery
  brachial, vasoactivity, endothelium-dependent, transient impairment after single high-fat meal, effect of antioxidant vitamins on, 241
  carotid, disease, 33
    asymptomatic, outcome of, 33
  coronary (see Coronary, artery)
Arthroscopic
  findings correlated with MRI findings in injured knees in children and adolescents, 188
Asbestos
  exposure and reduced FEV_1 in young men, and effectiveness of postal smoking cessation advice, 238
Ascorbic
  acid combined with d-α-tocopherol for protection against sunburn, 150
Aspirin
  atrial fibrillation patients using, stroke prevention in, 249
  combined with acetaminophen and caffeine for migraine, 257
  low-dose, in prevention of preeclampsia, 356
  use and colorectal cancer, 379
Asthma, 121
  allergic, skin sensitivity to allergen does not accurately predict airway response to allergen in, 125
  hospitalization for, risk of, and inhaled steroids, 121
  pulmonary function in, effect of inactivated influenza vaccine on, 124
  salmeterol improves quality of life in patients requiring inhaled corticosteroids, 122
Atherosclerosis
  carotid
    Asymptomatic Carotid Atherosclerosis Study, effect on carotid endarterectomy, 35
    bone changes in postmenopausal women and, 339
    progression and smoking, 231
Athletes
  high school, preparticipation cardiovascular screening for, 292

young, screening for hypertrophic cardiomyopathy in, 294
Atopic
   dermatitis and food hypersensitivity reactions, 159
Atopy
   development after brief neonatal exposure to cow's milk, 128
Atrial
   fibrillation
      aspirin use in, and stroke prevention, 249
      likelihood of spontaneous conversion to sinus rhythm, 25
Attention
   -deficit hyperactivity disorder, educational and occupational outcome of grown-up boys after, 306
Attitudes
   physicians'
      toward gatekeeping, 409
      vs. patients', toward pharmaceutical industry gifts, 383
Ayre spatula
   endocervical brush after, and quality of Pap smear, 327

B

Back
   pain, 176
      in children and adolescents, 177
      low, chronic, nortriptyline for, 176
      low, during pregnancy, follow-up, 178
Bacteremia
   risk for febrile young children in post-*Hemophilus influenzae* type b era, 272
Bacteriological
   examination in elderly women, urine sampling method for, 111
Barotrauma
   air travel-associated, oral pseudoephedrine vs. topical oxymetazoline in prevention of, 262
Barrett's esophagus
   screening for, 10 years' experience with, 135
Basal cell
   skin cancer, invasive cancers after, 160
Bedside
   rationing and patients' best interests, 385

Behavior(s)
   abusive, women's perceptions of defining, 205
Behavioral
   effects of gonadal steroids in premenstrual syndrome, 334
   vs. educational interventions for fibromyalgia, 179
Benzodiazepine
   use in nursing homes, effects of restraint intervention and OBRA '87 regulations on, 217
Benzydamine
   topical, effectiveness of, 186
Beta agonists
   in preterm labor, variations between family physicians and obstetricians in use of, 360
Beta-blockers
   cancer risk with, 26
Beta-carotene
   intake, low, and risk of breast cancer, 311
   in prevention of cardiovascular disease, 240
Biliary
   cirrhosis, primary, ursodeoxycholic acid delays onset of esophageal varices in, 144
Biofeedback
   for constipation, 137
      results of, 138
   for fecal incontinence, 137
Birth
   anxiety over, severe, and obstetric outcome, 372
   incontinence after, transient urinary, effect of pelvic muscle exercise on, 370
   outcomes and midwifery care, in U.S., 375
Bites
   tick, and Lyme disease in endemic setting, 93
Blacks
   energy expenditure in, resting, in overweight females, 57
   headache in, tension-type, 254
Bleeding
   as predictor of endometrial hyperplasia in postmenopausal women on hormone replacement therapy, 344
   vaginal, unexpected, with cyclic vs. continuous postmenopausal hormone replacement therapy, 346
Block
   nerve, dorsal penile

EMLA cream prior to, for circumcision, in children, 170
  vs. ring block and topical anesthesia for neonatal circumcision, 171
  ring, *vs.* dorsal penile nerve block and topical anesthesia for neonatal circumcision, 171
Blood
  chemistries of morbidly obese adolescents, effect of high-protein, low-fat ketogenic diet on, 59
  glucose, high, as risk factor for mortality in nondiabetic middle-aged men, 78
  pressure
    in diabetics, insulin-dependent, on intensive therapy, effect of excessive weight gain on, 65
    exercise training and, 2
    monitoring, ambulatory, in pregnancy, 357
    pulse, as predictor of long-term cardiovascular mortality, 10
    sleep apnea and, obstructive, effect of avoidance of supine position during sleep on, 3
  urea nitrogen levels after short-term ibuprofen use in infants and children, 299
Body
  composition of morbidly obese adolescents, effect of high-protein, low-fat ketogenic diet on, 59
  fat, dietary fat as major determinant of, 54
Bone
  age progression, variation in healthy children, 297
  changes and carotid atherosclerosis in postmenopausal women, 339
Borrelia burgdorferi
  outer-surface lipoprotein A, recombinant, with adjuvant, vaccination against Lyme disease with, 95
  outer-surface protein A, recombinant, vaccine with, to prevent Lyme disease, 94
Botulinum
  toxin for palmar hyperhidrosis, 155
Bowel
  cancer and Turner syndrome, 88
Brachial
  artery vasoactivity, endothelium-dependent, transient impairment after single high-fat meal, effect of antioxidant vitamins on, 241

BRCA1
  mutations and breast cancer, 313
Breakfast
  cereal fortified with folic acid, reduction of plasma homocysteine levels in coronary heart disease patients with, 28
Breast
  cancer (*see* Cancer, breast)
  cysts, oil, sonographic features of, 320
  development, marked, at puberty, evaluation of boys with, 303
  -fed infants, multiple food allergy in, 127
Bronchiolitis
  albuterol in, in hospitalized infants, 277
  otitis media in children with, acute, 274
Brush
  endocervical
    after Ayre spatula, and quality of Pap smear, 327
    use after endocervical curettage, 323
Budesonide
  vs. mesalamine for active Crohn's disease, 141
BUN
  levels after short-term ibuprofen use in infants and children, 299
Bupropion
  sustained-release, for smoking cessation, 235

C

Caffeine
  combined with aspirin and acetaminophen for migraine, 257
  intake, heavy, during pregnancy, and sudden infant death syndrome, 286
  supplementation, long-term effect on weight maintenance, 58
Calcium
  carbonate in premenstrual syndrome, 332
  channel blockers and risk of cancer, 26
Canada
  physician supply in, and class of 1989, 413
Cancer, 378
  bowel, and Turner syndrome, 88
  breast, 310
    BRCA1 mutations and, 313
    risk, and diet, nutrition, and physical exercise, 310
    risk, dual effects of weight and weight gain on, 311
    surgery for, effect of Nancy Reagan's mastectomy on choice of, 317

survival from, and treatment in health maintenance organization and fee-for-service settings, 318
survival from, 5-year, and hospital volume, 316
survivors, vitamin E for hot flashes in, 315
tamoxifen in, uterine side effects of, 314
cervix, 320
screening among women with and without hysterectomies, 320
childhood, risk of cancer in offspring of survivors of, 381
colorectal, and aspirin use, 379
incidence and mortality, 20-year report card of, in U.S., 378
lung, and prolonged cough, 382
patients treatment preferences and prognosis, 380
prostate
detection, early, by serendipity, 170
incidence and patient mortality, effects of screening and early detection on, 168
risk and calcium channel blockers, 26
skin
basal cell, invasive cancers after, 160
sunscreens in prevention of, 149
Carbohydrate
diet, high preparatory, no effect on 3-hour oral glucose tolerance test in pregnancy, 362
supplementation, long-term effect on weight maintenance, 58
Carbon-13
urea breath test for *Helicobacter pylori* and abdominal symptoms, in children, 275
Carcinoma (*see* Cancer)
Cardiac (*see* Heart)
Cardiomyopathy
hypertrophic, screening young athletes for, 294
Cardiovascular
disease, 1
prevention with antioxidant vitamins, 239
events
after myocardial infarction, effect of pravastatin on, in women, 24
in patients with hypertension and type 2 diabetes, effects of fosinopril *vs.* amlodipine on, 70
mortality, long-term, pulse pressure as predictor of, 10

risk from childhood to young adulthood in offspring of parents with coronary artery disease, longitudinal changes in, 8
screening, preparticipation, for high school athletes, 292
Care
Alzheimer's disease special care units, residence in, effects on functional outcomes, 195
day care center, child, postlicensure effectiveness of varicella vaccine during outbreak in, 266
gynecologic, associated with unexpected vaginal bleeding with cyclic *vs.* continuous postmenopausal hormone replacement therapy, 346
health (*see* Health, care)
managed, expense of unlimited mental health care coverage under, 210
medical, sabotaging one's own, 221
obstetric, why family physicians provide, 374
patient, effect of consumer reports in health care on, 417
primary (*see* Primary care)
quality of, reliability and validity of peer review of, 418
Carotid
artery disease, 33
asymptomatic, outcome of, 33
atherosclerosis
Asymptomatic Carotid Atherosclerosis Study, effect on carotid endarterectomy, 35
bone changes in postmenopausal women and, 339
endarterectomy
effect of Asymptomatic Carotid Atherosclerosis Study on, 35
indications, outcomes, and provider volumes for, 34
Carpal
tunnel syndrome
treatment for, conservative medical *vs.* chiropractic, 185
work-related, measuring functional outcomes in, 183
Carpet
removal in bedroom for house dust mite reduction, efficacy of, 124
shampoo, anti-mite, long-term efficacy of reduction of house dust mites, 123
Case
management programs in primary care, 404

Subject Index / 427

manager, electronic, for diabetes control, 83
Cashew
 allergy and atopic dermatitis, 159
Catfish
 allergy and atopic dermatitis, 159
Catheterization
 cardiac, on-site, long-term outcome in myocardial infarction patients admitted to facilities with and without, 20
CD4+
 cell count and plasma viral load as prognostic indicators for AIDS and infectious disease death in HIV-infected injection drug users, 109
CD11b
 expression as diagnostic marker for early-onset neonatal infection, 279
Cell
 basal cell skin cancer, invasive cancer after, 160
 CD4+, count, and plasma viral load, as prognostic indicators for AIDS and infectious disease death in HIV-infected injection drug users, 109
Cephalic
 version, external, terbutaline for, 365
Cephalohematoma
 neonatal, from vacuum extraction, 366
Cephalosporin
 allergy, diagnosis of, 129
Cereal
 breakfast, fortified with folic acid, reduction of plasma homocysteine levels in coronary heart disease patients with, 28
Cerebral
 hemorrhage and hypertension, 248
Cervicovaginal
 cytology, false positive, 325
Cervix
 cancer, 320
  screening among women with and without hysterectomies, 320
 endocervical brush use after endocervical curettage, 323
 lesions, squamous intraepithelial, cost-effectiveness analysis of diagnosis and management of, 321
 order of endocervical and ectocervical cytologic sampling and quality of Pap smear, 327
 smears, PAPNET-assisted rescreening of, 328
Cesarean section
 diabetes and, gestational, 373
 perinatal transmission of papillomavirus in infants and, 282
 rate, rising, in New Zealand, 369
 vaginal delivery after, admission scoring system to predict, 367
Chest
 pain, acute, in diabetics, rate and mode of death during 5-year follow-up, 82
Chickenpox (see Varicella)
Children
 acetaminophen doses in, multiple, hepatotoxicity after, 300
 adenoidal obstruction in, 301
 adenotonsillar hypertrophy in, chronic, amoxicillin/clavulanate for, 273
 adolescent (see Adolescent)
 allergy in, penicillin, amoxicillin, and cephalosporin, diagnosis of, 129
 asthma in, inhaled steroids in, and risk of hospitalization, 121
 back pain in, 177
 cancer in, risk of cancer in offspring of survivors of, 381
 cardiovascular risk from childhood to young adulthood in offspring of parents with coronary artery disease, longitudinal changes in, 8
 circumcision in, EMLA cream prior to dorsal penile nerve block for, 170
 dermatitis in, atopic, and food hypersensitivity reactions, 159
 febrile young, bacteremia risk in, in post-*Hemophilus influenzae* type b era, 272
 fibromyalgia syndrome in, 180
 fractures and Turner syndrome in, 88
 gastroenteritis in, early feeding in, 281
 health of, 265
 healthy, variation of bone age progression in, 297
 Helicobacter pylori and abdominal symptoms in, 275
 house dust mite reduction strategies in, efficacy of, 123
 hyperactivity in, educational and occupational outcome of grown-up boys after, 306
 immunization in, 266
 infant (see Infant)
 infectious diseases in, 272
 injury in, 288
  mortality of, predictors in early childhood, 288
  trampoline-related, in U.S., 290
 knee injuries in, correlation of arthroscopic and clinical findings with MRI findings in, 188

Munchausen syndrome by proxy in, procedures, placement, and risks of further abuse after, 220
newborn (see Newborn)
otitis media in, acute, with bronchiolitis, 274
poisoning in, nonaccidental, procedures, placement, and risks of further abuse after, 220
preschool, speech and language screening in, 296
psychosocial problems in, recognition of, and insurance status, 212
pubertal boys, marked breast development in, 303
renal function after short-term ibuprofen use in, 299
respiratory illnesses in, medical expenditures for, and maternal smoking, 233
rheumatic diseases in, antinuclear antibody testing to screen for, 395
school age, with uncertain history of chickenpox, varicella serology among, 267
suffocation after, nonaccidental, procedures, placement, and risks of further abuse after, 220
urinalysis in, screening dipstick, 110
Chinese herbal cream
potent topical steroid in, 157
Chips
olestra potato, gastrointestinal symptoms after consumption of, 140
Chiropractic
treatment of carpal tunnel syndrome, 185
Chlorthalidone
long-term effects on sexual function, in men and women, 6
Cholesterol
high-density lipoprotein, plus C-reactive protein in determining risk of first myocardial infarction, 52
levels, average, lovastatin for primary prevention of acute coronary events in men and women with, 49
-lowering effects of fat-restricted diets in hypercholesterolemia and combined hyperlipidemia, in men, 48
metabolism, effect of garlic oil preparation on, 243
total, plus C-reactive protein in determining risk of first myocardial infarction, 52

Chromium
supplementation, long-term effect on weight maintenance, 58
Ciclopirox
anti-inflammatory activity of, 153
Cigarette
smoking (see Smoking)
Ciprofloxacin
oral, efficacy and safety for chronic suppurative otitis media in adults, 114
Circumcision, 170
EMLA cream prior to dorsal penile nerve block for, 170
neonatal, comparison of ring block, dorsal penile nerve block, and topical anesthesia for, 171
Cirrhosis
biliary, primary, ursodeoxycholic acid delays onset of esophageal varices in, 144
Class of 1989
physician supply in Canada and, 413
Clavulanate
/amoxicillin for chronic adenotonsillar hypertrophy, in children, 273
Clinical
findings correlated with MRI findings in injured knees in children and adolescents, 188
issues, 377
Clobetasol
Chinese herbal cream containing, 157
vs. testosterone for severe vulvar lichen sclerosus, 156
Cod
allergy and atopic dermatitis, 159
Codeine
acetaminophen with, after misoprostol for early abortion, 338
Cold-
and hot-pack contrast therapy, 187
Colorectal
cancer and aspirin use, 379
Colposcopy
for cervical squamous intraepithelial lesions, cost-effectiveness of, 322
Coma
reduction after insulin lispro in insulin-dependent diabetics, 64
Community
-based ambulatory encounters involving medical students, 397
dimensions of primary care practice, 402
Compensation
of primary care physicians in medical groups, 408

Complementary
  medicine, 391
Compliance
  patient (see Patient, compliance)
Computed tomography
  of appendix, effect on treatment and
    use of hospital resources, 148
Computer
  program GIDEON for diagnosis of
    fever in hospitalized patients, 112
Condom
  availability program, high school,
    students' acquisition and use of
    condoms in, 305
  use by urban adolescents, effect of HIV
    counseling and testing on, 104
Condylomata
  acuminata
    imiquimod for, 99
    isotretinoin for, oral, 101
Conium
  maculatum D3 in homeopathic
    preparation for vertigo, 261
Connective tissue
  disease, mixed, antinuclear antibody
    testing to screen for, in children,
    396
Consent
  informed, and prostate-specific antigen
    screening in elderly men, 167
Constipation
  biofeedback for, 137
  results of, 138
Consumer
  reports in health care, effect on patient
    care, 417
Contraception
  emergency, 336
  self-administering, effects of, 336
Contrast
  therapy, cold- and hot-pack, 187
Coronary
  artery disease
    (See also Heart, disease, coronary)
    parents with, longitudinal changes in
      cardiovascular risk from childhood
      to young adulthood in offspring of,
      8
    patients, aerobic and myocardial
      demands of lawn mowing in, 228
    prevention, secondary, 24
    risk, 7
  events, acute, primary prevention with
    lovastatin in men and women with
    average cholesterol levels, 49
  heart disease (see Heart, disease,
    coronary)
Corticosteroids
  inhaled, in asthma
    risk of hospitalization and, 121
    salmeterol improves quality of life in
      patients requiring, 122
  prescribing by nondermatologists vs.
    dermatologists for cutaneous fungal
    infections, 158
Cost
  -analysis model of tacrine treatment of
    Alzheimer's disease, 196
  -effectiveness
    analysis of diagnosis and management
      of cervical squamous intraepithelial
      lesions, 321
    of mandatory vs. voluntary screening
      for HIV in pregnancy, 105
    of test-treatment strategies in
      suspected Lyme disease, 92
  of health services for enrollees in
    managed care organizations, effect
    of primary care physician
    compensation method in medical
    groups on, 408
  of nurse specialist anticoagulant service,
    41
Cough
  prolonged, and lung cancer, 382
Counseling
  HIV, effect on sexually transmitted
    diseases and condom use in urban
    adolescents, 104
  parents to reduce risk of sudden infant
    death syndrome, 284
Couple
  interventions for marital distress and
    adult mental health problems, 209
Cow's milk
  neonatal exposure to, brief, and
    development of atopy, 128
Cramps
  muscle, hydroquinine in, 184
Crash
  -related factors, effect on prognosis of
    whiplash, 189
C-reactive protein
  value in determining risk of first
    myocardial infarction, 52
Creatinine
  levels after short-term ibuprofen use in
    infants and children, 299
Creativity
  mental illness and, 218
Crohn's disease
  active, budesonide vs. mesalamine for,
    141

CT
   of appendix, effect on treatment and use of hospital resources, 148
Curettage
   elective, *vs.* expectant management for spontaneous abortion, 337
   endocervical, endocervical brush use after, 323
Cutaneous (*see* Skin)
Cyclobenzaprine
   in fibromyalgia syndrome in children and adolescents, 182
Cysts
   mammary oil, sonographic features of, 320
Cytochrome P-450 3A
   interactions with dermatologic therapies, 153
Cytologic
   sampling, endocervical and ectocervical, order of, and quality of Pap smear, 327
Cytology
   cervicovaginal, false positive, 325

D

Day care center
   child, postlicensure effectiveness of varicella vaccine during outbreak in, 266
Death
   (*See also* Mortality)
   cardiac, sudden, risk of, and fish consumption, 12
   in diabetics with acute chest pain during 5-year follow-up, 82
   infant, sudden (*see* Sudden infant death syndrome)
   infectious disease, in HIV-infected injection drug users, prognostic indicators for, 109
Decision
   analysis of mandatory *vs.* voluntary HIV testing in pregnancy, 107
   making, end of life, patient and physician roles in, 386
Delivery, 365
   of babies, why family physicians deliver, 374
   cesarean (*see* Cesarean section)
   mode and perinatal transmission of papillomavirus in infants, 282
   vaginal
      after cesarean delivery, admission scoring system to predict, 367
      vacuum extraction, neonatal cephalohematoma after, 366

Dementia, 194
   diagnosis in general practice, limits of Mini-Mental State Examination in, 194
   ginkgo biloba for, 197
Demographic
   factors, socio-, effect on prognosis of whiplash, 189
Depressive
   symptoms
      in affluent older population, 212
      in premenstrual dysphoric disorder, effect of sertraline on, 332
Dermatitis
   atopic, and food hypersensitivity reactions, 159
Dermatologic
   therapies, interactions with cytochrome P-450 3A, 153
Dermatologists
   prescribing for cutaneous fungal infections by, 158
Diabetes mellitus
   control, electronic case manager for, 83
   foot ulcers in, topical hyperbaric oxygen and low energy laser for, 84
   gestational, 361
      diagnosis of, self-perceived health status of women 3 to 5 years after, 364
      glucose tolerance test in diagnosis of, 3-hour oral, no effect of high carbohydrate preparatory diet on, 362
      postnatal diabetes after, 363
      postnatal diabetes after, prevalence and predictors of, 363
      pregnancy outcomes and, 373
      selective screening for, 361
   glycemic control in, and fish oil, 80
   insulin-dependent, 61
      insulin lispro in, and reduced frequency of severe hypoglycemia and coma, 64
      intensive therapy in, and effect of excessive weight gain on lipid levels and blood pressure, 65
      microalbuminuria in, association with dietary saturated fat intake and dietary protein intake, 62
      renal failure in, prevention with ACE inhibitors, 61
   non–insulin-dependent, 66
      albumin excretion rate in, long-term effects of simvastatin on, 75
      dietary-treated, acarbose *vs.* metformin in, 73

hypertension and, fosinopril *vs.*
  amlodipine for, 70
insulin therapy in, effectiveness,
  complications, and resource
  utilization, 71
metformin/troglitazone in, 68
newly diagnosed, comparison of
  sulfonylurea, insulin, and
  metformin therapy in, 66
renal function in, effect of enalapril
  on, 69
stroke in, serum uric acid as predictor
  of, 250
troglitazone and insulin in, 67
postnatal, after gestational diabetes, 363
  prevalence and predictors of, 363
Turner syndrome and, 88
type 1 *(see* insulin-dependent *above)*
type 2 *(see* non–insulin-dependent
  above)
unrecognized
  among hospitalized patients, 76
  prepregnancy, estimation of
    prevalence of, 363
Diarrhea
after sertraline in premenstrual
  dysphoric disorder, 332
Didanosine
-based treatment of HIV infection,
  improved survival after, 108
Diet
breast cancer risk and, 310
carbohydrate, high preparatory, no
  effect on 3-hour oral glucose
  tolerance test in pregnancy, 362
fat from *(see* Fat, dietary*)*
fat-restricted, long-term
  cholesterol-lowering effects in
  hypercholesterolemia and combined
  hyperlipidemia, in men, 48
folate from, and risk of coronary heart
  disease in women, 14
ketogenic, high-protein, low-fat, effects
  on morbidly obese adolescents, 59
protein in, association with
  microalbuminuria in
  insulin-dependent diabetics, 62
sodium from, and mortality, 11
soy supplementation in, effect on hot
  flushes, 340
-treated type 2 diabetes, acarbose *vs.*
  metformin in, 73
vitamin B_6 from, and risk of coronary
  heart disease in women, 14
Digital
rectal examination as part of routine
  pelvic exam, diagnostic utility of,
  347

Diphtheria
vaccine response in extremely premature
  infants, 269
Dipstick
urinalysis, screening, 110
Disasters
natural, suicide after, 215
Dislocation
trampoline-related, in children, 291
Distress
marital, 205
  interventions for, couple and family,
    209
Domestic
abuse, management guidelines when
  male and female partners are
  patients of same physician, 206
violence, 205
  screening men in primary care setting
    for, 208
Dong quai
estrogenic effects in postmenopausal
  women, 341
Dosage
frequency and patient compliance, 389
Doxazosin
long-term effects on sexual function, in
  men and women, 6
Drinking
problem, screening for, 198
Drug(s)
antifungal
  anti-inflammatory activity of, 152
  prescribing by nondermatologists *vs.*
    dermatologists, 158
antihypertensive
  effects on sexual function, long-term,
    in men and women, 6
  intracerebral hemorrhage and, 249
anti-inflammatory, nonsteroidal *(see*
  Anti-inflammatory, drugs,
  nonsteroidal)
company gifts, physicians' *vs.* patients'
  attitudes toward, 383
dosage frequency and patient
  compliance, 389
psychoactive, use in nursing homes,
  effects of restraint reduction
  intervention and OBRA '87
  regulations on, 217
reactions, adverse, incidence in
  hospitalized patients, 394
use, 198
users, injection, HIV-infected,
  prognostic indicators for AIDS and
  infectious disease death in, 109

Dust
  mite, house, reduction strategies, long-term efficacy of, 123
Dyspepsia
  after sildenafil for erectile dysfunction, 174
Dysphoric
  disorder, premenstrual, sertraline in, 331
Dystocia
  shoulder, and gestational diabetes, 373

E

Ear
  conditions, 259
Earthquakes
  suicide rates after, 216
Eating
  habits and weight change in men, 56
Econazole
  anti-inflammatory activity of, 153
Economics, 401
Ectocervical
  and endocervical cytologic sampling, order of, and quality of Pap smear, 327
Ectopic
  pregnancy, repeat, epidemiology of, 349
Education
  for physicians, impact on patient outcomes, 414
Educational
  level and tension-type headache, 254
  outcome of hyperactive boys grown up, 306
  vs. behavioral interventions for fibromyalgia, 179
Efficacy
  trials, randomized, effect of statistical significance of results on time to completion and publication of, 396
EGb 761
  for dementia, 197
Egg
  allergy and atopic dermatitis, 159
El Niño
  cycles of malaria associated with, in Venezuela, 118
Elderly
  affluent, depressive symptoms among, 212
  alcohol consumption and mortality among, in U.S., 200
  Alzheimer's disease in (see Alzheimer's disease)
  community-dwelling, physical fitness and functional limitations in, 224
  constipation in, biofeedback for, 138
    results of, 139
  dementia in, limitations of Mini-Mental State Examination in diagnosis in general practice, 194
  frail, reliability and validity of peer review of quality of care for, 418
  garlic intake in, chronic, effect on aortic elasticity, 244
  incontinence in, fecal, biofeedback for, 138
  prostate-specific antigen screening in, and preferences and informed consent, 167
  in public housing, physical activity and health promotion for, 226
  retired men, nonsmoking, effects of walking on mortality among, 229
  urine sampling method for bacteriological examination in, in women, 111
Electrical
  stimulation, pelvic floor, for stress incontinence, 172
Electrocautery
  ovarian, in polycystic ovary syndrome, late endocrine effects of, 329
Electronic
  case manager for diabetes control, 83
Embolism
  pulmonary, 37
    prevention in patients with proximal deep vein thrombosis, vena caval filters for, 38
    syncope as emergency department presentation of, 39
Emergency
  department presentation of pulmonary embolism, syncope as, 39
EMLA cream
  prior to dorsal penile nerve block for circumcision in children, 170
  vs. ring block and dorsal penile nerve block for neonatal circumcision, 171
Emotional
  abuse, effects on health indicators, in women, 205
  difficulties, non-directive psychotherapy vs. routine general practitioner care for, 216
Empowerment
  patient, no effect on pain in seriously ill hospitalized adults, 393
Enalapril
  effect on renal function in type 2 diabetics, 69

long-term effects on sexual function, in men and women, 6
End of life
  decision making, patient and physician roles in, 386
  issues, 383
Endarterectomy
  carotid
    effect of Asymptomatic Carotid Atherosclerosis Study on, 35
    indications, outcomes, and provider volumes for, 34
Endocervical
  brush use after endocervical curettage, 323
  and ectocervical cytologic sampling, order of, and quality of Pap smear, 327
Endocrine
  abnormality causing marked breast development in boys at puberty, 305
  effects
    late, of ovarian electrocautery in polycystic ovary syndrome, 329
    of metformin in polycystic ovary syndrome, 330
Endocrinology, 45
Endometrial
  hyperplasia in postmenopausal women on hormone replacement therapy, bleeding as predictor of, 344
Endometriosis
  leuprolide depot and hormonal add-back in, 350
  nafarelin in, 351
Endothelium
  -dependent brachial artery vasoactivity, transient impairment after single high-fat meal, effect of antioxidant vitamins on, 241
Energy
  expenditure
    evolutionary perspective, 225
    resting, in African American *vs.* Caucasian overweight females, 57
Enteral
  vs. parenteral nutrition in severe acute pancreatitis, 143
Environmental
  tobacco smoke exposure and ischemic heart disease, 232
Enzyme
  inhibitors, angiotensin-converting
    cancer risk with, 26
    for prevention of renal failure in insulin-dependent diabetics, 61

Equity
  in allocating resources to primary care, 407
Erectile
  dysfunction
    effects of antihypertensive drugs on, long-term, 6
    sildenafil for, 173
Esophagogastroduodenoscopy
  performed by family physician, 131
Esophagus
  Barrett's, screening for, 10 years' experience with, 135
  gastroesophageal reflux disease, omeprazole in diagnosis of, 136
  varices in primary biliary cirrhosis, ursodeoxycholic acid delays onset of, 144
Estradiol
  plus leuprolide in premenstrual syndrome, behavioral effects of, 335
Estrogen
  conjugated equine, and norethindrone with leuprolide in endometriosis, 351
  replacement therapy, postmenopausal (*See also* Hormone, replacement therapy, postmenopausal)
    vasodilator effects of, no effect of androgen on, 341
  therapy in premenstrual syndrome, behavioral effects of, 334
Estrogenic
  effects of dong quai in postmenopausal women, 341
Ethical
  considerations in provision of controversial screening tests, 384
Ethics, 383
Euthanasia
  physician-assisted, in U.S., 387
Evolutionary
  perspective on physical activity, energy expenditure and fitness, 225
Examination
  digital rectal, diagnostic utility as part of routine pelvic exam, 347
  preparticipation, 292
    Mayo Clinic experience with, 293
Exercise
  (*See also* Physical, activity)
  advice, written, provided by general practitioners, 227
  breast cancer risk and, 310
  pelvic muscle, effect on transient incontinence during pregnancy and after birth, 370

training
  blood pressure and, 2
  effect on aerobic fitness, immune indices, and quality of life in HIV-positive patients, 103
  vigorous, and weight change in men, 56
Expectant management
  vs. elective curettage for spontaneous abortion, 337
Expenditures
  health care, related to primary care vs. specialty physicians as personal physicians, 406
  medical, for childhood respiratory illnesses, and maternal smoking, 233
Expense
  of unlimited mental health care coverage under managed care, 210
Extraction
  vacuum, neonatal cephalohematoma after, 366
Extremity
  lower
    cramps, hydroquinine in, 184
    trampoline-related injuries of, in older children, 290
  upper
    trampoline-related injuries of, in young children, 290–291
    Upper Extremity Function Scale, development and validation of, 182
    work-related disorders, measuring functional outcomes in, 182
Eye
  conditions, 259

F

Family
  interventions for marital distress and adult mental health problems, 209
  physician (*see* Physician, family)
  practice, physician practice styles and patient outcomes in, vs. general internal medicine, 405
Fat
  body, dietary fat as major determinant of, 54
  dietary
    coronary heart disease risk in women and, 46
    as major determinant of body fat, 54
    obesity and, epidemiologic study, 54
  high-fat meal, single, effect of antioxidant vitamins on transient impairment of endothelium-dependent brachial artery vasoactivity after, 241
  low-fat, high-protein ketogenic diet, effects on morbidly obese adolescents, 59
  -restricted diets, long-term cholesterol-lowering effects in hypercholesterolemia and combined hyperlipidemia, in men, 48
  saturated, dietary intake associated with microalbuminuria in insulin-dependent diabetics, 62
Fatigue
  general, in fibromyalgia syndrome in children and adolescents, 180
Fear
  of violence in workplace, psychosocial correlates of, 214
Febrile
  children, young, bacteremia risk in, in post-*Hemophilus influenzae* type b era, 272
Fecal
  incontinence, biofeedback for, 137
Feedback
  no effect on pain in seriously ill hospitalized adults, 393
Feeding
  early, in childhood gastroenteritis, 281
Fee-for-service
  practice, physician satisfaction with, 411
  setting, breast cancer treatment and survival in, 318
Felbinac
  topical, effectiveness of, 186
FEV_1
  reduced, and asbestos exposure in young men, and effectiveness of postal smoking cessation advice, 238
Fever
  diagnosis in hospitalized patients, computer program GIDEON for, 112
Fiber
  supplementation, long-term effect on weight maintenance, 58
Fibrillation
  atrial
    aspirin use in, and stroke prevention, 249
    likelihood of spontaneous conversion to sinus rhythm, 25

Fibrolamellar
  hepatocarcinoma and marked breast development in boys at puberty, 305
Fibromyalgia, 175, 179
  interventions for, behavioral vs. educational, 179
  syndrome in children and adolescents, 180
Filters
  vena caval, in prevention of pulmonary embolism in patients with proximal deep vein thrombosis, 38
Financial
  incentives to enhance patient compliance, 388
Finasteride
  in prostatic hyperplasia, benign, 163
Fish
  consumption and risk of sudden cardiac death, 12
  oil and glycemic control in diabetes, 80
Fitness, 224
  aerobic, of HIV-positive patients, effect of exercise training on, 103
  evolutionary perspective, 225
  physical, and functional limitations in older adults, 224
Floods
  suicide rates after, 215
Fluorescence
  spectroscopy of cervical squamous intraepithelial lesions, cost-effectiveness of, 322
Flushing
  after sildenafil for erectile dysfunction, 174
Folate
  intake and risk of coronary heart disease in women, 14
Folic acid
  breakfast cereal fortified with, reduction of plasma homocysteine levels in coronary heart disease patients with, 28
Food
  allergy, multiple, in breastfed infants, 127
  hypersensitivity reactions and atopic dermatitis, 159
  intolerance to dietary soy supplementation for hot flushes, 340
Foot
  ulcers, diabetic, topical hyperbaric oxygen and low energy laser for, 84

Fosinopril
  vs. amlodipine in hypertensive type 2 diabetics, 70
Fracture
  trampoline-related, in children, 291
  Turner syndrome and, 88
Functional
  limitations and physical fitness in older adults, 224
  outcomes
    effects of residence in Alzheimer disease special care units on, 195
    in work-related upper extremity disorders, measuring, 182
Fungal
  skin infections, nondermatologists are more likely than dermatologists to prescribe antifungal/corticosteroid products for, 158

G

Gallstone
  disease, symptomatic, risk for, relation to physical activity, in men, 142
Garlic, 243
  intake, chronic, effect on aortic elasticity, in elderly, 244
  oil preparation, effect on serum lipoproteins and cholesterol metabolism, 243
Gastroenteritis
  childhood, early feeding in, 281
Gastroenterology, 131
Gastroesophageal
  reflux disease, omeprazole in diagnosis of, 136
Gastrointestinal
  complaints after acarbose in dietary-treated type 2 diabetics, 74
  problems
    lower, 137
    upper, 131
  side effects of dietary soy supplementation for hot flushes, 340
  symptoms after consumption of olestra potato chips, 140
Gatekeeping
  physicians' attitudes toward, 409
Gene
  BRCA1, mutations, and breast cancer, 313
General practice
  diagnosing dementia in, limitations of Mini-Mental State Examination in, 194

General practitioners
  care, routine, *vs.* non-directive psychotherapy, 216
  written exercise advice provided by, 227
Generalist
  role of specialty physicians, 403
Genital
  herpes virus type 2, in U.S., 97
  warts
    imiquimod for, 99
    isotretinoin for, oral, 101
Gestational
  diabetes mellitus (*see* Diabetes mellitus, gestational)
GIDEON
  computer program for diagnosis of fever in hospitalized patients, 112
Gifts
  pharmaceutical industry, physicians' *vs.* patients' attitudes toward, 383
Ginkgo
  biloba for dementia, 197
Glaucoma
  quality of life and, 259
Globulin
  sex hormone-binding, increase after ovarian electrocautery for polycystic ovary syndrome, 329
Glucose
  blood, high, as risk factor for mortality in nondiabetic middle-aged men, 78
  tolerance test, 3-hour oral, in pregnancy, no effect of high carbohydrate preparatory diet on, 362
Glycemic
  control in diabetes, and fish oil, 80
Gonadal
  steroids in premenstrual syndrome, behavioral effects of, 334
Gonadotropin(s)
  decrease after ovarian electrocautery for polycystic ovary syndrome, 329
  -releasing hormone agonist leuprolide
    behavioral effects in premenstrual syndrome, 335
    depot, and hormonal add-back in endometriosis, 350
Gonorrhea
  single-dose therapy of, trovafloxacin *vs.* ofloxacin for, 96
Gowning
  effects on patient satisfaction, 398
Graduates
  medical school, in 1989, and physician supply in Canada, 413

Graves' ophthalmopathy
  course of, relation to therapy for hyperthyroidism, 85
Guidelines
  for managing domestic abuse when male and female partners are patients of same physician, 206
Gynecologic
  care, associated with unexpected vaginal bleeding with cyclic *vs.* continuous postmenopausal hormone replacement therapy, 346
Gynecomastia
  in adolescent boys, 303

H

Happiness
  can money buy? 212
Harassment
  in workplace, psychosocial correlates of, 214
Headache, 254
  in fibromyalgia syndrome in children and adolescents, 180
  migraine
    acetaminophen, aspirin, and caffeine in, 257
    homeopathic prophylaxis of, 255
  after sildenafil for erectile dysfunction, 174
  tension-type, epidemiology of, 254
Health
  care
    consumer reports in, effect on patient care, 417
    expenditures related to primary care *vs.* specialists as personal physicians, 406
    insurance or regular physician as most powerful predictor of, 412
  children's, 265
  indicators, effects of emotional abuse on, in women, 205
  maintenance organization
    breast cancer treatment and survival in, 318
    practice, physician satisfaction with, 411
  mental (*see* Mental, health)
  plans, physicians' views of, 410
  policy, 401
  promotion for older adults in public housing, 226

services for enrollees in managed care organizations, effect of primary care physician compensation method in medical groups on use and cost of, 408
status, self-perceived, of women 3 to 5 years after gestational diabetes, 364
system issues, 409
women's, 309
Heart
catheterization, on-site, long-term outcome in myocardial infarction patients admitted to facilities with and without, 20
death, sudden, risk of, and fish consumption, 12
disease, coronary
(See also Coronary, artery disease)
homocysteine levels in patients with, plasma, reduction by breakfast cereal fortified with folic acid, 28
prediction using risk factor categories, 7
risk, and dietary fat intake in women, 46
risk, and folate and vitamin B_6 intake in women, 14
risk, and hyperinsulinemia, 15
risk factors for, and *Helicobacter pylori* infection, 17
disease, ischemic
mortality of, and *Helicobacter pylori* infection, 16
nitrate tolerance in, effect of vitamin E supplementation on, 242
risk factors for, fasting insulin and apolipoprotein B levels and low-density lipoprotein particle size as, 51
tobacco smoke exposure and, environmental, 232
Turner syndrome and, 88
Helicobacter pylori
abdominal symptoms and, in children, 275
infection and mortality from ischemic heart disease, 16
infection and risk factors for coronary heart disease, 17
seropositivity and hyperemesis gravidarum, 357
Heme
component in iron supplementation in pregnancy, 354
Hemophilus influenzae
type b vaccine use, risk of bacteremia for febrile young children in era after, 272
vaccine response in extremely premature infants, 269
Hemorrhage
intracerebral, and hypertension, 248
Heparin
low-molecular-weight, in prevention of pulmonary embolism in patients with proximal deep vein thrombosis, 38
subcutaneous, for deep venous thrombosis, algorithm for administration of, 40
Hepatitis
B
vaccination, immune responses of prematurely born infants to, 270
vaccine response in extremely premature infants, 269
Hepatocarcinoma
fibrolamellar, and marked breast development in boys at puberty, 305
Hepatotoxicity
of acetaminophen after multiple doses, in children, 300
Herbal
cream, Chinese, potent topical steroid in, 157
Herpes
simplex virus type 2, in U.S., 97
High school
athletes, preparticipation cardiovascular screening for, 292
condom availability program, students' acquisition and use of condoms in, 305
HIV
(See also AIDS)
counseling and testing, effect on sexually transmitted diseases and condom use in urban adolescents, 104
infection, 102
advanced, declining morbidity and mortality among patients with, 102
antiretroviral therapy in, improved survival after initiation of, 108
in injection drug users, prognostic indicators for, 109
-positive patients, effect of exercise training on aerobic fitness, immune indices, and quality of life in, 103
screening in pregnancy, voluntary *vs.* mandatory
cost-effectiveness of, 105

decision analysis of, 107
HMG
  CoA reductase inhibitors, effect on stroke, 252
HMO
  breast cancer treatment and survival in, 318
  practice, physician satisfaction with, 411
Home(s)
  nursing, psychoactive drug use in, effects of restraint reduction intervention and OBRA '87 regulations on, 217
Homeopathic
  prophylaxis of migraine, 255
  treatment of vertigo, 261
Homocysteine
  levels, plasma, in coronary heart disease patients, reduction by breakfast cereal fortified with folic acid, 28
Hormone
  add-back and leuprolide depot in endometriosis, 350
  gonadotropin-releasing hormone agonist leuprolide
    behavioral effects in premenstrual syndrome, 335
    depot, and hormonal add-back in endometriosis, 350
  replacement therapy, postmenopausal, 341
    bleeding as predictor of endometrial hyperplasia after, 344
    cyclic vs. continuous, unexpected vaginal bleeding and associated gynecologic care with, 346
    patient-specific decisions about, 343
    sex hormone-binding globulin increase after ovarian electrocautery for polycystic ovary syndrome, 329
Hospital
  with cardiac catheterization facilities, long-term outcome in myocardial infarction patients admitted to, 20
  resource use, effect of CT of appendix on, 148
  volume and 5-year survival from breast cancer, 316
Hospitalization
  for asthma, risk of, and inhaled steroids, 121
Hospitalized
  adults, seriously ill, pain in, no effect of patient empowerment and feedback on, 393
  infants, albuterol for bronchiolitis in, 277

patients
  adverse drug reactions in, incidence of, 394
  diabetes among, unrecognized, 76
  fever diagnosis in, computer program GIDEON for, 112
  pneumonia in, community-acquired, time to clinical stability in, 116
Hot
  and cold-pack contrast therapy, 187
flashes
  in breast cancer survivors, vitamin E for, 315
  soy supplementation and, dietary, 340
House
  dust mite reduction strategies, long-term efficacy of, 123
Housing
  public, physical activity and health promotion for, 226
Human immunodeficiency virus (see AIDS)
Hurricanes
  suicide rates after, 215
Hydrocortisone
  anti-inflammatory activity of, 153
Hydroquinine
  in muscle cramps, 184
3-Hydroxy-3-methylglutaryl
  coenzyme A inhibitors, effect on stroke, 252
Hygienic
  treatment, nutritional, in hypertensive men and women, long-term effects on sexual function, 6
Hyperactivity
  educational and occupational outcome in grown-up boys after, 306
Hyperbaric
  oxygen, topical, for diabetic foot ulcers, 84
Hypercholesterolemia
  cholesterol-lowering effects of fat-restricted diet in, long-term, in men, 48
Hyperemesis
  gravidarum and *Helicobacter pylori* seropositivity, 357
Hyperhidrosis
  palmar, botulinum toxin for, 155
Hyperinsulinemia
  coronary heart disease risk and, 15
Hyperlipidemia
  combined, long-term
    cholesterol-lowering effects of fat-restricted diet in, in men, 48

Hyperplasia
  endometrial, in postmenopausal women on hormone replacement therapy, bleeding as predictor of, 344
  prostate, benign, finasteride in, 163
Hypersensitivity
  reactions, food, and atopic dermatitis, 159
Hypertension, 2
  airway resistance during sleep and, abnormal upper, 4
  diabetes and, type 2, fosinopril vs. amlodipine for, 70
  drug treatment of, long-term effects on sexual function, in men and women, 6
  intracerebral hemorrhage and, 248
  nutritional hygienic treatment of, long-term effects on sexual function, in men and women, 6
  Turner syndrome and, 88
Hyperthyroidism
  therapy related to course of Graves' ophthalmopathy, 85
Hypertrophic
  cardiomyopathy, screening young athletes for, 294
Hypertrophy
  adenotonsillar, chronic, amoxicillin/clavulanate for, in children, 273
Hypoglycemia
  severe, after insulin lispro in insulin-dependent diabetics, 64
Hysterectomy
  cervical cancer screening among women with and without, 320

I

Ibuprofen
  for carpal tunnel syndrome, 185
  after misoprostol for early abortion, 338
  topical, effectiveness of, 186
  use, short-term, renal function after, in infants and children, 299
Ileal
  -release budesonide vs. mesalamine for active Crohn's disease, 141
Illness
  serious, hospitalized adults with, no effect of patient empowerment and feedback on pain in, 393

Imaging
  magnetic resonance imaging findings correlated with arthroscopic and clinical findings in injured knees in children and adolescents, 188
Imiquimod
  for genital warts, 99
Immune
  indices in HIV-positive patients, effect of exercise training on, 103
  -response modifier for genital warts, 99
  responses of prematurely born infants to hepatitis B vaccination, 270
  system, effects of lovastatin on, 27
Immunization
  in children, 266
Immunodeficiency
  syndrome, acquired (see AIDS)
  virus, human (see AIDS)
Immunofluorescence
  antinuclear antibody test, indirect, to screen for rheumatic diseases, in children, 395
Incontinence
  fecal, biofeedback for, 137
  urinary
    stress, pelvic floor electrical stimulation for, 172
    transient, during pregnancy and after birth, effect of pelvic muscle exercise on, 370
Indomethacin
  topical, effectiveness of, 186
Infant
  allergy in, penicillin, amoxicillin, and cephalosporin, diagnosis of, 129
  breast-fed, multiple food allergy in, 127
  death, sudden (see Sudden infant death syndrome)
  hospitalized, albuterol for bronchiolitis in, 277
  papillomavirus transmission in, perinatal, 282
  premature
    extremely, vaccine response in, 269
    hepatitis B vaccination in, immune responses to, 270
    renal function after short-term ibuprofen use in, 299
Infarction
  myocardial (see Myocardial, infarction)
  ventricular, right, effect of reperfusion on biventricular function and survival after, 23
Infection
  newborn, early-onset, neutrophil CD11b expression as diagnostic marker for, 279

Infectious
　disease, 91
　　in children, 272
　　death in HIV-infected injection drug
　　　users, prognostic indicators for, 109
Influenza
　vaccine, inactivated, effect on
　　pulmonary function in asthma, 124
Informed consent
　prostate-specific antigen screening in
　　elderly men and, 167
Injection
　drug users, HIV-infected, prognostic
　　indicators for AIDS and infectious
　　disease death in, 109
Injuries
　in children, 288
　　trampoline-related, in U.S., 290
　　young, predictors of mortality of, 288
　knee, correlation of arthroscopic and
　　clinical examinations with MRI
　　findings of, in children and
　　adolescents, 188
Insulin
　-dependent diabetes mellitus (see
　　Diabetes mellitus,
　　insulin-dependent)
　levels, fasting, as risk factor for
　　ischemic heart disease, 51
　lispro in insulin-dependent diabetes, and
　　reduced frequency of severe
　　hypoglycemia and coma, 64
　sensitivity and intensity and amount of
　　physical activity, 77
　therapy
　　effectiveness, complications, and
　　　resource utilization, in type 2
　　　diabetes, 71
　　intensive, in type 1 diabetes, and
　　　effect of excessive weight gain on
　　　lipid levels and blood pressure, 65
　　with troglitazone in type 2 diabetes,
　　　67
　　vs. sulfonylurea and metformin in
　　　newly diagnosed type 2 diabetes,
　　　66
Insurance
　mental health, 210
　　unlimited, expense under managed
　　　care, 210
　status and recognition of psychosocial
　　problems, in children, 212
　vs. regular physician as most powerful
　　predictor of health care, 412
Internal medicine
　general, physician practice styles and
　　patient outcomes in, vs. family
　　practice, 405

Intracerebral
　hemorrhage and hypertension, 248
Intraepithelial
　cervical lesions, squamous,
　　cost-effectiveness analysis of
　　diagnosis and management of, 321
Intramuscular
　temperature, effect of cold- and hot-
　　pack contrast therapy on, 187
Iron
　supplementation in pregnancy, 354
Ischemia
　heart disease due to (see Heart, disease,
　　ischemic)
　myocardial, after nitroglycerin patch
　　removal, effects of intermittent
　　transdermal nitroglycerin on, 30
Isotretinoin
　oral, for condylomata acuminata, 101

K

Ketoconazole
　anti-inflammatory activity of, 153
Ketogenic
　diet, high-protein, low-fat, effects on
　　morbidly obese adolescents, 59
Ketoprofen
　topical, effectiveness of, 186
Kevorkian endocervical curette
　endocervical brush use after, 323
Kidney
　cancer risk and calcium channel
　　blockers, 26
　failure in insulin-dependent diabetics,
　　prevention with ACE inhibitors, 61
　function
　　in diabetics, type 2, effect of enalapril
　　　on, 69
　　after ibuprofen use, short-term, in
　　　infants and children, 299
Klinefelter's syndrome
　breast development in boys at puberty
　　and, marked, 305
Knee
　injuries, correlation of arthroscopic and
　　clinical examinations with MRI
　　findings of, in children and
　　adolescents, 188

L

Labor, 365
　preterm, variations between family
　　physicians and obstetricians in
　　evaluation and treatment of, 360

Laboratories
  physicians' office and other, quality comparison of, 416
Lamivudine
  regimen in HIV infection, improved survival after, 108
Language
  screening, preschool, 296
Laparoscopy
  ovarian electrocautery via, for polycystic ovary syndrome, late endocrine effects of, 329
Laser
  low energy, for diabetic foot ulcers, 84
Lawn
  mowing, aerobic and myocardial demands of, in coronary artery disease patients, 228
Leg
  cramps, hydroquinine in, 184
Leuprolide
  depot, and hormonal add-back in endometriosis, 350
  in premenstrual syndrome, behavioral effects of, 335
Libido
  decreased, after sertraline in premenstrual dysphoric disorder, 332
Lichen
  sclerosus, severe vulvar, clobetasol *vs.* testosterone for, 156
Life
  end of life
    decision making, patient and physician roles in, 386
    issues, 383
  quality of (*see* Quality, of life)
Light
  ultraviolet, causing premature skin aging, pathophysiology of, 151
Limb (*see* Extremity)
Lipid(s), 46
  levels in insulin-dependent diabetics on intensive therapy, effect of excessive weight gain on, 65
Lipoprotein
  A, recombinant *Borrelia burgdorferi* outer-surface, with adjuvant, vaccination against Lyme disease with, 95
  cholesterol, high-density, plus C-reactive protein, in prediction of first myocardial infarction, 52
  low-density, particle size, as risk factor for ischemic heart disease, 51
  serum, effect of garlic oil preparation on, 243

Lispro
  insulin, in insulin-dependent diabetes, and reduced frequency of severe hypoglycemia and coma, 64
Liver
  disease, end-stage, prognostic model for, 145
Lovastatin
  effects on immune system, 27
  for primary prevention of acute coronary events in men and women with average cholesterol levels, 49
Lung
  (*See also* Pulmonary)
  cancer and prolonged cough, 382
  function in asthma, effect of inactivated influenza vaccine on, 124
Lupus
  erythematosus, systemic, antinuclear antibody testing to screen for, in children, 396
Lyme disease, 92
  prevention with vaccine of recombinant *Borrelia burgdorferi* outer-surface protein A, 94
  suspected, test-treatment strategies for, 92
  tick bites and, in endemic setting, 93
  vaccination with recombinant *Borrelia burgdorferi* outer-surface lipoprotein A with adjuvant against, 95

M

Macrosomia
  gestational diabetes and, 373
Magnesium
  sulfate in preterm labor, variations between family physicians and obstetricians in use of, 360
Magnetic resonance imaging
  findings correlated with arthroscopic and clinical findings in injured knees in children and adolescents, 188
Malaria
  cycles associated with El Niño in Venezuela, 118
Mammary (*see* Breast)
Managed care
  expense of unlimited mental health care coverage under, 210
  organizations, use and cost of health services for enrollees in, effect of primary care physician compensation method in medical groups on, 408

Management
  case management programs in primary care, 404
Manager
  case, electronic, for diabetes control, 83
Marital
  distress, 205
    interventions for, couple and family, 209
Mastectomy
  Nancy Reagan's, effect on choice of surgery for breast cancer, 317
Maternal
  smoking and medical expenditures for childhood respiratory illnesses, 233
Mattress
  encasement for reduction of house dust mites, long-term efficacy of, 123
Maxillary
  sinuses of symptomless young men, radiology of, 260
Mayo Clinic
  experience with preparticipation examinations, 293
Meal
  high-fat, single, effect of antioxidant vitamins on transient impairment of endothelium-dependent brachial artery vasoactivity after, 241
Medical
  care, sabotaging one's own, 221
  expenditures for childhood respiratory illnesses and maternal smoking, 233
  groups, primary care physician compensation method in, 408
  risk factors, midwifery care, and birth outcomes, in U.S., 375
  school graduates in 1989 and physician supply in Canada, 413
  students, community-based ambulatory encounters involving, 397
  wards, general, vs. stroke units, survival in, 253
Medicine
  alternative, 391
    why patients use, 391
  complementary, 391
  internal, general, physician practice styles and patient outcomes in, vs. family practice, 405
  preventive, 223
Menopause, 339
Menstrual
  pattern after metformin therapy in polycystic ovary syndrome, 330
  symptoms in premenstrual syndrome, effect of calcium carbonate on, 332

Mental
  health, 193
    care coverage, unlimited, expense under managed care, 210
    insurance, 210
    problems, adult, couple and family interventions for, 209
    services, 210
  illness and creativity, 218
Mesalamine
  vs. budesonide for active Crohn's disease, 141
Metabolic
  effects of metformin in polycystic ovary syndrome, 330
Metabolism, 45
  cholesterol, effect of garlic oil preparation on, 243
Metformin
  in polycystic ovary syndrome, 330
  /troglitazone in type 2 diabetes, 68
  vs. acarbose in dietary-treated type 2 diabetics, 73
  vs. insulin therapy and sulfonylurea in newly diagnosed type 2 diabetes, 66
Methimazole
  in hyperthyroidism, effects on course of Graves' ophthalmopathy, 85
Mexican
  descent, women of, risk of neural tube defect-affected pregnancies in, 355
Microalbuminuria
  in diabetics
    type 1, association with dietary saturated fat intake and dietary protein intake, 62
    type 2, long-term effects of simvastatin on albumin excretion rate in, 75
Midwifery
  birth outcomes and, in U.S., 375
Migraine
  acetaminophen, aspirin, and caffeine in, 257
  homeopathic prophylaxis of, 255
Milk
  allergy and atopic dermatitis, 159
  cow's, brief neonatal exposure to, and development of atopy, 128
Mini-Mental State Examination
  limits in diagnosing dementia in general practice, 194
Miscarriage
  treatment, 359

Misoprostol
  action in early abortion, effect of nonsteroidal anti-inflammatory drugs on, 338
  vs. omeprazole for NSAID-related ulcers, 132
Mite
  house dust, reduction strategies, long-term efficacy of, 123
Mixed connective tissue disease
  antinuclear antibody testing to screen for, in children, 396
MMSE
  limitations in diagnosing dementia in general practice, 194
Model
  cost-analysis, of tacrine treatment of Alzheimer's disease, 196
  prognostic, for end-stage liver disease, 145
Money
  can it buy happiness? 212
Monitoring
  blood pressure, ambulatory, in pregnancy, 357
Morality
  of bedside rationing, 385
Morbidity
  of HIV infection, advanced, declining, 102
  in Turner syndrome, 87
Morning
  stiffness in fibromyalgia syndrome in children and adolescents, 180, 182
Mortality
  (See also Death)
  alcohol consumption and
    among middle-aged, in U.S. and Russia, 202
    among middle-aged and elderly, in U.S., 200
  cancer, 20-year report card of, in U.S., 378
  cardiovascular, long-term, pulse pressure as predictor of, 10
  heart disease, ischemic, and *Helicobacter pylori* infection, 16
  of HIV infection, advanced, declining, 102
  infant, and midwifery care, in U.S., 375
  injury, in early childhood, predictors of, 288
  prostate carcinoma, effects of screening and early detection on, 168
  related to primary care *vs.* specialty physicians as personal physicians, 406
  of retired men, nonsmoking, effects of walking on, 229
  risk factor, high blood glucose as, in nondiabetic middle-aged men, 78
  sodium intake and, dietary, 11
Mowing
  lawn, aerobic and myocardial demands of, in coronary artery disease patients, 228
MRI
  findings correlated with arthroscopic and clinical findings in injured knees in children and adolescents, 188
Munchausen syndrome
  by proxy, procedures, placement, and risks of further abuse after, 220
Muscle
  cramps, hydroquinine in, 184
  exercise, pelvic, effect on transient incontinence during pregnancy and after birth, 370
  intramuscular temperature, effect of cold- and hot-pack contrast therapy on, 187
Musculoskeletal
  conditions, 175
Myocardial
  demands of lawn mowing in coronary artery disease patients, 228
  infarction, 19
    first, risk, C-reactive protein adds to predictive value of total and HDL cholesterol in determining, 52
    non-Q-wave, outcome after invasive *vs.* conservative management, 19
    outcome, long-term, in patients admitted to hospitals with and without on-site cardiac catheterization facilities, 20
    pravastatin effects on cardiovascular events in women after, 24
  ischemia after nitroglycerin patch removal, effects of intermittent transdermal nitroglycerin on, 30

N

Nafarelin
  in endometriosis, 351
Naftifine
  anti-inflammatory activity of, 153
Naltrexone
  in alcohol dependence management, 204
Nancy Reagan's mastectomy
  effect on choice of surgery for breast cancer, 317

Nasal
  strips, sports, and airflow, 263
Nausea
  after sertraline in premenstrual dysphoric disorder, 332
Neoplasia
  skin, sunscreens in prevention of, 149
Nerve
  block, dorsal penile
    EMLA cream prior to, for circumcision, in children, 170
    vs. ring block and topical anesthesia for neonatal circumcision, 171
Neural
  tube defect, risk in pregnancies in women of Mexican descent, 355
Neuroleptics
  use in nursing homes, effects of restraint intervention and OBRA '87 regulations on, 217
Neurologic
  conditions, 247
  disorders and marked breast development in boys at puberty, 305
Neutrophil
  CD11b expression as diagnostic marker for early-onset neonatal infection, 279
Newborn
  cephalohematoma from vacuum extraction, 366
  circumcision, comparison of ring block, dorsal penile nerve block, and topical anesthesia for, 171
  exposure to cow's milk, brief, and development of atopy, 128
  infection, early-onset, neutrophil CD11b expression as diagnostic marker for, 279
Nicotine
  transdermal, and telephone support in smoking cessation, 234
Nifedipine
  in preterm labor, variations between family physicians and obstetricians in use of, 360
Nitrate
  tolerance and supplemental vitamin E, 242
Nitrogen
  levels, blood urea, after short-term ibuprofen use in infants and children, 299
Nitroglycerin
  intermittent transdermal, effects on occurrence of ischemia after patch removal, 30

Nocturnal
  leg cramps, hydroquinine in, 184
Nondermatologists
  prescribing for cutaneous fungal infections by, 158
Norethindrone
  /leuprolide in endometriosis, 351
Nortriptyline
  for back pain, chronic low, 176
  in fibromyalgia syndrome in children and adolescents, 182
Nose
  conditions, 259
NSAIDs (see Anti-inflammatory, drugs, nonsteroidal)
Nurse
  specialist anticoagulant service, cost and effectiveness of, 41
Nursing
  homes, psychoactive drug use in, effects of restraint reduction intervention and OBRA '87 regulations on, 217
Nutrition
  breast cancer risk and, 310
  enteral vs. parenteral, in severe acute pancreatitis, 143
Nutritional
  hygienic treatment in hypertensive men and women, long-term effects on sexual function, 6

O

Obesity, 54
  breast cancer risk and, in postmenopausal women, 311
  fat and, dietary, epidemiologic study, 54
  morbid
    in adolescents, effects of high-protein, low-fat, ketogenic diet on, 59
  pregnancy outcome and weight gain recommendations and, 371
  in offspring of parents with coronary artery disease, 9
  resting energy expenditure and, in African-American vs. Caucasian females, 57
OBRA '87 regulations
  effects on psychoactive drug use in nursing homes, 217
Obstetric
  care, why family physicians provide, 374
  outcomes (see Pregnancy, outcomes)
Obstetricians
  variations between family physicians and obstetricians in evaluation and treatment of preterm labor, 360

Occupational
   outcome of hyperactive boys grown up, 306
Ofloxacin
   vs. trovafloxacin for single-dose therapy of gonorrhea, 96
Oil
   cysts, mammary, sonographic features of, 320
Olestra
   potato chips, gastrointestinal symptoms after consumption of, 140
Omeprazole
   in diagnosis of gastroesophageal reflux disease, 136
   for NSAID-related ulcers
      vs. misoprostol, 132
      vs. ranitidine, 134
Omnibus Budget Reconciliation Act
   '87 regulations, effects on psychoactive drug use in nursing homes, 217
Ophthalmopathy
   Graves', course of, relation to therapy for hyperthyroidism, 85
Oral
   challenge, reliability to diagnosis of penicillin, amoxicillin, and cephalosporin allergy, 129
Osteoporosis
   carotid atherosclerosis and, in postmenopausal women, 339
   fractures due to, and Turner syndrome, 88
Otitis media
   acute, in children with bronchiolitis, 274
   chronic suppurative, in adults, efficacy and safety of oral ciprofloxacin for, 114
Outcomes, 414
   patient, impact of education for physicians on, 414
Ovary
   electrocautery of, in polycystic ovary syndrome, late endocrine effects of, 329
   polycystic ovary syndrome (see Polycystic, ovary syndrome)
Overlap syndrome
   antinuclear antibody testing to screen for, in children, 396
Over-the-counter
   status, switching oral acyclovir from prescription to, 113
Overweight females
   differences in resting energy expenditure in African-Americans vs. Caucasians, 57

Oxiconazole
   anti-inflammatory activity of, 153
Oxygen
   hyperbaric, topical, for diabetic foot ulcers, 84
Oxymetazoline
   topical, vs. oral pseudoephedrine in prevention of air travel-associated barotrauma, 262

P

P-450 3A
   cytochrome, interactions with dermatologic therapies, 153
Pain
   back (see Back, pain)
   chest, acute, in diabetics, rate and mode of death during 5-year follow-up, 82
   diffuse, in fibromyalgia syndrome in children and adolescents, 180
   in seriously ill hospitalized adults, no effect of patient empowerment and feedback on, 393
Palmar
   hyperhidrosis, botulinum toxin for, 155
Pancreatitis
   acute, severe, enteral vs. parenteral nutrition in, 143
Papanicolaou smear
   among women with and without hysterectomies, 321
   PAPNET-assisted rescreening of, 328
   quality of, and order of endocervical and ectocervical cytologic sampling, 327
   results, abnormal, efforts to improve follow-up after, 324
Papillomavirus
   transmission, perinatal, in infants, 282
PAPNET
   -assisted rescreening of cervical smears, 328
Parent(s)
   with coronary artery disease, longitudinal changes in cardiovascular risk from childhood to young adulthood in offspring of, 8
   counseling of, to reduce risk of sudden infant death syndrome, 284
Parenteral
   vs. enteral nutrition in severe acute pancreatitis, 143
Paroxetine
   for social phobia, generalized, 219

Partner
  violence, screening men in primary care setting for, 208
Patient
  best interests of, and bedside rationing, 385
  cancer treatment preferences and prognosis of, 380
  care, effect of consumer reports in health care on, 417
  compliance, 388
    dosage frequency and, 389
    financial incentives to enhance, 388
  empowerment, no effect on pain in seriously ill hospitalized adults, 393
  outcomes
    impact of education for physicians on, 414
    physician practice styles and, 405
  role in end of life decision making, 386
  satisfaction, effects of gowning on, 398
  -specific decisions about hormone replacement therapy in postmenopausal women, 343
  vs. physician attitudes toward pharmaceutical industry gifts, 383
  why patients use alternative medicine, 391
Pediatricians
  education for, impact on patient outcomes, 414
  reactions to recommendation for universal varicella vaccination, 268
Peer review, 414
  of quality of care, reliability and validity of, 418
Pelvic
  examination, routine, digital rectal exam as part of, diagnostic utility of, 347
  floor electrical stimulation for stress incontinence, 172
  muscle exercise, effect on transient incontinence during pregnancy and after birth, 370
  prolapse, simplified protocol for pessary management of, 348
Penicillin
  allergy, diagnosis of, 129
Penile
  nerve block, dorsal
    for circumcision, EMLA cream prior to, in children, 170
    vs. ring block and topical anesthesia for neonatal circumcision, 171
Perinatal
  transmission of papillomavirus in infants, 282

Pertussis
  vaccine response in extremely premature infants, 269
Pessary
  management, simplified protocol for, 348
Petroleum
  rectificatum D8 in homeopathic preparation for vertigo, 261–262
Pharmaceutical
  industry gifts, physicians' vs. patients' attitudes toward, 383
Phobia
  social, generalized, paroxetine for, 219
Photoaging
  tretinoin and, topical, 161
Physical
  activity, 224
    (See also Exercise)
    evolutionary perspective, 225
    intensity and amount, relation to insulin sensitivity, 77
    for older adults in public housing, 226
    relation to risk for symptomatic gallstone disease in men, 142
  fitness and functional limitations in older adults, 224
  symptoms in premenstrual dysphoric disorder, effect of sertraline on, 332
Physician(s)
  -assisted suicide and euthanasia, in U.S., 387
  attitudes
    toward gatekeeping, 409
    vs. patients' attitudes toward pharmaceutical industry gifts, 383
  education for, impact on patient outcomes, 414
  family
    esophagogastroduodenoscopy performed by, 131
    preterm labor treatment and evaluation by, variations between obstetricians and, 360
    why they delivery babies, 374
  general
    care, routine, vs. non-directive psychotherapy, 216
    written exercise advice provided by, 227
  laboratories of, quality comparison with commercial laboratories, 416
  management guidelines for domestic abuse when both partners are patients, 206

personal, primary care physicians vs. specialists as, expenditures and mortality related to, 406
practice styles and patient outcomes, 405
prescribing for cutaneous fungal infections, differences in nondermatologists and dermatologists for, 158
primary care
  compensation method in medical groups for, 408
  as personal physicians, expenditures and mortality related to, 406
  regular, vs. insurance as most powerful predictor of health care, 412
  role in end of life decision making, 386
  satisfaction with HMO and fee-for-service practices, 411
specialty
  generalist role of, 403
  as personal physicians, expenditures and mortality related to, 406
  supply in Canada, and class of 1989, 413
views of health plans, 410
Piroxicam
  topical, effectiveness of, 186
Plans
  health, physicians' views of, 410
Pneumonia
  community-acquired, time to clinical stability in patients hospitalized with, 116
Poisoning
  non-accidental, procedures, placement, and risk of further abuse after, 220
Polio
  vaccine response in extremely premature infants, 269
Polycystic
  ovary syndrome, 329
  electrocautery in, ovarian, late endocrine effects of, 329
  metformin in, 330
Position
  supine, during sleep, avoidance of, effect on blood pressure in obstructive sleep apnea patients, 3
Postal
  smoking cessation advice, effectiveness in young men with reduced FEV_1 and asbestos exposure, 238
Postmenopausal women
  bone changes and carotid atherosclerosis in, 339
  breast cancer in
    risk of, and obesity, 311

risk of, and weight, 312
tamoxifen in, uterine side effects of, 314
dong quai in, estrogenic effects of, 341
estrogen replacement therapy in (See also Hormone, replacement therapy, postmenopausal)
  vasodilator effects of, effect of androgen on, 341
hormone replacement therapy in (see Hormone, replacement therapy, postmenopausal)
lichen sclerosus in, severe vulvar, clobetasol vs. testosterone for, 156
lovastatin for primary prevention of acute coronary events in women with average cholesterol levels, 49
myocardial infarction in, effect of pravastatin on cardiovascular events after, 24
Postnatal
  diabetes mellitus after gestational diabetes, 363
  prevalence and predictors of, 363
Potato
  chips, olestra, gastrointestinal symptoms after consumption of, 140
Practice
  fee-for-service, physician satisfaction with, 411
  general, diagnosing dementia in, limitations of Mini-Mental State Examination in, 194
  HMO, physician satisfaction with, 411
  primary care, community dimensions of, 402
  styles, physician, and patient outcomes, 405
Practitioner (see Physician)
Pravastatin
  effect on cardiovascular events in women after myocardial infarction, 24
Prednisone
  /radioiodine therapy for hyperthyroidism, relation to course of Graves' ophthalmopathy, 85
Preeclampsia
  prevention with low-dose aspirin, 356
Preemption
  in tobacco control, 237
Pregnancy, 353
  back pain during, low, follow-up, 178
  blood pressure monitoring in, ambulatory, 357
  caffeine intake during, heavy, and sudden infant death syndrome, 286

diabetes in (see Diabetes mellitus, gestational)
ectopic, repeat, epidemiology of, 349
glucose tolerance test in, 3-hour oral, no effect of high carbohydrate preparatory diet on, 362
HIV screening in, voluntary vs. mandatory
  cost-effectiveness of, 105
  decision analysis of, 107
iron supplementation in, 354
neural tube defect-affected, risk in women of Mexican descent, 355
outcomes, 370
  in anxious women, 372
  after diabetes, gestational, 373
  incontinence during, transient urinary, effect of pelvic muscle exercise on, 370
  in morbidly obese women, 371
Premature infants
  extremely, vaccine response in, 269
  hepatitis B vaccination in, immune responses to, 270
Premenopausal
  women, breast cancer risk in, and alcohol and β-carotene intake, 311
Premenstrual
  dysphoric disorder, sertraline in, 331
  syndrome, 331
    calcium carbonate in, 332
    steroids in, gonadal, behavioral effects of, 334
Prenatal
  issues, 354
Preparticipation
  examinations, 292
    Mayo Clinic experience with, 293
  screening
    cardiovascular, for high school athletes, 292
    for hypertrophic cardiomyopathy in young athletes, 294
Preschool
  speech and language screening, 296
Prescribing
  for cutaneous fungal infections, differences in nondermatologists and dermatologists for, 158
Prescription
  switching oral acyclovir from prescription to over-the-counter status, 113
Preterm
  labor, variations between family physicians and obstetricians in evaluation and treatment of, 360

Preventive medicine, 223
Primary care
  case management programs in, 404
  equity in allocating resources to, 407
  hidden system of? 403
  issues in, 402
  physicians
    compensation method in medical groups for, 408
    as personal physicians, expenditures and mortality related to, 406
  practice, community dimensions of, 402
  providers, naltrexone in management of alcohol dependence by, 204
  respiratory tract illness in, acute lower, effect of antibiotics on, 117
  sabotaging one's own medical care in, 221
  setting, screening men for partner violence in, 208
Progesterone
  therapy in premenstrual syndrome, behavioral effects of, 334
Prone sleeping
  abandoning, effect on sudden infant death syndrome, 283
Prostate
  cancer
    detection, early, by serendipity, 170
    incidence and patient mortality, effects of screening and early detection on, 168
  disease, 163
  hyperplasia, benign, finasteride in, 163
  -specific antigen screening in elderly men, and preferences and informed consent, 167
Prostatitis
  chronic, α-blockers combined with antibiotics in, 166
Protease
  inhibitor in HIV infection, and declining morbidity and mortality, 103
Protein
  A, recombinant *Borrelia burgdorferi* outer-surface, in vaccine for prevention of Lyme disease, 94
  C-reactive, value in determining risk of first myocardial infarction, 52
  high-protein, low-fat ketogenic diet, effects on morbidly obese adolescents, 59
  intake, dietary, association with microalbuminuria in insulin-dependent diabetics, 62

Proteus
  mirabilis in chronic suppurative otitis media in adults, efficacy and safety of oral ciprofloxacin for, 114
Provider
  volumes and outcomes for carotid endarterectomy, 34
Pseudoephedrine
  oral, *vs.* topical oxymetazoline in prevention of air travel-associated barotrauma, 262
Pseudomonas
  aeruginosa in chronic suppurative otitis media in adults, efficacy and safety of oral ciprofloxacin for, 114
Psychiatry, 193
Psychoactive
  drug use in nursing homes, effects of restraint reduction intervention and OBRA '87 regulations on, 217
Psychosocial
  correlates of harassment, threats and fear of violence in workplace, 214
  problems
    back pain and, in children and adolescents, 177
    recognition of, and insurance status, in children, 212
Psychotherapy
  non-directive, *vs.* routine general practitioner care, 216
Puberty
  breast development at, marked, evaluation of boys with, 303
Public
  housing, physical activity and health promotion for, 226
  perception of stroke warning signs, 247
Publication
  of randomized efficacy trials, effect of statistical significance of results on time to, 396
Pulmonary
  (*See also* Lung)
  embolism (*see* Embolism, pulmonary)
  tuberculosis, directly observed therapy for treatment completion of, 115
Pulse
  pressure as predictor of long-term cardiovascular mortality, 10

Q

Quality, 414
  of care, reliability and validity of peer review of, 418
  comparison of physicians' office and commercial laboratories, 416

of life
  of asthma patients requiring inhaled corticosteroids, salmeterol improves, 122
  glaucoma and, 259
  of HIV-positive patients, effect of exercise training on, 103

R

Radioiodine
  therapy for hyperthyroidism, effects on course of Graves' ophthalmopathy, 85
Radiology
  findings in adenoidal obstruction, in children, 301
  of maxillary sinuses of symptomless young men, 260
Randomized efficacy trials
  effect of statistical significance of results on time to completion and publication of, 396
Ranitidine
  vs. omeprazole for NSAID-related ulcers, 134
Rationing
  bedside, and patients' best interests, 385
Reconsultation
  for respiratory tract illness, acute lower, effect of antibiotics on, 117
Rectal
  cancer and aspirin use, 379
  examination, digital, as part of routine pelvic exam, diagnostic utility of, 347
Reflux
  gastroesophageal, omeprazole in diagnosis of, 136
Renal (*see* Kidney)
Reperfusion
  after right ventricular infarction, effect on biventricular function and survival, 23
Reports
  consumer, in health care, effect on patient care, 417
Residence
  in Alzheimer disease special care units, effects on functional outcomes, 195
Resource(s)
  allocation to primary care, equity in, 407
  hospital, use of, effect of CT of appendix on, 148
  utilization and insulin therapy in type 2 diabetes, 71

Respiratory
  illnesses, childhood, medical expenditures for, and maternal smoking, 233
  tract illness, acute lower, effect of antibiotics on reconsultation for, 117
Restraint
  intervention, effects on psychoactive drug use in nursing homes, 217
Retired men
  nonsmoking, effects of walking on mortality among, 229
Review
  peer, 414
  of quality of care, reliability and validity of, 418
Rheumatic
  diseases, antinuclear antibody testing to screen for, in children, 395
Ring block
  vs. dorsal penile nerve block and topical anesthesia for neonatal circumcision, 171

S

Salmeterol
  improves quality of life in asthma patients requiring inhaled corticosteroids, 122
School
  children with uncertain history of chickenpox, varicella serology among, 267
  high
    athletes, preparticipation cardiovascular screening for, 292
    condom availability program, students' acquisition and use of condoms in, 305
  medical school graduates in 1989 and physician supply in Canada, 413
  preschool speech and language screening, 296
Scoring system
  admission, to predict vaginal delivery after cesarean delivery, 367
Screening
  tests, controversial, ethical considerations in provision of, 384
Sentence Repetition Screening Test
  in preschoolers, 296
Serendipity
  early prostate cancer detection by, 170

Seriously ill
  hospitalized adults, pain in, no effect of patient empowerment and feedback on, 393
Serology
  testing for tick bites and Lyme disease, 93
  varicella, among school age children with uncertain history of chickenpox, 267
Sertraline
  in premenstrual dysphoric disorder, 331
Sex
  hormone-binding globulin increase after ovarian electrocautery for polycystic ovary syndrome, 329
Sexual
  function, long-term effects of antihypertensive drugs and nutritional hygienic treatment in hypertensive men and women on, 6
Sexually
  transmitted disease, 96
    effect of HIV counseling and testing on, in urban adolescents, 104
Shampoo
  anti-mite carpet, long-term efficacy in reduction of house dust mites, 123
Shoulder
  dystocia and gestational diabetes, 373
SIDS (see Sudden infant death syndrome)
Sildenafil
  for erectile dysfunction, 173
Simvastatin
  long-term, effect on albumin excretion rate in type 2 diabetics, 75
Sinus(es)
  maxillary, of symptomless young men, radiology of, 260
  rhythm, likelihood of spontaneous conversion of atrial fibrillation to, 25
Skin
  aging, premature, ultraviolet light-induced, pathophysiology of, 151
  cancer
    basal cell, invasive cancers after, 160
    sunscreens in prevention of, 149
  conditions, 149
    therapeutics, 152
  infections, fungal, nondermatologists are more likely than dermatologists to prescribe antifungal/corticosteroid products for, 158

sensitivity to allergen does not accurately predict airway response to allergen, 125
testing, reliability to diagnosis of penicillin, amoxicillin, and cephalosporin allergy, 129
Sleep
  abnormalities, effects of high-protein, low-fat ketogenic diet in morbidly obese adolescents on, 59
  airway resistance during, abnormal upper, and hypertension, 4
  apnea, obstructive, and blood pressure, effect of avoidance of supine position during sleep on, 3
  disturbances in fibromyalgia syndrome in children and adolescents, 180
  position
    prone, abandoning, effect on sudden infant death syndrome, 283
    supine, avoidance of, effect on blood pressure in obstructive sleep apnea patients, 3
Smear
  cervical, PAPNET-assisted rescreening of, 328
  Papanicolaou (see Papanicolaou smear)
Smoke
  tobacco, environmental exposure, and ischemic heart disease, 232
Smoking, 231
  atherosclerosis progression and, 231
  cessation
    advice, postal, effectiveness in young men with reduced FEV_1 and asbestos exposure, 238
    bupropion for, sustained-release, 235
    telephone support as adjunct to transdermal nicotine in, 234
    counseling parents to reduce risk of sudden infant death syndrome and, 285
  effect on course of Graves' ophthalmopathy after hyperthyroidism therapy, 85
  hypertension and intracerebral hemorrhage, 249
  maternal, and medical expenditures for childhood respiratory illnesses, 233
Social
  phobia, generalized, paroxetine for, 219
  risk factors, midwifery care, and birth outcomes, in U.S., 375
Sociodemographic
  factors, effect on prognosis of whiplash, 189
Sodium
  intake, dietary, and mortality, 11

Sonographic
  features of mammary oil cysts, 320
Soy
  allergy and atopic dermatitis, 159
  supplementation, dietary, effect on hot flushes, 340
Spatula
  Ayre, endocervical brush after, and quality of Pap smear, 327
Specialists
  as personal physicians, expenditures and mortality related to, 406
Specialty
  physicians, generalist role of, 403
Spectroscopy
  fluorescence, of cervical squamous intraepithelial lesions, cost-effectiveness of, 322
Speech
  screening, preschool, 296
Sports
  nasal strips and airflow, 263
Squamous
  intraepithelial cervical lesions, cost-effectiveness analysis of diagnosis and management of, 321
Staphylococcus
  aureus in chronic suppurative otitis media in adults, efficacy and safety of oral ciprofloxacin for, 114
Statistical
  significance of results of randomized efficacy trials, effect on time to completion and publication of, 396
Stavudine
  regimen in HIV infection, improved survival after, 108
Steroid(s)
  corticosteroids (see Corticosteroids)
  gonadal, in premenstrual syndrome, behavioral effects of, 334
  topical, potent, in Chinese herbal cream, 157
Stiffness
  morning, in fibromyalgia syndrome in children and adolescents, 180, 182
Stress
  incontinence, pelvic floor electrical stimulation for, 172
Stroke, 247
  in diabetics, non–insulin-dependent, serum uric acid as predictor of, 250
  effect of HMG CoA reductase inhibitors of, 252
  prevention in patients with atrial fibrillation using aspirin, 249
  risk factors, potential, knowledge of, 247

Turner syndrome and, 88
units *vs.* general medical wards, survival in, 253
warning signs, public perception of, 247
Students
  medical, community-based ambulatory encounters involving, 397
Subcutaneous
  temperature, effect of cold- and hot-pack contrast therapy on, 187
Sudden cardiac death
  risk of, and fish consumption, 12
Sudden infant death syndrome, 283
  caffeine intake during pregnancy and, heavy, 286
  risk of
    counseling parents to reduce, 284
    effect of abandoning prone sleeping on, 283
  weather temperatures and, 287
Suffocation
  nonaccidental, procedures, placement, and risk of further abuse after, 220
Suicide
  after natural disasters, 215
  physician-assisted, in U.S., 387
Sulfonylurea
  vs. insulin and metformin therapy in newly diagnosed type 2 diabetes, 66
Sun
  exposure, 149
Sunburn
  protective effect of combined vitamin C and E on, 150
Sunscreens
  in prevention of actinic damage and neoplasia, 149
Supine
  position during sleep, avoidance of, effect on blood pressure in obstructive sleep apnea patients, 3
Syncope
  as emergency department presentation of pulmonary embolism, 39

T

Tacrine
  in Alzheimer's disease, 196
Tamoxifen
  uterine side effects of, 314
Telephone
  support as adjunct to transdermal nicotine in smoking cessation, 234
Television
  watching and weight change in men, 56

Temperature
  subcutaneous and intramuscular, effect of cold- and hot-pack contrast therapy on, 187
  weather, and sudden infant death syndrome, 287
Tension
  -type headache, epidemiology of, 254
Terazosin
  /antibiotics for chronic prostatitis, 166
Terbinafine
  anti-inflammatory activity of, 153
Terbutaline
  for cephalic version, external, 365
Test(s)
  screening, controversial, ethical considerations in provision of, 384
Testicular
  failure, primary, and marked breast development in boys at puberty, 305
Testosterone
  levels in polycystic ovary syndrome, transitory effects of metformin on, 330
  vs. clobetasol for severe vulvar lichen sclerosus, 156
Tetanus
  vaccine response in extremely premature infants, 269
Therapeutic
  touch, close look at, 392
Threats
  of violence in workplace, psychosocial correlates of, 214
Throat
  conditions, 259
Thrombosis
  vein, deep, 37
    does this patient have deep vein thrombosis? 37
    heparin for, subcutaneous, algorithm for administration of, 40
    proximal, vena caval filters in prevention of pulmonary embolism in patients with, 38
Tick
  bites and Lyme disease in endemic setting, 93
Tissue
  mixed connective tissue disease, antinuclear antibody testing to screen for, in children, 396
Tobacco
  control, preemption in, 237
  smoke exposure, environmental, and ischemic heart disease, 232
  smoking (*see* Smoking)

Tocolytics
  in preterm labor, variations between family physicians and obstetricians in use of, 360
d-α-Tocopherol
  combined with ascorbic acid for protection against sunburn, 150
Tomography
  computed, of appendix, effect on treatment and use of hospital resources, 148
Tonsillar
  hypertrophy, chronic, amoxicillin/clavulanate for, in children, 273
Touch
  therapeutic, close look at, 392
Toxicity
  hepatotoxicity of multiple doses of acetaminophen, in children, 300
Toxin
  botulinum, for palmar hyperhidrosis, 155
Training
  exercise
    blood pressure and, 2
    effect on aerobic fitness, immune indices, and quality of life in HIV-positive patients, 103
Trampoline
  -related injuries in children, in U.S., 290
Transdermal
  nicotine and telephone support in smoking cessation, 234
  nitroglycerin, intermittent, effects on occurrence of ischemia after patch removal, 30
Travel
  air travel-associated barotrauma, oral pseudoephedrine vs. topical oxymetazoline in prevention of, 262
Treatment
  preferences and prognosis of cancer patients, 380
Tretinoin
  topical, and photoaging, 161
Trials
  randomized efficacy, effect of statistical significance of results on time to completion and publication of, 396
Triglyceride
  level decrease after fish oil in diabetics, 80
  potato chips, regular, gastrointestinal symptoms after consumption of, vs. olestra chips, 140

Troglitazone
  in insulin-treated type 2 diabetics, 67
Trovafloxacin
  vs. ofloxacin for single-dose therapy of gonorrhea, 96
Tube
  neural tube defect, risk in pregnancies in women of Mexican descent, 355
Tuberculosis
  pulmonary, directly observed therapy for treatment completion of, 115
Turner syndrome
  morbidity in, 87
TV
  watching and weight change in men, 56

U

Ulcer
  foot, diabetic, topical hyperbaric oxygen and low energy laser for, 84
  NSAID-related, omeprazole for
    vs. misoprostol, 132
    vs. ranitidine, 134
Ultraviolet
  light-induced premature skin aging, pathophysiology of, 151
Upper Extremity Function Scale
  development and validation of, 182
Urban
  adolescents, effect of HIV counseling and testing on sexually transmitted diseases and condom use in, 104
Urea
  breath test, carbon-13, for *Helicobacter pylori* and abdominal symptoms, in children, 275
  nitrogen levels, blood, after short-term ibuprofen use in infants and children, 299
Uric acid
  serum, as predictor of stroke in non–insulin-dependent diabetics, 250
Urinalysis
  screening dipstick, 110
Urinary
  incontinence
    stress, pelvic floor electrical stimulation for, 172
    transient, during pregnancy and after birth, effect of pelvic muscle exercise on, 370
  retention in benign prostatic hyperplasia, effect of finasteride on risk of, 163
  tract infection, 110

Urine
  sampling method for bacteriological examination in elderly women, 111
Urological
  conditions, 163
Ursodeoxycholic acid
  delays onset of esophageal varices in primary biliary cirrhosis, 144
Uterine
  side effects of tamoxifen, 314

V

Vaccination
  hepatitis B, immune responses of prematurely born infants to, 270
  against Lyme disease with recombinant *Borrelia burgdorferi* outer-surface lipoprotein A with adjuvant, 95
  varicella, universal, pediatricians reactions to recommendation for, 268
Vaccine
  Hemophilus influenzae type b, era after, risk of bacteremia for febrile young children in, 272
  influenza, inactivated, effect on pulmonary function in asthma, 124
  recombinant *Borrelia burgdorferi* outer-surface protein A, to prevent Lyme disease, 94
  response in extremely premature infants, 269
  varicella, postlicensure effectiveness during outbreak in child care center, 266
Vacuum
  extraction, neonatal cephalohematoma after, 366
Vaginal
  bleeding, unexpected, with cyclic *vs.* continuous postmenopausal hormone replacement therapy, 346
  cervicovaginal cytology, false positive, 325
  delivery
    after cesarean delivery, admission scoring system to predict, 367
    perinatal transmission of papillomavirus in infants and, 282
    vacuum extraction, neonatal cephalohematoma after, 366
Vaginitis
  after trovafloxacin *vs.* ofloxacin single-dose therapy of gonorrhea, 97

Varicella
  serology among school age children with uncertain history of chickenpox, 267
  vaccination, universal, pediatricians reactions to recommendation for, 268
  vaccine, postlicensure effectiveness during outbreak in child care center, 266
Varices
  esophageal, in primary biliary cirrhosis, ursodeoxycholic acid delays onset of, 144
Vascular
  disease, 33
Vasoactivity
  brachial artery, endothelium-dependent, transient impairment after single high-fat meal, effect of antioxidant vitamins on, 241
Vasodilator
  effects of estrogen are not diminished by androgen in postmenopausal women, 341
Vein
  thrombosis (*see* Thrombosis, vein)
Vena caval
  filters in prevention of pulmonary embolism in patients with proximal deep vein thrombosis, 38
Ventricle
  right, infarction, effect of reperfusion on biventricular function and survival after, 23
Version
  cephalic, external, terbutaline for, 365
Vertigo
  homeopathic treatment of, 261
Viagra
  for erectile dysfunction, 173
Violence
  domestic, 205
  partner, screening men in primary care setting for, 208
  threats and fear of, in workplace, psychosocial correlates of, 214
Virus
  herpes simplex type 2, in U.S., 97
  immunodeficiency, human (*see* AIDS)
  load, plasma, and CD4+ cell count as prognostic indicators for AIDS and infectious disease death in HIV-infected injection drug users, 109
  papillomavirus, perinatal transmission in infants, 282
Vitamin(s)
  antioxidant

Subject Index / 455

effect on transient impairment of endothelium-dependent brachial artery vasoactivity after single high-fat meal, 241
in prevention of cardiovascular disease, 239
B_6 intake and risk of coronary heart disease in women, 14
C
combined with vitamin E for protection against sunburn, 150
after high-fat meal, 241
in prevention of cardiovascular disease, 240
E
combined with vitamin C for protection against sunburn, 150
after high-fat meal, 241
for hot flashes in breast cancer survivors, 315
intake, low, and risk of breast cancer, 311
in prevention of cardiovascular disease, 240
supplemental, and nitrate tolerance, 242
Vulvar
lichen sclerosus, severe, clobetasol vs. testosterone for, 156

W

Walking
effects on mortality among nonsmoking retired men, 229
Wards
general medical, vs. stroke units, survival in, 253
Warfarin
anticoagulation, excessive, acetaminophen and other risk factors for, 43
Warts
genital
imiquimod for, 99
isotretinoin for, oral, 101
Weather
temperatures and sudden infant death syndrome, 287
Weight
change, predictors of, in men, 56
gain
excessive, effect on lipid levels and blood pressure in insulin-dependent diabetics on intensive therapy, 65
recommendations in pregnancy in morbidly obese women, 371
maintenance, effect of long-term supplementation of carbohydrate, chromium, fiber and caffeine on, 58
weight gain and, dual effects on breast cancer risk, 311
Wheat
allergy and atopic dermatitis, 159
Whiplash
prognosis, effect of sociodemographic and crash-related factors on, 189
Women
abuse of
domestic, management guidelines when male and female partners are patients of same physician, 206
emotional, effects on health indicators, 205
coronary heart disease risk in
fat intake and, dietary, 46
folate and vitamin B_6 intake and, 14
elderly
alcohol consumption and mortality among, in U.S., 200
urine sampling method for bacteriological examination in, 111
headache in, tension-type, 254
health of, 309
incontinence in, stress urinary, pelvic floor electrical stimulation for, 172
lovastatin for primary prevention of acute coronary events in women with average cholesterol levels, 49
middle-aged, alcohol consumption and mortality among
in U.S., 200
in U.S. and Russia, 202
myocardial infarction in, pravastatin effects on cardiovascular events after, 24
overweight, differences in resting energy expenditure in African-Americans vs. Caucasians, 57
postmenopausal (see Postmenopausal women)
premenopausal, breast cancer risk and alcohol and β-carotene intake in, 311
Work
-related upper extremity disorders, measuring functional outcomes in, 182
Workplace
psychosocial correlates of harassment, threats and fear of violence in, 214
Wrist
supports for carpal tunnel syndrome, 185

Written exercise advice
   provided by general practitioners, 227

X

XX
   46,XX maleness and marked breast development in boys at puberty, 305

Z

Zalcitabine
   -based treatment of HIV infection, improved survival after, 108
Zidovudine
   -based treatment of HIV infection, improved survival after, 108

Author Index

A

Aalberse RC, 128
Abernathy J, 202
Ackermann RJ, 131
Ahmed AH, 124
Albert CM, 12
Albertazzi P, 340
Albisser AM, 83
Alderman MH, 11
Allen TL, 39
Anand SS, 37
Anderson MB, 325
Andrade MA, 274
Armstrong D, 113
Arroll B, 227
Astin JA, 391
Atherly AJ, 418
Atkinson JH, 176

B

Bagatella P, 40
Baird D, 336
Bakker A, 389
Baldwin L-M, 403
Balkau B, 78
Bao W, 8
Baptiste MS, 316
Barbacci MB, 300
Barbalias GA, 166
Barry MJ, 170
Bartalena L, 85
Barton DL, 315
Baskett TF, 348
Bass DA, 125
Basso C, 294
Baucom DH, 209
Baum J, 180
Beischer NA, 363
Bell DM, 30
Bell RM, 305
Bellamy P, 145
Benetos A, 10
Benso L, 297
Berezovskaya M, 103
Berger M, 3
Berkovitz GD, 303
Berlière M, 314
Bernard BS, 301
Bernardi E, 40
Berry SH, 305
Bertakis KD, 405
Berthold HK, 243
Bessler A, 306
Beutner KR, 99

Bevan G, 407
Bianco AT, 371
Bickell NA, 316
Bingham BJG, 263
Black SB, 267
Blake PA, 266
Block B, 324
Bloom SL, 365
Blouch DL, 383
Blumenthal D, 409
Bobula JA, 374
Bode G, 275
Boden WE, 19
Bofill JA, 366
Bogazzi F, 85
Bonaccorsi G, 340
Bornstein J, 156
Borowsky SJ, 410
Boudoulas H, 244
Bouma MJ, 118
Bowers TR, 23
Bowton DL, 125
Bowyer L, 357
Brady-Fryer B, 171
Branham RA, 324
Brasseux C, 104
Brawley OW, 168
Breithaupt-Grögler K, 244
Brenner H, 275
Brizzi P, 75
Broderick J, 247
Brorsson B, 259
Brosh D, 69
Brown J, 287
Brown MA, 357
Brynhildsen J, 178
Bucher HC, 252
Buchner DM, 226
Buckner S-B, 328
Bulger T, 369
Buntinx F, 382
Burchfiel CM, 229
Burks AW, 159
Burstin HR, 412
Buske L, 413
Byington RP, 70

C

Callahan EJ, 405
Campbell KA, 347
Cantor SB, 321
Capezuti E, 217
Caritis S, 356
Carol J, 237
Carroll D, 186

Carroll JL, 284
Casey BM, 373
Caskey PM, 177
Caulfield TA, 25
Causino N, 409
Cebul RD, 34
Charles A, 314
Chaulk CP, 115
Cheadle A, 408
Chen E, 364
Cheskin LJ, 140
Childs GE, 212
Ciccarese M, 75
Clark LR, 104
Clark NM, 414
Coakley EH, 56
Cohen H, 11, 41
Col NF, 343
Colborn DK, 301
Colditz G, 56
Colditz GA, 311
Cole LL, 214
Coleston-Shields DM, 255
Collins MM, 170
Combs JA, 177
Conrad DA, 408
Cook DA, 122
Cook EF, 380
Cooper GS, 145
Cordain L, 225
Corey L, 113
Corey PN, 394
Cornoni-Huntley J, 224
Corrado D, 294
Corretti MC, 241
Creinin MD, 338
Cuddeback JK, 35

D

D'Agostino RB, 7
Daling JR, 313
Danaceau MA, 334
Danesh J, 17
D'Angio CT, 269
Danias PG, 25
Datta SC, 151
Davis MK, 410
Davis P, 220
Davis PT, 185
Davis Y, 371
Dawson NV, 145
de Boissieu D, 127
Decarli A, 310
Decousus H, 38
Deev A, 202

de Jong MH, 128
Dennis DT, 92
Desbiens NA, 393
Devera-Sales A, 198
Devidas M, 366
Dobson JV, 277
Donahue JG, 121
Doukas DJ, 384
Downs JR, 49
Duell PB, 28
Durrant E, 187
Dwyer T, 62
Dye C, 118

E

Eaker ED, 320
Eaton SB, 225
Eberlein-König B, 150
Eckman MH, 343
Eeg-Olofsson KE, 138
Eide GE, 238
Eisenberger D, 327
Emmons C-A, 387
Entrekin K, 362
Eriksson N, 349
Eskeland B, 354
Eskelin M, 260
Ettinger B, 346
Every NR, 20

F

Farmer KC, 149
Farrell SA, 348
Farren CK, 204
Fasano MB, 125
Feig DS, 364
Feld LG, 110
Feldman SR, 158
Fergie N, 263
Ferguson JA, 404
Fernandez CO, 365
Ferris LE, 206
Fetters M, 384
Feuerstein M, 182
Fihn SD, 20
Fine MJ, 116
Finucane P, 2
Fiscella K, 406
Fisher GJ, 151, 161
Fix AD, 93
Flamm BL, 367
Fleischer AB Jr, 158
Fleming DT, 97
Fleming MF, 208
Flory JD, 27

Ford RPK, 286, 287
Frank SH, 397
Franks P, 406
Friedberg CE, 80
Friedli K, 216
Frigo P, 356
Funk SG, 296

G

Galant C, 314
Gehanno P, 114
Geiger AM, 367
Georgiou S, 101
Geurs FJC, 111
Gibbons RV, 383
Gildengorin GL, 212
Ginsburg J, 273
Giovannucci EL, 142
Giuffrida A, 388
Gjønnæss H, 329
Glasier A, 336
Glover DW, 292
Glover ED, 235
Glustein J, 274
Glynn RJ, 52, 379
Goertz C, 410
Goldberg RB, 83
Goldstein I, 173
Gong M, 414
Goold S, 385
Gotshall RW, 225
Graham N, 109
Grant J, 93
Gravholt CH, 87
Gray A, 41
Gray B, 233
Green JA, 296
Griffith LE, 252
Grimm RH Jr, 6
Grines C, 23
Grubb PL, 214
Guldvog B, 253
Guyatt GH, 252

H

Hadgu A, 349
Hakim AA, 229
Halbert JA, 2
Hállden M, 138
Halm EA, 116, 409
Hankinson SE, 311
Hansson Å, 178
Harder S, 189
Harper MB, 272
Hart LG, 403

Harvey JA, 320
Haskin-Popp C, 228
Hawes C, 195
Hawkey CJ, 132
Hayward RA, 71
Heath KV, 108
Heifetz S, 156
Heiman H, 43
Heine RJ, 80
Helms LJ, 405
Hemminki E, 359
Hennekens CH, 12, 52
Herlitz J, 82
Hernandez E, 327
Hess DL, 28
Heubi JE, 300
Hiegel A, 159
Hilborne LH, 416
Hill DJ, 123
Himmelstein J, 182
Hirata JD, 342
Hoberman A, 274
Hoffman J, 73
Hoffmann RG, 317
Hogg RS, 108
Hokanson JE, 65
Holleman F, 64
Holmes WF, 117
Hoogendam A, 382
Hoover D, 109
Hornstein MD, 350
Hougham AJ, 99
Howard G, 231
Howden-Chapman P, 369
Howell-Pelz A, 317
Hu FB, 14, 46
Huang Z, 311
Huber TS, 35
Hueston WJ, 360
Hulbert JR, 185
Humerfelt S, 238
Hunt D, 37
Hurd WW, 337
Hurst J, 416
Hurt RD, 235
Hylek EM, 43

I

Incaudo GA, 122
Ioannidis JPA, 396
Isolauri E, 281
Izurieta HS, 266

J

Jablonski K, 76

Author Index / 459

Jakicic JM, 57
James JM, 159
Janeway D, 180
Jansen PHP, 184
Janssen MJEM, 80
Jarrett RJ, 78
Jindal KK, 61
Johnson RE, 97
Johnston SC, 386
Jones BA, 325
Jones JS, 262
Jones RB, 96
Jordan J, 237
Jorgensen RA, 144
Jousimies-Somer H, 260
Juul S, 87

K

Kakihana M, 242
Kalfarentzos F, 143
Kane RL, 418
Kang S, 161
Kaplan RE, 110
Kaplan SH, 71
Karas RH, 343
Karlbom U, 138
Karlson BW, 82
Karlsson G, 196
Kassak KM, 185
Kehagias J, 143
Kelleher KJ, 212
Kellner Y, 156
Kemp JP, 122
Kesler K, 270
Khalak R, 269
Kiberd BA, 61
King MB, 216
Klein P, 261
Klein R, 346
Klein RG, 306
Klevan D, 234
Klinkenberg-Knol EC, 136
Knopp RH, 48
Ko CY, 137
Koivunen RM, 330
Konitzer KA, 320
Kothari R, 247
Kresnow M-J, 215
Krug EG, 215
Kuipers EJ, 136
Kvåle G, 238

L

Laakso M, 15
Lamarche B, 51

Land G, 417
Landau Z, 84
Lander J, 171
Lando HA, 234
Landry FJ, 383
Lang C, 357
Langa D, 397
Laskowski ER, 293
La Vecchia C, 160, 310
Law MR, 16, 232
Lazarou J, 394
Le Bars PL, 197
Lee GM, 272
Lee I-M, 379
Lehman RE, 137
Lehto S, 250
Leitzmann MF, 142
Lesko SM, 299
Levetan CS, 76
Levi F, 160
Levi Z, 69
Levy D, 7
Lewis SJ, 24
Li D-K, 346
Liang C-C, 282
Liatsikos EN, 166
Liebowitz MR, 219
Liedekerken BMJ, 381
Lieu TA, 267
Lindor KD, 144
Lindqvist J, 82
Ling M, 244
Lipton RB, 257
Livingston JM, 121
Lloyd M, 216
Longenecker JC, 107
Longo DR, 417
Lonn EM, 239
Lopez AD, 200
Lopez LM, 30
Loprinzi CL, 315
Lucas MJ, 373
Lundström M, 259
Lydiard RB, 219

M

Macdonald CE, 135
MacDorman MF, 375
MacFarlane JT, 117
MacFarlane RM, 117
Mackey AE, 33
Mackinnon MJ, 395
Madhaven S, 11
Maislin G, 217
Maldonado Y, 279
Malinow MR, 28
Malleson PN, 395

Malone KE, 313
Malterud K, 354
Mandelberg A, 170
Manning WG, 71
Mannuzza S, 306
Manson JE, 46
Marcocci C, 85
Marcovina SM, 65
Markestad T, 283
Maron BJ, 292
Marrie TJ, 116
Marsland A, 27
Martin ML, 226
Matarazzo P, 127
Maurer EJ, 320
Mauriège P, 51
Mayer-Davis EJ, 77
Maynard C, 408
McClure RJ, 220
McConnell JD, 163
McIntire DD, 373
McMahon SR, 277
McQuillan GM, 97
Mead N, 143
Measom G, 187
Meier DE, 387
Meit SS, 398
Mencken FC, 398
Meneghini LF, 83
Merrill RM, 318
Metcalfe JB, 171
Mezzetti M, 310
Michielsen WJS, 111
Miday R, 140
Miettinen H, 15
Migeon CJ, 303
Miller JM, 370
Mims BL, 370
Mitchel EF Jr, 288
Mitchell AA, 299
Mitchell MF, 321
Moberg DP, 411
Monastirli A, 101
Mongan PF, 205
Moore RA, 186
Moran RE, 320
Morey MC, 224
Morild I, 283
Morin-Papunen LC, 330
Morris JK, 16, 232
Mueser KT, 209
Muldoon MF, 27
Myers ER, 105
Myrer JW, 187

N

Naeraa RW, 87

Nakchbandi IA, 107
Nasenbeny J, 270
Nattinger AB, 317
Naylor CD, 361, 364
Naylor MF, 149
Nazareno D, 228
Newman RD, 268
Nguyen-Van-Tam JS, 124
Nicassio PM, 179
Nichol G, 92
Nicholson KG, 124
Nickel K, 416
Nicola RM, 226
Nieman LK, 334
Nikiforidis G, 166
Niskanen L, 250
Nordberg A, 196
Novelline RA, 148

O

O'Brien WA, 103
O'Connor PG, 204
O'Day SJ, 380
O'Donnell CJ, 12
Oexmann MJ, 59
Ohtsuka S, 242
Oksenberg A, 3, 4
O'Leary TJ, 328
O'Neill WW, 23
Orengo I, 152
Oriel KA, 208
Owen J, 362

P

Paes AHP, 389
Pahor M, 70
Palella FJ Jr, 102
Palmer JR, 26
Pancioli AM, 247
Pansini F, 340
Paradise JL, 301
Parsons LS, 20
Pasman WJ, 58
Passaro M, 76
Pastorin L, 297
Pathman DE, 402
Peddicord JP, 215
Pepine CJ, 30
Persson A, 178
Peto R, 17, 200
Petrovitch H, 229
Phillips CD, 195
Pichichero DM, 129
Pichichero ME, 129, 269
Pickar JH, 344

Pieper CF, 224
Pierzchajlo RPJ, 131
Pine R, 34
Placzek M, 150
Playford RJ, 135
Plotnick GD, 241
Pomeranz BH, 394
Potosky AL, 318
Prandoni P, 40
Pransky G, 182
Przybilla B, 150
Purnell JQ, 65
Pyörälä M, 15

Q

Quella SK, 315

R

Rabin RL, 279
Radojevic V, 179
Randolph JF Jr, 337
Ransohoff DF, 170
Rao PM, 148
Rao S, 26
Ravid M, 69
Ray WA, 288
Reed DM, 212
Reisenberger K, 357
Retzlaff BM, 48
Rhea JT, 148
Richmond D, 104
Ridker PM, 52
Ries LAG, 378
Riley GF, 318
Riley MD, 62
Rimm EB, 14, 56, 142
Risksecker MA, 107
Roberts RG, 374
Robinson A, 357
Rocchiccioli F, 127
Rolfe K, 220
Rolnick S, 234
Rönnemaa T, 250
Rønning OM, 253
Roohan PJ, 316
Rosa E, 392
Rosa L, 392
Rosen T, 152
Rosenberg HM, 378
Rosenberg L, 26
Rosenblatt RA, 403
Ross JJ, 112
Rothenbacher D, 275
Rottiers R, 64
Rounsaville BJ, 204

Rudnichi A, 10
Ruffin MT IV, 384
Ruokonen A, 330
Rust OA, 366
Ryan RE Jr, 257
Ryten E, 413

S

Sachs DPL, 235
Safar M, 10
Sailer M, 395
Sakakibara R, 172
Sampselle CM, 370
Sande MA, 113
Sandhu BK, 281
Sankila R, 381
Sansone LA, 221
Sansone RA, 221
Saris WHM, 58
Sarner L, 392
Sarrel PM, 341
Sauter SL, 214
Savolainen S, 260
Scharp-van der Linden VTM, 128
Scheckler WE, 411
Schell BJ, 152
Schellevis FG, 194
Schenk BE, 136
Schiavon M, 294
Schluter PJ, 287
Schmidt PJ, 334
Schmitt H, 64
Scholer SJ, 288
Schork MA, 414
Schorling JB, 167
Schramm W, 417
Schulz R, 411
Schuster MA, 305
Schwartz BS, 254
Schwartz S, 67
Sclafani AP, 273
Seidell JC, 54
Serour F, 170
Shah MK, 273
Shapiro DS, 112
Shapiro LE, 153
Shaughnessy AF, 347
Shaw GM, 355
Shear NH, 153
Sheedy MT, 363
Sheffield W, 262
Shelley ED, 155
Shelley WB, 155
Sher ES, 303
Shestov D, 202
Shipley M, 78

Author Index / 461

Shoham V, 209
Shulman T, 338
Siegel DM, 180
Siegel M, 237
Siegler EL, 217
Sigal LH, 94
Silagy CA, 2
Silverberg DS, 3, 4
Simon D, 254
Simpson K, 105
Singer MI, 153
Singh GK, 375
Siska ES, 284
Sjögren B, 372
Skadberg BT, 283
Skates SJ, 43
Skjeldestad FE, 349
Slater MA, 176
Sloane PD, 195
Smilen SW, 371
Smith ES, 158
Smith GA, 290
Smith J, 293
Smith MA, 418
Smulian JC, 365
Snow RJ, 34
Soe-Agnie CJ, 389
Soong Y-K, 282
Sox CM, 412
Spengler M, 73
Sporik R, 123
Springate JE, 110
Spruance SL, 99
Srinivasan SR, 8
Stampfer MJ, 46
Stange KC, 397
Stanitski CL, 188
Steere AC, 92, 95
Stein MB, 219
Steiner BD, 402
Steiner TJ, 255
Stephens-Groff SM, 277
Stewart WF, 254, 257
Stoddard JJ, 233
Stone P, 369
Strebel PM, 266
Strickland GT, 93
Strickland JL, 323
Stringer WW, 103
Strösser W, 261
Sturm R, 210
Stürmer T, 379
Sturner RA, 296
Sudhop T, 243
Suissa S, 189
Swartz K, 412
Sweirsz LM, 342
Swinburn BA, 227

T

Taj N, 198
Takahashi H, 267
Talanin NY, 155
Tate KM, 323
Tatti P, 70
Taylor FC, 41
Taylor JA, 268
Tchernof A, 51
Te V-C, 160
Tellado M, 328
Tener T, 327
Therneau TM, 144
Thomassen P, 372
Thompson JD, 313
Thompson JW, 105
Thompson PJ, 123
Thomsen OØ, 141
Thrift AG, 248
Thun MJ, 200
Thurber AD, 413
Thys-Jacobs S, 332
Tong J, 137
Tonolo G, 75
Torgerson DJ, 388
Tortolero-Luna G, 321
Tramèr MR, 186
Tsambaos D, 101
Tseng C-J, 282

U

Ubel PA, 385
Ulvik RJ, 354
Uyama O, 339

V

Valdez R, 8
Vannelli S, 297
Veenhuizen KCW, 184
Veilleux M, 189
Velie EM, 355
Verschraegen GLC, 111
Vierkant RA, 320
Vinson DC, 198
Vlahov D, 109
Vogel RA, 241
Vogel RL, 131

von Bergmann K, 243
Voorhees JJ, 161

W

Waddell C, 218
Wagner PJ, 205
Wainwright R, 270
Wald NJ, 16, 232
Walden CE, 48
Walker-Smith JA, 281
Wallenstein S, 387
Walter LG, 227
Wändell PE, 259
Wang ZQ, 151
Wasserman CR, 355
Wasserman RC, 212
Watanabe H, 242
Weeks JC, 380
Wegner J, 228
Weigner MJ, 25
Wein P, 363
Weinberger M, 404
Weirich E, 279
Weiser M, 261
Weisman MH, 179
Weiss ST, 121
Wells PS, 37
Wesseling AIM, 184
West CG, 212
Westerterp-Plantenga MS, 58
Wheeler KG, 35
White LJ, 262
Whitfield RR, 337
Whitmarsh TE, 255
Wicks AC, 135
Wiederman MW, 221
Wiita B, 341
Willett WC, 14, 54
Willi SM, 59
Williams D, 398
Williams E, 402
Williams RA, 176
Wilson PWF, 7
Wimo A, 196
Wind AW, 194
Wing RR, 57
Wingo PA, 378
Wishart J, 157
Wolf AMD, 167
Wolfe TR, 39
Wolkomir MS, 374
Wood B, 157
Work B, 362
Wright A, 66
Wright NM, 59

Wu AW, 393
Wu V, 348

Y

Yamamoto Y, 339
Yamanishi T, 172
Yasuda K, 172
Yasui Y, 393
Yeomans ND, 134
Yip B, 108
Yonkers KA, 331
Yoshimoto Y, 339
Yusuf S, 239

Z

Zabeeda D, 170
Zell B, 342
Zimmerman HJ, 300
Zorich N, 140